Nikolai N. Korpan (ed.)

Atlas of Cryosurgery

SpringerWienNewYork

Nikolai N. Korpan, MD, Ph D
Professor of Surgery
Head, Vienna International Institute
for Cryosurgery
Department of Surgery, Evangelical
Hospital Wien-Währing
Vienna, Austria

Active Membership in national, European and international societies: Austrian Society of Surgery, Ukrainian Society of Surgery, Swiss Society of Surgery, European Society for Clinical Investigation, Co-founder and Board Member of the European Society of Cryosurgery, Alumni Gold Club, European School of Oncology, Arbeitsgruppe 'Kryochirurgie- Deutschland', International Society of Cryosurgery, International College of Surgeons, International Society of Surgery, International College of Angiology, The New York Academy of Sciences, The American Association for the Advancement of Science, Founder and Head of the Vienna International Institute for Cryosurgery, Founder and President of the International Association of Inventors 'Perpetuus', Vice President of the European Society of Cryosurgery.

This work is subject to copyright.
All rights are reserved, whether the whole or part of the material is concerned, specifically those of translation, reprinting, re-use of illustrations, broadcasting, reproduction by photocopying machines or similar means, and storage in data banks.

Product Liability: The publisher can give no guarantee for all the information contained in this book. This does also refer to information about drug dosage and application thereof. In every individual case the respective user must check its accuracy by consulting other pharmaceutical literature. The use of registered names, trademarks, etc. in this publication does not imply, even in the absence of a specific statement, that such names are exempt from the relevant protective laws and regulations and therefore free for general use.

© 2001 Springer-Verlag/Wien
Printed in Slovenia

Typesetting: Scientific Publishing Services (P) Ltd., Madras
Printing: Gorenjski Tisk, Kranj

Printed on acid-free and chlorine-free bleached paper

SPIN: 10760725

With over 1200 mostly colored figures

CIP data applied for

ISBN 3-211-83449-4 Springer-Verlag Wien New York

Dedication

'Per aspera ad astra'

This Atlas is dedicated to surgeons and the many medical specialists throughout the world, who have contributed their knowledge, efforts and creativity towards developing modern, twenty-first century cryosurgery.

I also dedicate this book to my 'alma mater', the National Medical University of Kiev, as well as to all my teachers, who provided me with the best possible knowledge in the field of traditional medicine, and who greatly shaped my life and paved the way for me to become a doctor and a surgeon.

This book is further dedicated to my dear wife, Dr. Marta Korpan, and my daughter, Irina, who witnessed the emergence of the modern era of cryosurgery in the 1980s and the 1990s.

Nikolai N. Korpan

Foreword by Omar Maiwand

The therapeutic effects of low temperatures have been known for many years and the first successful treatment of malignant disease with cold was reported in 1855. Despite the enormous advances that have been made in medical science, the full potential of the use of extreme cold has not been fully explored. Dermatology was the first area to benefit substantially from the extensive use of cryosurgery, and cure rates of over 90% have been achieved for skin cancer. There is little doubt that low temperature treatment will destroy the cancer cells with excellent healing of the surrounding tissues. As a therapeutic agent cryosurgery is here to stay.

The use of cryosurgery for internal organs such as the trachea and bronchi, the prostate and the liver developed later. This is because of the difficulty of the controlled delivery of a low temperature to the treatment site without damaging the surrounding healthy tissue. For effective tissue destruction a temperature of at least $-30°C$ must be applied to the core and also to the extremities of the tumor. The future success of cryosurgery depends on the development of suitable probes, improved temperature monitoring techniques, and, more importantly, the use of new cryogens will be needed to provide practicable units delivering controllable lower temperatures.

Further laboratory and clinical research is required in the use of different cryogens and standardization of local temperature without damaging the surrounding tissues. Detailed study of the cryo-sensitivity of various tissues must be undertaken. Examination of the immunological effects of freezing may lead to improvements in tumoricidal responses of the host.

There is a lack of scientific literature on the subject and the publication of this book is greatly welcomed. I congratulate Professor Nikolai Korpan on the production of this much needed volume and have no doubt that it will be of enormous benefit to the international cryosurgery community.

Dr. Omar Maiwand
Consultant Thoracic Surgeon
President, European Society of Cryosurgery
Vice President and Co-Chairman of the International Society of Cryosurgery
Harefield, UK

Foreword by Jean-Paul Homasson

Cryosurgery is a therapeutic method using freezing temperatures for the purpose of destroying tissues in selected target areas. The hemostatic, analgesic and anti-inflammatory properties of ice have been known to man since the days of the Egyptian pharaohs; however the use of freezing techniques began in the mid-1850's, when iced saline solutions were used to treat carcinomas of the breast and of the uterine cervix. After an initial infatuation for the technique in different branches of medicine at the beginning of the 20th century, some uses of cryosurgery have fallen into disfavor, mostly because of alternative effective therapeutic methods. In other branches of medicine, cryosurgery has become an integral part of standard medical practice. Experimental studies over the past decade have provided improved knowledge of the mechanisms of injury to tissue as a result of freezing. Cryosurgery experienced a revival in the 1990's, due to important improvements in cryosurgical equipment, including the development of thin cryosurgical probes, which have widened out the potential scope and therapeutic uses of cryosurgery. New uses of cryosurgery, for example in treating liver tumors, and a renewed interest in its use in combating prostatic cancer, have been made possible by means of real-time intraoperative ultrasound; this new method of monitoring the freezing process guarantees precision of cryosurgical treatment. The scope of cryosurgery continues to widen out. The use of cryosurgery to treat dermatological benign or malignant lesions is well documented, and favorable results are regularly gotten in comparison to other techniques. Cryosurgery is widely used when lesions are easily accessible (proctology, gynecology, ophthalmology, ENT, maxillofacial surgery...). In other branches of medicine, the use of cryosurgery has been relatively recent, having been dependent on the miniaturization of the cryoprobes, which must be of a sufficiently narrow diameter in order to pass through the operative channel of the endoscopes (pulmonology). Other tumor sites, including those of the kidney, pancreas, brain, bones are relatively new indications, and an evaluation of the therapy is yet to be realized. Most commonly used as a palliative treatment of cancer, and at times of advanced external cancer, cryosurgery may also be medically indicated for the treatment of benign disorders. Some interesting works suggest a more intensive or synergistic effect if coupled with radiotherapy or chemotherapy, but the local immunological response to cryosurgery is still unclear and more experimental and clinical studies will be required to evaluate this response after freezing. The atlas of cryosurgery offers physicians an extensive overview of the different uses of cryosurgery, that should be regarded as one of the tools that may be chosen to treat a variety of benign or malignant lesions.

Dr. Jean-Paul Homasson
Immediate Past President
International Society of Cryosurgery
European Society of Cryosurgery
Paris, France

Editor's Preface

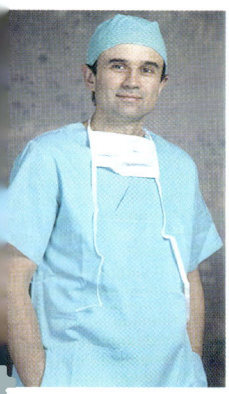

This is the first time that a book of this kind has ever been published in the history of global medicine and surgery. The *Atlas of Cryosurgery* is the first fundamental publication to document the modern era of cryosurgery which dawned in the mid-1960s. The revival of cryosurgery in the 1990s stimulated cryosurgical research. The use of sub-zero temperatures to destroy abnormal tissue, which is the basis of cryosurgery, is now successfully applied in many branches of medicine, especially to treat different malignancies. The aim of this Atlas is to present the fundamental aspects of modern cryosurgery and the advantages it offers cancer patients compared with conventional surgical approaches.

The Atlas lists definitions of the most frequently used terms, a short description of the historical and scientific background of cryosurgery, and gives an oversight of cryosurgical equipment and techniques. Moreover, the whole spectrum of experimental and clinical cryosurgery is outlined. For the first time, the results of the cryosurgical treatment of tumors of the liver, rectum, pancreas, lung, prostate, breast, uterus, oral cavity, bone, lymph nodes, heart and brain, as also of the veins and skin, are shown. Over 1200 illustrations, mostly in color, collected from a wide variety of international sources, serve to demonstrate the cryosurgical approach.

Each section contains a brief introductory text and a series of illustrations accompanied by clinical summaries and descriptive legends. Some of the slide collections contain a wide variety of selected light microscope micrographs from the authors' and other researchers' collections. They have been included to clarify pathological details. Particular attention has been given to the selection of illustrations that will be of great value to the student. They also contain sufficient cryosurgical detail to be of use to surgeons in training.

What is particularly important is that the Atlas reflects the wide experience gained by specialists in the twentieth century in the following fields: abdominal cryosurgery, cryosurgical proctology, cryosurgical dermatology, cryosurgical urology, cryosurgical gynecology, pulmonary cryosurgery, neurosurgery, cryosurgical otorhynolaryngology, cryosurgery for breast cancer, orthopedic cryosurgery, plastic cryosurgery and cardiovascular cryosurgery. This publication is the first to cover the fundamental aspects of modern cryosurgery, which will appear at the beginning of the third millennium, and will prove to be a vital contribution towards the further development of this particular branch of medicine, one that in future will come to be regarded as indispensable.

Prof. Dr. Nikolai N. Korpan
Vienna, Austria

List of Contributors

Boris I. Alperovich, M.D., Dr.Med.Sc.

Professor of Surgery
Siberia Medical University
Department of General Surgery
Tomsk
Russia

Joao A. Amaro, M.D.

Department of Dermatology
District Hospital of Santarem
Lisbon
Portugal

Nedjeljka Baldass, M.D.

Pharmaceutical Consultant
Janssen-Cilag Pharma GmbH
Austria

Franz Beer, M.D.

Consultant, Pathology and Histology
Pathologisch-Bakteriologisch-Humangenetisches Institut
SMZ-Ost Donauspital
Vienna
Austria

Jacob Bickels, M.D.

Department of Orthopedic Oncology
Tel-Aviv Sourasky Medical Center
Tel-Aviv
Israel

Vincent Dor, M.D.

Professor of Surgery
Monaco Cardio-Thoracic Center
Monte-Carlo
Monaco

Jean-Marc Frapier, M.D.

Chirurgie Thoracique et Cardio-vasculaire
Service du Professeur Chaptal
Hopital Arnaud de Villeneuve
Montpellier
France

Inderbir S. Gill, M.D., M.Ch.

Head, Section of Laparoscopic and Minimally Invasive Surgery
Department of Urology
The Cleveland Clinic Foundation
Cleveland, Ohio
USA

Jose Carlos d'Almeida Gonçalves, M.D.

President of the International Society of Cryosurgery
Head, Department of Dermatology
District Hospital of Santarem
Portuguese Institute of Oncology
Lisbon
Portugal

Gerhard Hochwarter, M.D.

Consultant, General Surgery
Department of Surgery
SMZ-Ost Donauspital
Vienna
Austria

Jean-Paul Homasson, M.D.

Immediate Past President of the European Society of Cryosurgery
International Society of Cryosurgery
Medical Chief, Centre Hospitalier Specialise en Pneumologie
Chevilly-Larue
France

Yoshiaki Hosaka, M.D.

Professor of Surgery
Chairman, Department of Plastic and Reconstructive Surgery
Showa University School of Medicine
Tokyo
Japan

Irina R. Khramova, M.D.

Department of Dermatology
   with Cosmetology
Orenburg State Hospital
Orenburg
Russia

Tatjana B. Komkova, M.D., Dr.Med.Sc.

Professor of Surgery
Siberia Medical University
Department of General Surgery
Tomsk
Russia

Nikolai N. Korpan, M.D., Ph.D., F.I.S.S., F.I.C.S.

Professor of Surgery
Vice President of the European
   Society of Cryosurgery
Chairman, Vienna International Institute
   for Cryosurgery
Consultant, General Surgery
Department of Surgery
Evangelical Hospital Wien-
   Währing
Vienna
Austria

Omar Maiwand, M.D.

Consultant Thoracic Surgeon
President of the European Society of
   Cryosurgery
Vice President and Co-Chairman of
   the International Society of
   Cryosurgery
Royal Brompton & Harefield NHS
   Trust
Harefield Hospital
Harefield
United Kingdom

Martin M. Malawer, M.D.

Professor of Orthopedic Surgery
Director, Orthopedic Oncology
George Washington University
School of Medicine
Washington Cancer Institute
Washington Hospital Center
National Cancer Institute
National Institutes of Health
Bethesda, Maryland
Sarcoma Consultant, Surgical Branch
USA

Sybren Meijer, M.D.

Professor of Surgery
Department of Surgical Oncology
Free University Hospital
Amsterdam
The Netherlands

Giuseppe Monfrecola, M.D.

Associate Professor of Dermatology
Department of Dermatology
University of Napoli "Federico II"
Napoli
Italy

Peter Nordin, M.D.

Läkarhuset Göteborg
Göteborg
Sweden

Patrick J.M. Le Pivert, M.D., Ph.D.

Chairman and Chief Medical Officer
Cryoflex, Inc.
West Palm Beach
Florida
USA

Yoed Rabin, Sc.D.

Associate Professor
Department of Mechanical
   Engineering
Carnegie Mellon University
Pittsburgh
USA

Daniel Luna Sabate, M.D.

Vice President of the European
Society of Cryosurgery
Neumologia
Hospital N.S.Aranzazu
San Sebastian
Spain

List of Contributors

Marco Scala, M.D.

Istituto nazionale per la ricerca sul cancro
Istituto scientifico per lo studio e la cura dei tumori
Division of Surgical Oncology
Genoa
Italy

Massimiliano Scalvenzi, M.D.

Assistant Dermatologist
Department of Dermatology
University of Napoli "Federico II"
Napoli
Italy

H.W.B. Schreuder, M.D., Ph.D.

Orthopedic Surgeon
Department of Orthopedics,
University Medical Center St. Radboud
Nijmegen
The Netherlands

Franz Sellner, M.D.

Associate Professor of Surgery
Department of Surgery
Kaiser-Franz-Josef-Spital
Vienna
Austria

Rodney Sinclair, M.D.

Senior Lecturer in Dermatology
The University of Melbourne
Department of Medicine (Dermatology)
St. Vincent's Hospital
Melbourne
Australia

Alberto Tajana, M.D.

Professor of Surgery
Director, Department of General Surgery
University of Milan
Milan
Italy

Shigeo Tanaka, M.D.

Tanaka Clinic
Obusemachi, Naganoken
Japan

Ved R. Tandan, M.D., M.Sc., F.R.C.S.C., F.A.C.S.

Assistant Professor
McMaster University
Department of Surgery
St. Joseph's Hospital
Surgical Oncology
Hepatobiliary and Pancreatic Surgery
Minimally Invasive Surgery
Hamilton, Ontario
Canada

Iwan S. Tchekman, M.D., Dr.Med.Sc.

Professor of Pharmacology
Head, Chair of General and Clinical Pharmacology
National Medical University of Kiev
Kiev
Ukraine

Laszlo Vizsy, M.D.

General Surgical Department
Country Legal City Hospital of Nagykanizsa
Hungary

James C. Wittig, M.D.

Orthopedic Oncology Fellow
Washington Cancer Institute
Washington Hospital Center
National Cancer Institute
National Institutes of Health
Bethesda, Maryland
Sarcoma Consultant, Surgical Branch
USA

Jaroslav V. Zharkov, Engineer, Designer

Director, Cryosurgical Research
"Pulse" Company
Kiev
Ukraine

Contents

Section A   **Fundamental Aspects of Cryosurgery**

3   *Chapter 1*
Definition and Terminology
Nikolai N. Korpan

7   *Chapter 2*
History of Cryosurgery
Nikolai N. Korpan

15   *Chapter 3*
Theoretical Aspects of Cryosurgery
Nikolai N. Korpan with contributions by Jaroslav V. Zharkov and Patrick J.M. Le Pivert

Section B   **Experimental Foundations of Cryosurgery**

21   *Chapter 4*
Experimental Basis of Cryosurgery
Nikolai N. Korpan with contributions by Jaroslav V. Zharkov

Section C   **Basis of Cryosurgical Equipment and Technology**

73   *Chapter 5*
Basic Aspects of Cryosurgical Equipment and Technology
Nikolai N. Korpan with contributions by Jaroslav V. Zharkov

81   *Chapter 6*
Technical Requirements for Cryosurgical Equipment
Jaroslav V. Zharkov

Section D   **Basic Cryosurgical Techniques**

85   *Chapter 7*
General Techniques of Cryosurgery
Nikolai N. Korpan

Chapter 8   95
Liver Cryosurgical Techniques
Nikolai N. Korpan

Experimental Aspects   **Section E**

Chapter 9   105
Liver Cryosurgery. An Animal Experiment
9.0. Introduction   105
9.1. Open Hepatic Cryosurgery   106
9.2. Laparoscopic Hepatic Cryosurgery   114
9.3. Ultrastructural Changes in Liver Tissue   116
9.4. Histological Study of the Liver   129
Nikolai N. Korpan with contributions by Iwan S. Tchekman, Jaroslav V. Zharkov, Franz Beer and Ved R. Tandan

Chapter 10   137
Pancreas Cryosurgery. An Animal Experiment
10.0. Introduction   137
10.1. Pancreatic Cryosurgery: Experimental Basis   138
10.2. The 'Lunar Eclipse' Phenomenon   144
10.3. Ultrastructural Changes in Pancreas Tissue   149
10.4. Morphological Study of the Pancreas   157
Nikolai N. Korpan with contributions by Iwan S. Tchekman, Jaroslav V. Zharkov and Franz Beer

Clinical Aspects   **Section F**

Chapter 11   165
Cryosurgical Dermatology
11.0. Introduction   165
11.1. Standard Cryosurgical Procedures of Cutaneous Lesions   168

172	11.2. Benign Tumors	*Jean-Paul Homasson,*	
186	11.3. Malignant Tumors	*Omar Maiwand*	
	Nikolai N. Korpan with	*and Daniel Luna Sabate*	
	contributions by Joao		
	A. Amaro, Jose Carlos	*Chapter 15*	319
	d'Almeida Gonçalves,	Anorectal Cryosurgery:	
	Giuseppe Monfrecola,	Curative and Palliative	
	Peter Nordin, Patrick J.M.	Cryosurgery	
	Le Pivert, Massimiliano	15.0. Introduction	319
	Scalvenzi and Rodney	15.1. Hemorrhoidal	
	Sinclair	Disease	321
		15.2. Anorectal Tumors	326
235	*Chapter 12*	*Nikolai N. Korpan with*	
	Abdominal Cryo-	*contributions by Sybren*	
	surgery: Hepatic Cryo-	*Meijer, Patrick J.M. Le*	
	surgery	*Pivert and Alberto Tajana*	
235	12.0. Introduction		
	12.1. Hepatic Cryo-	*Chapter 16*	343
	surgery for Small Liver	Breast Cancer	
236	Metastases	Cryosurgery	
	12.2. Hepatic Cryo-	16.0. Introduction	343
	surgery for Large Liver	16.1. Imaging of Breast	
	Metastatic Tumors	Cryosurgery	344
237	(Cancer)	16.2. Locally Advanced	
	12.3. Cryosurgical	Breast Cancer (LABC)	354
	Avascular Tumor	16.3. Local-Regional	
	Phenomenon (CAT-	Disease Recurrence	393
269	Phenomenon)	16.4. Skin Metastases	397
	12.4. Laparoscopic	*Nikolai N. Korpan with*	
273	Liver Cryosurgery	*contributions by Jose*	
	12.5. Cryosurgery for	*Carlos d'Almeida*	
	Echinococcal Cystic	*Gonçalves, Patrick J.M. Le*	
278	Disease of the Liver	*Pivert, Yoed Rabin*	
	12.6. Cryosurgery of	*and Shigeo Tanaka*	
284	Liver Alveococcosis		
	Nikolai N. Korpan with	*Chapter 17*	399
	contributions by Boris	Breast Cryosurgery:	
	I. Alperovich, Gerhard	Benign Disorders	
	Hochwarter, Franz Sellner	17.1. Papillary Lesions	399
	and Ved R. Tandan	*Nikolai N. Korpan*	
		Chapter 18	403
289	*Chapter 13*	Cryosurgical Urology	
	Abdominal Cryo-	18.0. Introduction	403
	surgery: Pancreas	18.1. Laparoscopic Renal	
	Cryosurgery	Cryoablation	405
289	13.0. Introduction	*Inderbir S. Gill*	
	13.1. Chronic		
291	Pancreatitis	*Chapter 19*	419
	13.2. Advanced	Orthopedic Cryosurgery	
296	Pancreatic Cancer	19.0. Introduction	419
	Nikolai N. Korpan with	19.1. Bone Tumors	421
	contributions by Gerhard	*Martin M. Malawer,*	
	Hochwarter, Tatjana	*H.W. Bart Schreuder,*	
	B. Komkova and Franz	*James C. Wittig*	
	Sellner	*and Jacob Bickels*	
303	*Chapter 14*	*Chapter 20*	445
	Pulmonary Cryosurgery	Cosmetic Cryosurgery	
303	14.0. Introduction	20.0. Introduction	445
	14.1. Bronchiogenic	20.1. Hypertrophic	
	Tumors and Endobron-	Scars (postoperative,	
304	chial Metastases	posttraumatic)	447

Contents

453   20.2. Skin Lesions
458   20.3. Nevus Ota
Nikolai N. Korpan with contributions by Yoshiaki Hosaka

475   *Chapter 21*
Cryosurgical Otorhynolaryngology
475   21.1. Benign Neoplasms
484   21.2. Malignant Tumors
Nikolai N. Korpan with contributions by Marco Scala

489   *Chapter 22*
Cryophlebology
489   22.0. Introduction
490   22.1. Cryo-Stripping
Patrick J.M. Le Pivert and Laszlo Vizsy

499   *Chapter 23*
Cryosurgical Gynecology
499   23.1. Advanced Cancer of the External Genital Organs
Jose Carlos d'Almeida Gonçalves

501   *Chapter 24*
Cardiovascular Cryosurgery
Vincent Dor and Jean-Marc Frapier

503   *Chapter 25*
Cryomassage

25.0. Introduction   503
25.1. Technique   504
Irina R. Khramova

Tumor Anemia   Section G

Chapter 26   507
Causes of Anemia in Cancer Patients
26.1. Introduction   507
26.2. Origin and Characteristics of ACD   507
26.3. The Erythropoietin Feedback Loop   508
26.4. Symptoms of Anemia   508
26.5. Risk Factors for Anemia in Cancer Patients   509
26.6. Anemia Associated with Platinum-Based Chemotherapy   509
26.7. Frequency of Anemia with Nonplatinum Chemotherapeutic Agents   509
26.8. Hb Level as a Risk Factor for Anemia— Skillings' Study   509
26.9. Hb Levels as a Risk for Anemia— Abels' Study   510
26.10. Management of Anemia   510
26.11. Patient Candidates for Epoetin Alpha Therapy   510
26.12. Titration   510
Nedjeljka Baldass

Subject Index   515

Section A

Fundamental Aspects of Cryosurgery

Definitions and Terminology

Nikolai N. Korpan

Synonyms for *cryo* are "cold", "frost" and "ice". In Greek "Kryos", (a derivative of which is "crystal") means "ice" or "cold", and thus combines both meanings. That is why one speaks of ice and cold therapy.

The operative separation of tissue, or the deliberate destruction of pathological tissue, by inducing necrosis through cold using a vacuum-insulated cryoinstrument (cryoprobe, cryoscalpel, cryoclamp), is termed cryosurgery (also known as cold surgery, more rarely as freeze surgery). Cryoinstruments filled with fluid liquid nitrogen or fluid carbon dioxide can reach sub-zero temperatures of $-196°C$ or $-160°C$ respectively. In most cases the tumors are not cut out but rather shock frozen.

The tissue is usually frozen to about $-20°C$. Sub-zero temperatures are achieved by means of a probe through which liquid nitrogen or carbon dioxide circulates.

Cryosurgery is thus an operation in which very low temperatures are applied to a lesion with the purpose of destroying the tissue *in situ* by the application of extreme cold. It is also the technique of exposing tissue to extreme cold so as to outline well-demarcated areas of cell injury and the area which is to be destroyed by surgical procedure.

One differentiates between a general lowering of body temperature (*hypothermia artificialis*) and a local temperature decline (*hypothermia localis* or *hypothermia regionalis*), as well as superficial local (*cryotherapy*) and deep local (*cryosurgery*) freezing.

According to how the temperatures are applied, these techniques are defined as follows:

Hypothermia – either hypothermia artificialis, or hypothermia localis, or hypothermia regionalis – is a method of deliberate therapeutic lowering of the body temperature, whereby the temperature of the body as a whole, or only a part of it is lowered down to, or not far above, freezing point.

Cryotherapy – means the use of a local, superficial temperature decline of maximally $(-10)–(-15)°C$ for treatment, whereby the tissue remains vital and the physio-biochemical processes are still reversible. Cryotherapy mostly involves the use of ice and other local applications of cold temperatures. It is therefore a form of therapy which uses cold packs to prevent tissue swelling.

Cold surgery, or freeze surgery, i.e. the implementation of extreme cold in cryotechnological practice, is a treatment involving the withdrawal of warmth by deliberate, local freezing of the tissue to approximately $-196°C$, whereby the tissue does not stay vital and the physio-biochemical processes are no longer reversible.

Other related definitions are as follows:

Cryoresection – the cryosurgical removal of a part of an organ, or of a complete structure or organ with pathological tissue (tumor) using cryoprobes, usually with the help of a cryogenic clamp or cryoscalpel or an instrument resembling a trocar (*or* the act of cutting out tissue by using low temperatures).

Chapter 1 Terminology

Cryoextirpation (cryoablation) – full (complete) removal of the tumor by freezing the tissue, usually using disk-shaped or trocar type cryoprobes.

Cryodestruction – partial removal of the tumor (diseased tissue) by freezing it in order to achieve reduction of the tumor mass, usually by applying disc-shaped cryoprobes (destruction = the action or process of destroying something).

For liver (hepatic) cryosurgery the definitions are as follows:

Liver (hepatic) cryoresection is the cryosurgical removal of pathological organ structures by means of a cold clamp or cryosurgical knife.

Liver (hepatic) cryoextirpation (cryoablation) is the full cryosurgical removal of the clearly demarcated focus or tumor in the healthy region by means of a trocar or disc-shaped *cryoinstrument* (cryoprobe, cryoneedle).

Liver (hepatic) cryodestruction involves performing an operation by applying cold to achieve partial removal of the tumor, thus reducing the entire tumor mass.

Laparoscopic liver (hepatic) cryosurgery or minimal invasive liver (hepatic) cryosurgery is a cryosurgical procedure, the purpose of which is to remove the liver tumor, or to achieve the reduction of the liver tumor mass, by applying laparoscopy and other minimal invasive techniques.

Further cryoterminology used in medical practice:

Cryometer [cryo + meter] – a thermometer for measuring low temperatures.

Cryoprobe – an instrument for applying extreme cold to tissue.

Cryoshaving – shaving off thin slices of pathological tissue by means of a cryosurgical instrument (such as a cryoapplicator).

Cryomassage – repeated short applications of superficial cold on healthy body tissue especially with a cryoinstrument to accelerate the process of stimulation and biological regeneration in the case of an anemic or hyperemic skin surface.

Cryoanalgesia – the relief of pain by application of cold by cryoprobe to peripheral nerves.

Cryoanesthesia [cryo + anesthesia] – local anesthesia obtained by refrigeration, i.e., by spraying rapidly evaporating substances on the desired part of the body; also termed frost or refrigeration anesthesia.

Cryoalgesia [cryo- + Greek algesis, pain] – the pain which is caused by contact with cold substances or due to the application of cold.

Cryoesthesia [cryo + Greek aisthesis, perception] – abnormal sensitivity to cold.

Cryoextraction – the application of low temperature to remove a cataract by means of a cryoinstrument. The extremely cold tip of which forms an "ice ball" on the lens, consequent to the thawing of which the lens is removed.

Cryoextractor [cryo + extractor] – a cryoprobe used in cryoextraction.

Cryocautery – [cryo + cautery] – cauterization by applying a particular substance, such as liquid nitrogen or carbon dioxide snow, or by using an instrument that destroys tissue by means of freezing; also termed cold cautery.

Cryoscopy – the study of the phenomena relating to the refrigeration of solutions or, in a more general sense, of a body fluid as compared to the freezing point of distilled water.

Crymo [Greek krymos, frost] – a related term denoting cold.

Crymotherapy = cryotherapy

Cryogen [cryo + Greek gennan, to produce] – a substance used for lowering temperatures.

Cryogenic – the science engaged in the development of freezing temperatures within a biological system and pertaining to or causing the production of low temperatures.

Cryohypophysectomy – destruction of the hypophysis by application of cold.

Cryothalamectomy – cryothalamotomy.

Cryothalamotomy – destruction of a portion of the thalamus by application of extreme cold.

Cryolymphadenectomy – removal of metastases from the lymph node by application of very low temperatures.

Cryolumpectomy – cryosurgical segment or quadrant resection of the breast.

Cryomastectomy – complete removal of the breast with the tumor by freezing, using a disk in the form of cryoprobes.

Cryovaricectomy or *cryo-stripping* involves removal of a too long or too short saphenous vein and localized removal of dilated collateral veins by using cryoangioprobes.

Cryoimmunology – a cryoimmunological reaction elicited by cryosurgical session and characterized by species-specificity and tissue- or organ-specificity; degenerative changes close to tissue destruction (cryosurgery) by cold injury may elicit a specific response of the host and induce production of specific autoantibodies.

Cryobiology – the study of the physical effects of low temperatures on living tissue.

Cryoglobulin – a serum globulin (invariably an immunoglobulin) that precipitates at low temperature (e.g., 4°C) and re-dissolves at 37°C. Cryoglobulins are classified as Type I, monoclonal immunoglobulins; Type II, immune complexes involving monoclonal immunoglobulins; or Type III, immune complexes involving polyclonal immunoglobulins; in most cases, there are globulin-antiglobulin immune complexes similar to Type II complexes.

Cryopreservation – the permanent cooling of living tissue, for example, blood, blood derivatives and semen, to preserve its use at a later time.

Cryotolerant – able to withstand unusually low temperatures.

Cryoglobulinemia – the presence of cryoglobulin in the blood, associated with a variety of clinical manifestations including Raynaud's phenomenon, vascular purpura, cold urticaria, vasculitis, etc.

History of Cryosurgery

Nikolai N. Korpan

The use of cold temperatures as a promising technique for medical purposes has been known for a long time. It was the anesthetizing properties of cold that were first used to treat a variety of medical conditions. In comparison, the history of cryosurgery is relatively short and, in the nineteenth and twentieth centuries, closely interwoven with developments in low-temperature physics, engineering and the refinement of the necessary instruments. A review of the history of cryosurgery will show that it has progressed in leaps and that each leap has usually been triggered by technological innovations which immediately preceded it. Thus the possibility of creating very low temperatures of less than −100°C was immediately followed by Schroeder's discovery in 1997 that the application of such low temperatures could induce cell death. The destruction of diseased tissue such as benign and malignant neoplasms by the application of exceedingly low temperatures is today known by the name of cryosurgery, and is generally accepted as a valuable optional treatment in several fields of medicine.

The damage that cold can do has been recognised from the earliest times and is referred to in both civilian and military sources. Historical accounts of the effect of cold climates on various body tissues foreshadow the far-reaching changes that modern cryosurgical methods have brought about (Shepherd and Dawber 1982).

Ancient Egypt

Already in 2500 BC, the use of cold compresses to treat compound skull fractures and infected wounds is mentioned in the Edwin Smith Surgical Papyrus (Breasted translation 1930).

Antiquity

In 460 BC, Greek medicine was concerned with the prevention and cure of illness caused by cold. Hippocrates, the father of medicine, noted the effects of cold on the inhabitants of countries with cold climates. He advocated the use of cold to control hemorrhages and reduce the swelling of painful joints (Zonnevylle 1981).

In 25 AD Celsus described the appearance of the skin after cold injury, and noted that if the injury was severe, dry gangrene supervened (Shepherd and Dawber 1982).

The loss of sensation which accompanies injury from cold is described by Galen in his treatise (70 AD) "Pain as a means of diagnosis" (Shepherd and Dawber 1982).

Military campaigns in the mountainous regions of the ancient world resulted in cold injuries of epidemic proportion. The Carthaginian mercenaries in Hannibal's army which crossed the Alps in 218 BC found that smearing their bodies with oil was an effective means of preventing frostbite, which nevertheless took a heavy toll (Shepherd and Dawson 1982). The forces of Alexander the Great found similar protection using sesame juice.

Eleventh Century

An unknown Anglo-Saxon monk (1050 AD) employed cold as a local anesthetic (Gratton and Singer 1952).

Sixteenth Century

Refrigeration anesthesia was known to Italian physicians by 1570 (Davison 1959).

Chapter 2 History

Seventeenth Century

In 1661 Thomas Bartholin of Copenhagen described the use of cold as a therapeutic for a variety of everyday illnesses (Bracco 1980).

In 1665 Robert Boyle published a monograph on the influence of cold on living animals (Breasted 1930).

Eighteenth Century

In 1714 Fahrenheit invented the mercury thermometer, which was later reinvented by Reaumur (1739) and Celsius (1742) (Walder 1966). The invention of the thermometer is of considerable importance because it was now possible to measure the actual "coldness" or temperature at which phenomena occurred. Furthermore, endeavors to generate lower and lower temperatures could now begin. Scientists were now able to standardize their experiments and exchange results (Schreuder 1997).

The effects a temperature of $-24°C$ had on insects, fish, amphibians, reptiles, birds and mammals was investigated by Spallanzani in 1787. He also established the existence of water at sub-zero temperatures without it becoming ice – a physical state later called "supercooling" (Walder 1966).

During the War of Independence (1775–1783), a medical diarist, Dr. James Thatcher, noted the serious losses of American forces due to cold injuries. He recorded that on one sortie five hundred troops were "slightly frozen" after a night in the open. In the Napoleonic Wars, Napoleon's surgeon-general, Von Larrey (1766–1842), made detailed observations of the effects of cold on his patients. He described erythema and blistering of the skin after freezing, and also noted that gangrene was not an inevitable consequence of freezing if exposure was not prolonged. Uneventful healing of wounds affected by cold was also described. Tissue cooling by surface application of snow and ice was used to facilitate amputation in Napoleon's Grand Army (Schechter and Sarot 1968). Casualties in later campaigns were numerous, amounting to 115 000 in World War I (Shepherd and Dawber 1982).

Nineteenth Century

The therapeutic effects of low temperatures have been known for many years. The first successful treatment of malignant disease in England was reported between 1845 and 1851 by Dr. James Arnott (1797–1883), who used iced saline solutions at temperatures of $-18°$ to $-24°C$ for the treatment of advanced breast and uterine cancer. He observed that "congelation arresting the accompanying inflammation and destroying the vitality of the cancer cell, is not only calculated to prolong life for a considerable period, but may, not improbably, in the early stage of the disease, exert a curative action" (Arnott 1850; Bird 1949). Thus Arnott is most probably the first doctor who used cold to treat malignancies. Although he did not cure them, he considerably reduced the morbidity of cancer, especially the pain, which is still sometimes a considerable problem. Most of his work focused on the application of cold in anesthesia.

The anesthetizing characteristics of low temperatures were already known by this time, but using low temperatures to destroy parts of a tumor was now recognized as an added effect of freezing. Although Arnott's contemporaries acknowledged the usefulness of applying cold and began to use freezing techniques locally, further developments in cryosurgery had to await technological advances, especially the development of better cryogenic agents (Gage 1998).

Esmarch's approach in 1862 was courageously outspoken: "The application of cold as a means of fighting hyperemic and inflammatory conditions is not given the recognition it deserves by a not inconsiderable number of contemporary physicians. Although the number of doctors who deny the antiphlogistic properties of cold is not great, many consider it dispensable. I therefore fully expect and am prepared to face forceful contradiction from many sides when I say that of all the means we have at our disposal to fight inflammatory processes, I consider cold to be the most important. Indeed, without this means, I would rather not be a surgeon."

In 1868 Samuel locally froze the ear of a rabbit by means of an ether spray and described the subsequent clinical and microscopic changes that occurred (Samuel 1868).

In 1883 Openchowski attempted to localize the physiological function of different areas within the cerebral cortex of dogs by local freezing. He obtained freezing temperatures by using the evaporation of ether in the form of a jet of warm air. Peripheral convulsions or paralyses produced by applying this method made functional mapping of the cortex possible.

The end of the nineteenth century witnessed several major discoveries in the field of cryogenics. Ether sprays described by Richardson (1866), and ethyl chloride described by Redard (1891) were used for cold analgesia but not for destructive freezing (Davison 1959).

In 1877 Cailletet in France and Pictet in Switzerland began developing adiabatic expansion systems for cooling gases. This led to the liquefaction of oxygen, air and nitrogen. Liquid air ($-190°C$) was first clinically used by Campbell-White in 1889 for the treatment of diverse skin diseases (White 1899, 1901). The liquid air was applied locally by means of a swab, spray or brass roller device.

Solidified carbon dioxide ($-78.5°C$) was first used by Pusey in 1907 and subsequently became an established therapeutic technique in dermatology and gynecology (Pusey 1907). After 1910, apparently, liquid air was little used. The most popular cryogenic agent in the early 1900s was solid carbon dioxide.

Twentieth Century

Until the beginning of the twentieth century, those who used the devices which generated cold had usually also invented them. After the turn of the century the two professions separated. Greater engineering know-how was required to improve the equipment for developing cryosurgical instruments and for the production of cryogenic media (Schreuder 1997).

In the 1920s liquid oxygen ($-182°C$) began to be used clinically as a cryogenic agent in the treatment of skin diseases. Liquid oxygen is potentially dangerous because it burns and explodes easily, and it has therefore never become a popular cryogen for cryosurgery (Kile and Welsh 1948).

In 1942 the development of chlorofluorocarbon refrigerants led to the first closed-cycle refrigeration system in cryosurgery. Temperatures as low as $-40°C$ could now be applied (Hall 1942). It was used for the treatment of chronic cervicitis. The device permitted rapid defrosting which released the applicator when required. These cryogens with closed refrigeration cycles never became popular. The temperatures which they can achieve are probably higher than those which can be achieved with the relatively less

Chapter 2 History

expensive solid carbon dioxide (Gage 1998).

Between 1936 and 1940 Temple Fay, an American neurosurgeon, used local and general refrigeration techniques to treat patients with advanced cancer, glioblastoma, Hodgkin's disease and other illnesses including large, symptomatic, inoperable cancers of the uterine cervix and the breast (Fay 1959).

In the early 1940s, Kapitsa in the Soviet Union and Collins in the United States began developing commercial techniques for the large-scale liquefaction of hydrogen and helium, with liquid nitrogen as an abundant and low-cost by-product. Liquid nitrogen ($-196°C$) became commercially available, and, in 1950, this cryogen was introduced to clinical practice by Allington (Allington 1950). The liquid nitrogen was applied with a cotton swab, and was soon commonly used to treat skin diseases and diverse non-neoplastic lesions. It was not commonly used for skin tumors because the swab technique produced only superficial freezing, perhaps 2 mm in depth (Gage 1998). Prior to the 1960s, the devices used for cryosurgery were not efficient and were only able to freeze to a depth of several millimeters. With a few exceptions, therefore, freezing was primarily used for the removal of superficial layers of undesirable tissue, most often in dermatology and gynecology.

The Era of Modern Cryosurgery

The development of cryosurgery as a therapeutic technique received a major stimulus from the introduction of the first cryosurgical system capable of delivering liquid nitrogen ($-196°C$) to trocar type probes with an insulated shaft and a conductive metal tip. This was the result of the combined work of Irving Cooper, a neurosurgeon, and Arnold Lee, an engineer (Cooper and Lee 1961). Their cryosurgery probe was in essence the prototype from which all future cryosurgical probes using liquid nitrogen were built (Gage 1998). The ability of the device to produce an avascular cryolesion in the liver was demonstrated on a cat (Cooper 1963). The design of the probes allowed surgeons for the first time to treat lesions deep within parenchymal organs with minimal trauma to the remaining organ. After the introduction of the new cryosurgical probe by Cooper and Lee, cryosurgery experienced a rapid growth which lasted to the end of the decade.

In the 1960s Zacarian and Adham attempted to achieve greater tissue depth penetration through the use of solid copper cylinder discs that were cooled by immersion in liquid nitrogen prior to their application to the skin (Zacarian and Adham 1966, 1967). The copper discs had a good thermal capacity and enhanced heat exchange characteristics in comparison to the cotton applications. They also provided an opportunity to exert pressure on the lesion. Tissue destruction to a depth of 7 mm became possible, which was certainly an improvement in technique, yet the freezing of large areas of tissue as needed to treat cutaneous malignancies was not easy (Kuflik et al. 2000).

In Kiev in the 1980s, Nikolai N. Korpan, a surgeon, began basic theoretical, experimental and clinical studies on modern cryosurgery, in co-operation with Jaroslav V. Zharkov, an engineer and designer. They developed new, highly-efficient universal cyrogenic techniques with liquid nitrogen that were designed especially for the treatment of a wide variety of malignant tumors, and have since been awarded numerous patents. Drawing on their extensive know-how, the two scientists formulated the basic clinical and technical requirements for modern cryosurgery, most importantly the need to freeze tissue at extremely low temperatures followed by deliberate thawing. The concepts underlying the design and production of the most technically advanced cryosurgical equipment used today in different fields of medicine were elaborated by Korpan and Zharkov (Korpan et al. 1985, 1987, 1996, 1997, 2000; Zharkov et al. 1985, 1997, 1998, 2000).

During the following twenty years, the cryosurgical treatment of tumors in various organs such as the liver (Korpan et al. 1985; Adam et al. 1997), pancreas (Korpan et al. 1985, 1997, 2000), rectum (Korpan 1985, 1996; Heberer et al. 1987; Yamamoto et al. 1989; Neijer et al. 1996), breast (Korpan 1981, 2000; Rand et al. 1987; Tanaka 1995; Staren et al. 1997), skin (Dawber et al. 1992; Gonçalves 1997; Nordin et al. 1997; Zouboulis 1998), lung (Katz 1989; Homasson et al. 1993; Maiwand 1999), brain (Stellar 1993), prostate (Wong et al. 1997; Chinn 1999), uterus (Andersen et al. 1988), oral cavity (Gage 1976; Pogrel et al. 1996), bone (Malawer et al. 1988; Aboulafia et al. 1994; Schreuder 1997), and cardiac surgery (Watanabe et al. 1996; Crawford and Gillette 1997) was reported.

In the 1990s the development of intraoperative ultrasound and its use to monitor the process of freezing renewed interest in cryosurgery (Marron et al. 1992; Onik et al. 1993; Crawford and Gillette 1997; Staren et al. 1997). The ultrasound image identified the site of the lesion, guided the placement of the cryoprobe into the lesion, and monitored the freezing process. This was a substantial advantage over the earlier techniques (Gage 1998). In addition, the development of an array of endoscopic and percutaneous access devices stimulated the use of cryosurgery in the treatment of visceral disease, especially for tumors.

Until recently, the devices used for cryosurgery were not efficient and were only able to freeze the lesions of superficial skin layers. The application of modern cryosurgery can only become possible if highly efficient cryotechnology is used. Experience in the use of cryosurgery to treat uterine fibroids and malignant tumors of the kidney, breast, pancreas and other organs is now beginning to be gathered (Marron et al. 1992; Staren et al. 1997; Uchida et al. 1995; Pitrof et al. 1994; Korpan and Hochwarter 1997).

References

Aboulafia, A.J., Rosenbaum, D.H., Sicard-Rosenbaum, L., Jelinek, J.S., Malawer, M.M. (1994): Treatment of large subchondral tumors of the knee with cryosurgery and composite reconstruction. Clin. Orthop. 307: 189–199

Adam, R., Akpinar, E., Johann, M. (1997): Place of Cryosurgery in the Treatment of Malignant Liver Tumors. An. Surg. 225(1): 39–50

Allington, H.V. (1950): Liquid nitrogen in the treatment of skin diseases. Calif. Med. 72: 153–155

Andersen, E.S., Thorup, K., Larsen, G. (1988): The results of cryosurgery for cervical intraepithelial neoplasia. Gynecol. Oncol. 30: 21–25

Arnott, J. (1850): Practical illustrations of the remedial efficacy of a very low or anaesthetic temperature. Lancet 2: 257–259

Bird, H.M. (1949): James Arnott, M.D. (Aberdeen) 1797–1883. A pioneer in refrigeration analgesia. Anaesthesia 4: 10–17

Bracco, D. (1980): Handbook on cryosurgery, Historical developments. New York, Marcel Dekker. 4

Breasted, J.H. (1930): The Edwin Smith Surgical Papyrus. Chicago, University of Chicago Oriental Institute Publications. III(1): 217–224

Chinn, D. (1999): Prostate cryosurgery: scientific and technical advancements. Urology. News. 3(4): 10–12

Cooper, I.S. (1963): Cryogenic surgery. A new method of destruction or extirpation of benign or malignant tissues. N. Engl. J. Med. 268: 743–749

Cooper, I.S., Lee, A. (1961): Cryostatic congelation: a system for producing a limited controlled region of cooling or freezing of biologic tissues. J. Nerv. Ment. Dis. 133: 259–263

Crawford, F.A., Gillette, P.C. (1997): Cryoablation of septal pathways in patients with supraventricular tachyarrhythmias. Updated in 1997. Ann. Thorac. Surg. 63(4): 1205–1206

Chapter 2
History

Davison, M.H.A. (1959): The evolution of anesthesia. Br. J. Anaesthesiol. 31: 134

Davison, M.M. (1959): The evolution of anaesthesia. Br. J. Anaesthesiol. 31: 134–137

Dawber, R., Colver, G., Jackson, A. (1992): Cutaneous Cryosurgery. Principles and Clinical Practice. London, Martin Dunitz

Esmarch, Fr. (1862): Die Anwendung der Kälte in der Chirurgie. Archiv für klinische Chirurgie. 275–333

Fay, T. (1959): Early experiences with local and generalized refrigeration of the human brain. J. Neurosurg. 16: 239–259

Gage, A.A. (1976): Five-year survival following cryosurgery for oral cancer. Arch. Surg. 111: 990–994

Gage, A.A. (1998): History of Cryosurgery. Sem. Surg. Oncol. 14: 99–109

Gonçalves, J.C. (1997): Fractional cryosurgery. A new technique for basal cell carcinoma of the eyelids and periorbital area. Dermatol. Surg. 23(6): 475–481

Gratton, J.H.G., Singer, C. (1952): Anglo-Saxon magic and medicine. London, Oxford University Press. 165

Hall, F.E. (1942): The use of quick freezing methods in gynecology practice. Am. J. Obstet. Gynecol. 43: 105–111

Heberer, G., Denecke, H., Demmel, N., Wirsching, R. (1987): Local procedures in the management of rectal cancer. World. J. Surg. 11: 499–503

Homasson, J.P., Bell, N.J. (1993): Cryotherapy in Chest Medicine. Paris, Springer Verlag

Katz, J. (1989): Cryoanalgesia for post-thoracotomy pain. Ann. Thorac. Surg. 48: 5

Kile, R.L., Welsh, A.L. (1948): Liquid oxygen in dermatologic practice. Arch. Dermatol. Syph. 57: 57–60

Korpan, N.N. (1996): Moeglichkeiten und Grenzen der modernen Kryochirurgie. In: Neugebauer H, ed. Was gibt es Neues in der Medizin, Vienna, Dr. Peter Mueller Verlag. 207–213

Korpan, N.N. (1997): Hepatic Cryosurgery for Liver Metastases. Long-Term Follow-Up. Ann. Surg. 225(2): 193–201

Korpan, N.N. (2000): Pancreas Cryosurgery. An Animal Study 2000. 1st European Congress of Cryosurgery (San Sebastian, Spain, March 29-April 2, 2000), Abstract Book, 7

Korpan, N.N., Hochwarter, G. (1997): Pancreatic cryosurgery – a new surgical procedure for pancreatic cancer. Eur. J. Clin. Invest. 27 (Suppl 1): A33

Korpan, N.N., Zharkov, J.V., Hochwarter, G. (1998): Concept of technical requirements for cryosurgical equipment. 10th World Congress of Cryosurgery (Orlando, Florida, USA, October 29–November 1, 1998), Abstract Book, 3–4

Korpan, N.N., Hochwarter, G., Sellner, F., Zharkov, J.V. (1997): Pancreatic cryosurgery – a new surgical strategy for pancreatic cancer. In: 37th World Congress of Surgery, International Surgical Week ISW97 (Acapulco, Mexico, August 24–30, 1997), Abstract Book, 156

Korpan, N.N., Muskin, J.N., Zemskov, V.S., Skiba, V.V. (1985): Abdomen cryosurgery. Vestn Surg. 9: 141–145

Korpan, N.N., Zemskov, V.S., Kolesnikov, E.B. (1985): Cryosurgery of liver and pancreas cancer. In: Ternovoi K, Gassanov G, eds. Low Temperatures in Medicine, Kiev, Naukova Dumka. 107–161

Kuflik, E.G., Gage, A.A., Lubritz, R.R., Graham, G.F. (2000): History of Dermatologic Cryosurgery. Dermatol. Surg. 26(8): 715–722

Maiwand, M.O. (1999): The role of cryosurgery in the palliation of tracheo-bronchial carcinoma. Eur. J. Cardio-Thoracic Surg. 15: 764–768

Malawer, M.M., Marks, M.R., McChesney, D., Piasio, M., Gunther, S.F., Schmookler, B.M. (1988): The effect of cryosurgery and polymethylmethacrylate in dogs with experimental bone defects comparable to tumor defects. Clin. Orthop. 226: 299–310

Marron, J.C., Onik, G., Quigley, M.R. (1992): Cryosurgery revisited for the removal and destruction of brain, spinal and orbital tumors. Neurol. Res. 14: 294–302

Meijer, S., Jas, B., de-Lange, E., Derksen, E.J. (1996): Palliative cryosurgery in rectal carcinoma. Ned. Tijdschr. Geneeskd. 140(35): 1766–1770

Nordin, P., Larko, O., Stenquist, B. (1997): Five-year results of curettage-cryosurgery of selected large primary basal cell carcinomas on the nose: an alternative treatment in a geographical area underserved by Mohs' surgery. Br. J. Dermatol. 136(2): 180–183

Onik, G., Cohen, J., Reyes, G., Rubinsky, B., Chang, Z., Baust, J. (1993): Transrectal ultrasound-guided percutaneous radical cryosurgical ablation of the prostate. Cancer. 72: 1291–1299

Openchowski, P. (1883): Sur l'action localisee du froid, applique a la surface de la region cortical du cerveau. CR Soc Biol, Paris. 35: 38

Pitrof, R., Majid, S., Murray, A. (1994): Transcervical endometrial cryoablation (ECA) for menorrhagia. Int. J. Gynecol. Obstet. 47: 135–140

Pogrel, M.A., Yen, C.K., Taylor, R. (1996): A study of infrared thermographic assessment of liquid nitrogen cryosurgery. Oral. Surg. Oral. Med. Oral. Pathol. Oral. Radiol. Endod. 81(4): 396–401

Pusey, W.A. (1907): The use of carbon dioxide snow in the treatment of nevi and other lesions of the skin. J. Am. Med. Assoc. 49: 1354–1356

Rand, R.W., Rand, R.P., Eggerding, F., Denbesten, L., King, W. (1987): Cryolumpectomy for carcinoma of the breast. Surg. Gynecol. Obstet. 165: 392–396

Samuel, S. (1868): Erstarrung und Entzündung. Virchows Arch. 43: 552

Schreuder, H.W.B. (1997): The cryosurgical treatment of benign and low-grade malignant bone tumors. Ponsen & Looijen. The Netherlands. 9–19

Shepherd, J., Dawber, R.P.R. (1982): The historical and scientific basis of cryosurgery. Clin. Experiment Dermatol. 7: 321–328

Staren, E.D., Sabel, M.S., Gianakakis, L.M., Wiener, G.A., Hart, V.M., Gorski, M., Dowlatshahi, K., Corning, B.F., Haklin, M.F., Koukoulis, G. (1997): Cryosurgery of breast cancer. Arch. Surg. 132(1): 28–33

Stellar, S. (1993): Intracranial cryosurgery in a canine model: a pilot study [letter]. Surg. Neurol. 39: 331–332

Tanaka, S. (1995): Cryosurgical treatment of advanced breast cancer. Skin Cancer. 10: 9–18

Uchida, M., Imaide, Y., Sugimoto, K. (1995): Percutaneous cryosurgery for renal tumors. Br. J. Urol. 75: 132–137

Walder, H.A.D. (1966): Toepassing van de bevriezingsmethode in de neurochirurgie. Thesis, Schriks' drukkerij N.V., Asten. 2

Watanabe, H., Eguchi, S., Miyamura, H., Hayashi, J., Aizawa, Y., Wakiya, Y., Igarashi, T. (1996): Histologic findings of long-term cryolesions in a patient with ventricular tachycardia. Cardiovasc. Surg. 4(3): 409–411

White, A.C. (1899): Liquid air: its application in medicine and surgery. Med. Rec. 56: 109–112

White, A.C. (1901): Possibilities of liquid air to the physician. J. Am. Med. Assoc. 36: 426–428

Wong, W.S., Chinn, D.O., Chinn, M., Chinn, J., Tom, W.L. (1997): Cryosurgery as a treatment for prostate carcinoma, results and complications. Cancer 79: 963–974

Yamamoto, Y., Sano, K., Kimoto, M. (1989): Cryosurgical treatment for anorectal cancer. A method of palliative or adjunctive treatment. Am. Surg. 55: 252–256

Zacarian, S., Adham, M. (1966): Cryotherapy of cutaneous malignancy. Cryobiol. 2: 212–218

Zacarian, S., Adham, M. (1967): Cryotherapy temperature studies of human skin. Temperature recordings at two millimeter human skin depth following application with liquid nitrogen. Cryobiol. 48: 7–10

Zharkov, J.V., Muskin, Y.N., Trushina, V.A. (1985): Experimental investigations of low temperatures influence on biological tissue. In: Ternovoi K, Gassanov G, eds. Low Temperatures in Medicine, Kiev, Naukova Dumka. 14–42

Zonnevylle, J.A. (1981): The influence of cryosurgery and electrocoagulation on the process of metastasizing. Thesis, Oegstgeest, Drukkerij de Kempenaer. 13

Zouboulis, Ch.C. (1998): Cryosurgery in dermatology. Eur. J. Dermatol. 8: 466–474

Chapter 3

Theoretical Aspects of Cryosurgery

*Nikolai N. Korpan[1]
with contributions by Jaroslav
V. Zharkov[1] and Patrick J.M. Le Pivert[2]*

1. Copper thermocouples
2. Device for the orientated fixation of the thermocouples
3. Ampervoltmeter
4. Accumulating device
5. Device for entering data
6. Thermostat

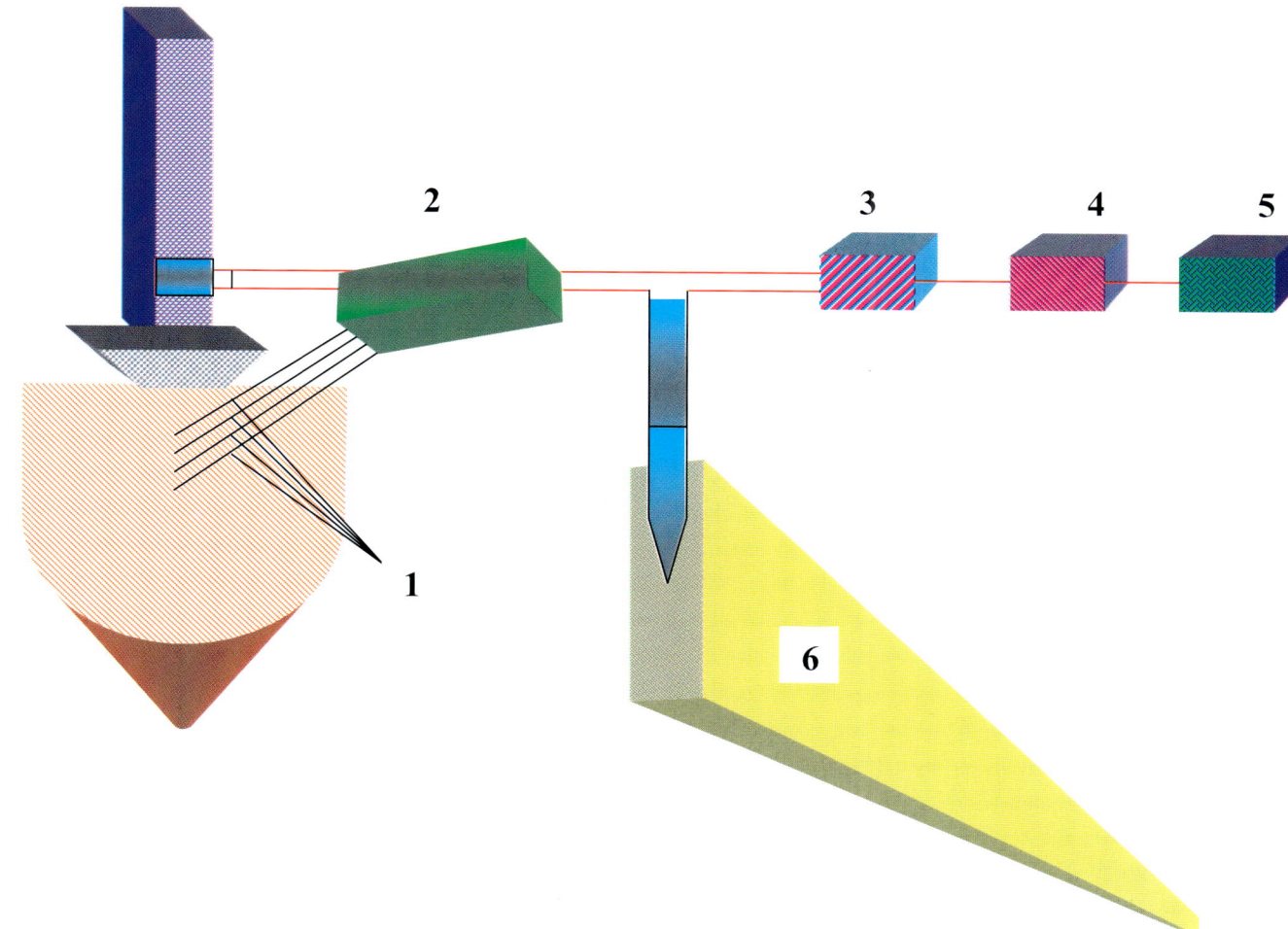

Fig. 3.1[1]. Block schema of the experimental model. Investigation of the dynamic temperature field of the frozen zone

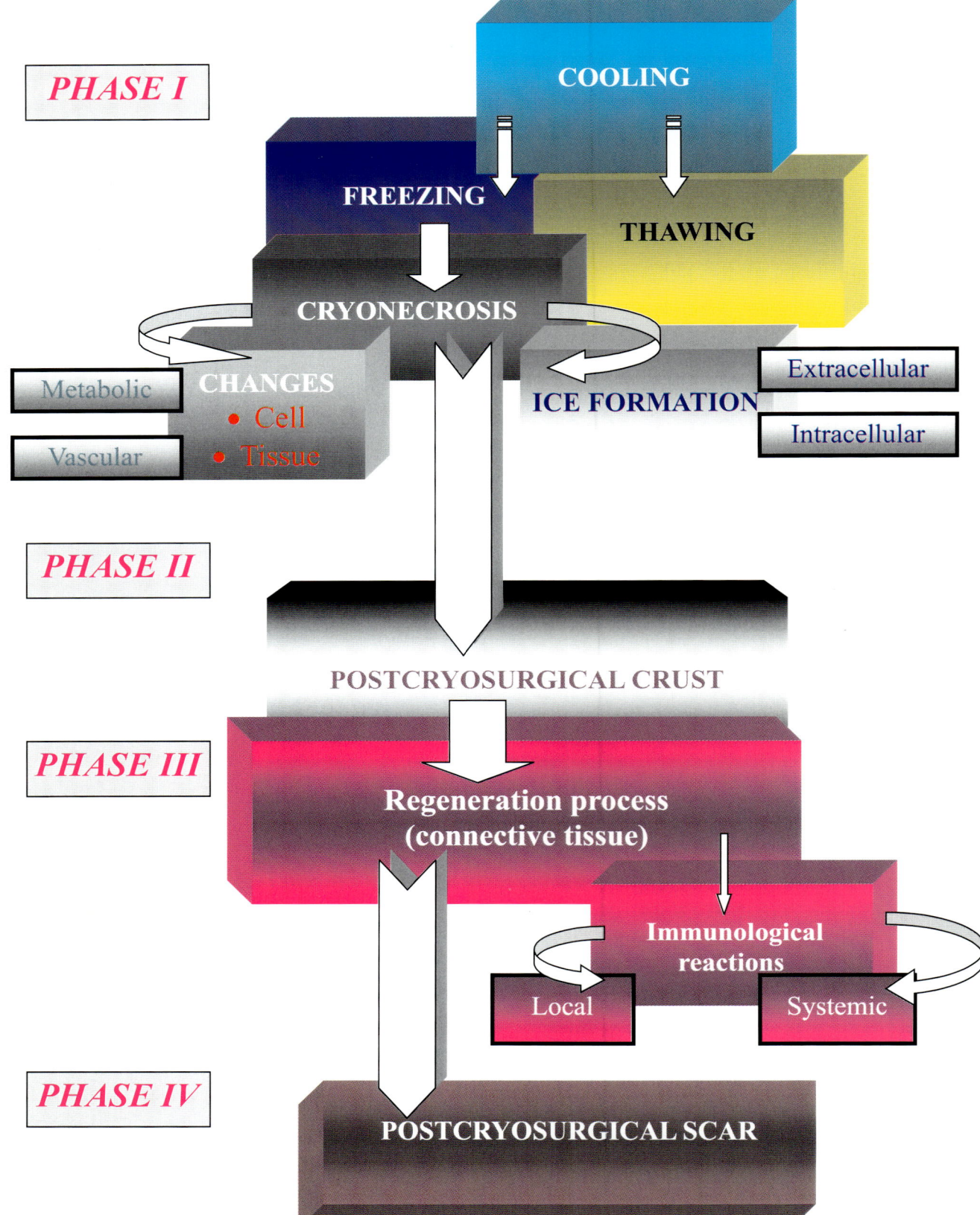

Fig. 3.2[1]. Effect of low temperatures on tissue, as observed in clinical practice

Section A   Fundamental Aspects

Chapter 3
Theory

1. Minimal temperature and high cooling velocity
2. Mild cooling regime
3. Slow cooling
4. Partial freezing of tissue
5. Cryoinstrument with cryoprobe
6. Cryosurgical device

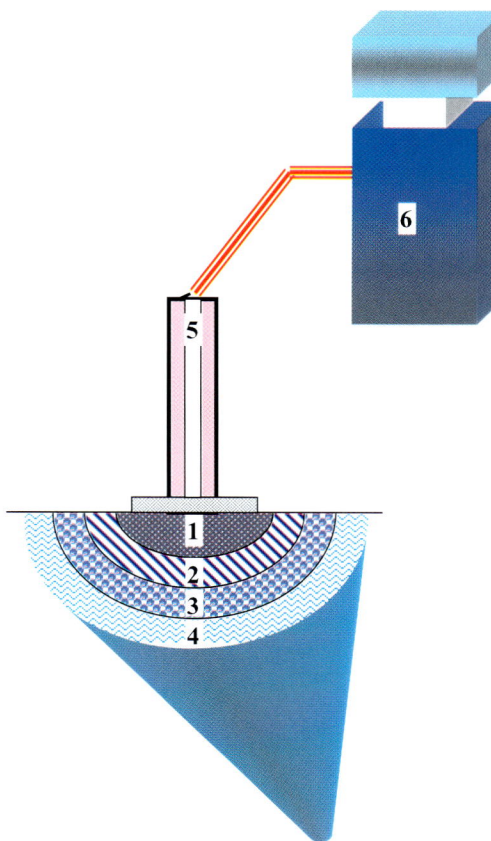

Fig. 3.3[1]. Temperature zones in the tissue during cryoexposure

Fig. 3.4[2]. The "Ice Ball" in Cryosurgery. Main characteristics of tissue crystallization resulting from thermal gradients around a cryoprobe: Theoretical model

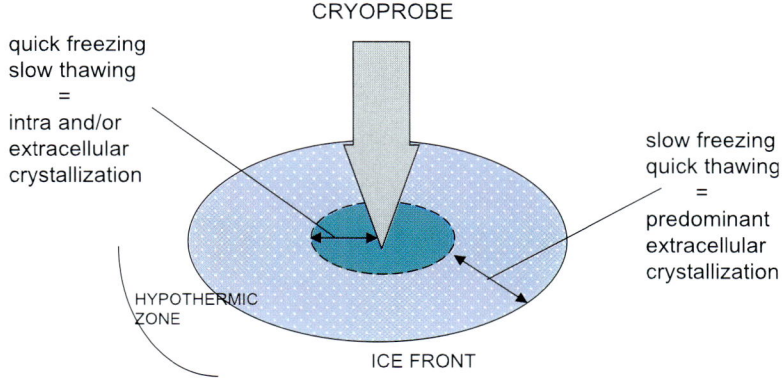

Chapter 3
Theory

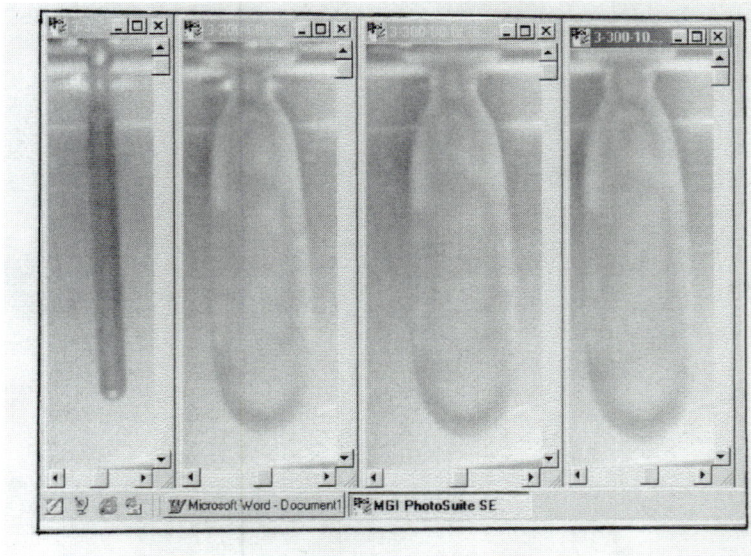

Fig. 3.5[2]. Electrical monitoring of cryosurgery. Ice ball growing around a cylindrical cryoprobe in a saline medium. Cylindrically-shaped nitrous oxide powered cryoprobe 3 mm in diameter, 30 mm in length. Photos taken at 0, 60, 80, and 100 seconds

Fig. 3.6[2]. Imaging Cryodestruction

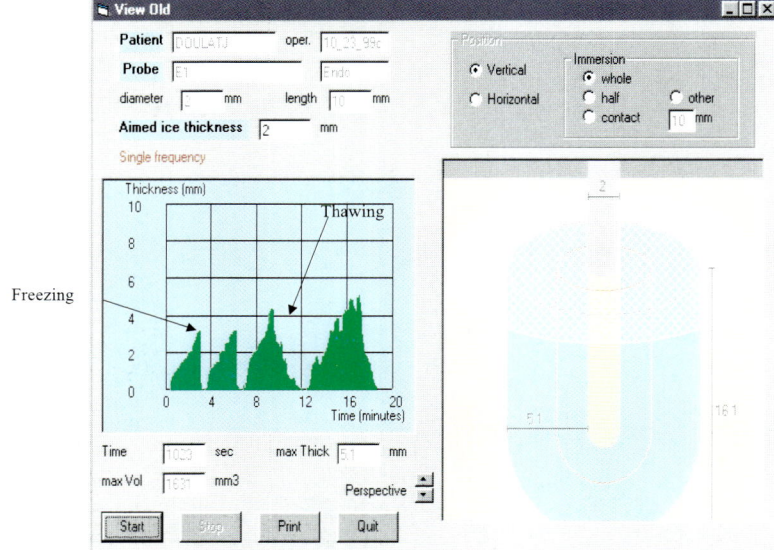

Section B

Experimental Foundations of Cryosurgery

Chapter 4

Experimental Basis of Cryosurgery

Nikolai N. Korpan
with contributions
by Jaroslav V. Zharkov

Introduction

Advances in cryosurgical technology have further stimulated interest in the use of cryosurgery to treat different diseases, first and foremost malignancies. The effect of different temperature applications on the freeze-thawing process *in vitro* to evaluate modern cryosurgical techniques as a treatment option for diseases of different organs, primarily for malignant tumors, has not yet been investigated. The effect of freeze-thawing processes using temperatures of varying intensity, and the cryosurgical response of a solution of 1.5% of gelatine in water kept at a constant temperature of +30°C, and continuously stirred, are described *in vitro* in this study. The investigations were performed at temperatures of −40°C, −80°C, −120°C, and −180°C by means of two disc-shaped cryoprobes with diameters of 5 to 50 mm respectively, and a laparoscopic needle with a diameter of 10 mm.

The cryoinstrument with disc-shaped, 5 mm to 50 mm cryoprobes was placed in a solution of 1.5% gelatine in water kept at a constant temperature of +30°C. An ice ball (hemispheric cryogenic zone) was generated without difficulty. During the freezing process, the diameter of the cryogenic zone was 28 to 58 mm larger than that of the cryoprobe throughout. Thawing after each freeze-thaw cycle took approximately 2.5 to 3.0 min in the automatic cryosurgical unit. The cryoprobe, too, was warmed up and removed from the gelatine-water solution. The one or two freeze-thaw cycles that were performed for each cryoformation in the course of this experimental cryosurgery showed an identical cryozone with an ice crater in the middle and an ice margin with a demarcation line immediately after the cryosurgical session was carried out.

The photograph analysis showed that during the 10 min cryogenic session at a temperature of −180°C by means of disc-shaped, 5 mm to 50 mm cryoprobes, different frozen cryozones developed. First, 10 min after a single freeze-thaw cycle, the hemispheric cryozone measured 28 mm in length and was 18 mm deep.

This is the first time that the effect of the freeze-thawing process using different temperatures, especially a temperature as low as −180°C, was investigated *in vitro* by means of disc-shaped cryoprobes measuring 5 mm to 50 mm and a laparoscopic needle 10 mm in diameter. It is the latest *in vitro* experimental study in the field of cryosurgery and shows a new cryozone formation which is dependent on the temperature and on the size of the cryoprobe.

This investigation is most important for the use of cryosurgery in clinical practice and for the development of modern cryosurgical technology. Two factors are of particular importance, temperature and exposure time. These two factors have a predominant influence on the formation of the cryozone and subsequently on the thorough destruction of the cancerous tissue. The investigation first of all shows that formation of the cryozone depends on the temperature factor. The lower the temperature, the larger the cryozone formed. Secondly, it is also evident that cryozone formation stops after five to seven minutes during

Chapter 4
Experiments

the cryogenic session. Thereafter, the cryozone stops growing and remains constant in size.

A problem associated with cryosurgery that has not been adequately addressed is that of identifying the mechanism by which damage is effected during the freezing process. This is important because, although cryosurgery is clinically used to treat parenchymal tumors, neither the freezing process, nor the damage mechanism involved, are fully understood. Research that elucidates the fundamental process of the freezing of parenchymal tissue must therefore concentrate on various experimental studies in modern cryosurgery, especially experimental studies devoted to refining the technology of modern cryosurgical equipment.

At the present time, our findings show that the elaboration of cryosurgical techniques make it possible to fulfill the main medical demands for the application of cryomethods. Such refinements in technique will increase their efficiency of use in different fields of medicine, primarily in the treatment of malignant tumors in the parenchymal organs.

Cryosurgery as an independent treatment, but also as a component of other treatments in the field of oncology, has been a success in medical practice. Tumors are not cut out but shock frozen. New scientific research on the application of freezing in the fields of biology and medicine, and numerous theoretical and experimental studies *in vitro* and *in vivo*, reveal the effect mechanisms of sub-zero temperatures have on the tissue as well as the impairment and destruction of cells under cryoinfluence. This new method can only be applied efficiently if the most technologically advanced instruments are used.

Section B

Cryoprobe

5 mm in diameter at a temperature of −**40°C** in a 1.5 l solution of 1.5% gelatine in water kept at a constant temperature of +30°C and continuously stirred

One picture per minute

Cryozone after 10 min freezing: diameter 8 mm, depth 7 mm

Chapter 4
Experiments

Start

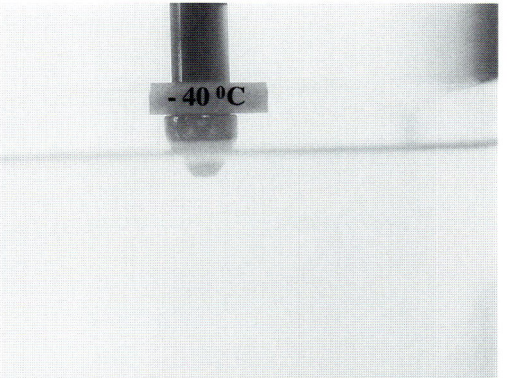

Fig. 4.1. Start of freezing

Fig. 4.2. Cryozone formation after exposure for 1 min

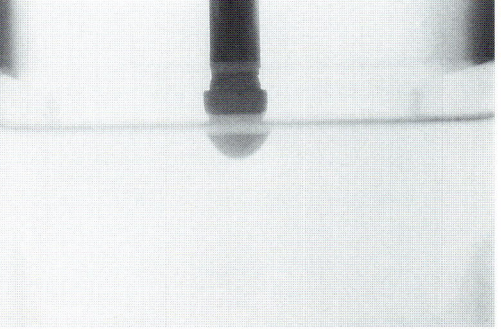

1 min

Chapter 4
Experiments

Cryoprobe

5 mm in diameter at a temperature of −40°C in a 1.5 l solution of 1.5% gelatine in water kept at a constant temperature of −30°C and continuously stirred

One picture per minute

Cryozone after 10 min freezing: diameter 8 mm, depth 7 mm

2 min

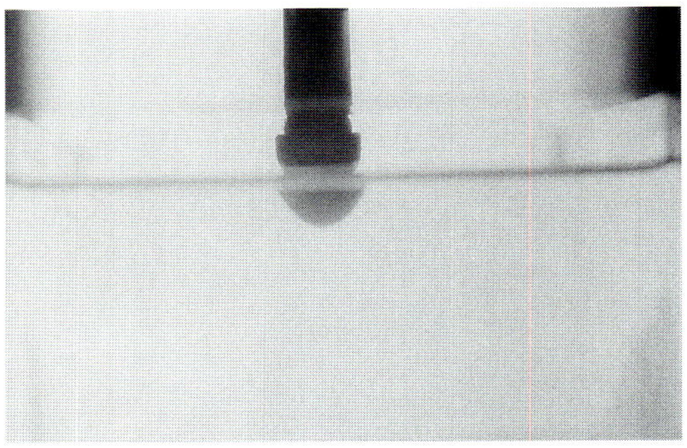

Fig. 4.3. Cryozone formation after exposure for 2 min

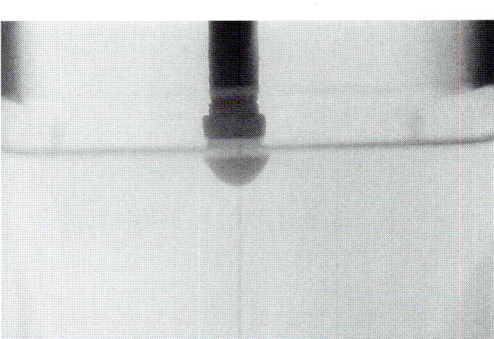

Fig. 4.4. Cryozone formation after exposure for 3 min

3 min

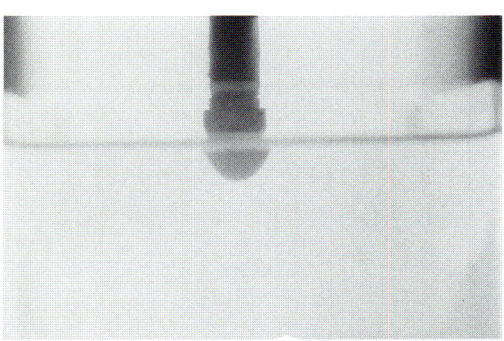

4 min

Fig. 4.5. Cryozone formation after exposure for 4 min

Section B

Cryoprobe

5 mm in diameter at a temperature of −40°C in a 1.5 l solution of 1.5% gelatine in water kept at a constant temperature of −30°C and continuously stirred

One picture per minute

Cryozone after 10 min freezing: diameter 8 mm, depth 7 mm

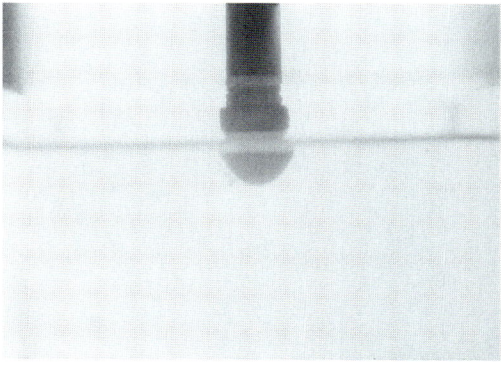

5 min

Fig. 4.6. Cryozone formation after exposure for 5 min

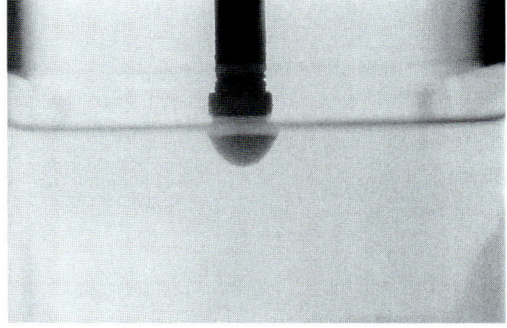

6 min

Fig. 4.7. Cryozone formation after exposure for 6 min

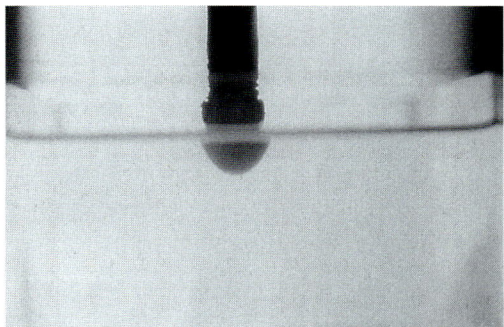

Fig. 4.8. Cryozone formation after exposure for 7 min

7 min

Chapter 4
Experiments

Cryoprobe

5 mm in diameter at a temperature of −40 °C in a 1.5 l solution of 1.5% gelatine in water kept at a constant temperature of −30 °C and continuously stirred

One picture per minute

Cryozone after 10 min freezing: diameter 8 mm, depth 7 mm

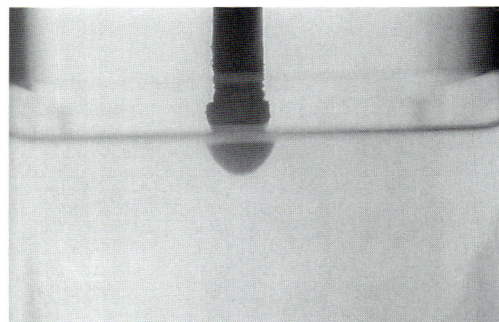

8 min

Fig. 4.9. Cryozone formation after exposure for 8 min

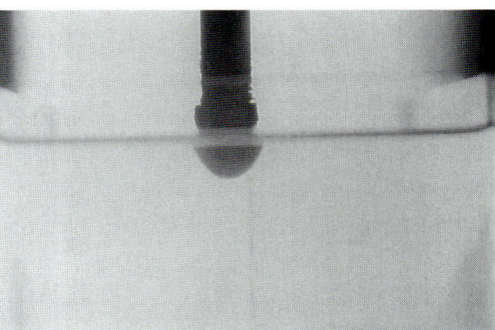

9 min

Fig. 4.10. Cryozone formation after exposure for 9 min

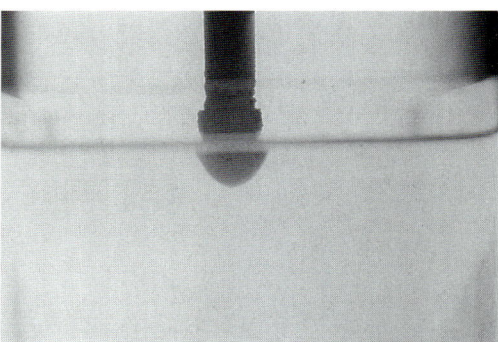

10 min

Fig. 4.11. Cryozone formation after exposure for 10 min

Section B Experimental Foundations

Cryoprobe

5 mm in diameter at a temperature of −**80°C** in a 1.5 l solution of 1.5% gelatine in water kept at a constant temperature of +30°C and continuously stirred

One picture per minute

Cryozone after 10 min freezing: diameter 11 mm, depth 9 mm

Chapter 4
Experiments

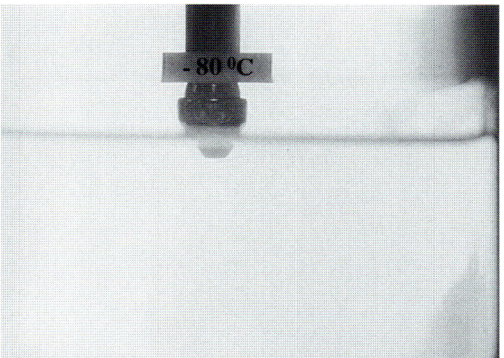

Start

Fig. 4.12. Start of freezing

Fig. 4.13. Cryozone formation after exposure for 1 min

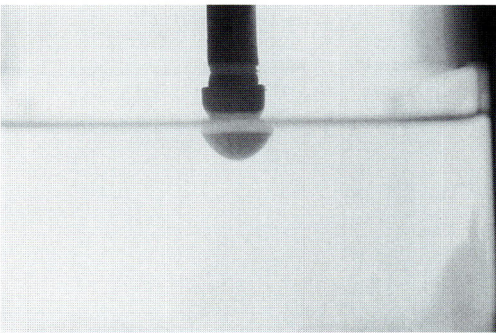

1 min

Chapter 4
Experiments

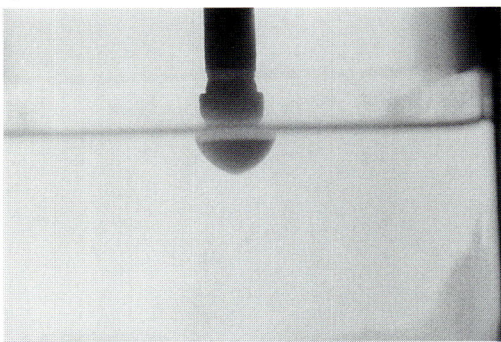

2 min

Fig. 4.14. Cryozone formation after exposure for 2 min

Cryoprobe

5 mm in diameter at a temperature of −80°C in a 1.5 l solution of 1.5% gelatine in water kept at a constant temperature of +30°C and continuously stirred

One picture per minute

Cryozone after 10 min freezing: diameter 11 mm, depth 9 mm

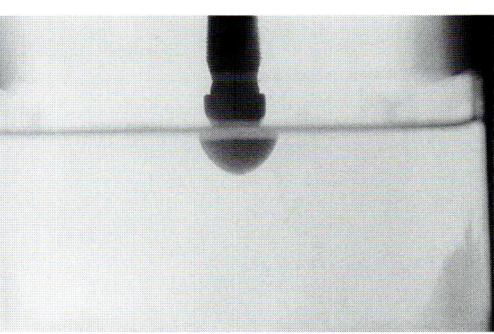

3 min

Fig. 4.15. Cryozone formation after exposure for 3 min

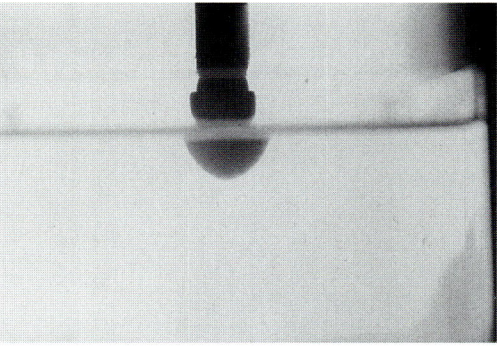

4 min

Fig. 4.16. Cryozone formation after exposure for 4 min

Section B Experimental Foundations

Cryoprobe

5 mm in diameter at a temperature of −80 °C in a 1.5 l solution of 1.5% gelatine in water kept at a constant temperature of −30 °C and continuously stirred

One picture per minute

Cryozone after 10 min freezing: diameter 11 mm, depth 9 mm

Chapter 4
Experiments

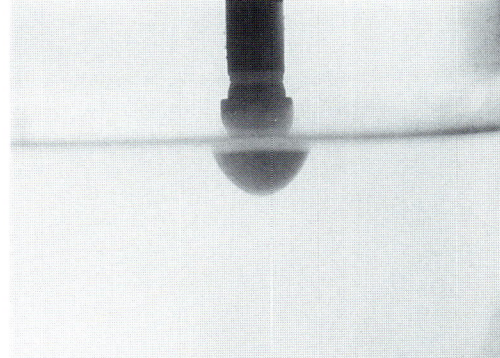

5 min

Fig. 4.17. Cryozone formation after exposure for 5 min

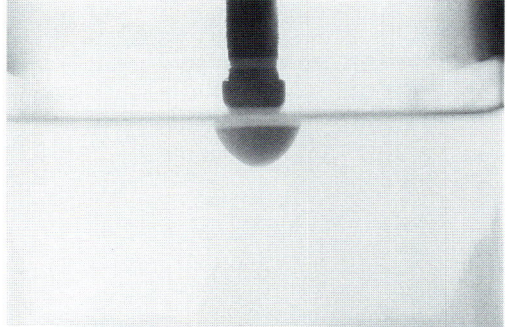

6 min

Fig. 4.18. Cryozone formation after exposure for 6 min

Fig. 4.19. Cryozone formation after exposure for 7 min

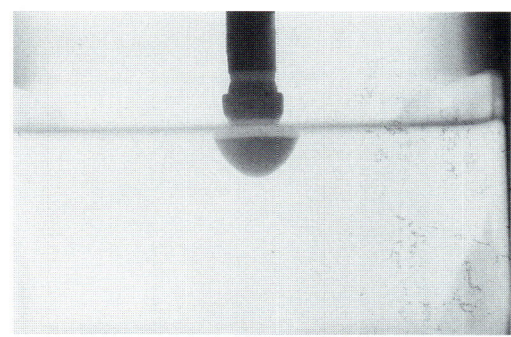

7 min

Chapter 4 Experiments

Fig. 4.20. Cryozone formation after exposure for 8 min

8 min

Fig. 4.21. Cryozone formation after exposure for 9 min

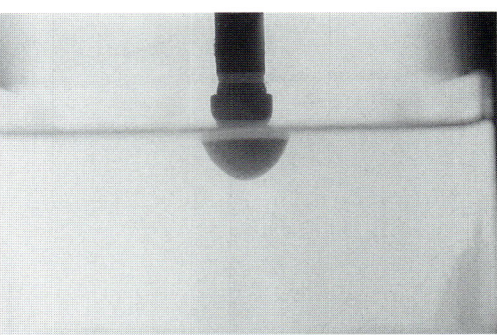

9 min

10 min

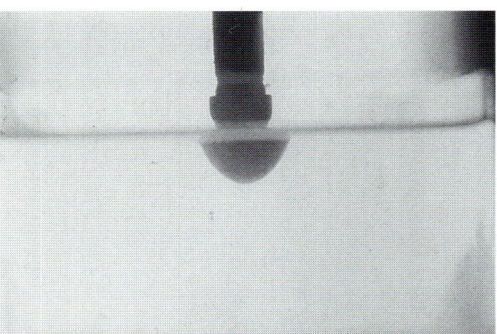

Fig. 4.22. Cryozone formation after exposure for 10 min

Cryoprobe

5 mm in diameter at a temperature of −80°C in a 1.5 l solution of 1.5% gelatine in water kept at a constant temperature of +30°C and continuously stirred

One picture per minute

Cryozone after 10 min freezing: diameter 11 mm, depth 9 mm

Section B — Experimental Foundations

Chapter 4
Experiments

Cryoprobe

5 mm in diameter at a temperature of −**120**°C in a 1.5 l solution of 1.5% gelatine in water kept at a constant temperature of +30°C and continuously stirred

One picture per minute

Cryozone after 10 min freezing: diameter 14 mm, depth 11 mm

Start

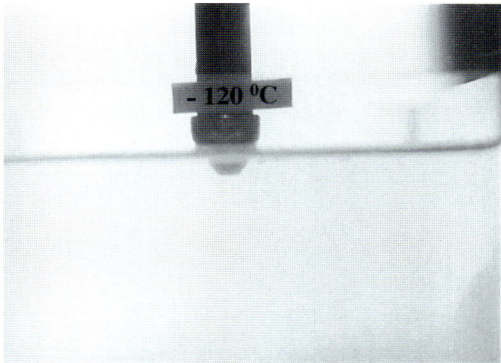

Fig. 4.23. Start of freezing

Fig. 4.24. Cryozone formation after exposure for 1 min

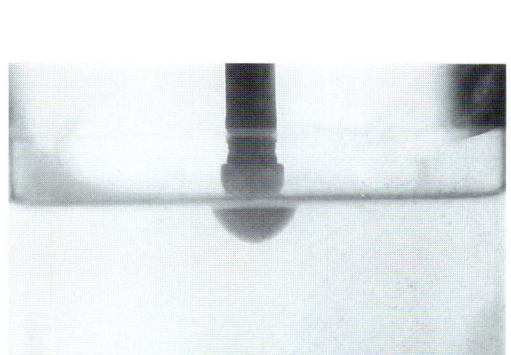

1 min

Chapter 4
Experiments

Cryoprobe

5 mm in diameter at a temperature of −120°C in a 1.5 l solution of 1.5% gelatine in water kept at a constant temperature of −30°C and continuously stirred

One picture per minute

Cryozone after 10 min freezing: diameter 14 mm, depth 11 mm

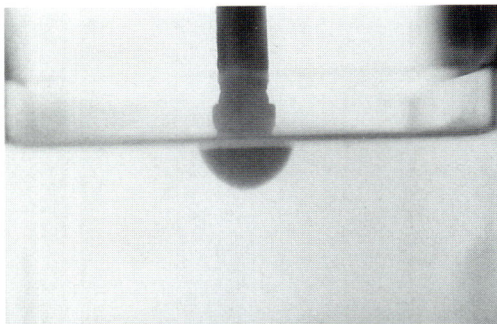

2 min

Fig. 4.25. Cryozone formation after exposure for 2 min

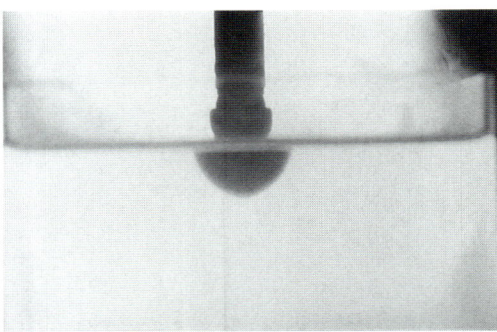

3 min

Fig. 4.26. Cryozone formation after exposure for 3 min

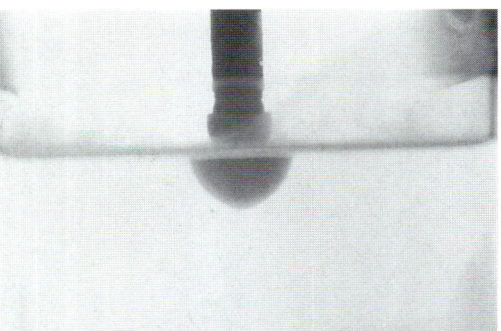

4 min

Fig. 4.27. Cryozone formation after exposure for 4 min

Section B

Cryoprobe

5 mm in diameter at a temperature of −120 °C in a 1.5 l solution of 1.5% gelatine in water kept at a constant temperature of −30 °C and continuously stirred

One picture per minute

Cryozone after 10 min freezing: diameter 14 mm, depth 11 mm

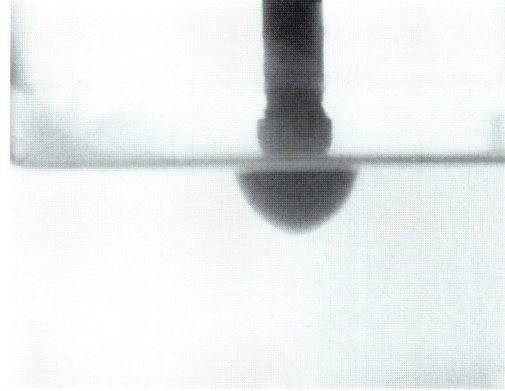

5 min

Fig. 4.28. Cryozone formation after exposure for 5 min

6 min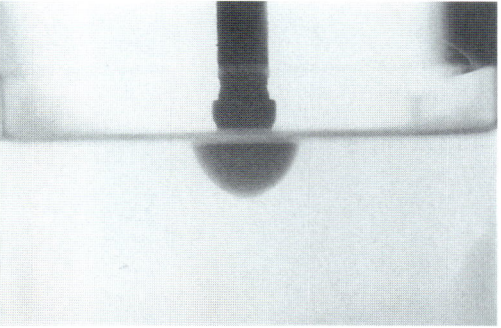

Fig. 4.29. Cryozone formation after exposure for 6 min

Fig. 4.30. Cryozone formation after exposure for 7 min

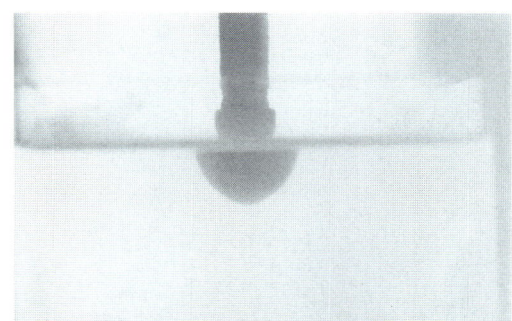

7 min

**Chapter 4
Experiments**

Cryoprobe

5 mm in diameter at a temperature of −120°C in a 1.5 l solution of 1.5% gelatine in water kept at a constant temperature of −30°C and continuously stirred

One picture per minute

Cryozone after 10 min freezing: diameter 14 mm, depth 11 mm

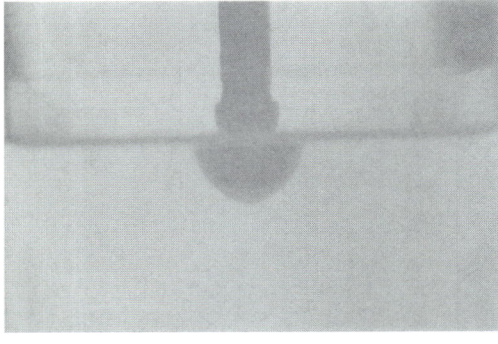

8 min

Fig. 4.31. Cryozone formation after exposure for 8 min

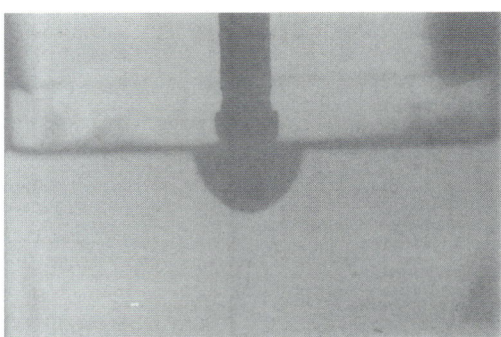

9 min

Fig. 4.32. Cryozone formation after exposure for 9 min

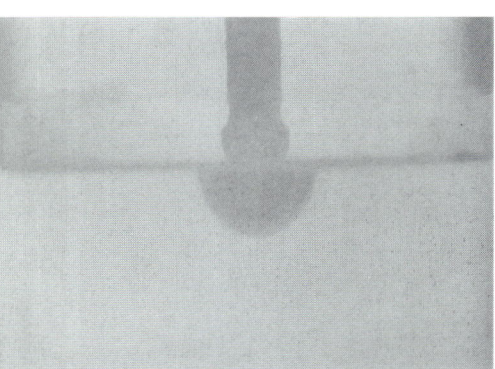

10 min

Fig. 4.33. Cryozone formation after exposure for 10 min

Section B

Cryoprobe

5 mm in diameter at a temperature of −**180**°C in a 1.5 l solution of 1.5% gelatine in water kept at a constant temperature of +30°C and continuously stirred

One picture per minute

Cryozone after 10 min freezing: diameter 28 mm, depth 18 mm

Experimental Foundations

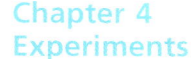
Chapter 4
Experiments

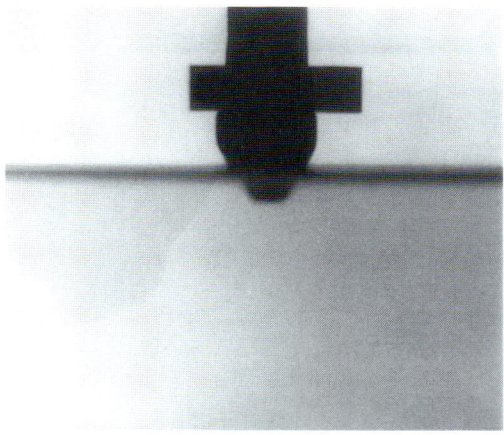

Start

Fig. 4.34. Start of freezing

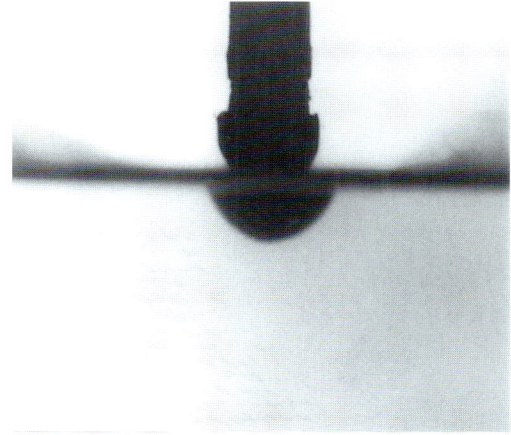

Fig. 4.35. Cryozone formation after exposure for 1 min

1 min

Chapter 4
Experiments

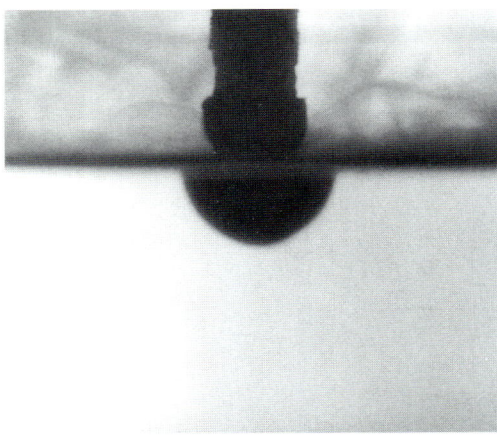

2 min

Fig. 4.36. Cryozone formation after exposure for 2 min

Fig. 4.37. Cryozone formation after exposure for 3 min

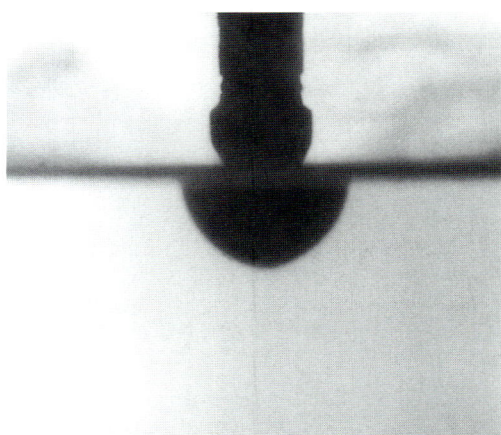

3 min

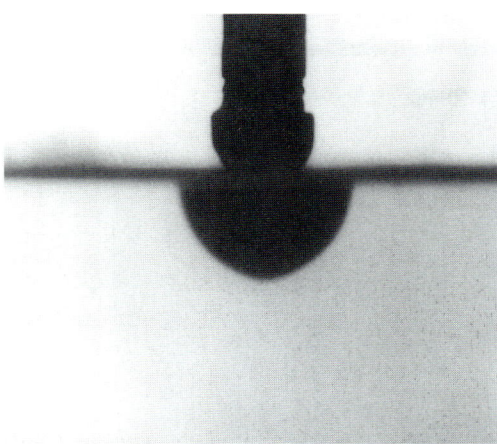

4 min

Fig. 4.38. Cryozone formation after exposure for 4 min

Cryoprobe

5 mm in diameter at a temperature of −180 °C in a 1.5 l solution of 1.5% gelatine in water kept at a constant temperature of −30 °C and continuously stirred

One picture per minute

Cryozone after 10 min freezing: diameter 28 mm, depth 18 mm

Section B

Cryoprobe

5 mm in diameter at a temperature of −180 °C in a 1.5 l solution of 1.5% gelatine in water kept at a constant temperature of −30 °C and continuously stirred

One picture per minute

Cryozone after 10 min freezing: diameter 28 mm, depth 18 mm

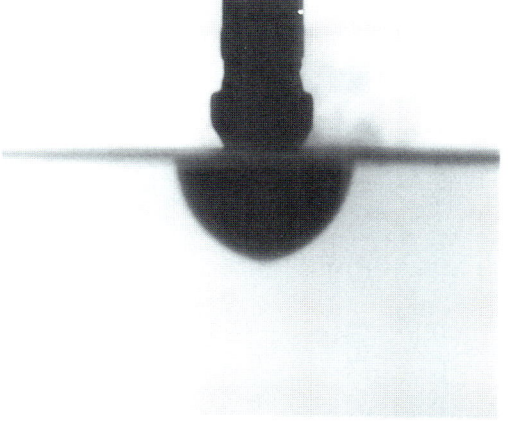

5 min

Fig. 4.39. Cryozone formation after exposure for 5 min

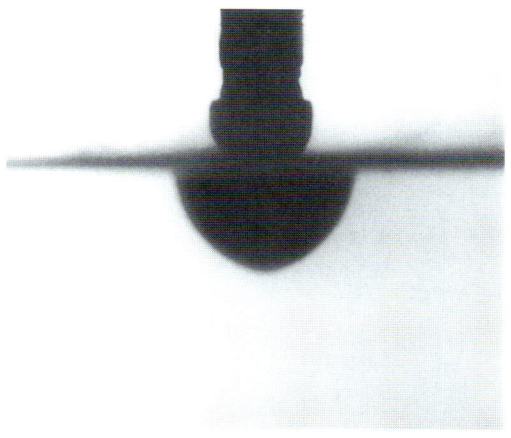

6 min

Fig. 4.40. Cryozone formation after exposure for 6 min

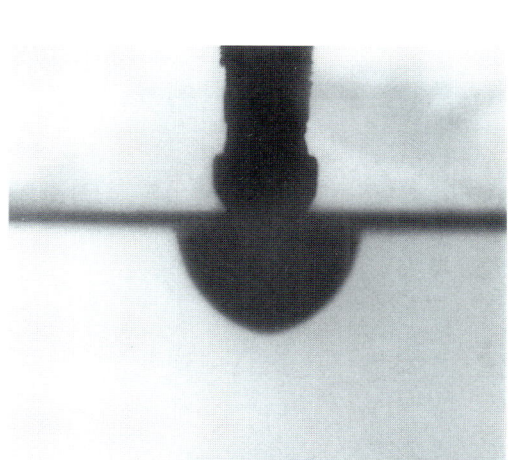

7 min

Fig. 4.41. Cryozone formation after exposure for 7 min

Chapter 4 Experiments

Cryoprobe

5 mm in diameter at a temperature of −180 °C in a 1.5 l solution of 1.5% gelatine in water kept at a constant temperature of +30 °C and continuously stirred

One picture per minute

Cryozone after 10 min freezing: diameter 28 mm, depth 18 mm

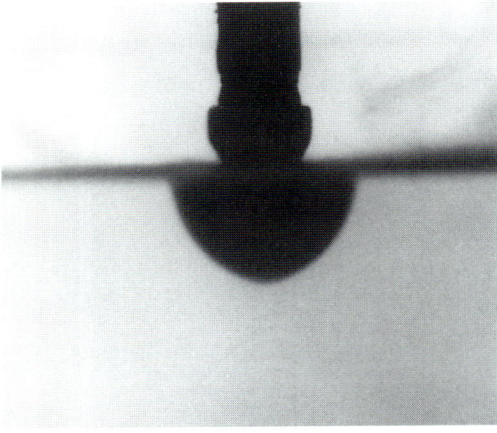

Fig. 4.42. Cryozone formation after exposure for 8 min

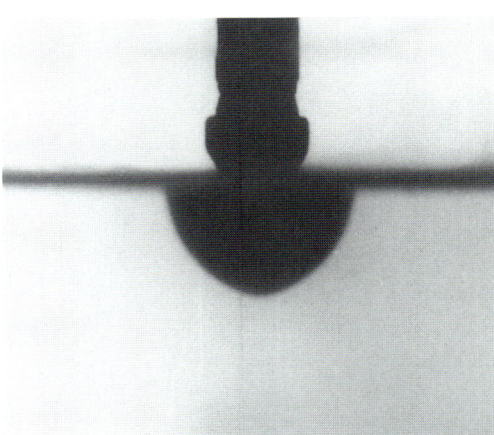

Fig. 4.43. Cryozone formation after exposure for 9 min

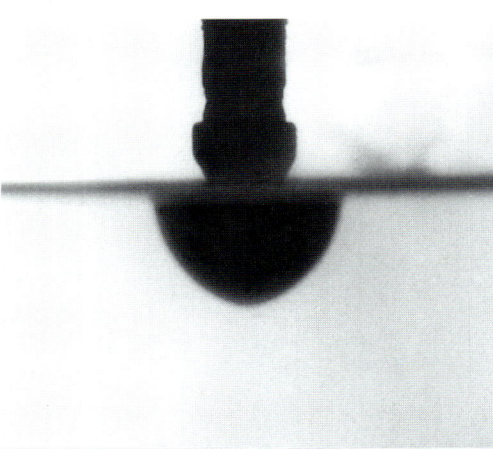

Fig. 4.44. Cryozone formation after exposure for 10 min

Section B

Cryoprobe

50 mm in diameter at a temperature of −40°C in a 1.5 l solution of 1.5% gelatine in water kept at a constant temperature of +30°C and continuously stirred

One picture per minute

Cryozone after 10 min freezing: diameter 51 mm, depth 10 mm

Chapter 4
Experiments

Start

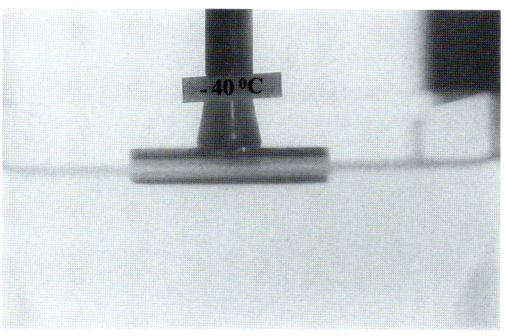

Fig. 4.45. Start of freezing

Fig. 4.46. Cryozone formation after exposure for 1 min

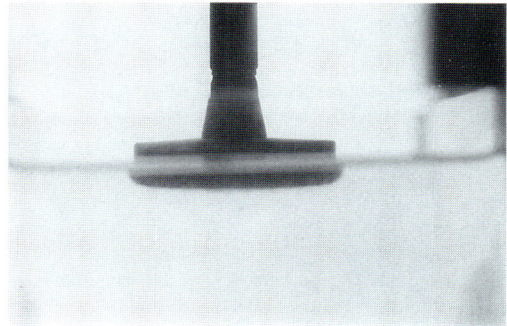

1 min

Chapter 4
Experiments

N. N. Korpan (ed.)

Atlas of Cryosurgery

Cryoprobe

50 mm in diameter at a temperature of −40 °C in a 1.5 l solution of 1.5% gelatine in water kept at a constant temperature of +30 °C and continuously stirred

One picture per minute

Cryozone after 10 min freezing: diameter 51 mm, depth 10 mm

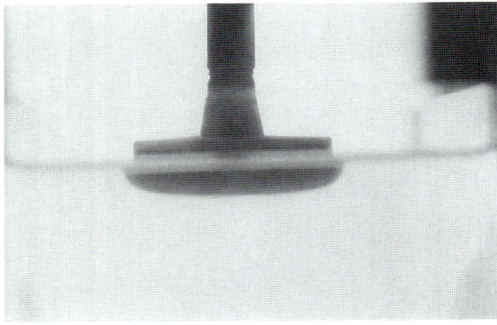

2 min

Fig. 4.47. Cryozone formation after exposure for 2 min

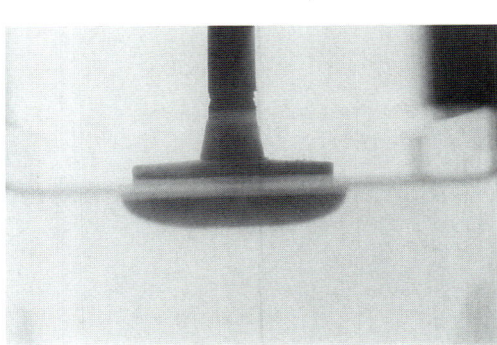

3 min

Fig. 4.48. Cryozone formation after exposure for 3 min

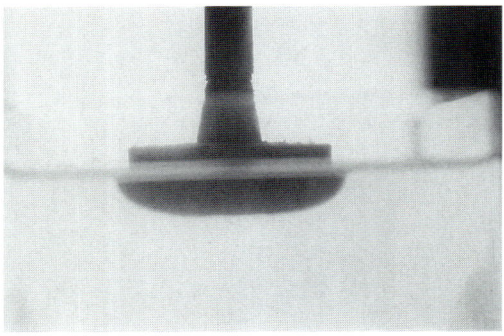

4 min

Fig. 4.49. Cryozone formation after exposure for 4 min

Section B

Cryoprobe

50 mm in diameter at a temperature of −40°C in a 1.5 l solution of 1.5% gelatine in water kept at a constant temperature of +30°C and continuously stirred

One picture per minute

Cryozone after 10 min freezing: diameter 51 mm, depth 10 mm

Experimental Foundations

Chapter 4
Experiments

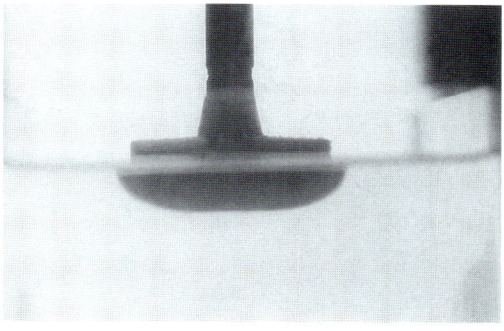

5 min

Fig. 4.50. Cryozone formation after exposure for 5 min

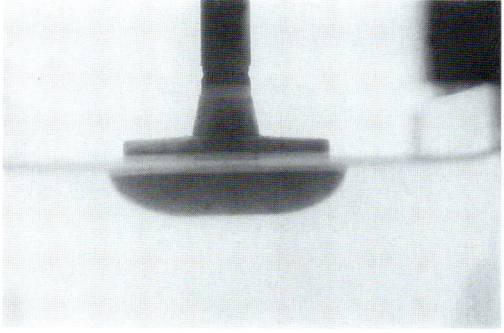

6 min

Fig. 4.51. Cryozone formation after exposure for 6 min

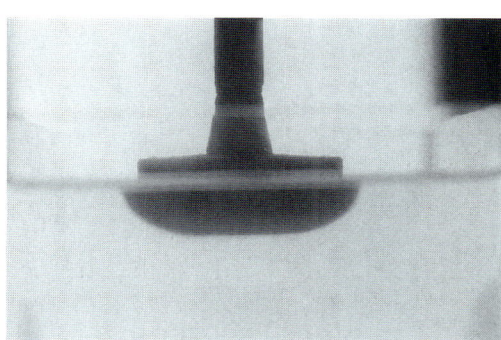

7 min

Fig. 4.52. Cryozone formation after exposure for 7 min

Chapter 4
Experiments

Cryoprobe

50 mm in diameter at a temperature of −40°C in a 1.5 l solution of 1.5% gelatine in water kept at a constant temperature of +30°C and continuously stirred

One picture per minute

Cryozone after 10 min freezing: diameter 51 mm, depth 10 mm

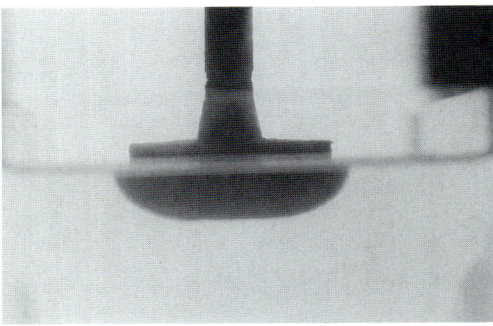

8 min

Fig. 4.53. Cryozone formation after exposure for 8 min

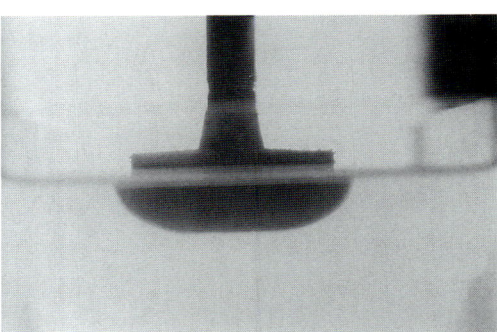

9 min

Fig. 4.54. Cryozone formation after exposure for 9 min

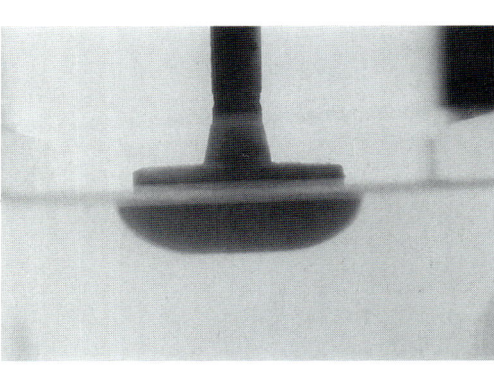

10 min

Fig. 4.55. Cryozone formation after exposure for 10 min

Section B | Experimental Foundations | **43**

Cryoprobe

50 mm in diameter at a temperature of $-80°C$ in a 1.5 l solution of 1.5% gelatine in water kept at a constant temperature of $+30°C$ and continuously stirred

One picture per minute

Cryozone after 10 min freezing: diameter 52 mm, depth 14 mm

Chapter 4
Experiments

Start

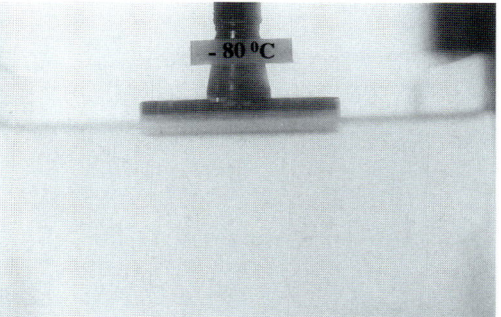

Fig. 4.56. Start of freezing

Fig. 4.57. Cryozone formation after exposure for 1 min

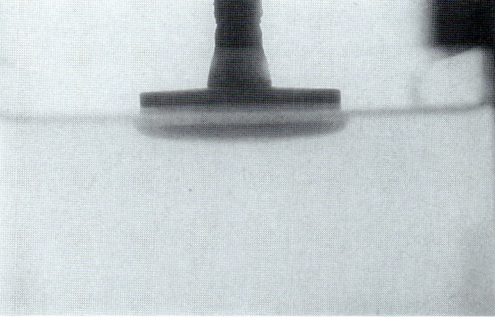

1 min

Chapter 4 Experiments

Cryoprobe

50 mm in diameter at a temperature of −80°C in a 1.5 l solution of 1.5% gelatine in water kept at a constant temperature of +30°C and continuously stirred

One picture per minute

Cryozone after 10 min freezing: diameter 52 mm, depth 14 mm

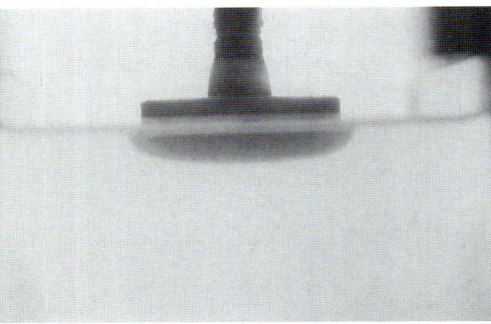

2 min

Fig. 4.58. Cryozone formation after exposure for 2 min

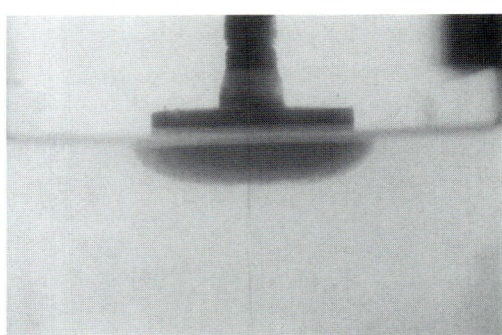

3 min

Fig. 4.59. Cryozone formation after exposure for 3 min

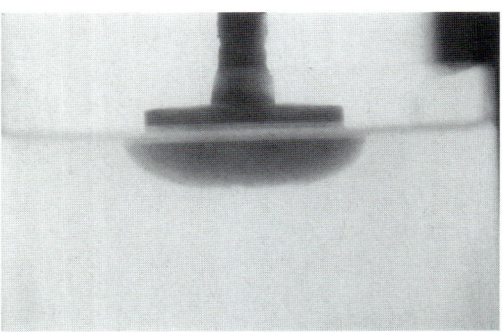

4 min

Fig. 4.60. Cryozone formation after exposure for 4 min

Section B

Cryoprobe

50 mm in diameter at a temperature of −80°C in a 1.5 l solution of 1.5% gelatine in water kept at a constant temperature of +30°C and continuously stirred

One picture per minute

Cryozone after 10 min freezing: diameter 52 mm, depth 14 mm

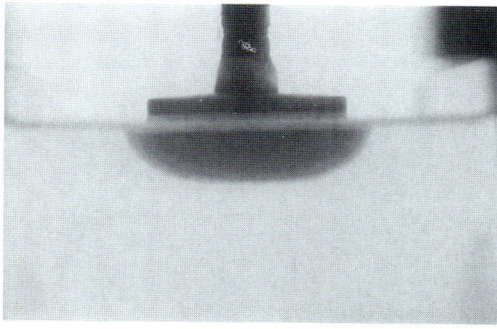

5 min

Fig. 4.61. Cryozone formation after exposure for 5 min

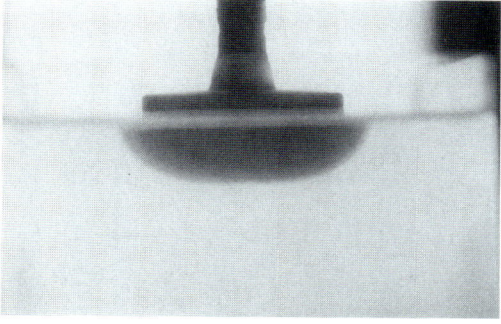

6 min

Fig. 4.62. Cryozone formation after exposure for 6 min

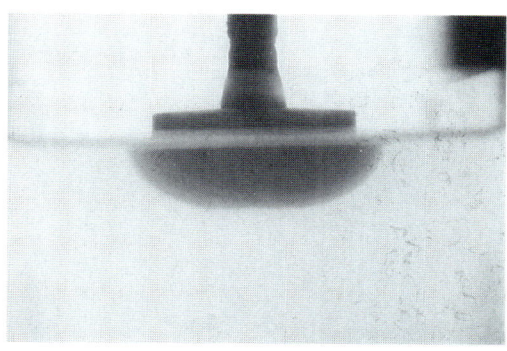

7 min

Fig. 4.63. Cryozone formation after exposure for 7 min

Chapter 4
Experiments

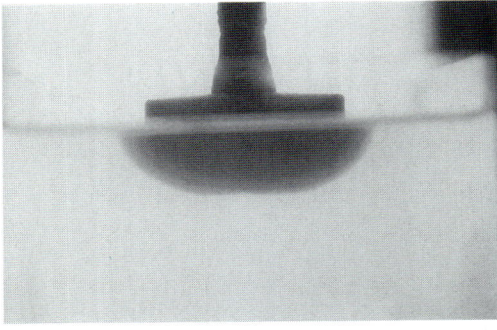

8 min

Fig. 4.64. Cryozone formation after exposure for 8 min

Cryoprobe

50 mm in diameter at a temperature of −80°C in a 1.5 l solution of 1.5% gelatine in water kept at a constant temperature of +30°C and continuously stirred

One picture per minute

Cryozone after 10 min freezing: diameter 52 mm, depth 14 mm

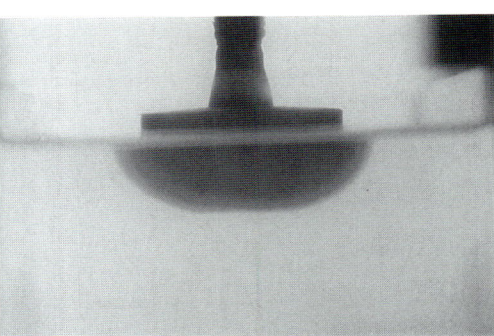

9 min

Fig. 4.65. Cryozone formation after exposure for 9 min

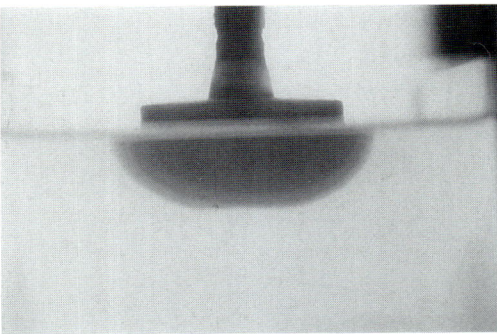

10 min

Fig. 4.66. Cryozone formation after exposure for 10 min

Section B   Experimental Foundations

Chapter 4
Experiments

Cryoprobe

50 mm in diameter at a temperature of −120°C in a 1.5 l solution of 1.5% gelatine in water kept at a constant temperature of +30°C and continuously stirred

One picture per minute

Cryozone after 10 min freezing: diameter 53 mm, depth 19 mm

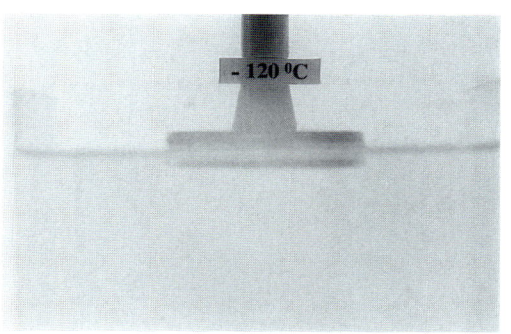

Start

Fig. 4.67. Start of freezing

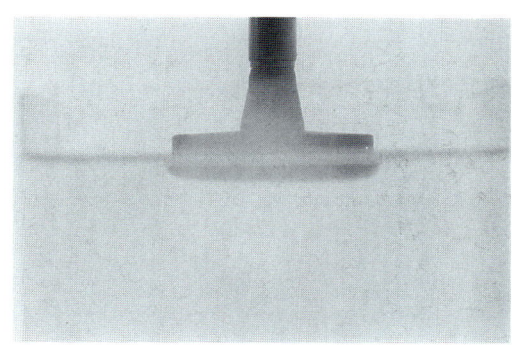

Fig. 4.68. Cryozone formation after exposure for 1 min

1 min

Chapter 4 Experiments

Cryoprobe

50 mm in diameter at a temperature of −120°C in a 1.5 l solution of 1.5% gelatine in water kept at a constant temperature of +30°C and continuously stirred

One picture per minute

Cryozone after 10 min freezing: diameter 53 mm, depth 19 mm

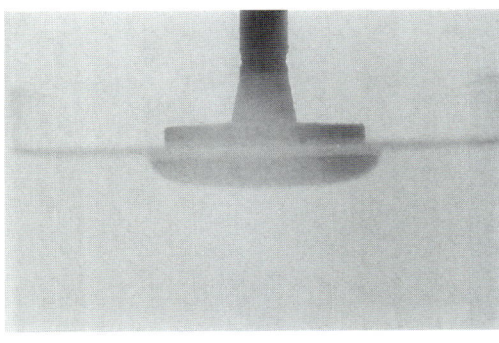

2 min

Fig. 4.69. Cryozone formation after exposure for 2 min

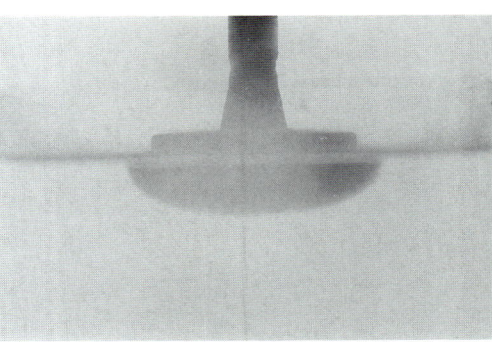

3 min

Fig. 4.70. Cryozone formation after exposure for 3 min

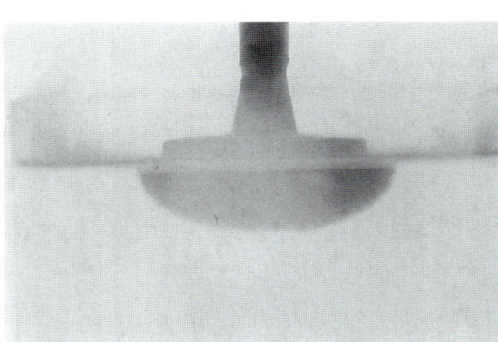

4 min

Fig. 4.71. Cryozone formation after exposure for 4 min

Section B

Cryoprobe

50 mm in diameter at a temperature of −120°C in a 1.5 l solution of 1.5% gelatine in water kept at a constant temperature of +30°C and continuously stirred

One picture per minute

Cryozone after 10 min freezing: diameter 53 mm, depth 19 mm

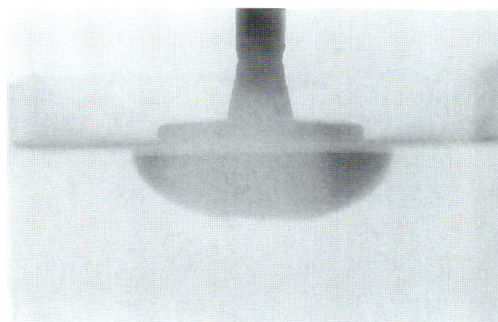

5 min

Fig. 4.72. Cryozone formation after exposure for 5 min

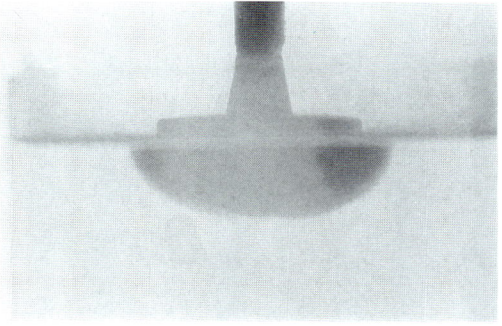

6 min

Fig. 4.73. Cryozone formation after exposure for 6 min

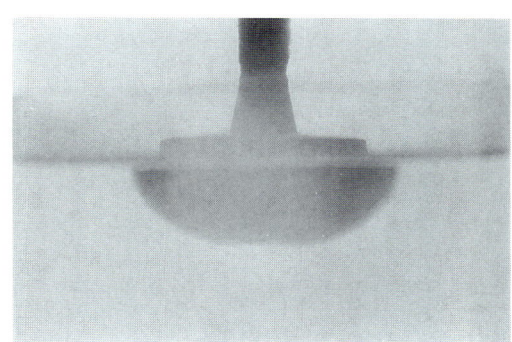

7 min

Fig. 4.74. Cryozone formation after exposure for 7 min

Chapter 4 Experiments

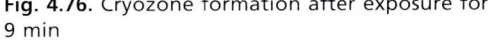

8 min

Fig. 4.75. Cryozone formation after exposure for 8 min

Cryoprobe

50 mm in diameter at a temperature of −120°C in a 1.5 l solution of 1.5% gelatine in water kept at a constant temperature of +30°C and continuously stirred

One picture per minute

Cryozone after 10 min freezing: diameter 53 mm, depth 19 mm

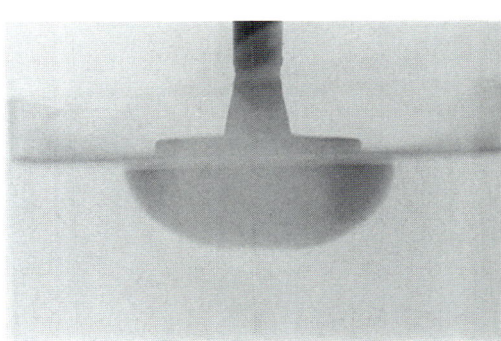

Fig. 4.76. Cryozone formation after exposure for 9 min

9 min

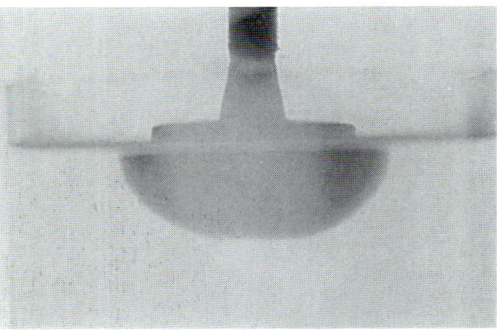

10 min

Fig. 4.77. Cryozone formation after exposure for 10 min

Section B   Experimental Foundations   **51**

Cryoprobe

Chapter 4
Experiments

50 mm in diameter at a temperature of −**180**°C in a 1.5 l solution of 1.5% gelatine in water kept at a constant temperature of +30°C and continuously stirred

One picture per minute

Cryozone after 10 min freezing: diameter 58 mm, depth 27 mm

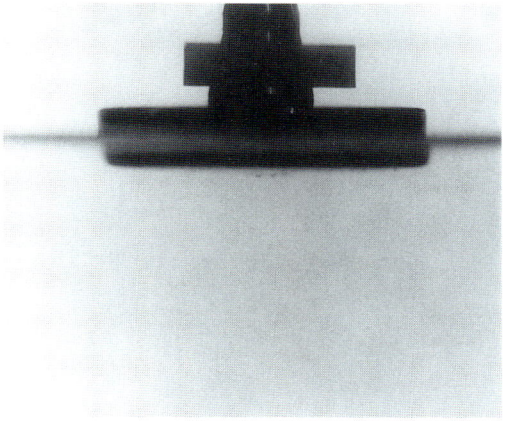

Start

Fig. 4.78. Start of freezing

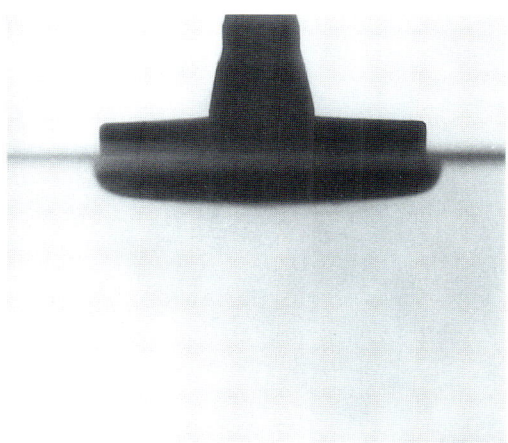

Fig. 4.79. Cryozone formation after exposure for 1 min

1 min

**Chapter 4
Experiments**

Cryoprobe

50 mm in diameter at a temperature of −180°C in a 1.5 l solution of 1.5% gelatine in water kept at a constant temperature of +30°C and continuously stirred

One picture per minute

Cryozone after 10 min freezing: diameter 58 mm, depth 27 mm

2 min

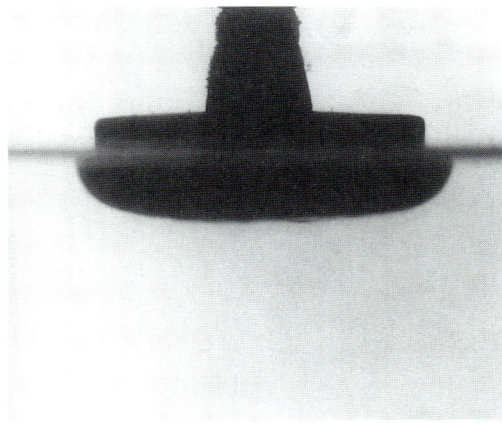

Fig. 4.80. Cryozone formation after exposure for 2 min

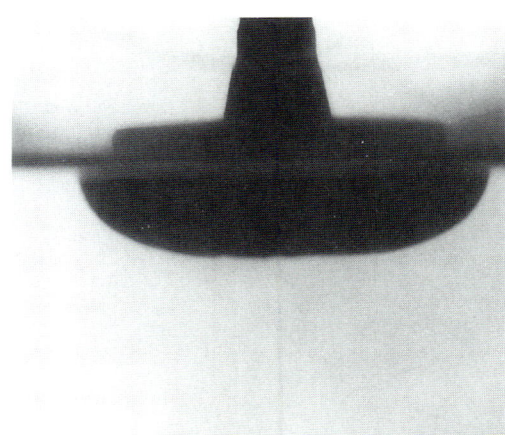

Fig. 4.81. Cryozone formation after exposure for 3 min

3 min

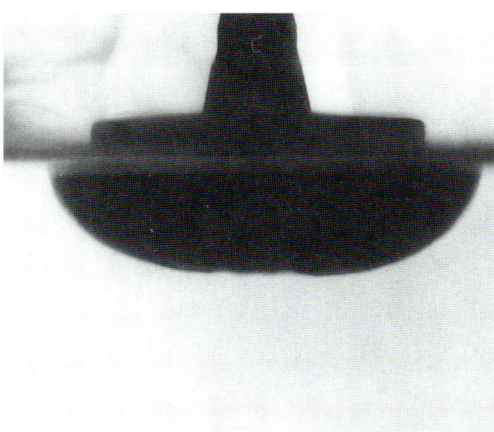

Fig. 4.82. Cryozone formation after exposure for 4 min

4 min

Section B Experimental Foundations

Cryoprobe

50 mm in diameter at a temperature of −180°C in a 1.5 l solution of 1.5% gelatine in water kept at a constant temperature of +30°C and continuously stirred

One picture per minute

Cryozone after 10 min freezing: diameter 58 mm, depth 27 mm

Chapter 4
Experiments

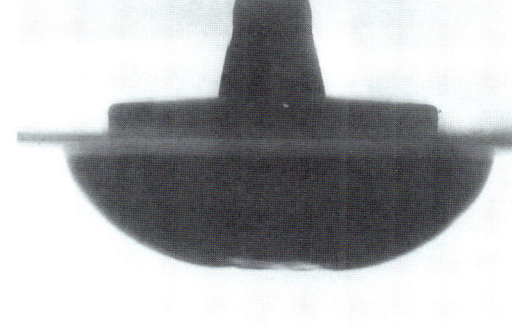

5 min

Fig. 4.83. Cryozone formation after exposure for 5 min

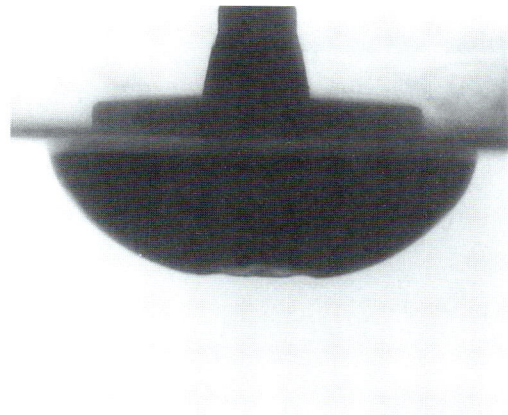

6 min

Fig. 4.84. Cryozone formation after exposure for 6 min

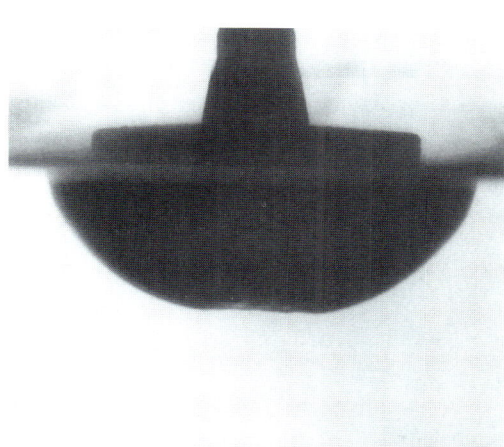

Fig. 4.85. Cryozone formation after exposure for 7 min

7 min

**Chapter 4
Experiments**

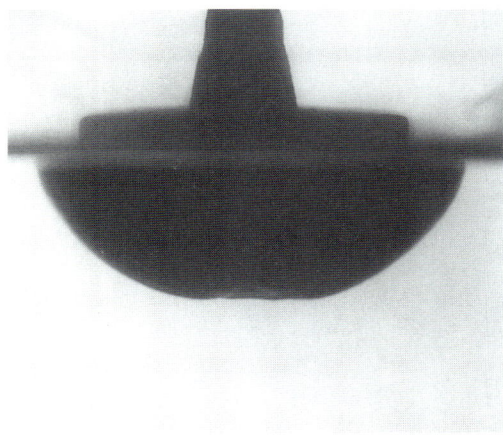

8 min

Fig. 4.86. Cryozone formation after exposure for 8 min

Cryoprobe

50 mm in diameter at a temperature of −180°C in a 1.5 l solution of 1.5% gelatine in water kept at a constant temperature of +30°C and continuously stirred

One picture per minute

Cryozone after 10 min freezing: diameter 58 mm, depth 27 mm

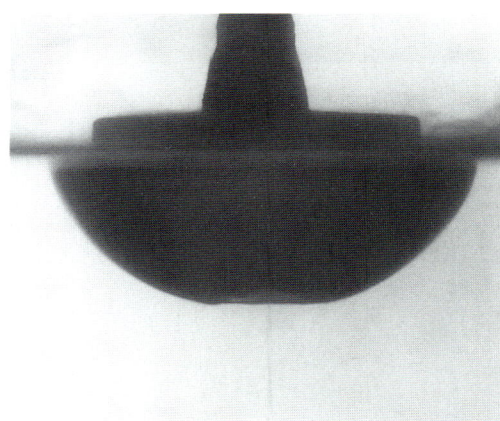

9 min

Fig. 4.87. Cryozone formation after exposure for 9 min

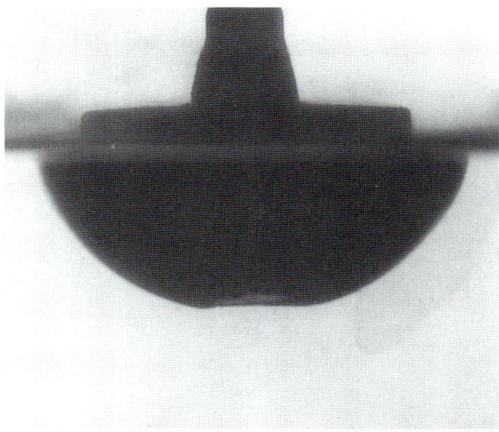

10 min

Fig. 4.88. Cryozone formation after exposure for 10 min

Section B Experimental Foundations 55

Laparoscopic Cryoprobe

Chapter 4
Experiments

10 mm in diameter 80 mm in length at a temperature of −**40°C** in a 1.5 l solution of 1.5% gelatine in water kept at a constant temperature of +30°C and continuously stirred

One picture per minute

Cryozone after 10 min freezing: diameter 11 mm, depth 82 mm

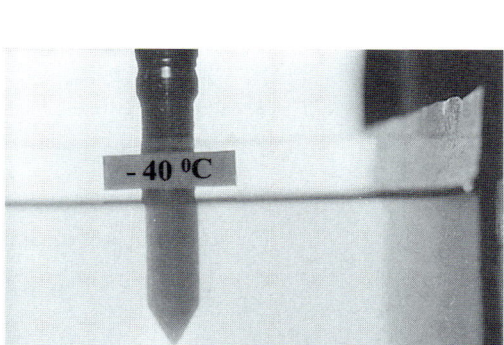

Start

Fig. 4.89. Start of freezing

Fig. 4.90. Cryozone formation after exposure for 1 min

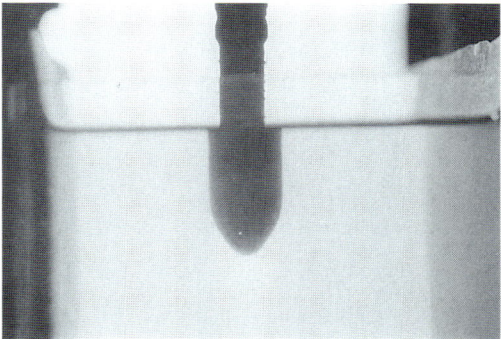

1 min

**Chapter 4
Experiments**

Laparoscopic Cryoprobe

10 mm in diameter 80 mm in length at a temperature of –40°C in a 1.5 l solution of 1.5% gelatine in water kept at a constant temperature of +30°C and continuously stirred

One picture per minute

Cryozone after 10 min freezing: diameter 11 mm, depth 82 mm

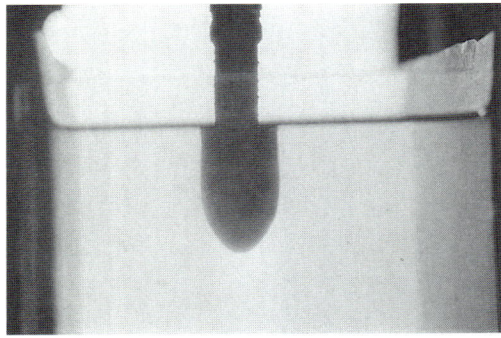

2 min

Fig. 4.91. Cryozone formation after exposure for 2 min

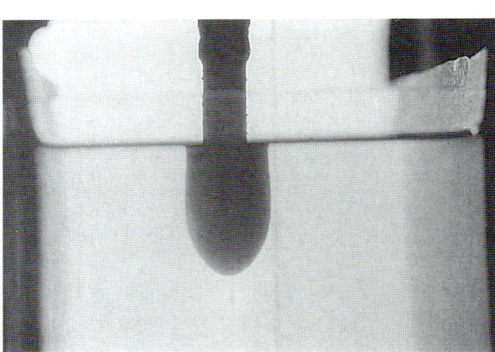

3 min

Fig. 4.92. Cryozone formation after exposure for 3 min

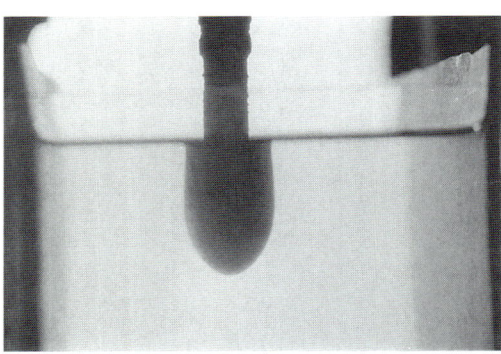

4 min

Fig. 4.93. Cryozone formation after exposure for 4 min

Section B

Laparoscopic Cryoprobe

10 mm in diameter 80 mm in length at a temperature of −40°C in a 1.5 l solution of 1.5% gelatine in water kept at a constant temperature of +30°C and continuously stirred

One picture per minute

Cryozone after 10 min freezing: diameter 11 mm, depth 82 mm

Experimental Foundations

Chapter 4
Experiments

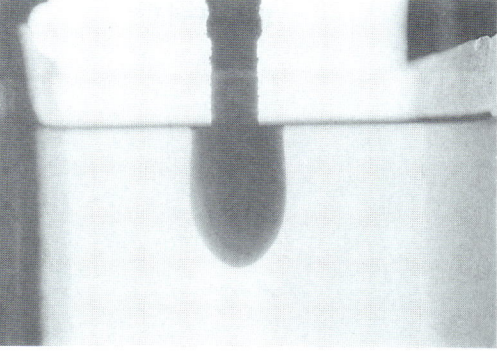

5 min

Fig. 4.94. Cryozone formation after exposure for 5 min

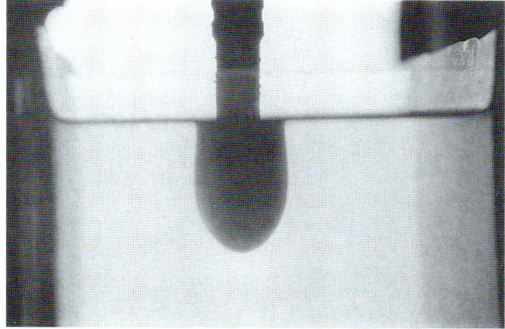

6 min

Fig. 4.95. Cryozone formation after exposure for 6 min

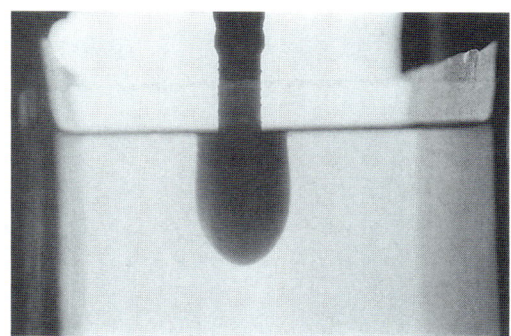

Fig. 4.96. Cryozone formation after exposure for 7 min

7 min

Chapter 4
Experiments

Laparoscopic Cryoprobe

10 mm in diameter 80 mm in length at a temperature of −40°C in a 1.5 l solution of 1.5% gelatine in water kept at a constant temperature of +30°C and continuously stirred

One picture per minute

Cryozone after 10 min freezing: diameter 11 mm, depth 82 mm

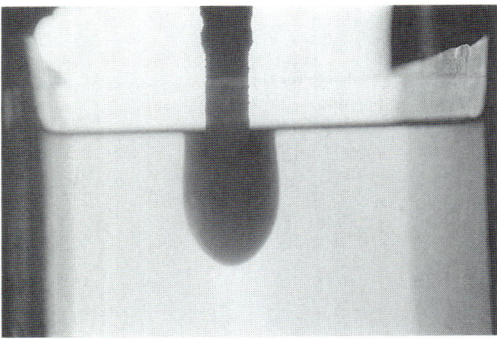

8 min

Fig. 4.97. Cryozone formation after exposure for 8 min

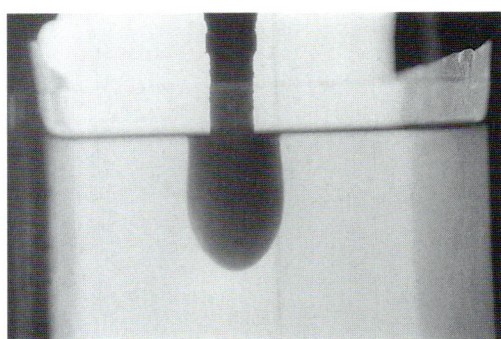

9 min

Fig. 4.98. Cryozone formation after exposure for 9 min

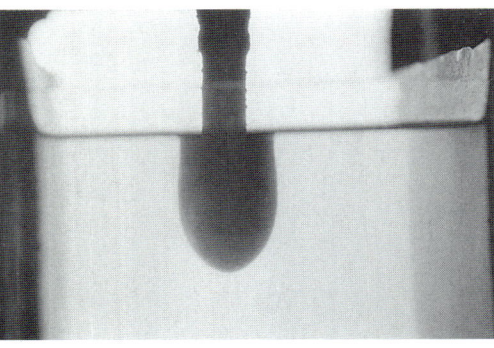

10 min

Fig. 4.99. Cryozone formation after exposure for 10 min

Section B Experimental Foundations 59

Laparoscopic Cryoprobe

Chapter 4
Experiments

10 mm in diameter 80 mm in length at a temperature of $-80°C$ in a 1.5 l solution of 1.5% gelatine in water kept at a constant temperature of $+30°C$ and continuously stirred

One picture per minute

Cryozone after 10 min freezing: diameter 12 mm, depth 84 mm

Start

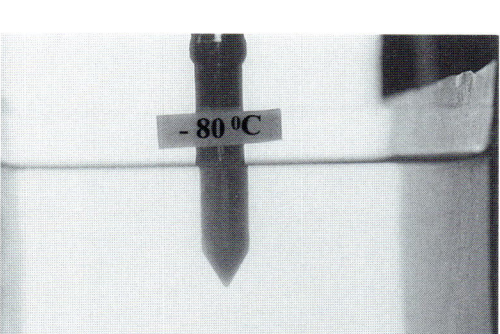

Fig. 4.100. Start of freezing

Fig. 4.101. Cryozone formation after exposure for 1 min

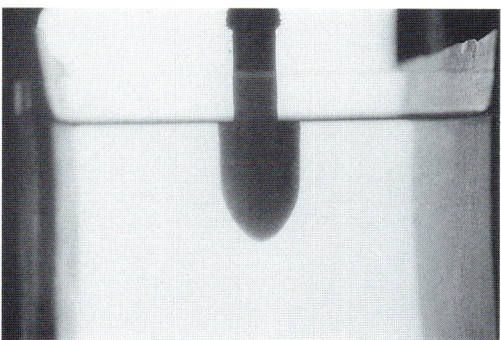

1 min

**Chapter 4
Experiments**

Laparoscopic Cryoprobe

10 mm in diameter 80 mm in length at a temperature of −80°C in a 1.5 l solution of 1.5% gelatine in water kept at a constant temperature of −30°C and continuously stirred

One picture per minute

Cryozone after 10 min freezing: diameter 12 mm, depth 84 mm

2 min

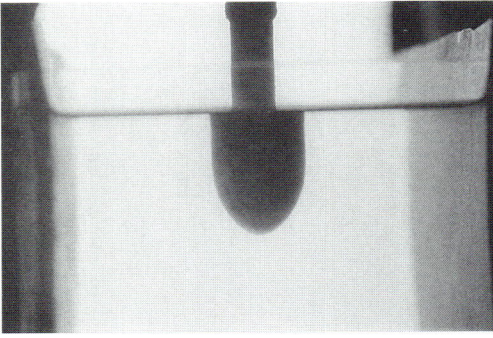

Fig. 4.102. Cryozone formation after exposure for 2 min

Fig. 4.103. Cryozone formation after exposure for 3 min

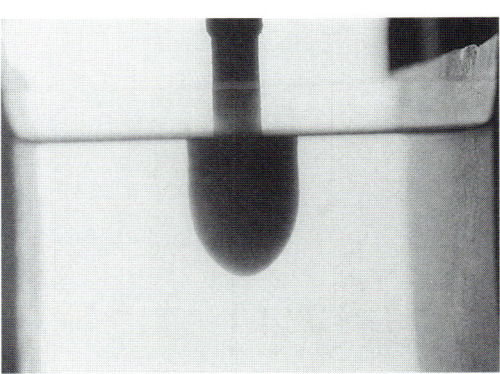

3 min

4 min

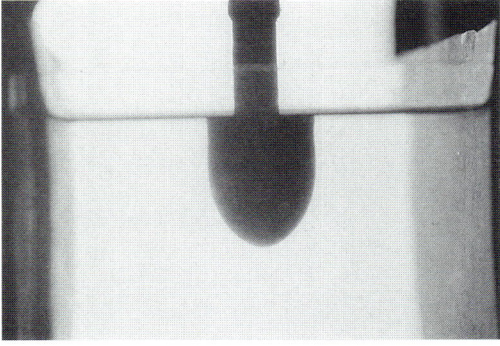

Fig. 4.104. Cryozone formation after exposure for 4 min

Section B Experimental Foundations

Laparoscopic Cryoprobe

10 mm in diameter 80 mm in length at a temperature of –80°C in a 1.5 l solution of 1.5% gelatine in water kept at a constant temperature of +30°C and continuously stirred

One picture per minute

Cryozone after 10 min freezing: diameter 12 mm, depth 84 mm

Chapter 4
Experiments

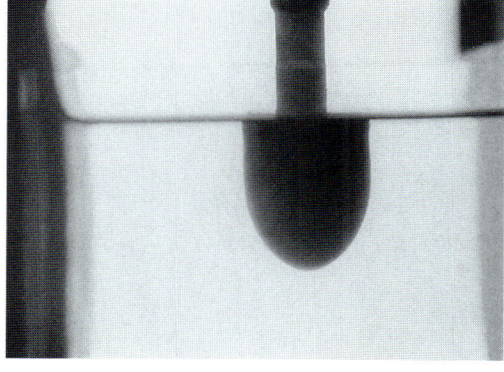

5 min

Fig. 4.105. Cryozone formation after exposure for 5 min

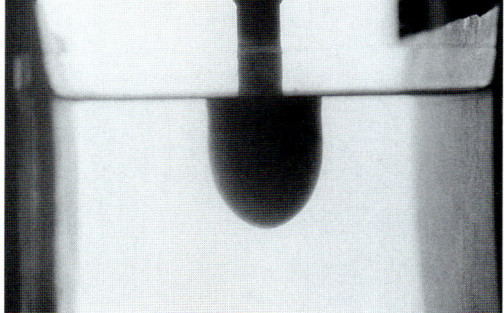

6 min

Fig. 4.106. Cryozone formation after exposure for 6 min

Fig. 4.107. Cryozone formation after exposure for 7 min

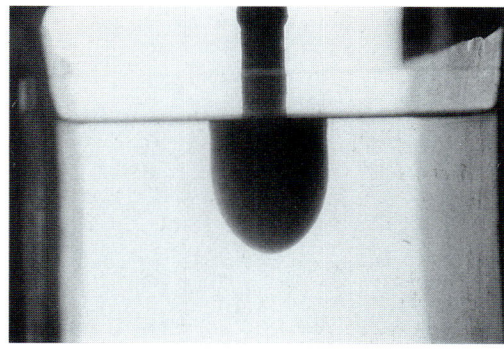

7 min

Chapter 4
Experiments

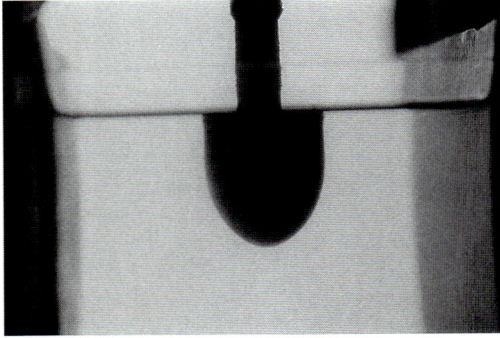

8 min

Fig. 4.108. Cryozone formation after exposure for 8 min

Laparoscopic Cryoprobe

10 mm in diameter 80 mm in length at a temperature of −80°C in a 1.5 l solution of 1.5% gelatine in water kept at a constant temperature of +30°C and continuously stirred

One picture per minute

Cryozone after 10 min freezing: diameter 12 mm, depth 84 mm

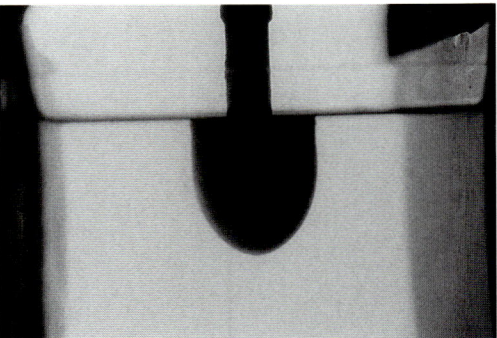

Fig. 4.109. Cryozone formation after exposure for 9 min

9 min

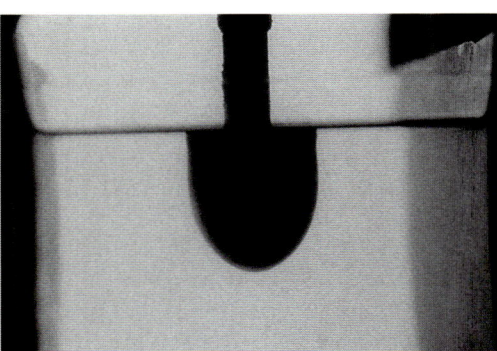

10 min

Fig. 4.110. Cryozone formation after exposure for 10 min

Section B   Experimental Foundations

Chapter 4
Experiments

Laparoscopic Cryoprobe

10 mm in diameter 80 mm in length at a temperature of $-120°C$ in a 1.5 l solution of 1.5% gelatine in water kept at a constant temperature of $+30°C$ and continuously stirred

One picture per minute

Cryozone after 10 min freezing: diameter 14 mm, depth 86 mm

Start

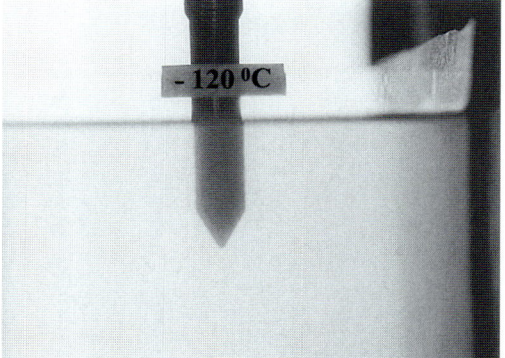

Fig. 4.111. Start of freezing

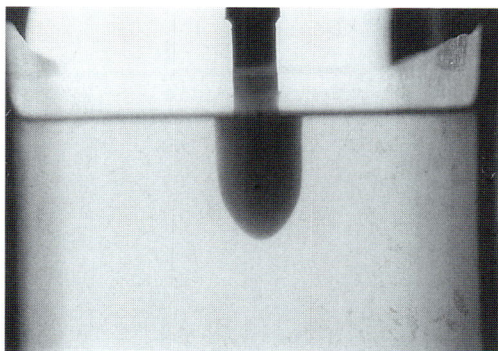

Fig. 4.112. Cryozone formation after exposure for 1 min

1 min

**Chapter 4
Experiments**

Laparoscopic Cryoprobe

10 mm in diameter 80 mm in length at a temperature of −120°C in a 1.5 l solution of 1.5% gelatine in water kept at a constant temperature of +30°C and continuously stirred

One picture per minute

Cryozone after 10 min freezing: diameter 14 mm, depth 86 mm

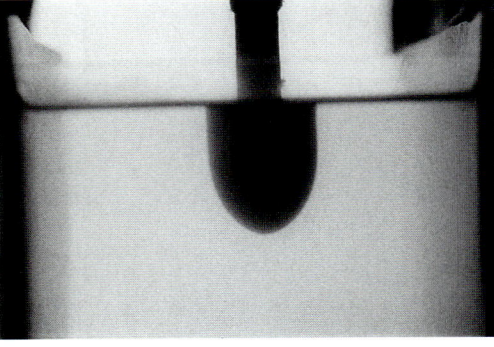

2 min

Fig. 4.113. Cryozone formation after exposure for 2 min

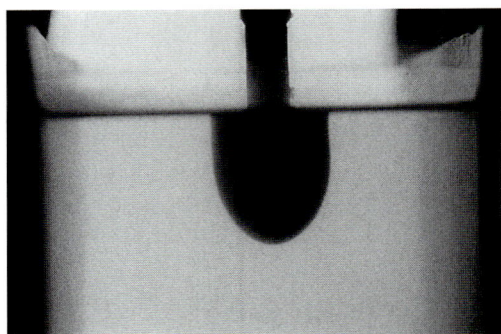

Fig. 4.114. Cryozone formation after exposure for 3 min

3 min

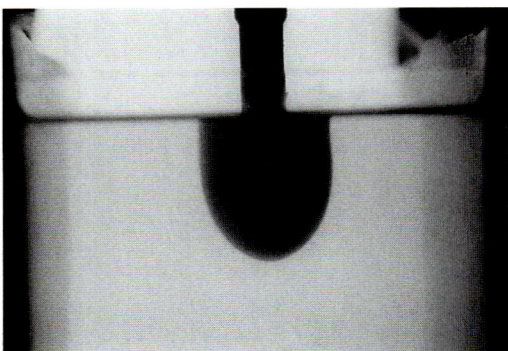

4 min

Fig. 4.115. Cryozone formation after exposure for 4 min

Section B Experimental Foundations

Laparoscopic Cryoprobe

10 mm in diameter 80 mm in length at a temperature of −120°C in a 1.5 l solution of 1.5% gelatine in water kept at a constant temperature of +30°C and continuously stirred

One picture per minute

Cryozone after 10 min freezing: diameter 14 mm, depth 86 mm

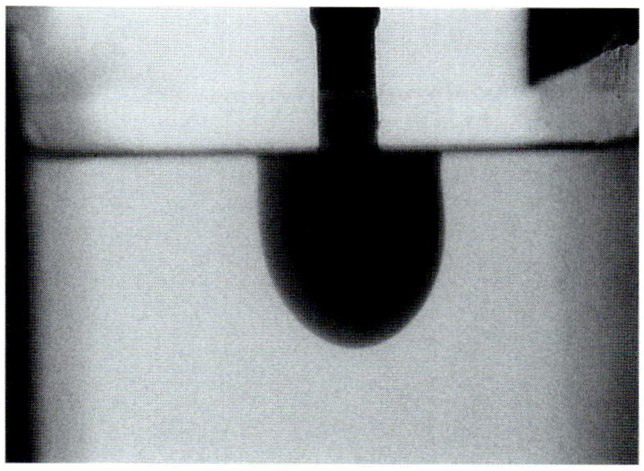

Chapter 4 Experiments

5 min

Fig. 4.116. Cryozone formation after exposure for 5 min

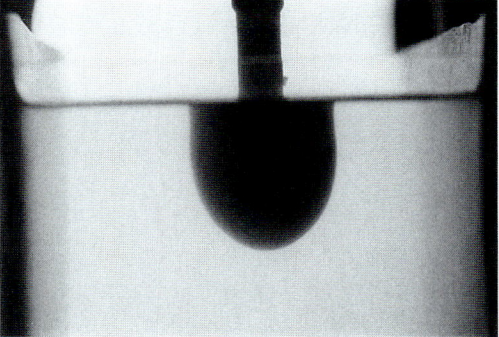

6 min

Fig. 4.117. Cryozone formation after exposure for 6 min

Fig. 4.118. Cryozone formation after exposure for 7 min

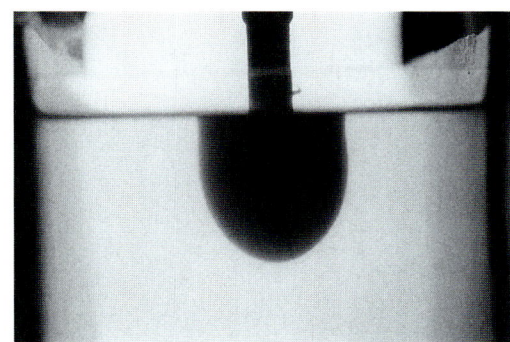

7 min

Laparoscopic Cryoprobe

10 mm in diameter 80 mm in length at a temperature of −120°C in a 1.5 l solution of 1.5% gelatine in water kept at a constant temperature of +30°C and continuously stirred

One picture per minute

Cryozone after 10 min freezing: diameter 14 mm, depth 86 mm

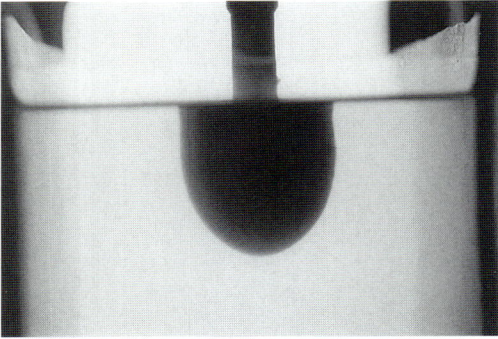

8 min

Fig. 4.119. Cryozone formation after exposure for 8 min

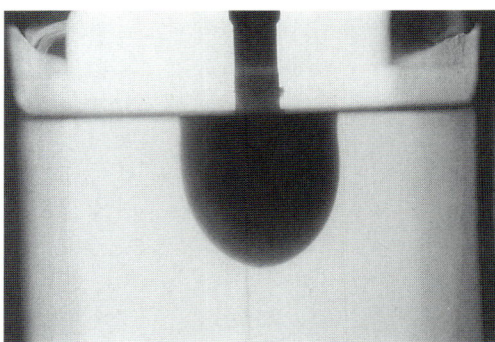

9 min

Fig. 4.120. Cryozone formation after exposure for 9 min

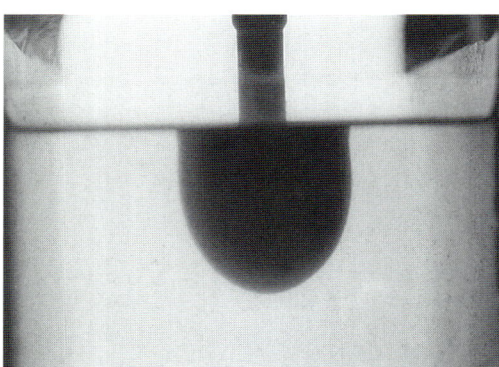

10 min

Fig. 4.121. Cryozone formation after exposure for 10 min

Section B · Experimental Foundations · Chapter 4 Experiments

Laparoscopic Cryoprobe

10 mm in diameter 80 mm in length at a temperature of −**180**°C in a 1.5 l solution of 1.5% gelatine in water kept at a constant temperature of +30°C and continuously stirred

One picture per minute

Cryozone after 10 min freezing: diameter 23 mm, depth 89 mm

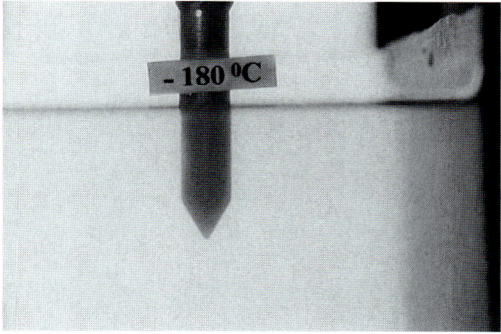

Start

Fig. 4.122. Start of freezing

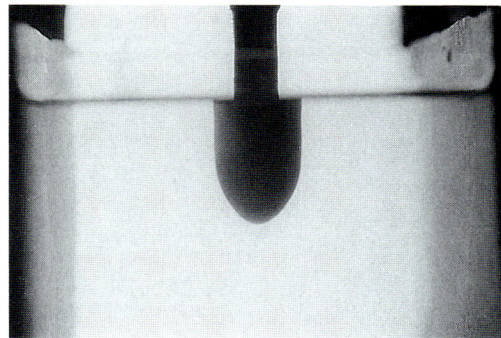

Fig. 4.123. Cryozone formation after exposure for 1 min

1 min

Chapter 4 Experiments

Laparoscopic Cryoprobe

10 mm in diameter 80 mm in length at a temperature of −180°C in a 1.5 l solution of 1.5% gelatine in water kept at a constant temperature of +30°C and continuously stirred

One picture per minute

Cryozone after 10 min freezing: diameter 23 mm, depth 89 mm

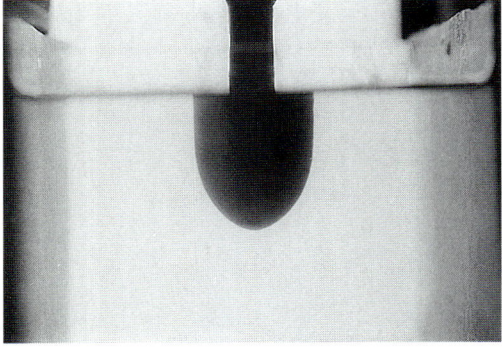

2 min

Fig. 4.124. Cryozone formation after exposure for 2 min

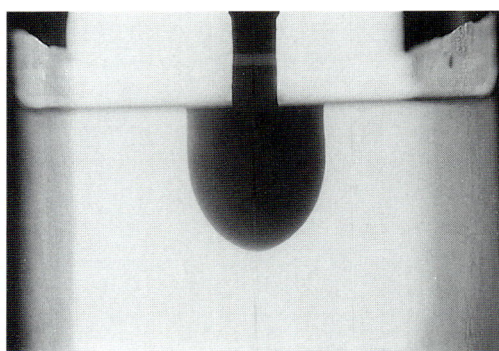

3 min

Fig. 4.125. Cryozone formation after exposure for 3 min

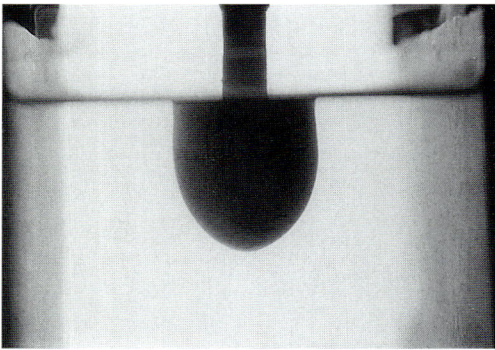

4 min

Fig. 4.126. Cryozone formation after exposure for 4 min

Section B · Experimental Foundations

Laparoscopic Cryoprobe

10 mm in diameter 80 mm in length at a temperature of –180°C in a 1.5 l solution of 1.5% gelatine in water kept at a constant temperature of +30°C and continuously stirred

One picture per minute

Cryozone after 10 min freezing: diameter 23 mm, depth 89 mm

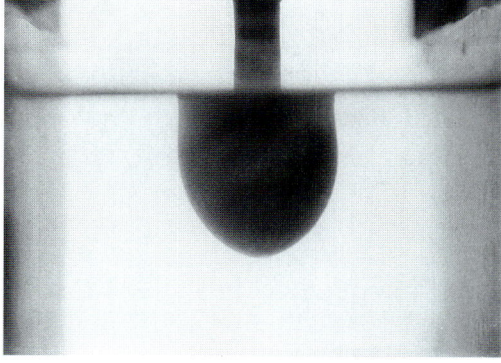

5 min

Fig. 4.127. Cryozone formation after exposure for 5 min

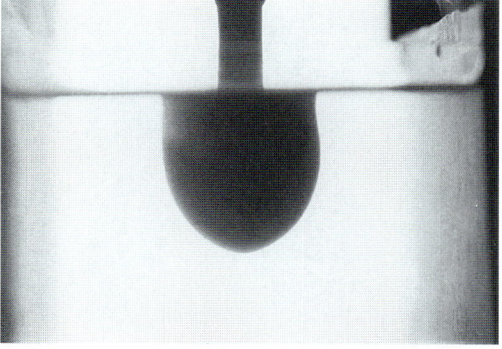

6 min

Fig. 4.128. Cryozone formation after exposure for 6 min

Fig. 4.129. Cryozone formation after exposure for 7 min

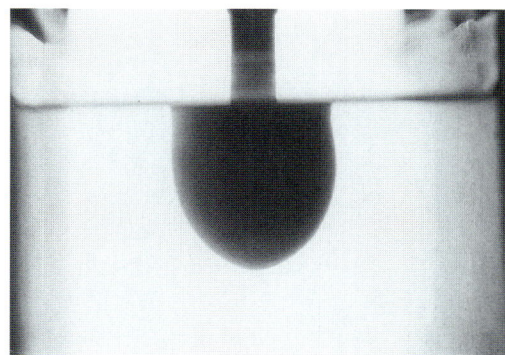

7 min

Chapter 4
Experiments

Laparoscopic Cryoprobe

10 mm in diameter 80 mm in length at a temperature of −180°C in a 1.5 l solution of 1.5% gelatine in water kept at a constant temperature of +30°C and continuously stirred

One picture per minute

Cryozone after 10 min freezing: diameter 23 mm, depth 89 mm

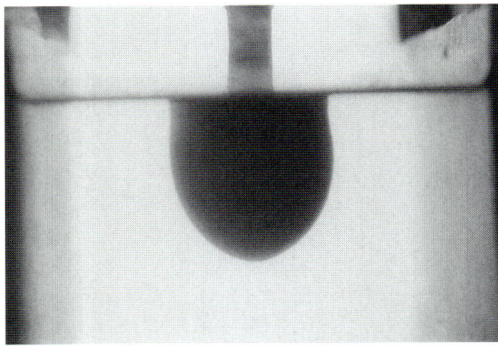

8 min

Fig. 4.130. Cryozone formation after exposure for 8 min

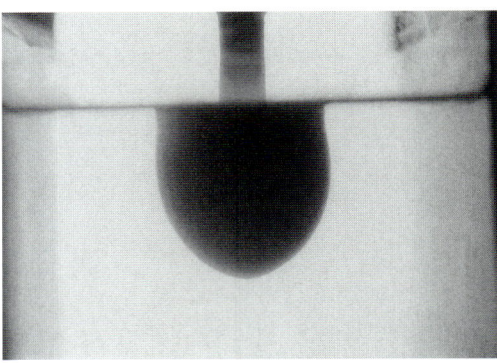

9 min

Fig. 4.131. Cryozone formation after exposure for 9 min

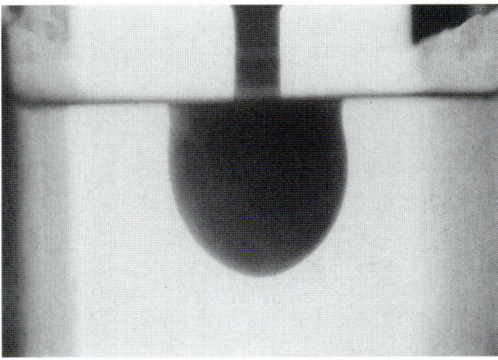

10 min

Fig. 4.132. Cryozone formation after exposure for 10 min

Section C

Basis of Cryosurgical Equipment and Technology

Chapter 5

Basic Aspects of Cryosurgical Equipment and Technology

Nikolai N. Korpan
with contributions by
Jaroslav V. Zharkov

One of the crucial factors which have influenced the development of cryosurgery is the standard and the technical competence of cryosurgical devices; the efficiency of cryosurgery in curative practice first of all depends on the technical proficiency of the cryosurgical devices used to perform cryooperations.

On the basis of our own theoretical, experimental and practical experience, and after examining the work of cryosurgery schools the world over, but also on the basis of our own know-how (21 national patents, including 3 world-wide patents), we have elaborated a concept of modern cryosurgical technology which can be used universally. It is produced by an automated system known as "Universal Cryosurgical Complex" (UCC). It will make it possible to apply the main advantages of the cryosurgical method in all fields of medicine. The UCC is illustrated below and consists of the following three cryosurgical systems:

a) "Cryosurgical System, Mobile" – CSM (Figs. 5.1–5.7)
b) "Cryosurgical System, Stationary" – CSS (Fig. 5.8)
c) "Cryosurgical System, Ambulatory" – CSA (Fig. 5.9)

The *mobile cryosurgical unit* (Figs. 5.1–5.7) is produced as a compact installation with a cryogenic system, and an automatic steering block which activates the cryogenic process. Storage of the cryoagent (10 l) provides uninterrupted cryoactivity for 3–4 hours and makes it possible to perform cryooperations in surgery, gynecology, urology, proctology, dermatology, etc. at out-patient clinics.

The *stationary cryogenic unit* (Fig. 5.8) is new and an absolute must in any modern operating theatre. The unit, with a complete set of cryosurgical instruments, is situated above the operating table and fixed at the required angle so as to fully relieve the surgeon's hand during operations which can last several hours.

The *ambulatory (portable) cryosurgical unit* (Fig. 5.9) is in a case and consists of a steering block and a small cryoblock (weighing 1.5 kg, plus 400 ml of liquid nitrogen), a set of cryodevices and applicators. It is easy to transport and can be used for performing a single cryodestruction of not more than 40 cm^3 of tissue volume. The set can be used during transport of the patient, or on site, from the electric network of an automobile, as it can run on a car battery.

All the above-mentioned units have a block in the centre to which the various cryodevices and applicators for use in the different fields of medicine can be attached. All these cryosystems contain the unique cryoelements (heat-exchangers, cryodevices and applicators, electromagnetic valves, heaters, cryopipelines, etc.), which satisfy all the above-mentioned requirements. Mechanized cryosystems allow the realization of variable parameters of cryoactivity, make it possible to conduct cryobiological investigations with the very best technology and under optimal conditions.

Chapter 5
Equipment Technology

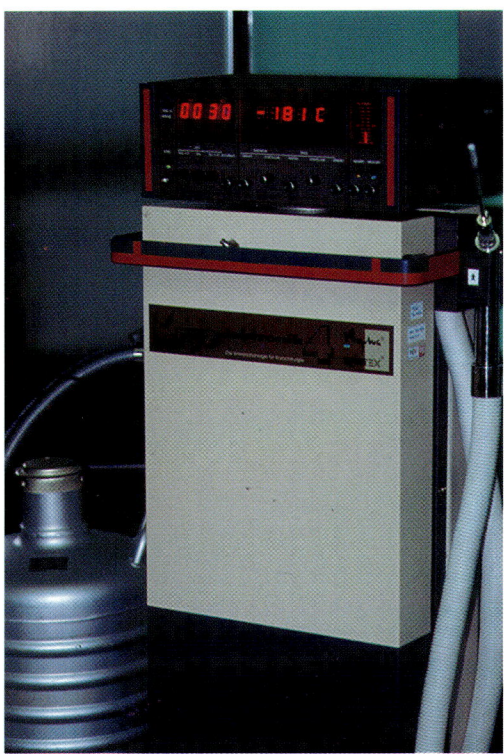

Fig. 5.1. Mobile Cryosurgical System. General view

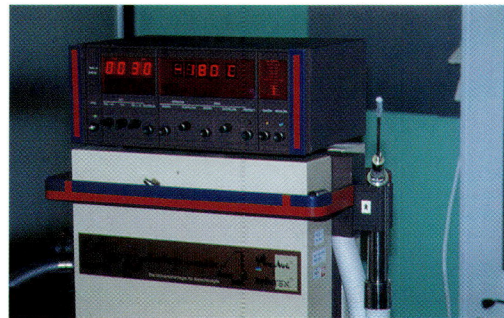

Fig. 5.2. Mobile Cryosurgical System. Display

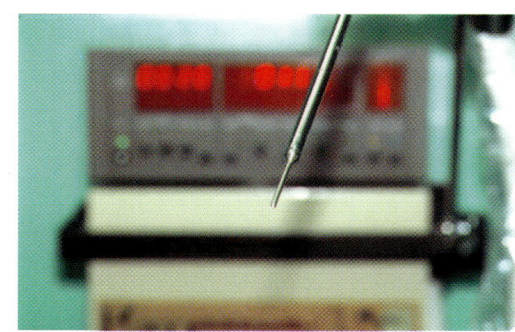

Fig. 5.3. Mobile Cryosurgical System with the needle for laparoscopic cryosurgery

Section C   Basic Equipment and Technology   75

Chapter 5
Equipment
Technology

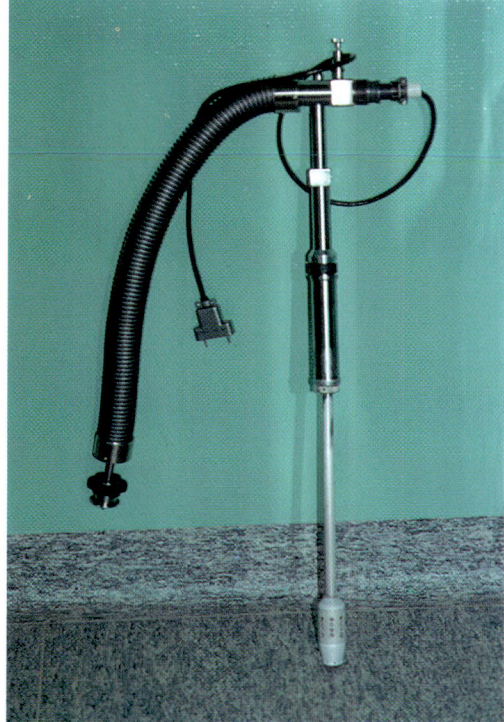

Fig. 5.4. Mobile Cryo-surgical System. Unit for filling with cryogen

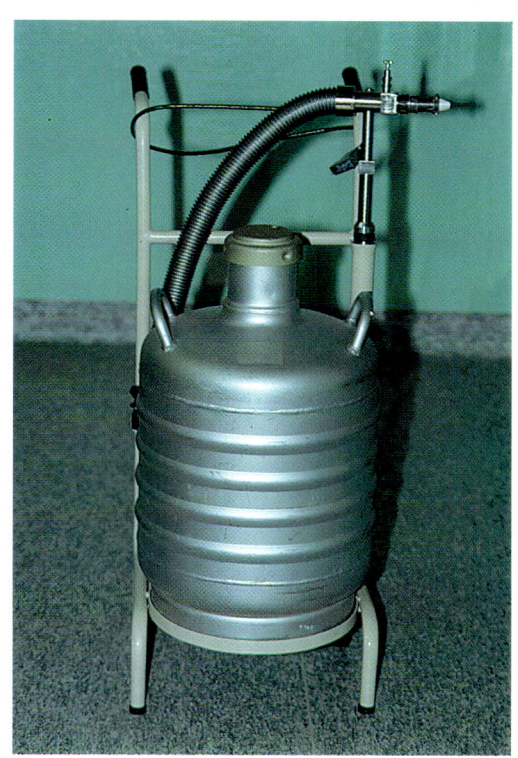

Fig. 5.5. Mobile Cryo-surgical System. Cryogenic vessel

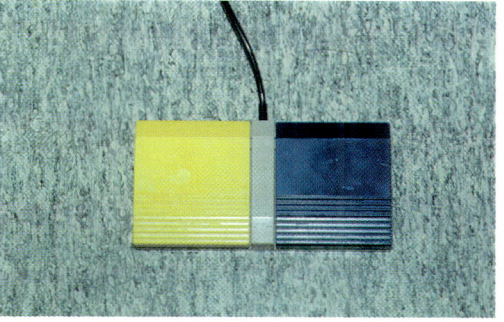

Fig. 5.6. Mobile Cryo-surgical System. Blue pedal for freezing and yellow one for heating

**Chapter 5
Equipment
Technology**

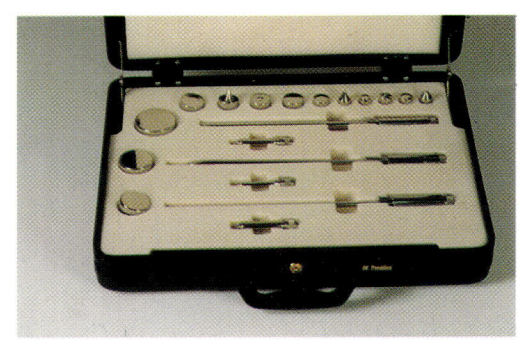

Fig. 5.7. Mobile Cryosurgical System. Set of the basic cryosurgical instruments

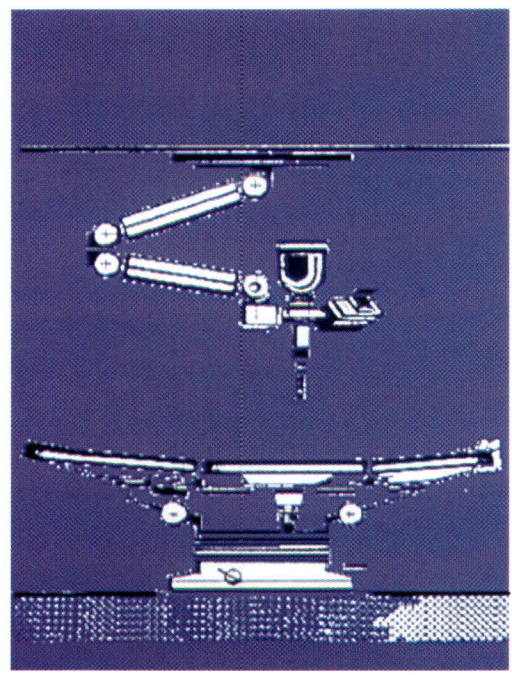

Fig. 5.8. Schematic view of the Stationary Cryosurgical System

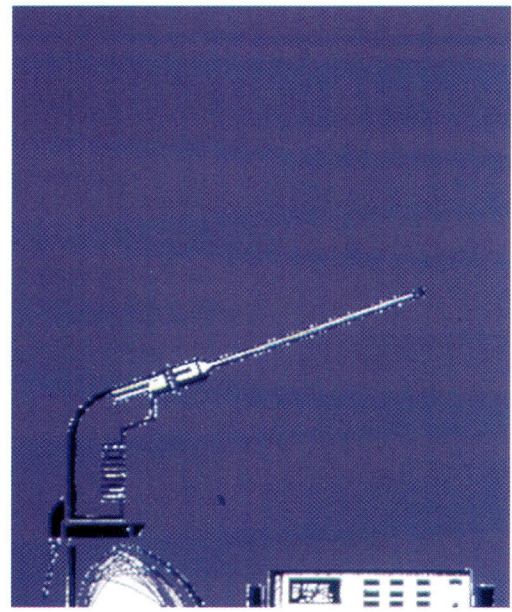

Fig. 5.9. Schematic view of the Ambulatory Cryosurgical System (Portable Cryosurgical Unit)

The way the cryosurgical complex is constructed has made it possible to increase the number of the various cryodevices and applicators for the three cryosystems, usable in all branches of medicine.

All the cryosystems mentioned above are based on the latest achievements in the field of cryo-heat-exchange, cryomaterial-science and mechanization of the cryo-processes.

The *new cryosurgical automated systems "Universal Cryosurgical Complex"* (UCC) has been constructed on our basic know-how, which includes the design and manufacture of porous heat-exchangers, the technology of electron-vacuum welding for thin-wall components, the design of electromagnetic valves for cryogenic liquids, and the results of clinical investigations of the new system in different fields of medicine.

Technical Data are as follows (Fig. 5.10):

- volume of the cryodestruction zone 1–180 cm^3
- liquid nitrogen capacity 10 litres
- freezing temperature range 20–190°C
- time needed to reach working temperature a max. of 5 min
- thawing time 2–3 min
- power consumed a max. of 600 W
- voltage 220 V 50 Hz
- weight 10 kg

The *main advantages* of the system referred to as the universal cryosurgical complex "UCC" are (Figs. 5.11–5.14):

1. high cooling capacity
2. quarantining the cryodestruction of the specified volume
3. enabling a choice for different oncological operations:

   a) high accuracy of measurement
   b) stabilization of the temperature required for cryosurgery, and the provision of a specially developed mathematical formula for

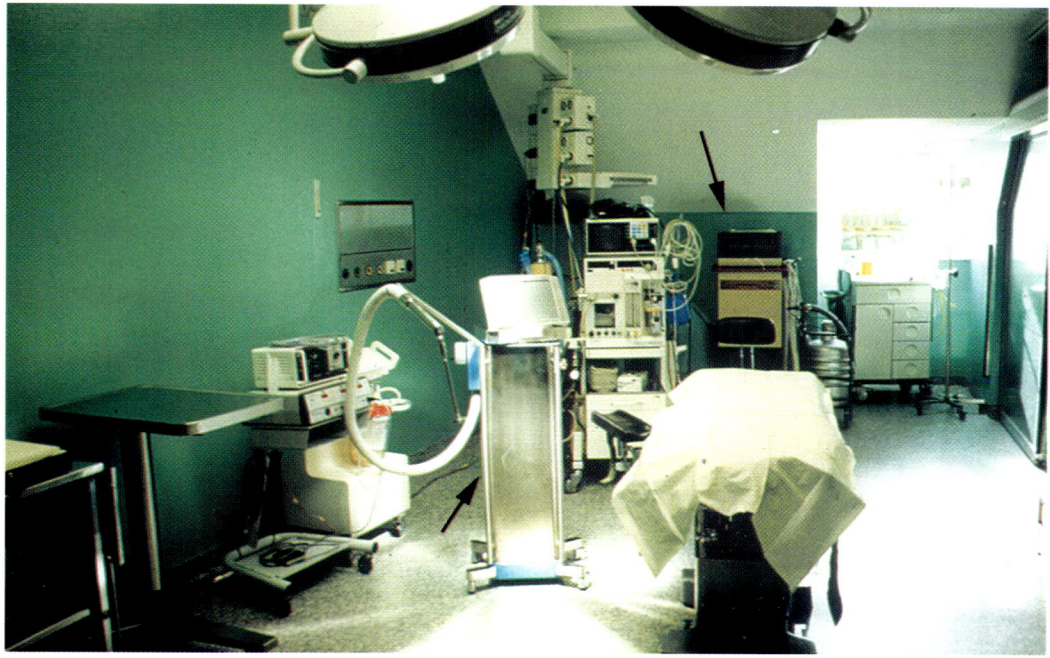

Fig. 5.10. Universal Cryosurgical Complex. Operating theatre (arrows point to cryosurgical units)

Chapter 5
Equipment Technology

evaluating the cryodestruction which is symmetrical around the axis, in order to predict the cryodestruction zone

c) the availability of three kinds of cryosystems, different cryoinstruments and applicators make it possible to realize various cryosurgical procedures (application, penetration, spraying, clamp) which can be used in almost all fields of medicine

d) the high reliability of vacuum and cryogenic equipment provided by the use of the advanced technologies of the electronic beam and of laser welding

When one analyzes the technical facilities of the cryosurgical systems in the suggested complex and compares them to those on the market today, it is possible to conclude that, as far as their technical standard is concerned, the cryosystems described here are three to five years ahead of their potential competitors.

In this study we have analyzed one of the most essential factors which influences the development of cryosurgery, namely the condition and standard of the cryosurgical appliances and their influence on the development of the method in general, and we have put forward our own conception of cryosurgical techniques.

Findings in cryobiological investigations, which have described the mechanisms of cryodestroying biological cells, have made it possible to formulate the main technical requirements for cryosurgical devices. *Our recommendations for the further development of cryosurgical techniques are based on various experimental and clinical results of the application of the cryomethod in different branches of medicine. We have used our own extensive experimental and clinical material.*

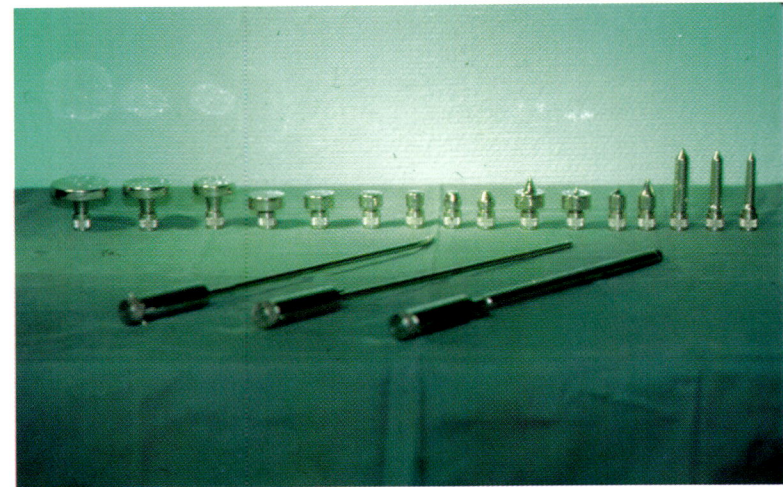

Fig. 5.11. The new cryosurgical instruments

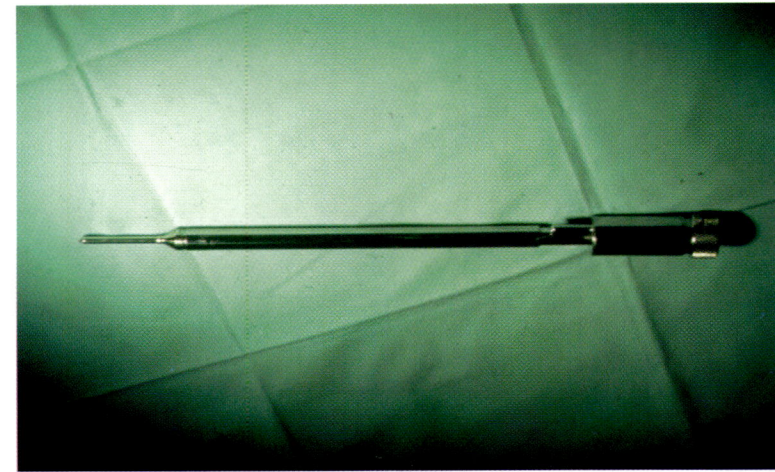

Fig. 5.12. The new laparoscopic cryosurgical needle

Section C Basic Equipment and Technology

Chapter 5
Equipment
Technology

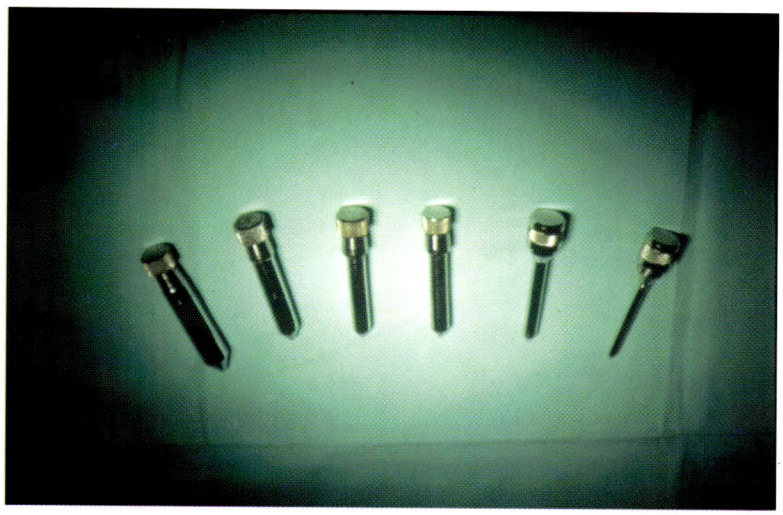

Fig. 5.13. Set of the new universal needles for cryosurgery

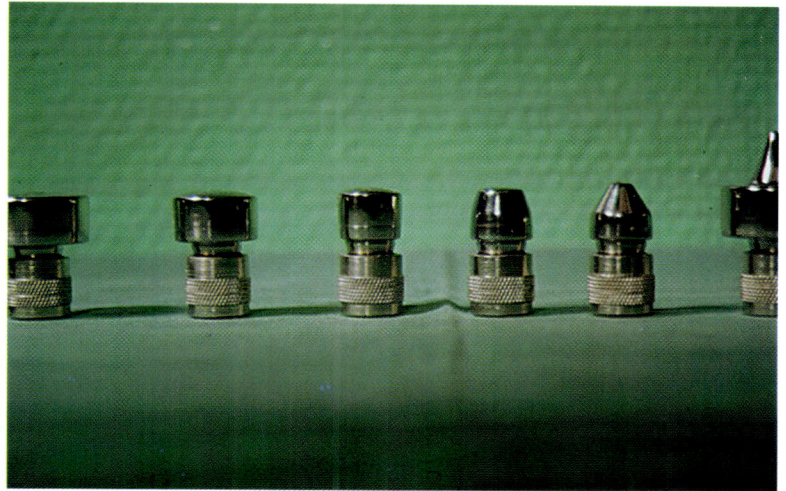

Fig. 5.14. The new cryosurgical probes

Technical Requirements for Cryosurgical Equipment

Jaroslav V. Zharkov

Findings in cryobiological investigations which describe cryodestructive mechanisms make it possible to formulate the main technical requirements of cryosurgical devices. The elaboration and improvement of any medical technique begins by trying to satisfy the main technical requirements so that the appliance will prove efficient in medical practice (Fig. 6.1).

Having studied the construction of many cryosurgical instruments made in different countries and based on various ways of attaining very low temperatures, one can now say that cryosurgical techniques have been going in the wrong direction. The first simple appliances appeared long before the main mechanisms for cryodestruction of biological cells was known. Technical requirements which could perhaps have been realized had not yet been established. Thus, for a long time, many scientists, who had applied the simple techniques without effect, no longer believed that cryosurgery had a future and stopped promoting it.

The main technical parameter for effective cryodestruction is the provision of a sufficiently low, sub-zero temperature in the biological tissue, followed by deliberate thawing. This very low temperature, in turn, is defined by the temperature of the working surface of the cryoinstrument which is in contact with the bulk tissue to be frozen. The results of experimental studies show that if the cryosurgical device provides temperatures of −170°C to −190°C on the working surface of the cryoinstrument which is in contact with the bulk of the tissue to be frozen, then in this case most of the cells die. If the temperature is not lowered quickly enough in the course of the cryosurgical procedure, there is an increasing probability that cells will be preserved in the bulk of the tissue which is to be frozen, and recurrences of malignant malformations become possible. Thus, during cryoactivity the temperature of the working surface of the cryodevice which is in contact with the tissue should not be higher than −170°C.

Another condition which must be fulfilled is the provision of great accuracy in measuring and stabilizing the correct temperature at which cryoactivity is carried out.

Our new cryosurgical technology is able to create sub-zero temperatures down to −196°C where they are required, that is, where the cryosurgical instrument makes contact with

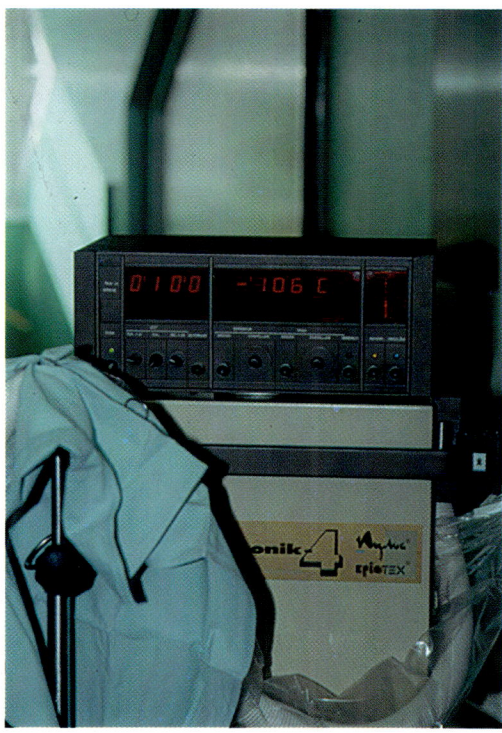

Fig. 6.1. Mobile Cryosurgical System, which is the universal cryosurgical unit and can be used in all fields of modern medicine

Chapter 6
Equipment Requirements

the tissue, and this accurate freezing procedure can, moreover, be repeated again and again. Although essential for cryosurgery to be effective, repeated lowering of the temperature to such a degree has up to now not been possible.

Simplicity, reliability, efficiency and safety are, of course, also essential qualities of this new technology.

Stability and the possibility of repeating several freeze-thaw cycles accurately, as well as the other above-mentioned requirements are provided by the construction of the cryosurgical unit and the all-important peculiarities of its functional structure, especially the accuracy of the steering.

In recent decades cryosurgical devices invented by different firms have appeared on the market. Although they are reasonably complicated automatic systems, they do not satisfy the main requirement, namely the very low temperatures required for cryoactivity. Because of their construction, devices currently on the market cannot produce a temperature lower than $-120°C$ on the working surface of the cryodevice which is in contact with the human organ and cannot, therefore, guarantee cryodestruction. This is doubtless why the cryosurgical method has not spread more extensively and why its possibilities have been neglected.

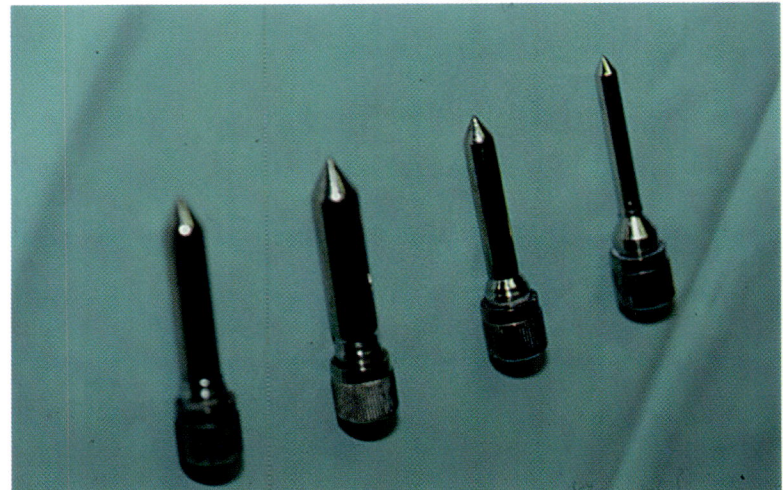

Fig. 6.2. Modern cryosurgical needles based on current know-how

Section D

Basic Cryosurgical Techniques

General Techniques of Cryosurgery

Nikolai N. Korpan

Introduction

It is evident that only very few patients with malignant tumors requiring extended surgery survive the operation. Most patients require interventional or (at least) minimally invasive, palliative therapy that guarantees a good quality of life and only short stays in hospital for the remaining survival time.

New scientific investigations in fundamental biology and experimental surgery, plus modern technological developments have opened up an important and at the same fascinating perspective for treatment strategies of malignant tumors which are in an advanced stage. Patients with primary or secondary parenchymal tumors which are inoperable, or who cannot undergo conventional surgery, are strongly advised to undergo cryosurgical treatment as it is both promising and highly motivating.

Cryosurgery, a particularly gentle operational technique, has begun to attract widespread notice internationally. Theoretical, clinical and experimental experience with modern cryosurgery, has been gathered since the 1960's. Due to the lack of the necessary technical apparatus, however, cryosurgery was not widely used. Successful application of this method, especially for various kinds of cancer, is now possible because the necessary technical devices have in the meanwhile become available.

By means of the various cryoprobes, it is now possible to apply and focus cold evenly. It has thus become possible to operate on different kinds of cancer using both open and minimally invasive cryosurgical techniques. We here define different general cryosurgical techniques.

Chapter 7 Techniques

I. Mode of Cryosurgical Application

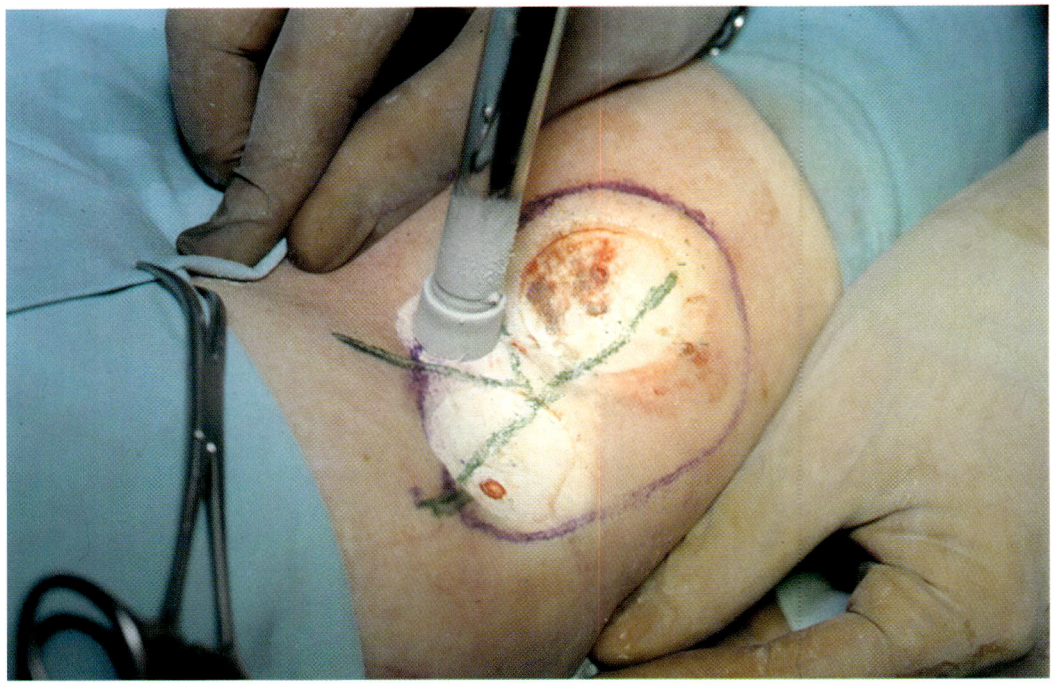

Fig. 7.1. Mode of cryosurgical application. Female, 48 years of age. A disc probe is placed on the skin tumor. For cryoexposure a temperature range of −40°C, −80°C, −120°C, −170°C and −196°C in contact with the skin tumor mass is selected with a temperature variation of ±1%

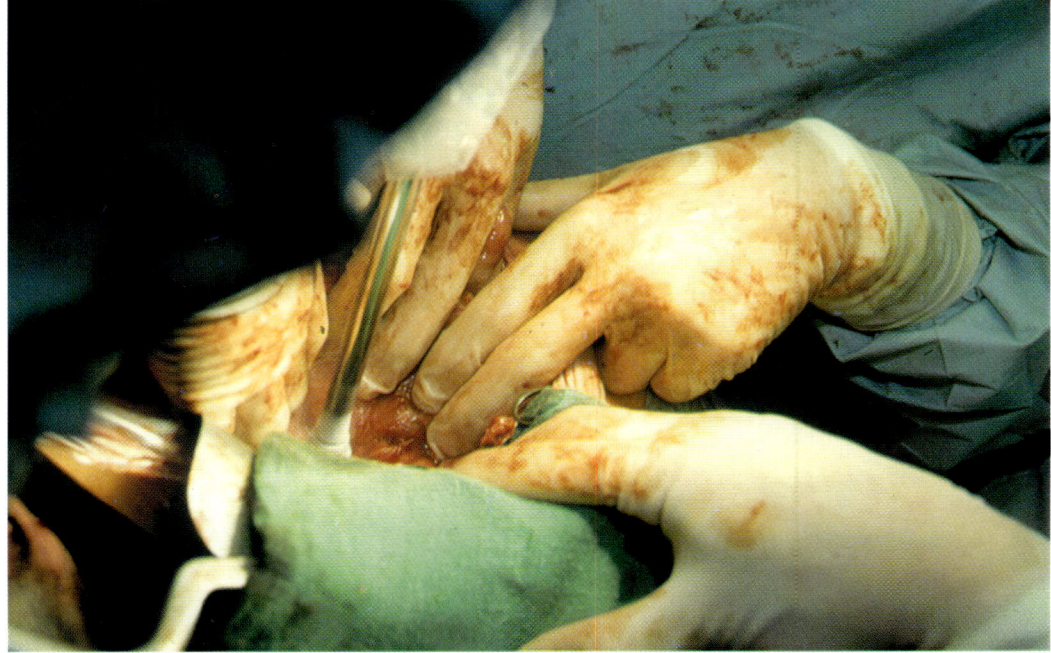

Fig. 7.2. Mode of cryosurgical application. Male, 59 years old. A disc probe 15 mm in diameter is placed on the pancreas head carcinoma. A 9 min freeze, followed by complete thawing of the pancreas is used for each freeze-thaw cycle. Each cryolesion is observed for 7–10 min after thawing

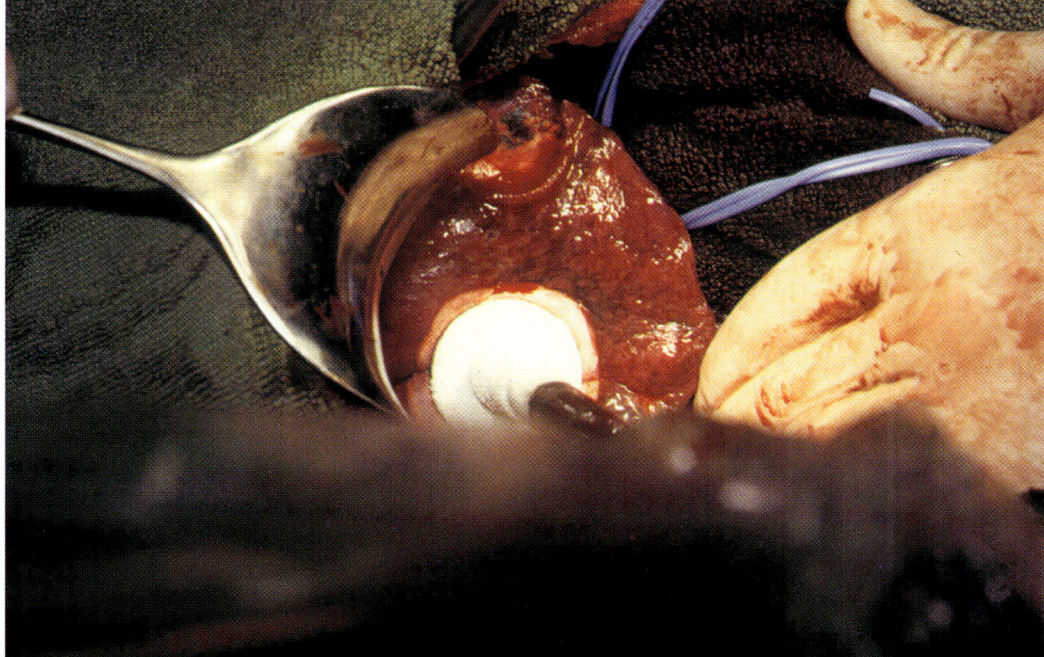

Fig. 7.3. Mode of cryosurgical application. Male, 64 years old. A disc probe is placed on the liver metastasis at a temperature of −180°C in contact with the tumor mass

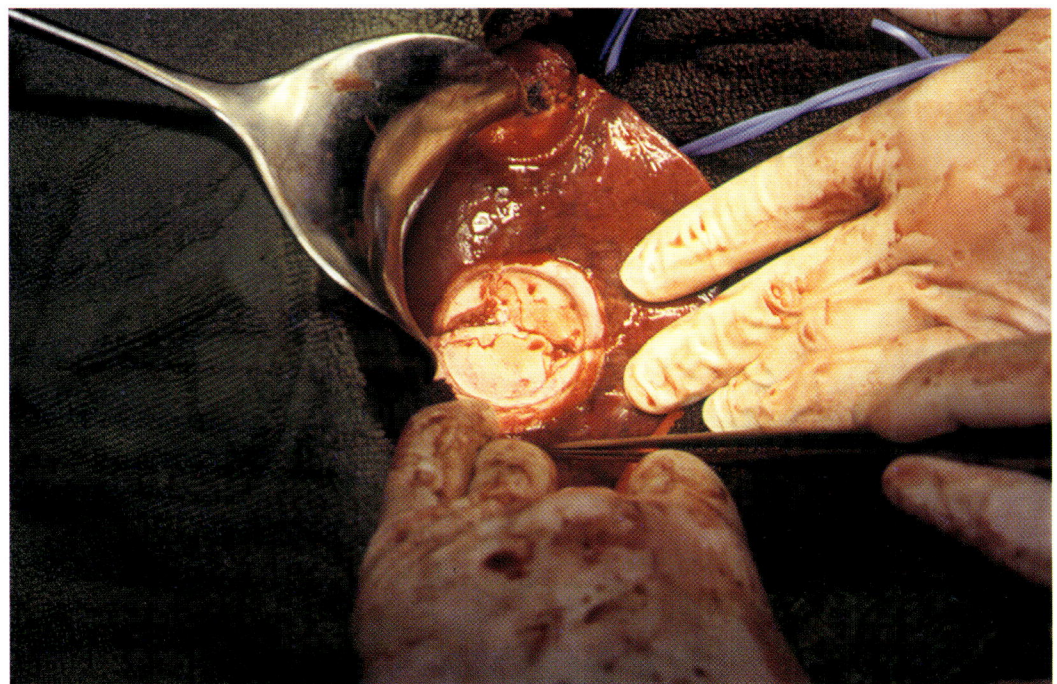

Fig. 7.4. Same patient. Appearance of the post-cryosurgical zone immediately after the cryosurgical exposure

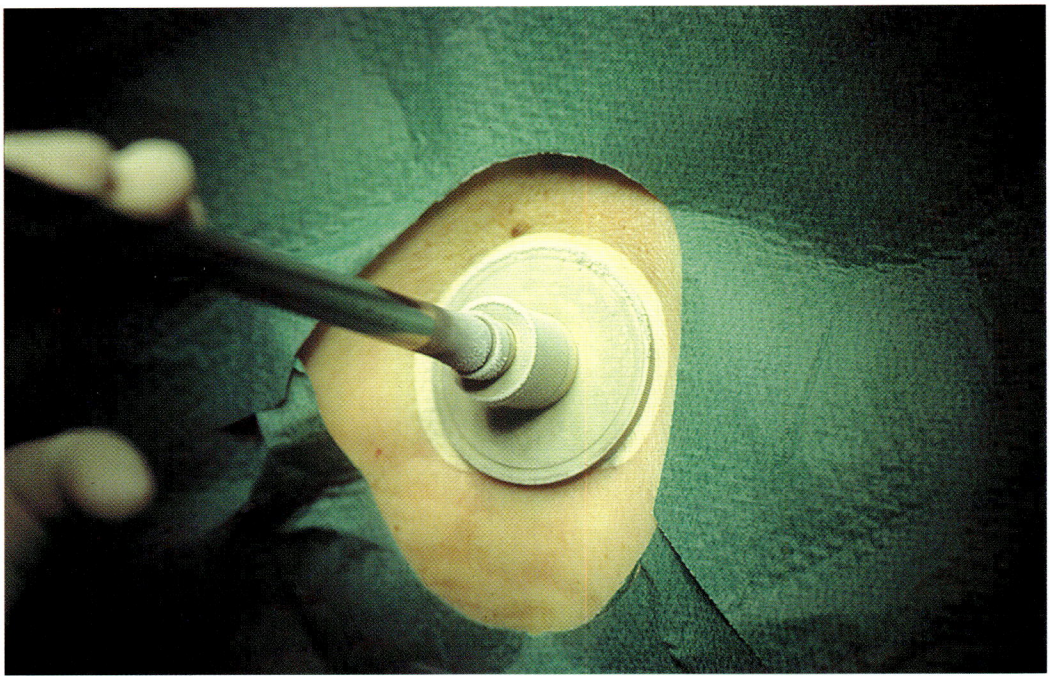

Fig. 7.5. Mode of cryosurgical application. Female, 72 years old. A disc probe is placed on the large skin metastasis after conventional melanoma extirpation

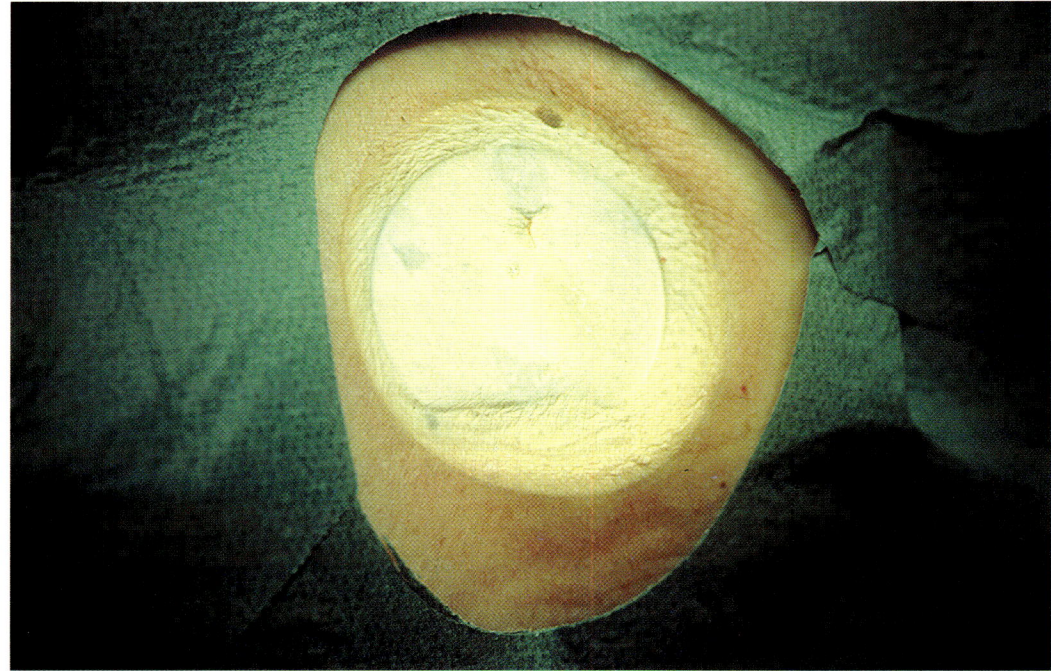

Fig. 7.6. View of the cryozone in the same patient immediately after the single freeze-thaw cycle

Section D Basic Techniques

II. Percutaneous Cryosurgical Extirpation

Chapter 7
Techniques

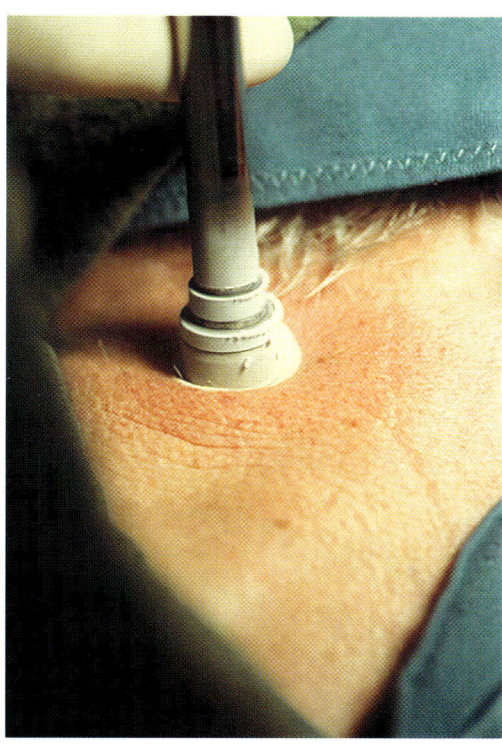

Fig. 7.7. Percutaneous cryosurgical extirpation of the lymph node. Male, 73 years old. Patient with multiple cervical lymph node metastases after conventional melanoma extirpation

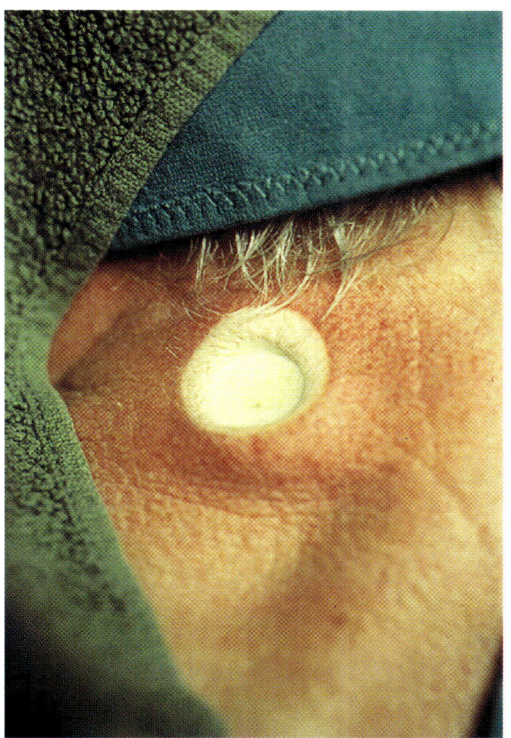

Fig. 7.8. View of the cryozone in the same patient immediately after the single freeze-thaw cycle

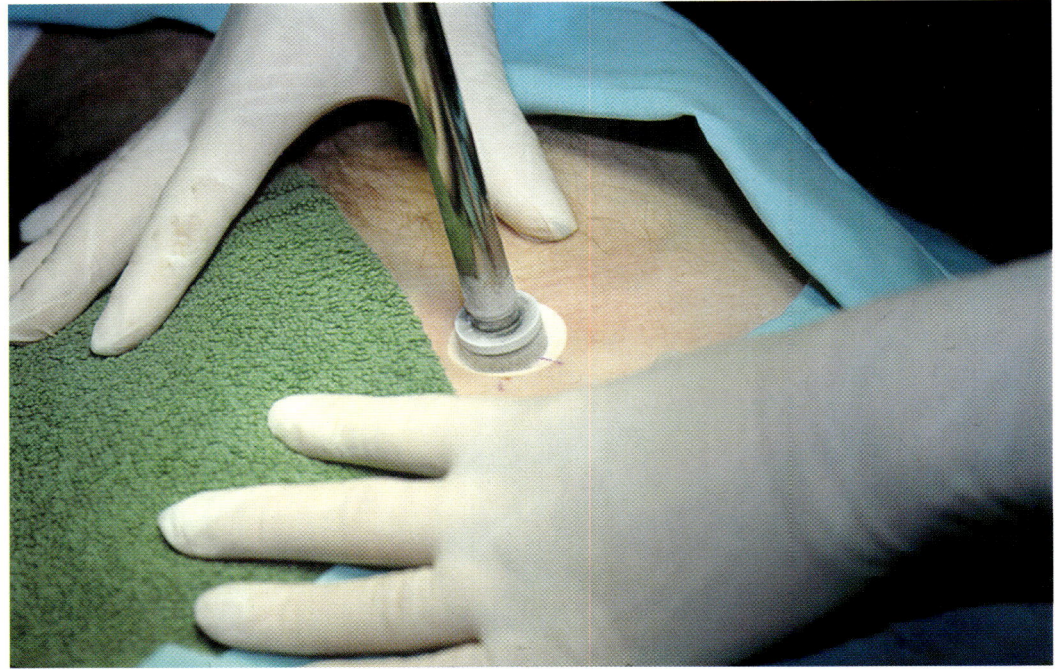

Fig. 7.9. Percutaneous cryosurgical lymph node extirpation. Male, 23 years of age. Patient with multiple inguinal lymph node metastases after conventional melanoma extirpation

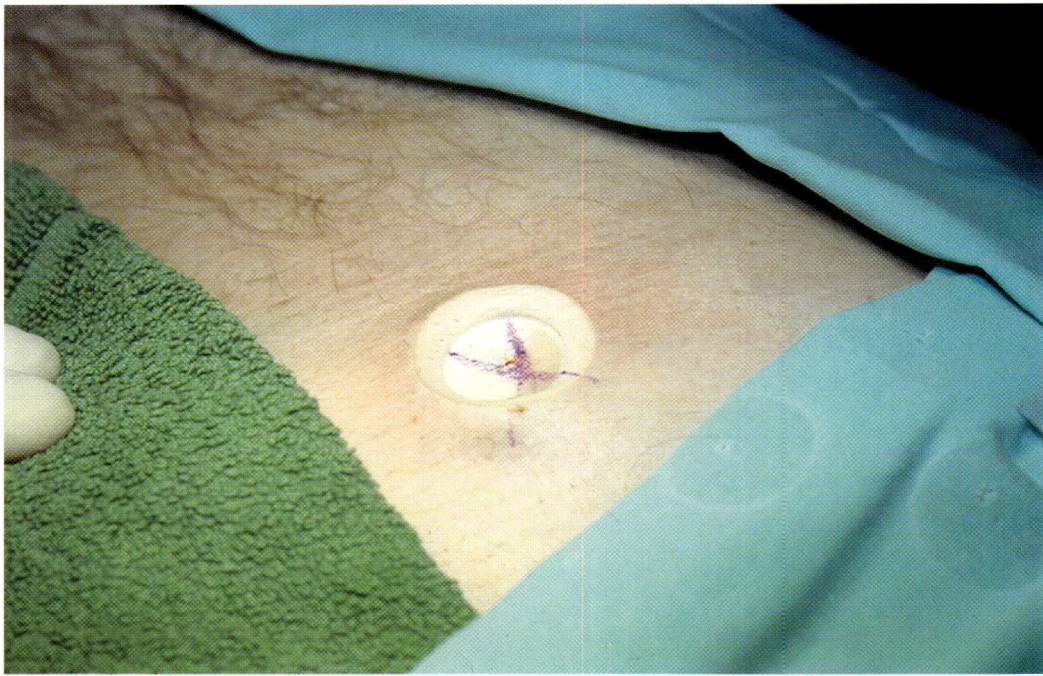

Fig. 7.10. Appearance of the cryozone in the same patient immediately after the single freeze-thaw cycle

III. Subcutaneous Cryosurgical Extirpation

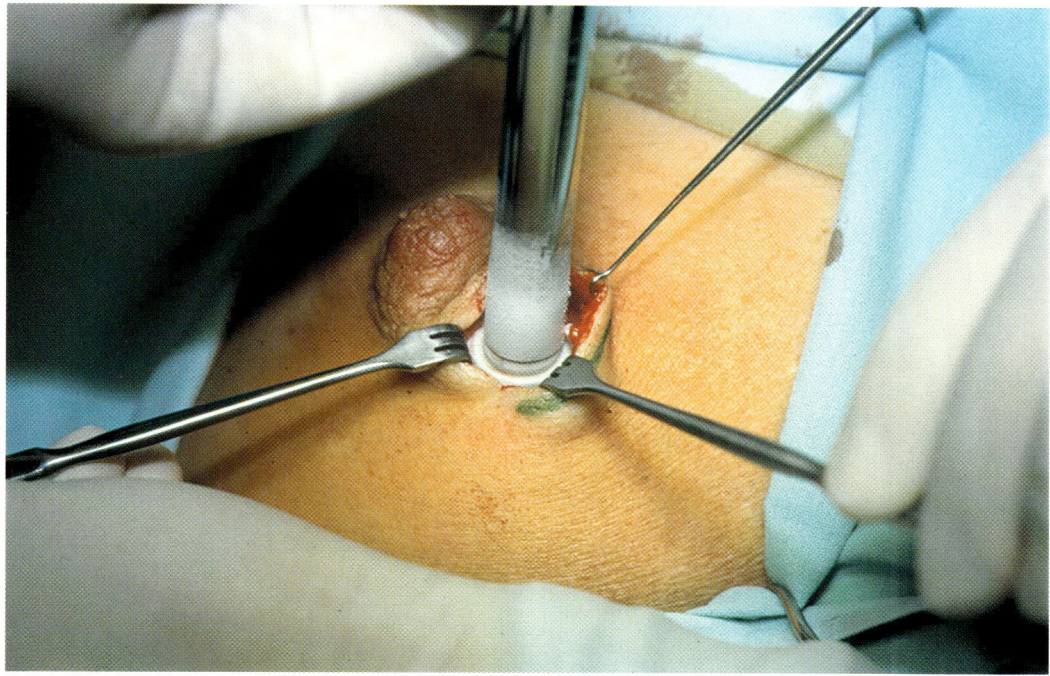

Fig. 7.11. Subcutaneous cryosurgical extirpation. Female, 37 years old. Primary breast cancer patient. The standard operation had been suggested, but the patient refused it

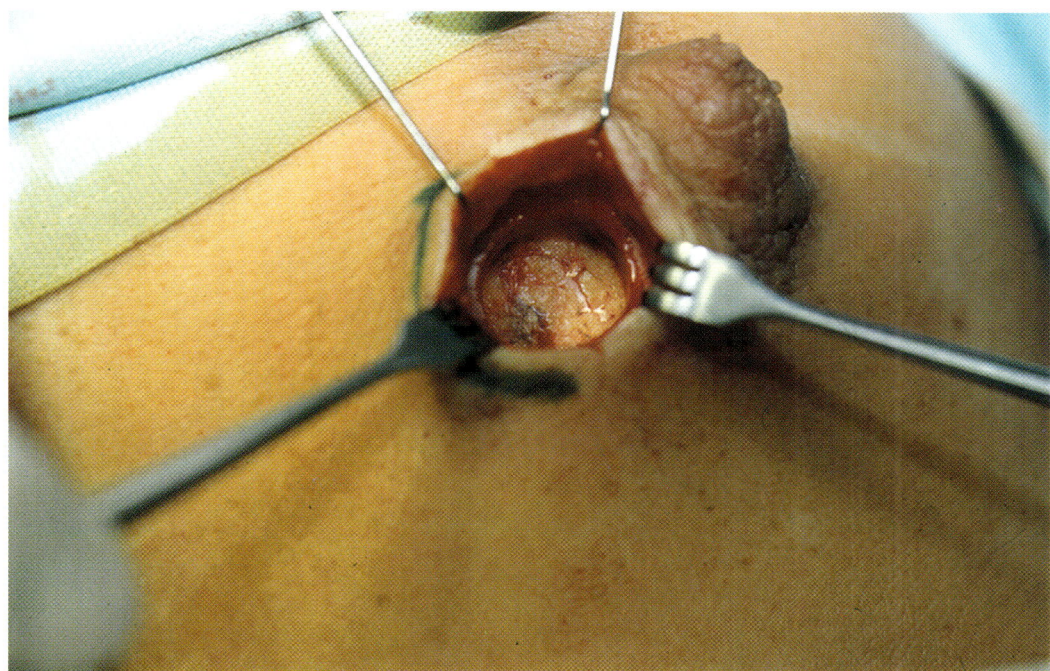

Fig. 7.12. Same patient. Appearance of the cryozone with demarcation line immediately after the single freeze-thaw cycle

Chapter 7
Techniques

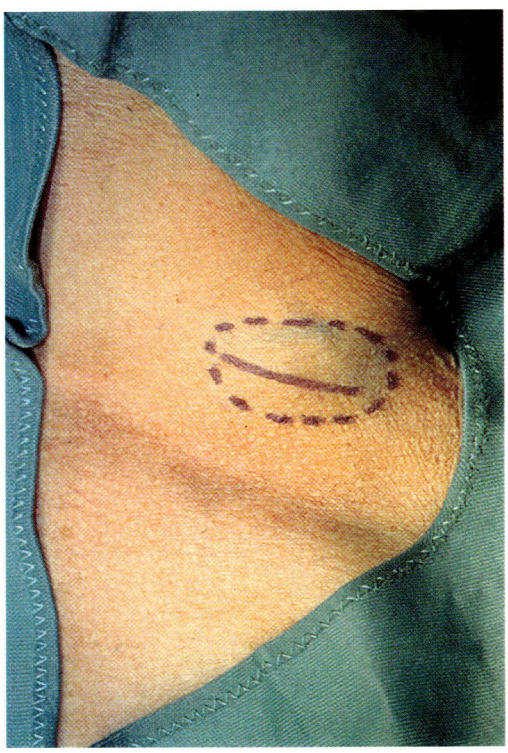

Fig. 7.13. Subcutaneous cryosurgical extirpation. Male, 53 years old. Patient with cervical lymph node metastases after conventional hypernephroma extirpation. View of the marked cervical lymph node metastases preoperatively

Fig. 7.14. Subcutaneous cryosurgical extirpation in the same patient

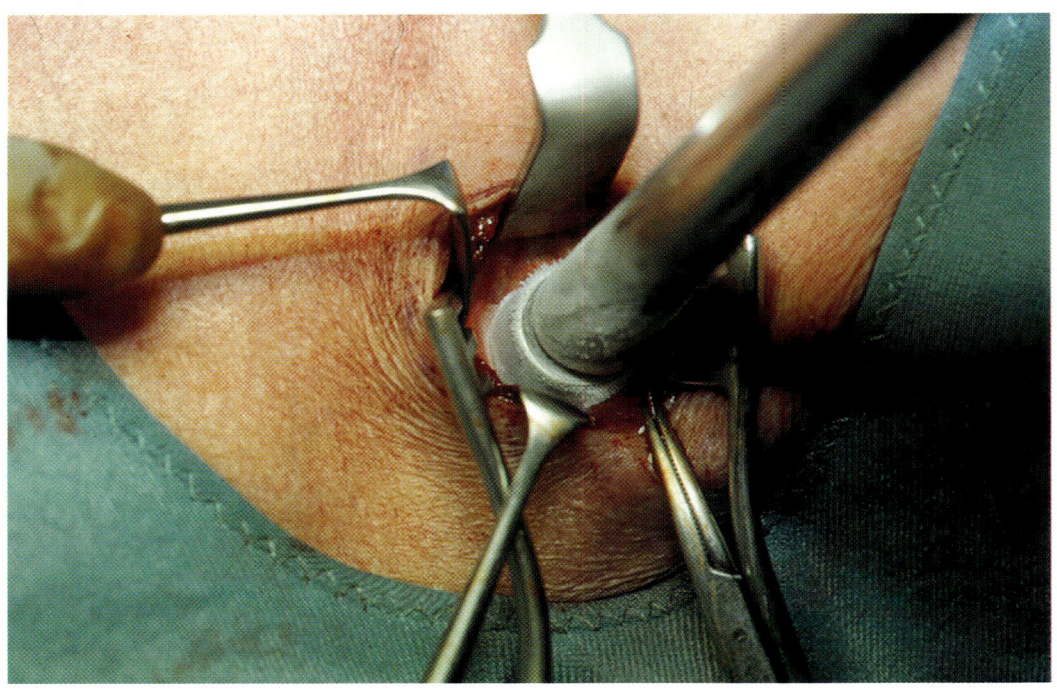

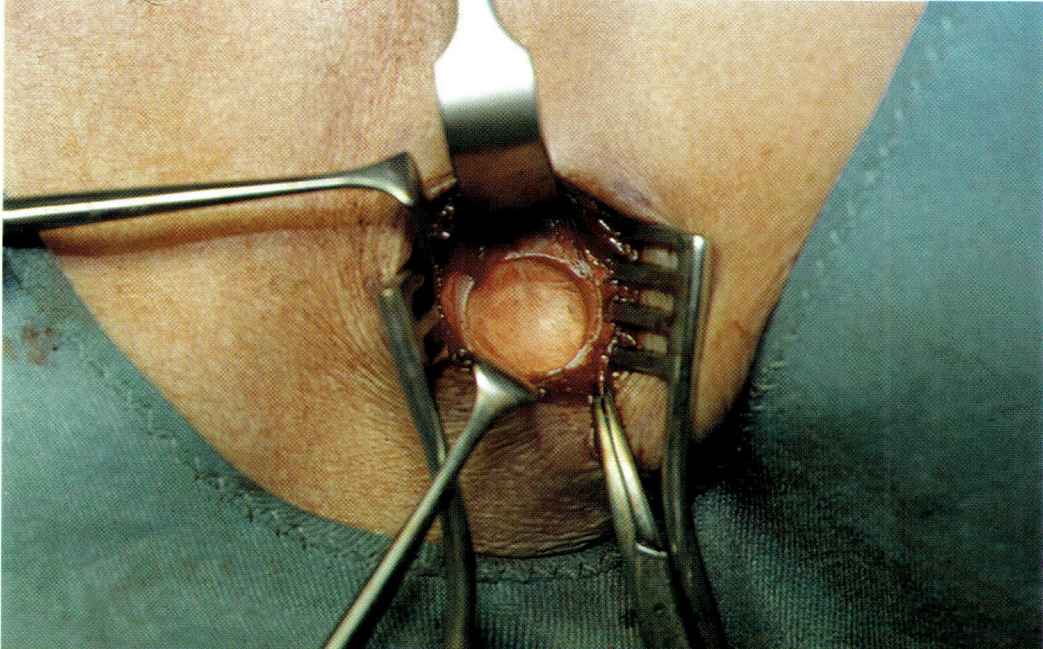

Fig. 7.15. View of the post-cryosurgical zone with demarcation line in the same patient immediately after the single freeze-thaw cycle

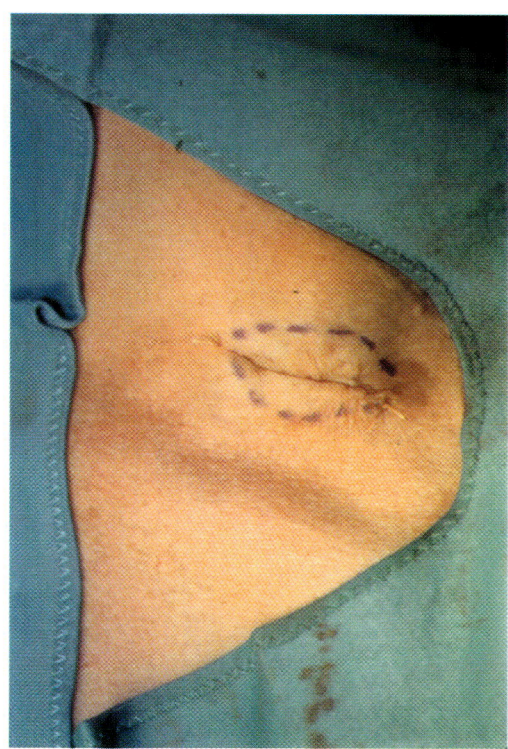

Fig. 7.16. Same patient. Appearance of wound immediately after the double freeze-thaw cycle

Chapter 7
Techniques

IV. Transanal Cryosurgical Extirpation

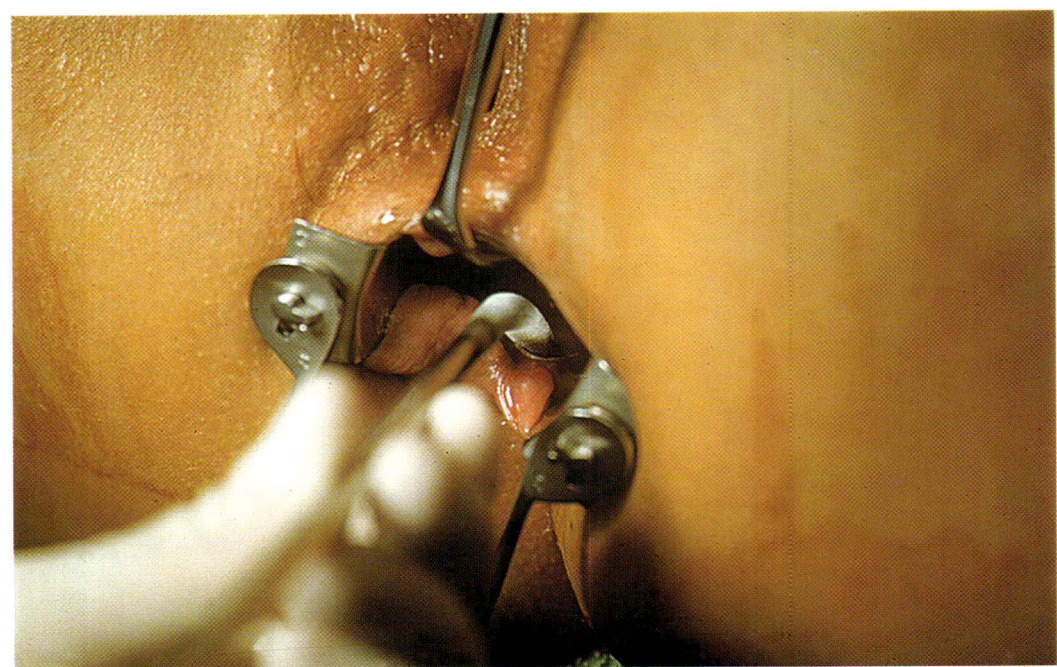

Fig. 7.17. Transanal cryosurgical extirpation. Female, 51 years old. Patient with multiple internal hemorrhoids at the dentate line. The single freeze-thaw cycle is performed at a temperature of −80°C

V. Intrarectal Cryosurgical Extirpation

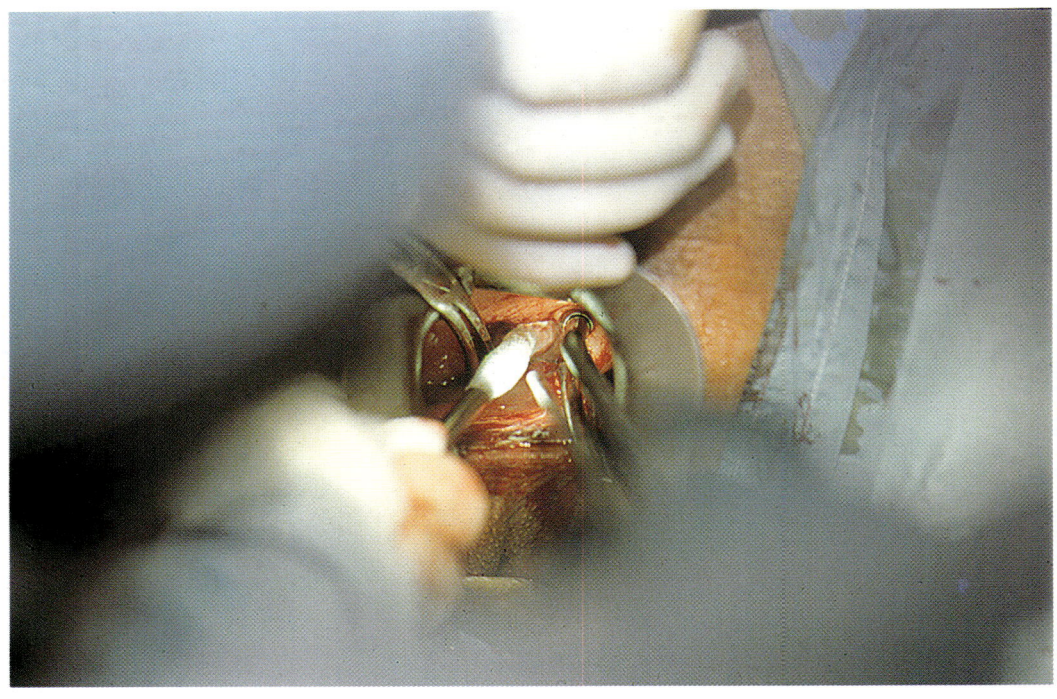

Fig. 7.18. Intrarectal cryosurgical extirpation. Male, 56 years of age. Patient with secondary, locally advanced, unresectable rectal cancer after conventional primary rectal cancer resection

Liver Cryosurgical Techniques

Nikolai N. Korpan

8.0 Introduction

Several years of extensive experience in the use of cryosurgery in advanced stages of liver cancer have demonstrated the possibilities and limitations of this method. Gentle conventional and minimally invasive (laparoscopic) cryosurgical procedures with the latest, highly efficient cryosurgical devices can be used on operable and inoperable liver tumors with a curative intent. Above all, the great efficiency, the uncomplicated surgical results, the high cure rate, the short period of hospitalization, and the patients' improved quality of life, all contribute to the fact that patients with operable and inoperable liver carcinoma and metastases experience a huge improvement in a relatively short time.

New perspectives for a minimally invasive treatment of malignant tumors have thus opened up. Cryosurgery is of great importance for patients with liver cancer, as it can improve their quality of life and their chance of survival. The possibility of destroying larger areas of tissue in the human organism by the application of extreme cold led to the development of modern technical devices for cryosurgery, as the method of "freezing" diseased tissue by exposing it to rays of extreme sub-zero temperatures is known. At first it was difficult to maintain a constant temperature of $-170°C$ to $190°C$ at the contact end of the probe for any length of time and at the same time not to damage healthy tissue. But with the latest generation of cryosurgical devices, produced by individual companies and used in various fields of medicine, this has become possible and modern, gentle cryosurgery can now be carried out.

Few doubts remain that both conventional and laparoscopic cryosurgery will in the future be the standard method for treating liver tumors.

A number of cryosurgical liver operations are described and illustrated below.

8.1. Open Liver Cryosurgery

8.1.1. Cryosurgical Placement Procedure

In conventional surgical procedures, cryoextirpation of the operable liver tumor (liver metastasis) or cryodestruction of the inoperable carcinoma (liver metastasis) is carried out en bloc by applying a round cryoprobe to the tumor mass in the liver parenchyma. Various cryoprobes of 2 to 50 mm in diameter are used. The cryosurgical operation is generally carried out in one to three sessions. Each session can last from 20 seconds to 9 minutes. The freeze-thaw cycle is carried out automatically and lasts for approximately 1.1 to 2.7 minutes. During this process, a cryozone with a volume of 40-80 cm^3 develops. The cryozone is clearly outlined by a demarcation line which separates it from the surrounding tissue. The exposure time and the amount of treatment cycles must, therefore, be adjusted for each individual clinical case. The cancerous tissue is destroyed by means of a cold shock of between $-170°C$ and $-190°C$, but healthy tissue is not affected, as the application of sub-zero temperatures can be exactly regulated both in size and time exposure.

Chapter 8
Liver Cryosurgery

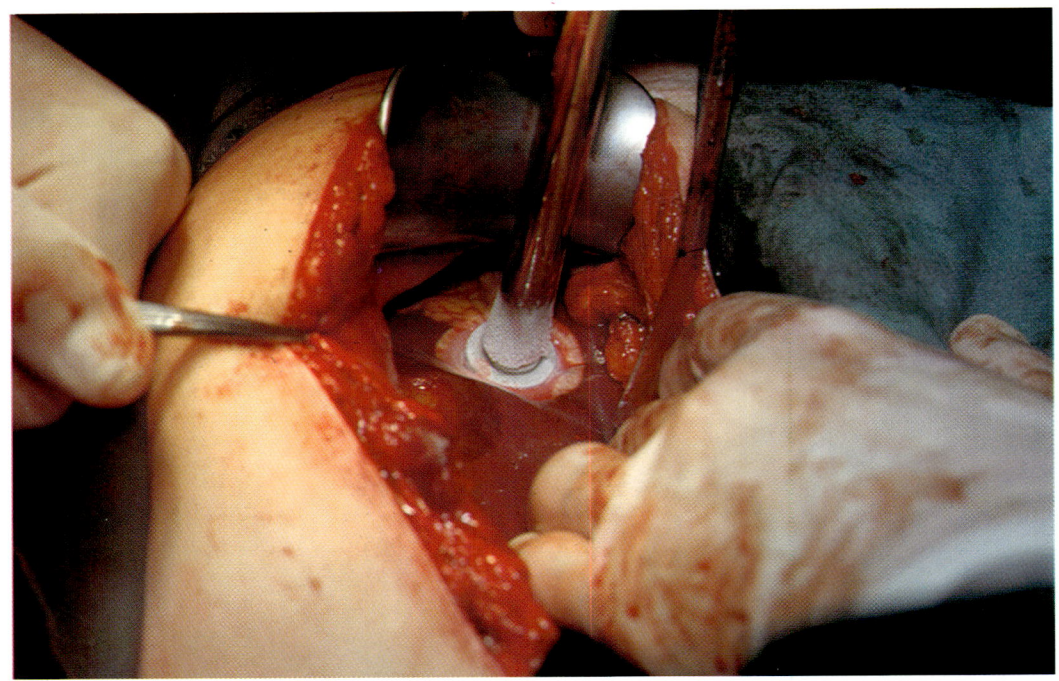

Fig. 8.1.1.1. Cryosurgical procedure for open liver cryosurgery placement. Male, 64 years old. Typical multiple liver metastases resulting from colorectal cancer. The tip of a disc-shaped cryoprobe measuring 20 mm in diameter is inserted into the center of a liver metastasis

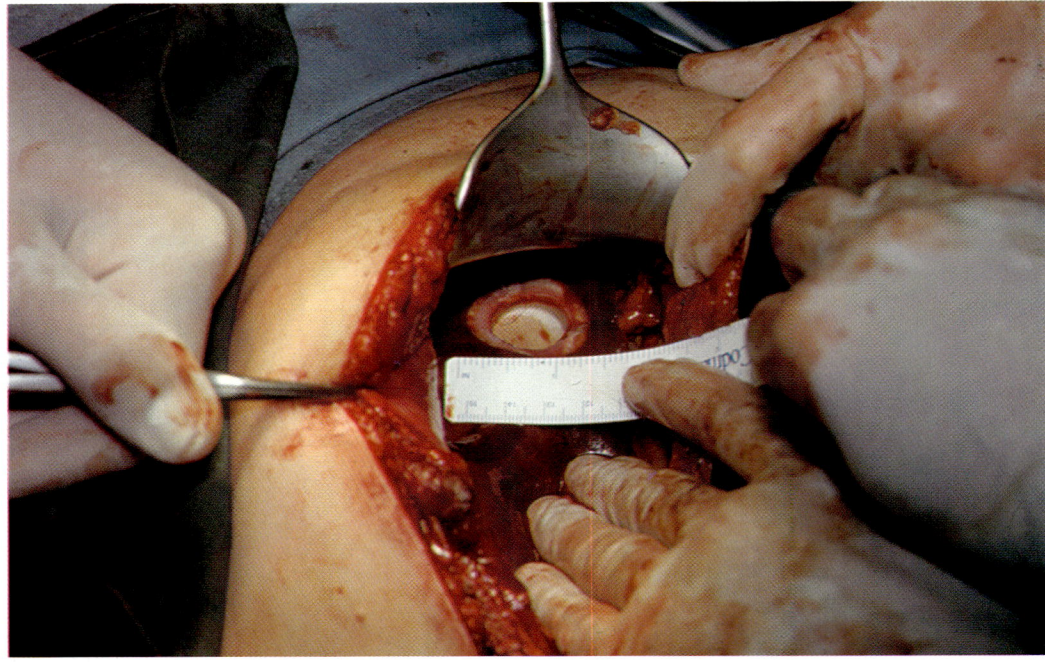

Fig. 8.1.1.2. Same patient. Typical view of the post-cryosurgical zone which measures 38 mm in diameter

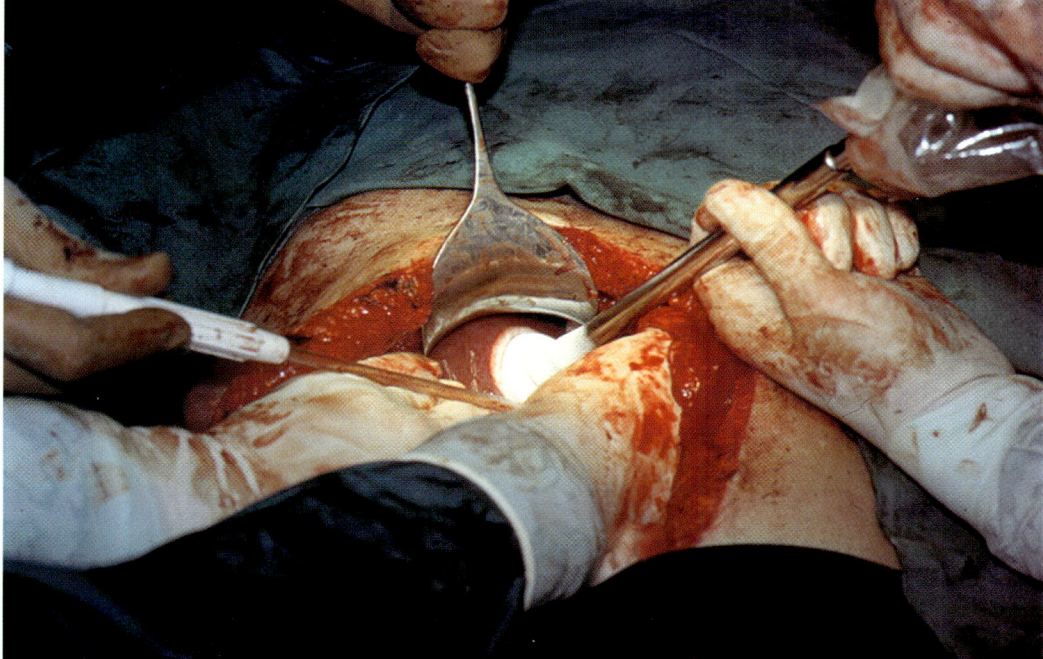

Fig. 8.1.1.3. Cryosurgical procedure for open liver cryosurgery placement. Female, 59 years old. Typical multiple liver metastases resulting from breast cancer. The tip of a disc-shaped cryoprobe 35 mm in diameter is inserted into the center of a liver metastasis

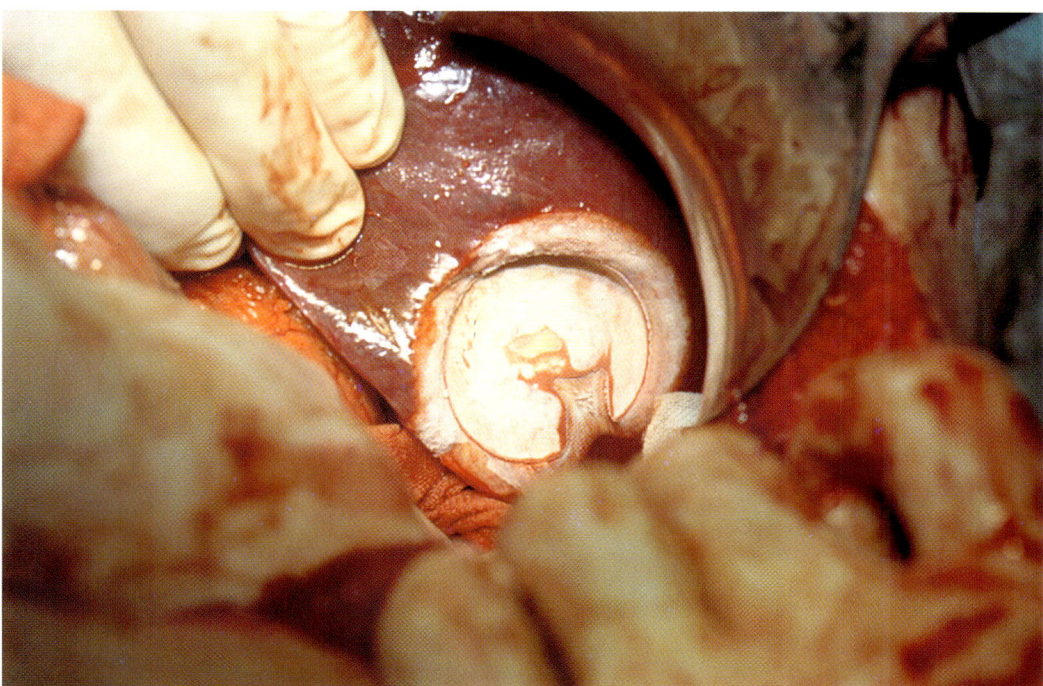

Fig. 8.1.1.4. Same patient. Typical view of the post-cryosurgical zone which is 53 mm in diameter

8.1.2. Needle Cryosurgical Technique

The smallest possible cryoneedles are required so that as little damage as possible is done to the healthy parenchyma. The needle is inserted directly into the tumor mass. Individual needles measuring at least 2 mm to maximally 2.2 cm are used (Fig. 8.1.2.1.). For larger liver tumors several cryoneedles can be used simultaneously to synergize, and thus increase, the effect of the cold. When two or more needles are used in liver cryosurgery, the distance between the needles plays an important role (Fig. 8.1.2.2.).

The liver tumor (liver metastasis) is pierced with a well-aimed thin needle and a cryoneedle is placed right next to it by the Seldinger approach (Fig. 8.1.2.3a–f). Then one to three freeze cycles are carried out on a small metastasis. In the case of a large liver metastasis, several thin needles are inserted in the tumor mass two to three centimeters apart in the form of an equilateral triangle with the help of ultra-sound monitoring. Parallel to this, cryoprobes are inserted into the liver parenchyma. Subsequently the usual freeze-thaw cycle is carried out. After thawing, the cryoneedles are removed and the abdominal wall closed in layers.

As conventional cryosurgical procedure is less invasive than liver resection, complications are less likely and postoperative morbidity rates very low. The postoperative phase for patients who have undergone cryosurgery for liver cancer and metastases is usually unproblematic and free of complications. Complications associated with conventional liver resection do not arise. Patients usually spend 5–7 days in the hospital.

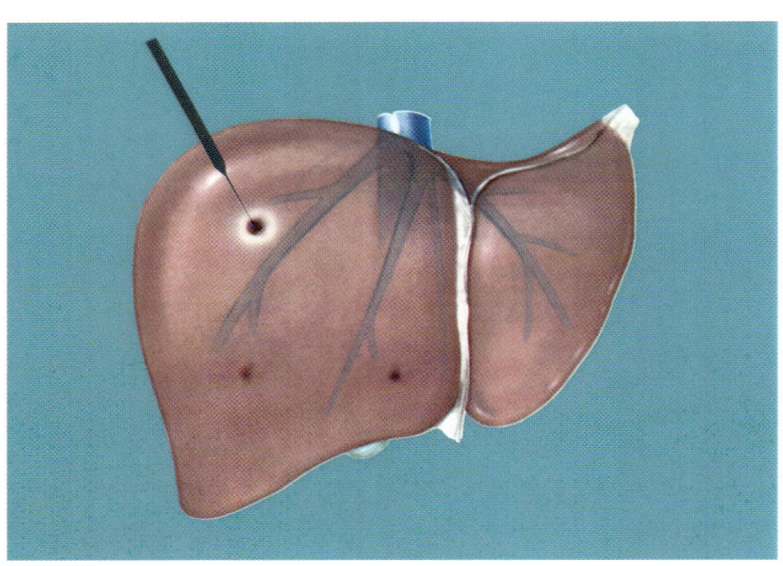

Fig. 8.1.2.1. The single needle is directly inserted into the tumor mass

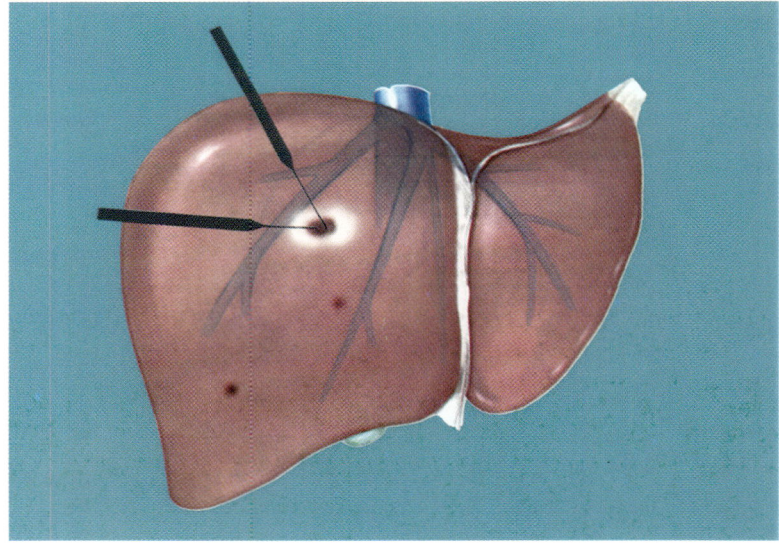

Fig. 8.1.2.2. Using 2 or more cryoneedles for liver cryosurgery

Section D Basic Techniques

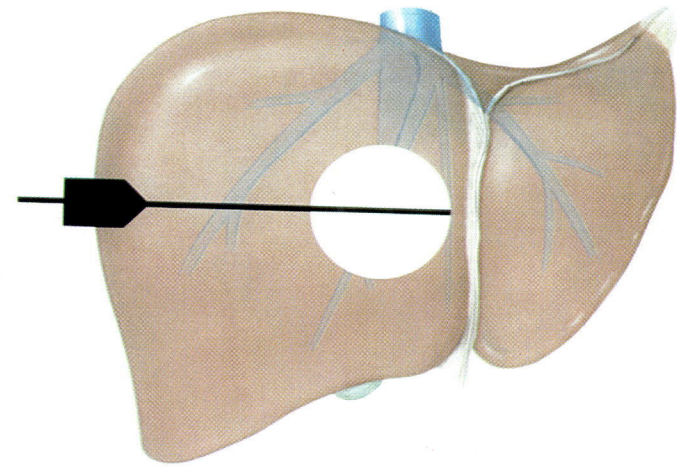

Fig. 8.1.2.3a. Single cryoneedle

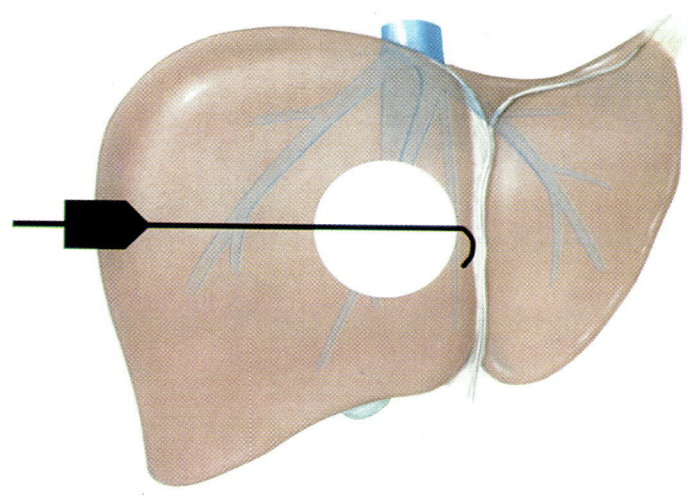

Fig. 8.1.2.3a–f. Set of schematic diagrams showing insertion of the cryoneedle into the tumor mass by the Seldinger technique

Fig. 8.1.2.3b. Cryo-needle with a wire

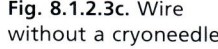

Fig. 8.1.2.3c. Wire without a cryoneedle

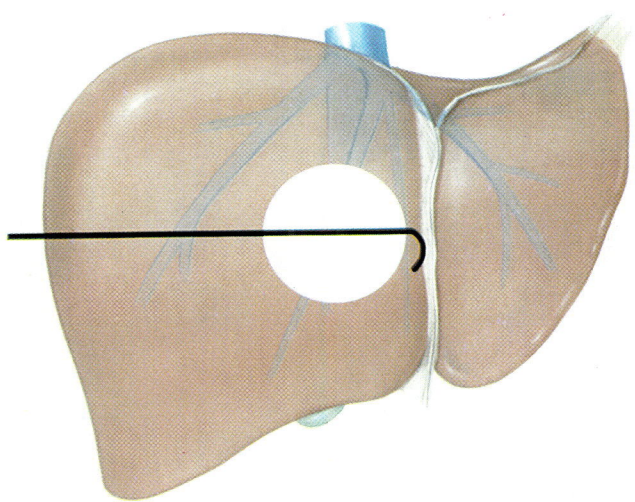

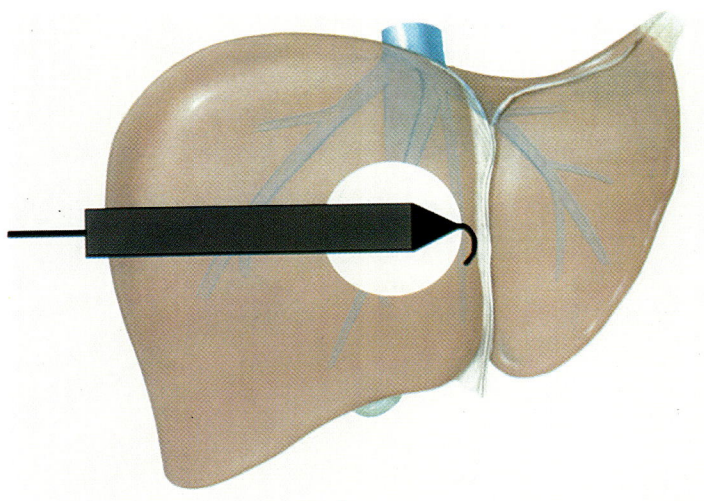

Fig. 8.1.2.3d. Cannula with a dilatator

Fig. 8.1.2.3a–f. Set of schematic diagrams showing insertion of the cryoneedle into the tumor mass by the Seldinger technique

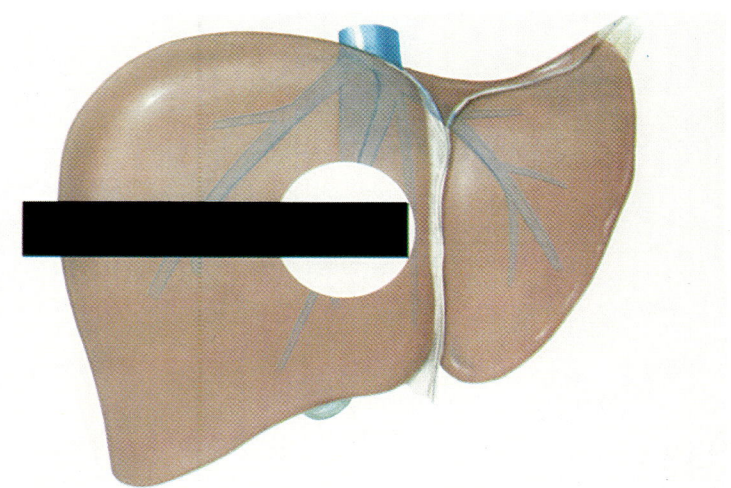

Fig. 8.1.2.3e. Cannula without a dilatator

Fig. 8.1.2.3f. Cryoneedle implantation

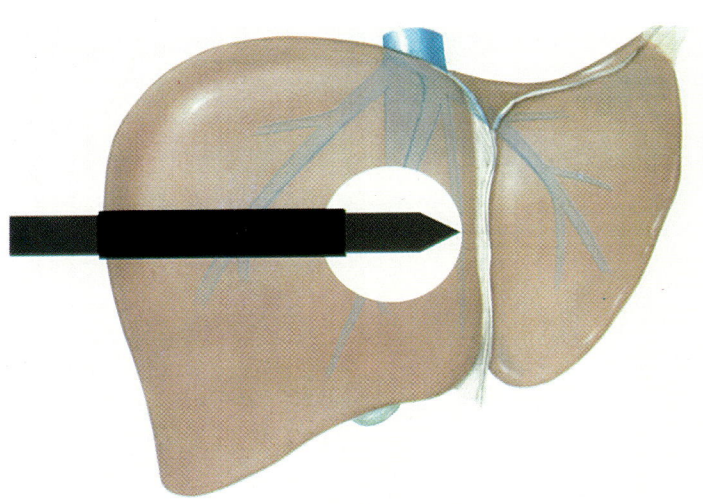

8.2. Laparoscopic Liver Cryosurgery

The pneumoperitoneum is applied under intubation anesthesia by means of the Veress needle and the optic endoscope is introduced into the peritoneal cavity. As a next step, after the abdominal cavity has been inspected, an incision is made in the epigastrium or right subcostal area and the 12 mm trocar used in laparoscopy is inserted with the help of an endoscope. A laparoscopic cryoprobe is then applied to the liver parenchyma in the tumor area. And finally the liver tumor (liver metastasis) is cryoextirpated in the usual manner by lowering the temperature to between −170°C and −190°C and then thawing.

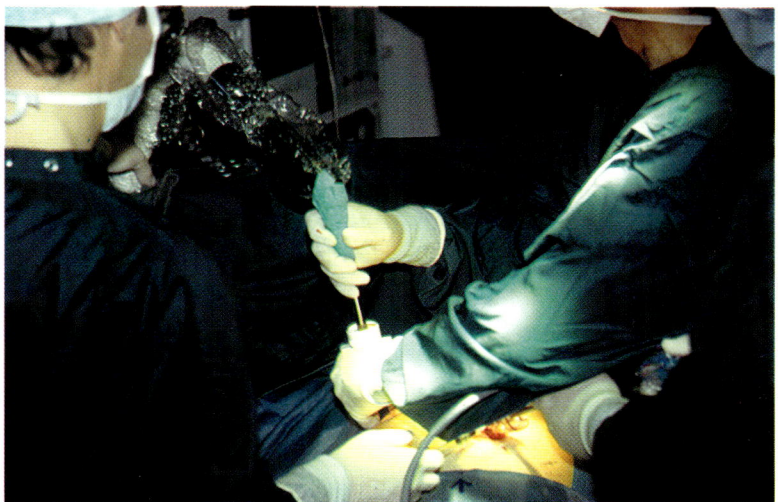

Fig. 8.2.1. Laparoscopic cryoneedle is inserted with the Veress needle into the peritoneal cavity

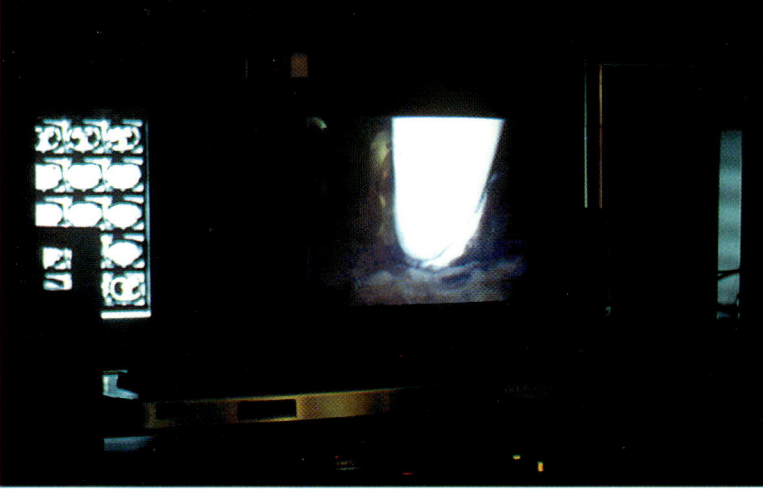

Fig. 8.2.2. Laparoscopic cryoneedle is inserted into the liver metastasis

Chapter 8 Liver Cryosurgery

8.3. Liver Cryosurgery by Minilaparotomy

A minimal subcostal incision is made on the right-hand side. The cryoprobe is applied to the liver tumor, that is, a cryoneedle is inserted into the tumor mass. At present this procedure is at the experimental stage.

8.4. Percutaneous Liver Cryosurgery

Monitored by ultrasound, the cryoneedle is inserted subcutaneously into the cancerous liver parenchyma, after which the usual cryosurgical procedure is carried out. The freeze-thaw cycle can last for 9 minutes.

8.5. Liver Cryosurgical Resection

The cryogenic clamp is used for hepatic cryoresection with preliminary freezing of the resection margin. The clamp's working surfaces are frozen by means of liquid nitrogen. The cryosurgical unit makes it possible to circulate the liquid nitrogen through the probe at $-196°C$. The cryogenic clamp is applied across the desired incision line of the liver and gradually frozen by liquid nitrogen refrigeration (Fig. 8.5.1.). When, at a temperature of $-196°C$, the incision line in the liver is completely frozen, freezing is stopped and the resection can then be performed without any blood or bile loss. The small capillaries and venules as well as the biliary ducts measuring $\varnothing \leqslant 1.5$ mm within the cryogenically frozen zone are thus destroyed. The large arteries and veins or biliary ducts measuring $\varnothing \geqslant 1.5$ mm which pass across the suture line are not destroyed.

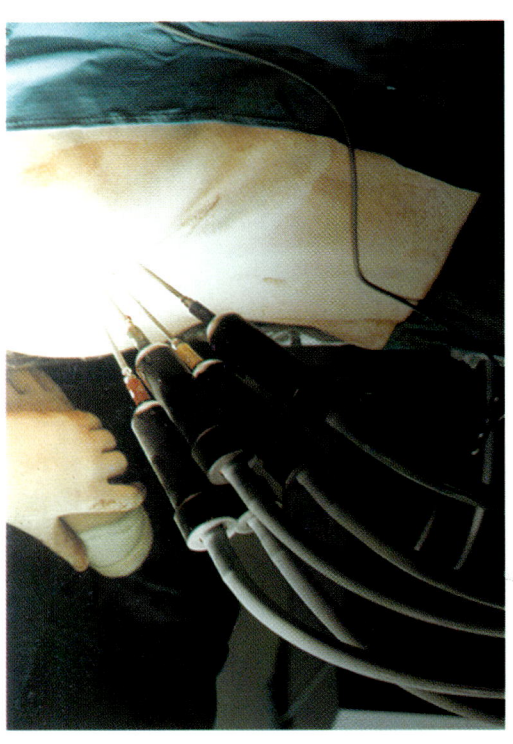

Fig. 8.4.1. Cryoneedles are placed percutaneously in the center of the liver with ultrasonographic guidance

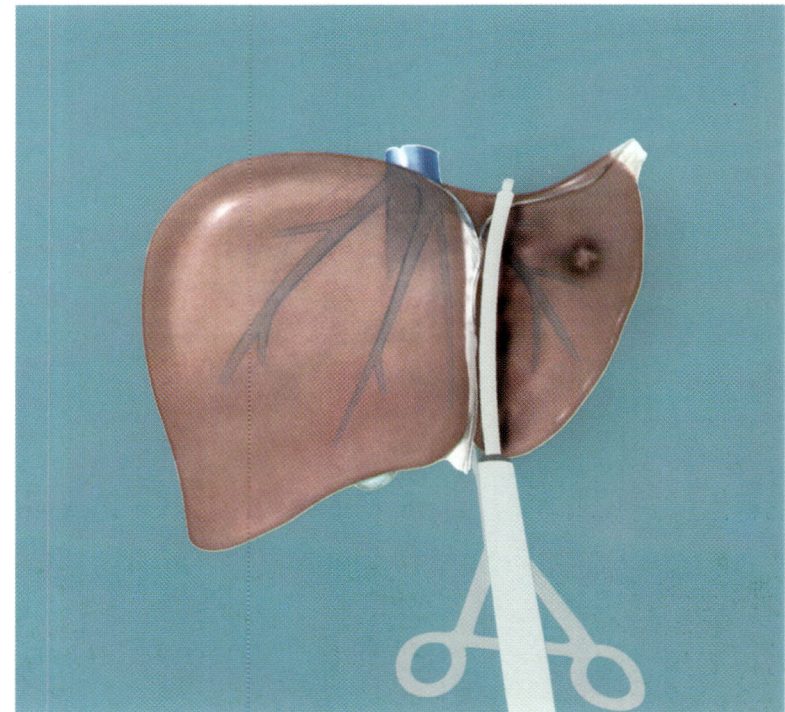

Fig. 8.5.1. Schematic demonstration of hepatic cryosurgical resection using a cryogenic clamp in a patient with liver metastases

Section E

Experimental Aspects

Chapter 9

Liver Cryosurgery. An Animal Experiment

Nikolai N. Korpan[1]
with contributions by Iwan S. Tchekman[1], Jaroslav V. Zharkov[1], Franz Beer[1] and Ved R. Tandan[2]

9.0 Introduction

In vitro and *in vivo* experiments paved the way for cryosurgical clinical investigations and for the development of different cryosurgical methods of treating primary liver tumors and liver metastases. The advances in cryosurgical technology have also aroused interest in the use of cryosurgery to treat hepatic malignancies.

The behavior and morphology of living tissue when subjected to low temperatures has been studied since the early twentieth century. Numerous reports in cryosurgical literature indicate that the application of cryogenic techniques for *in situ* ablation of tumors and the resection of parenchymal organs using subzero temperatures can be successful in treating liver malignancies. Experimental observations with regard to freezing *in vitro* cell lines and fluid systems eventually led to the application of cryosurgery to *in vivo* biological systems, and this in turn led to the emergence of hepatic cryosurgery as a viable therapeutic option in treating liver tumors.

One problem in cryosurgery that has not been adequately addressed is that of identifying the mechanism by which damage is effected during the freezing process. This is important because, although cryosurgery is clinically used to treat liver tumors, the freezing mechanism by which cells are destroyed in the course of the treatment is not as yet fully understood. It is this shortcoming which keeps surgeons from using cryosurgery with maximal effectiveness. Research which elucidates the fundamental freezing process in the case of liver tissue has, therefore, been a focal point of various experimental studies.

An experiment-based discussion of hepatic cryosurgery deals with the following four issues: 1) studies of the mechanism of tissue destruction in respect to liver freezing; 2) investigations focusing on the viability and safety of applying freezing to the liver; 3) the biological perspectives of freezing liver tumors; and 4) experimental studies devoted to refining the technology of the cryosurgical equipment needed for liver operations.

Since the advent of the laparoscopic era, the development of new cryoprobes and ultrasound devices has made laparoscopic hepatic cryosurgery a reality. Experiments using laparoscopic hepatic cryosurgery on animals demonstrate the effectiveness of this method and the possibility of using it in patients with liver tumors. The data gained from *in vivo* experiments using the laparoscopic method underline its great potential, especially with regard to repeated treatments, as it reduces both the length of hospital stays and morbidity.

Chapter 9
Animal Experiment

9.1. Open Hepatic Cryosurgery

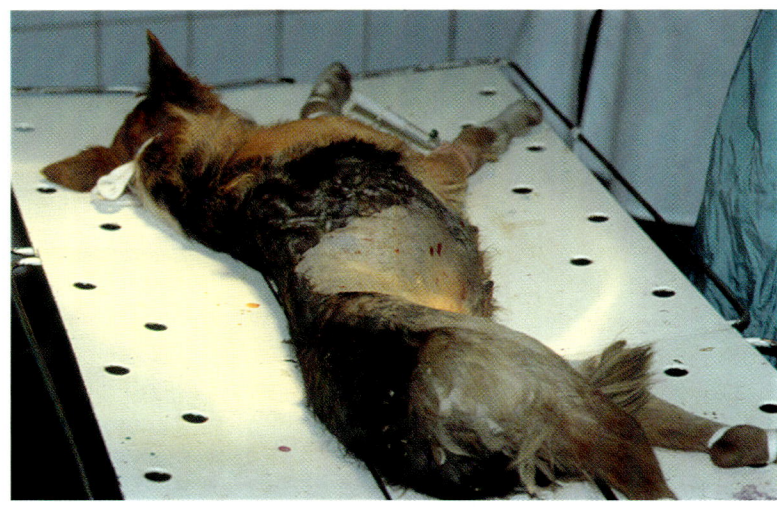

Fig. 9.1.1[1]. After a twelve hour fast, the dogs are given an anesthetic, of, for example, 50 mg/ml of ketalar (0.2 mg/kg body weight) and of xyla (xylazine base, 0.2 mg/kg body weight) at a ratio of 1:1 by intravenous injection

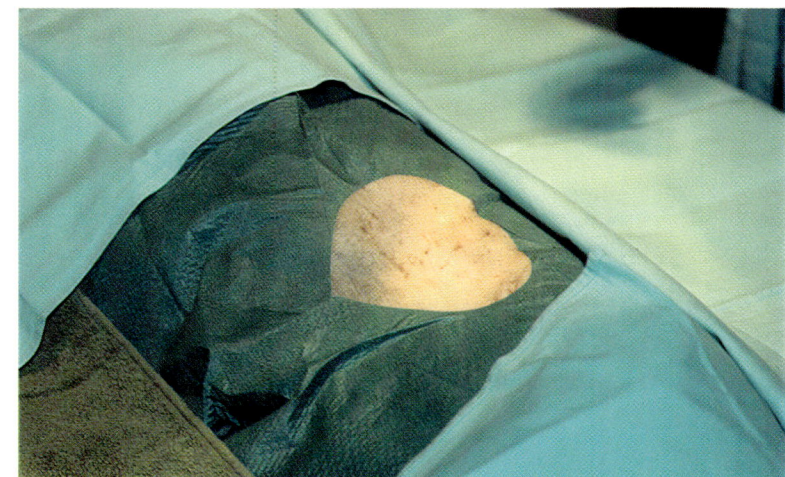

Fig. 9.1.2[1]. Operative field. After antiseptic prep solution is applied, the operative field is draped to ensure sterility without obscuring anatomic landmarks

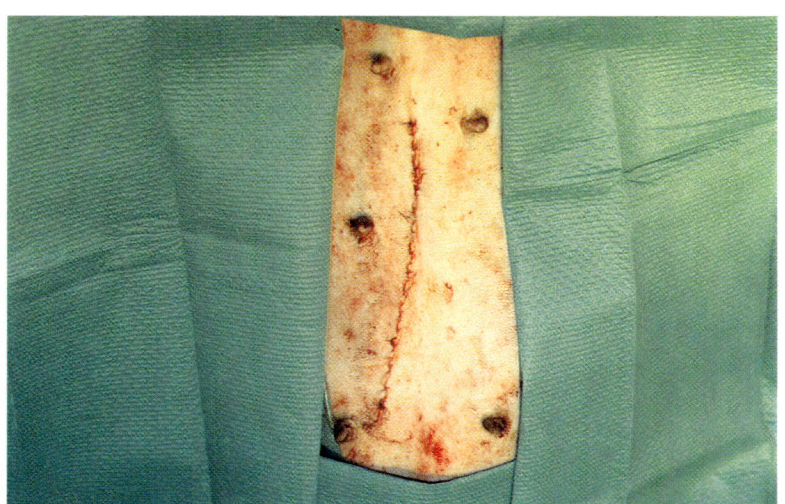

Fig. 9.1.3[1]. The liver is exposed to laparotomy using an oblique abdominal section through the vertical access

Section E — Experimental Aspects

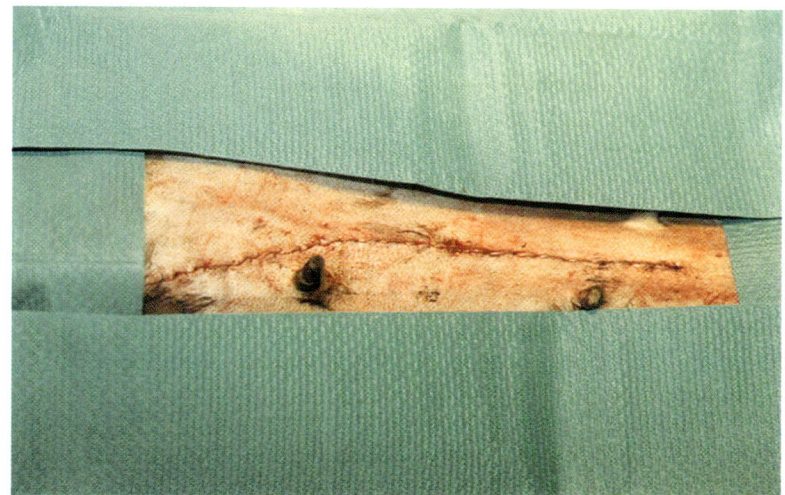

Fig. 9.1.4[1]. The liver can be exposed by laparotomy using an incision angled like a hockey-stick in the direction of the left costal arch

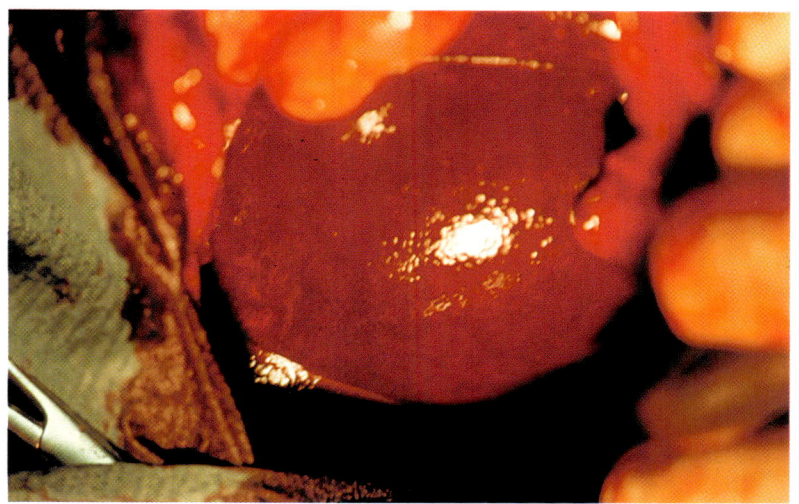

Fig. 9.1.5[1]. View of a dog liver before cryosurgery

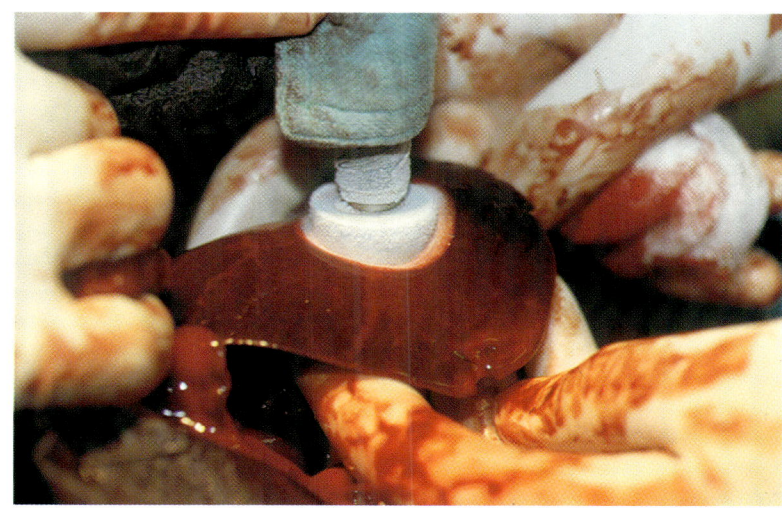

Fig. 9.1.6[1]. Cryosurgical application. The technique of cryosurgery, showing a disc probe with a diameter of 20 mm which is placed on the liver at a temperature of −180°C for 9 min using a single freeze-thaw cycle to induce aseptic cryonecrosis (tissue destruction)

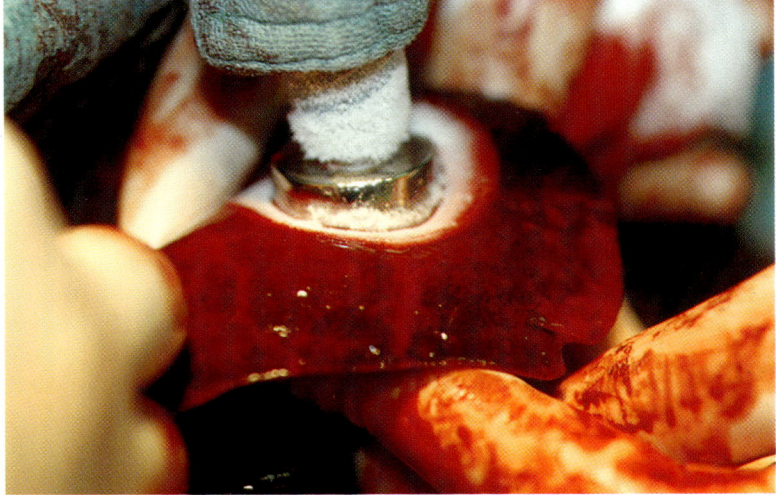

Fig. 9.1.7[1]. Cryosurgical application. The technique of cryosurgery, showing a disc probe and an ice ball (cryogenic zone) which is generated without difficulty. The cryozone is sharply outlined by its rim which forms the demarcation line between the area of cryodestruction (which is followed by cryogenic necrosis) and the healthy liver parenchyma

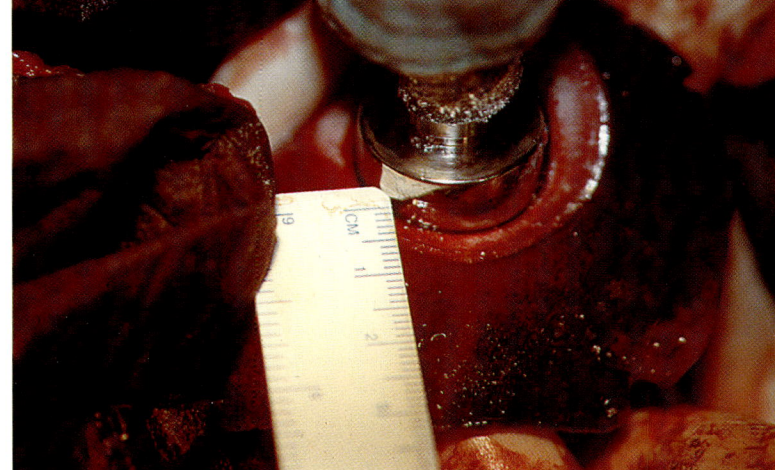

Fig. 9.1.8[1]. Cryosurgical application. The technique of cryosurgery, showing a disc probe and a cryozone with a 5 mm margin which surrounds the normal-appearing liver parenchyma after a 9-min single freeze-thaw cycle at a temperature of −60°C

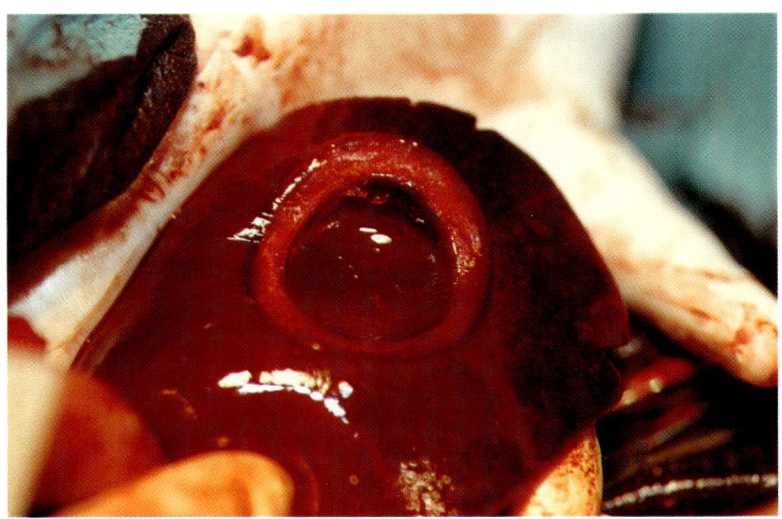

Fig. 9.1.9[1]. Cryosurgical application. The cryozone is clearly outlined by a demarcation line with a 5 mm margin which surrounds the normal-appearing liver parenchyma after a single 9-min freeze-thaw cycle at a temperature of −60°C. This cryozone measures 30 mm in diameter

Section E Experimental Aspects

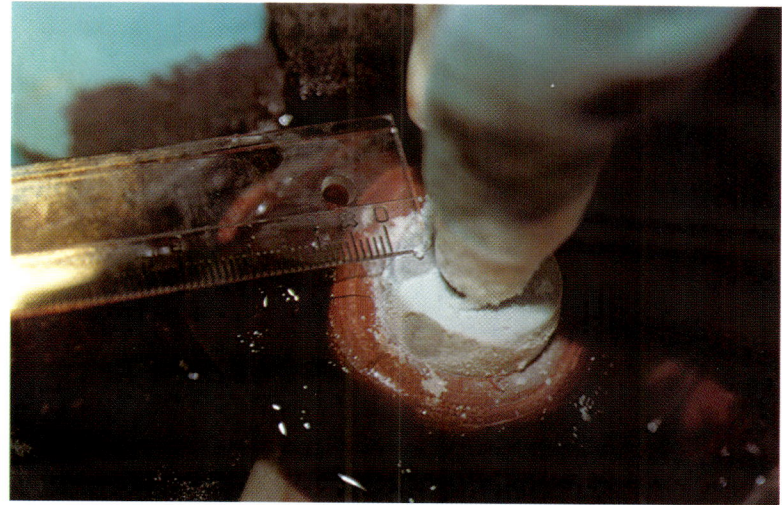

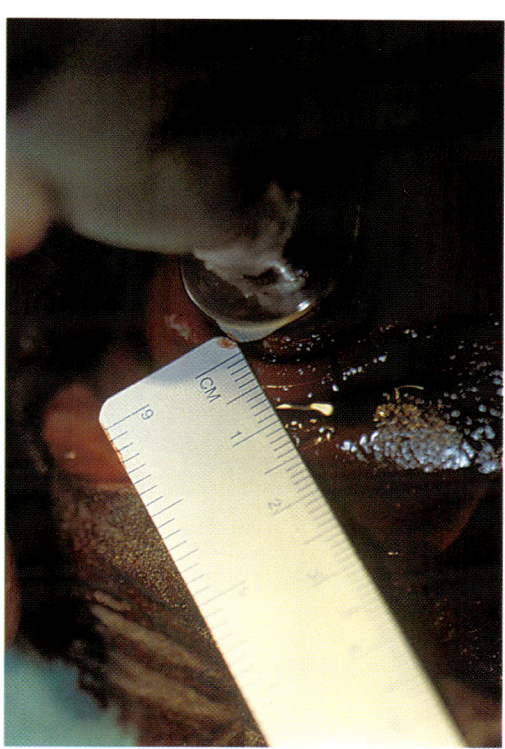

Fig. 9.1.10[1] (A[1], B[1]). Cryosurgical application. The technique of cryosurgery, showing a disc probe and a cryozone with a 12 mm margin which surrounds the normal-appearing liver parenchyma after a single 9-min freeze-thaw cycle at a temperature of $-180°C$

Fig. 9.1.11[1]. Cryosurgical application. Ice ball. View of a cryozone with the icecrater in the middle, and of the ice margin with the line of demarcation around the cryoprobe, immediately after the cryosurgical session, performed at a temperature of $-180°C$ for 9 min during a single freeze-thaw cycle. The cryozone includes a margin of 12 mm in the normal-appearing liver parenchyma, and measures 44 mm in diameter. The disc probe had a diameter of 20 mm

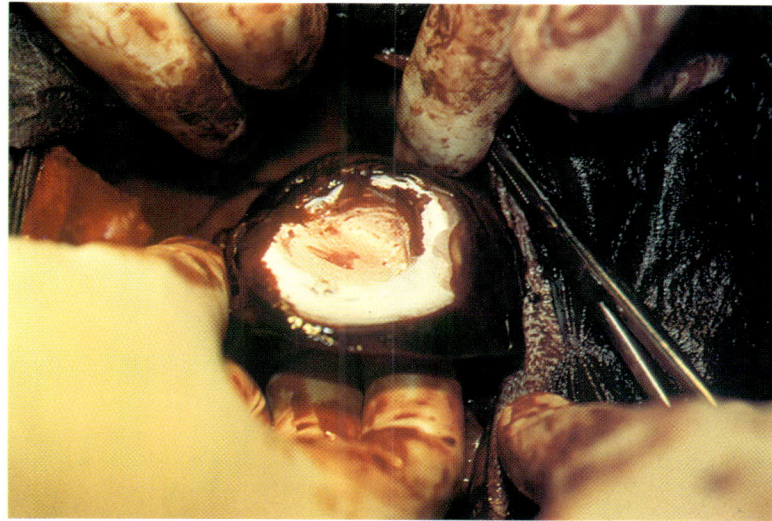

Chapter 9 Animal Experiment

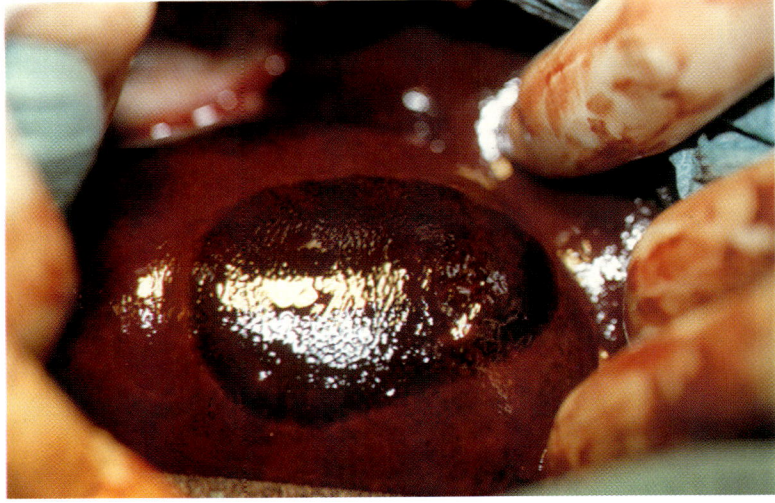

Fig. 9.1.12[1]. Post-cryosurgical view. Immediately after the full thawing of the liver parenchyma cryozone

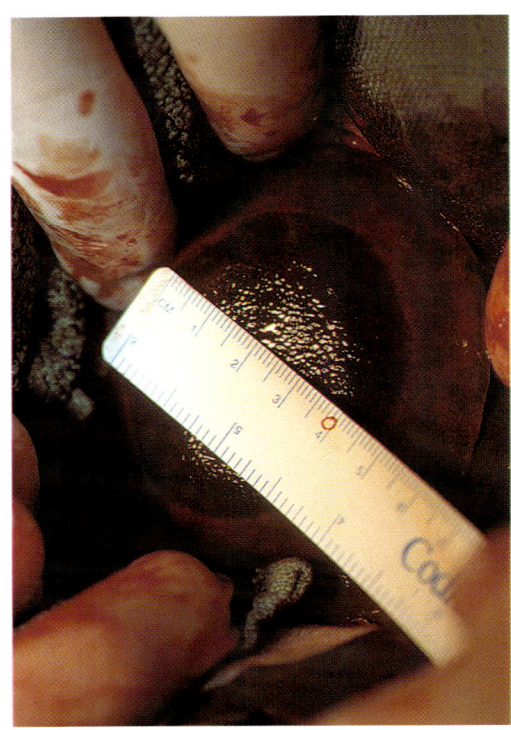

Fig. 9.1.13[1]. Post-cryosurgical view. Immediately after the full thawing of the liver parenchyma cryozone. The cryozone measures 44 mm in diameter, the disc probe had a diameter of 20 mm, the temperature was −180°C applied for 9 min using a single freeze-thaw cycle

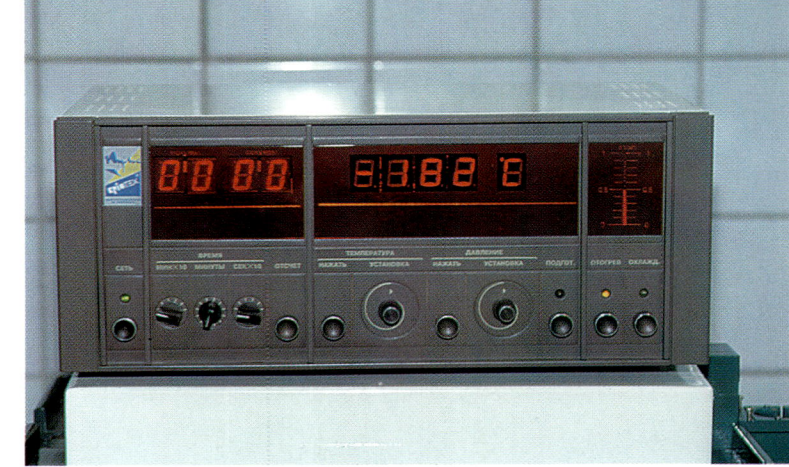

Fig. 9.1.14[1]. The liquid nitrogen is propelled by the universally applied cryosurgical system, for example, *mobile cryosurgical unit* (Cryotechnological Research Company "Pulse", Kiev, Ukraine), which circulates liquid nitrogen through the probe at −196°C

Section E Experimental Aspects

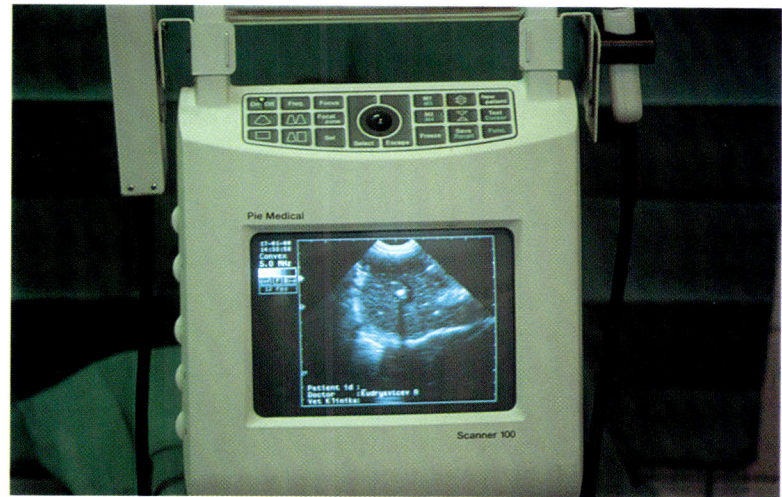

Fig. 9.1.15[1]. Guided by continuous intraoperative ultrasonographic monitoring, the liver tissue is frozen to −180°C to achieve complete tissue destruction

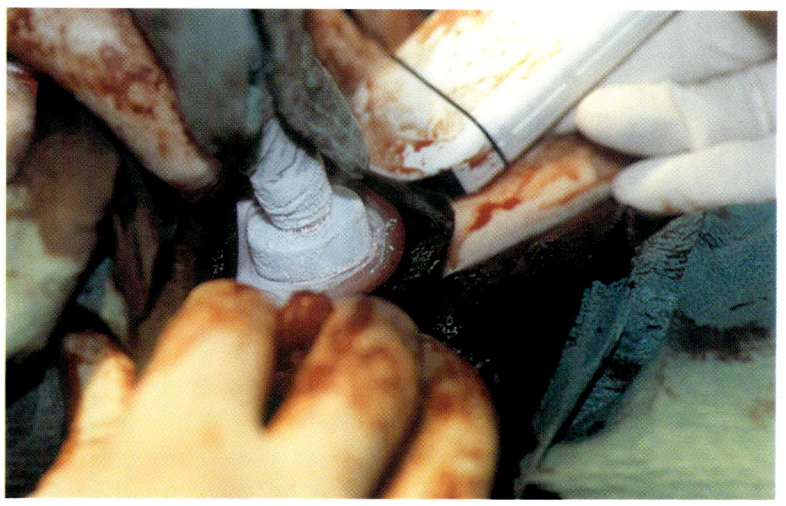

A

B

Fig. 9.1.16[1]. The monitoring process of the freeze-thaw cycle is carried out by intraoperative ultrasound before, during (**A[1]**) and after (**B[1]**) cryosurgery

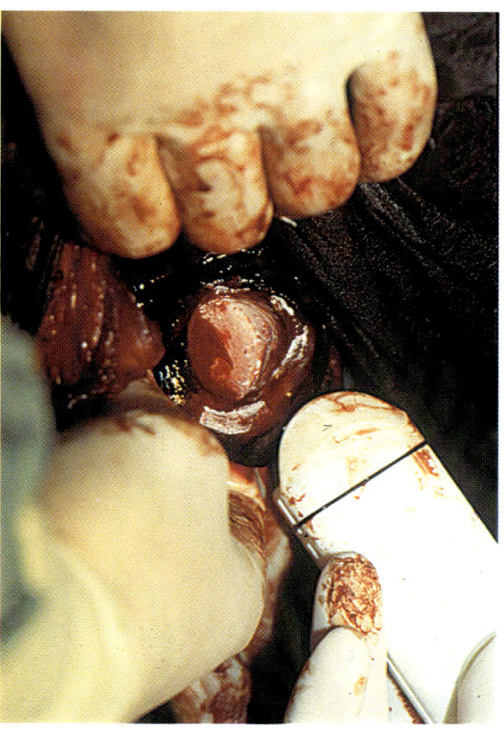

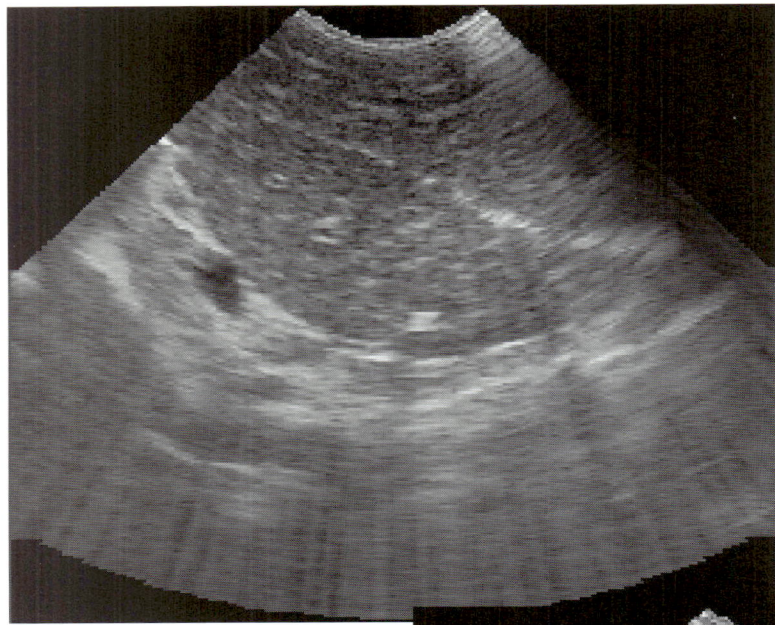

A[1]. The cryozone measures ±20 mm in diameter at start of freezing. The results comparing diameter of cryozone, duration of application, probe size, and temperature are statistically significant

B[1]. The cryozone measures ±29 mm in diameter for 7 min using a single freeze cycle

C[1]. The cryozone measures ±30 mm in diameter for 9 min using a single freeze cycle

Fig. 9.1.17[1]. Intraoperative ultrasound during freeze cycle on the dog liver using a disc probe with a diameter of 20 mm at a temperature of −60°C. Ice ball. Cryozone formation after exposure: at the start of freezing (**A[1]**), for 7 min (**B[1]**), and for 9 min (**C[1]**)

Section E   Experimental Aspects   **113**

**Chapter 9
Animal
Experiment**

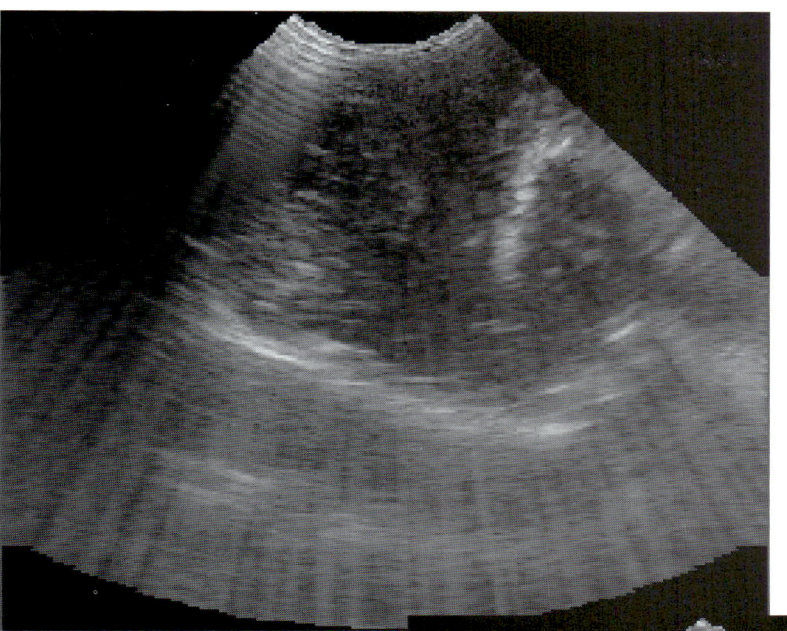

A¹. The cryozone measures ±24 mm in diameter at start of freezing

B¹. The cryozone measures ±42 mm in diameter for 7 min using a single freeze cycle

C¹. The cryozone measures ±44 mm in diameter for 9 min using a single freeze cycle

Fig. 9.1.18¹. Intraoperative ultrasound during freeze cycle on the dog liver using a disc probe with a diameter of 20 mm at a temperature of −180°C. Ice ball. Cryozone formation after exposure: at start of freezing (**A¹**), and for 7 min (**B¹**), and for 9 min (**C¹**)

Chapter 9
Animal Experiment

9.2. Laparoscopic Hepatic Cryosurgery

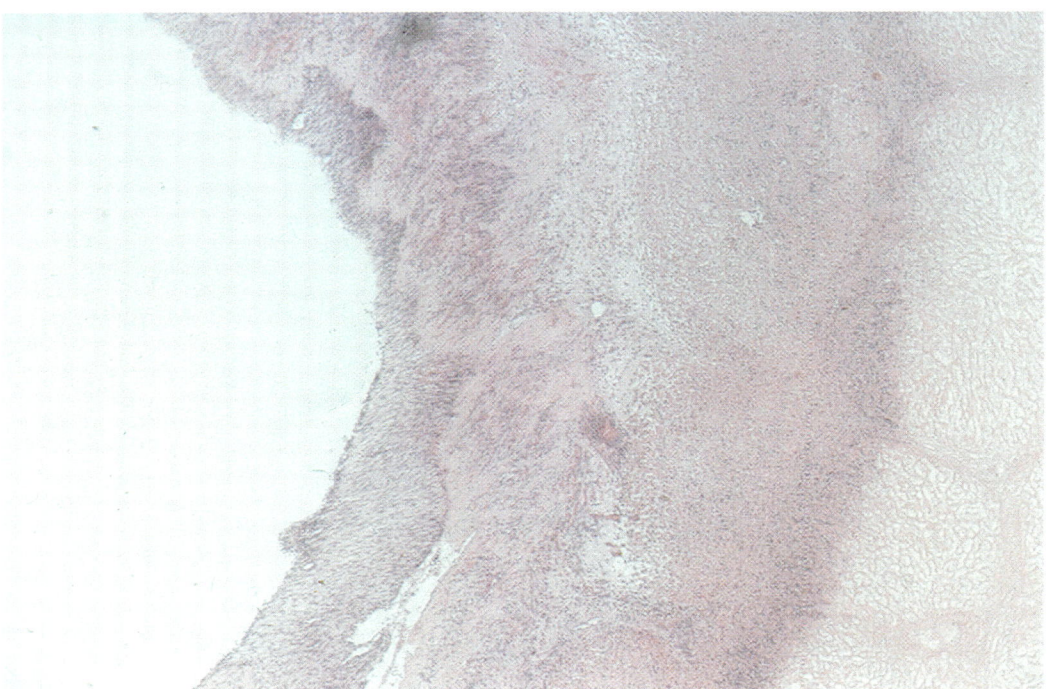

Fig. 9.2.1[2]. A photomicrograph, made during the cryosurgery, of a histologic section of a pig liver through the inferior vena cava following laparoscopic cryosurgery of occlusion of the vena cava inferior. The purpose of this experiment was to determine whether lesions immediately adjacent to the vena cava could be frozen without compromising the integrity of the cava or causing clotting. The picture shows normal parenchyma and various zones of necrosis up to the vena cava with necrosis at the level of the cava, but no damage in the vascular endothelium and no clot in the cava

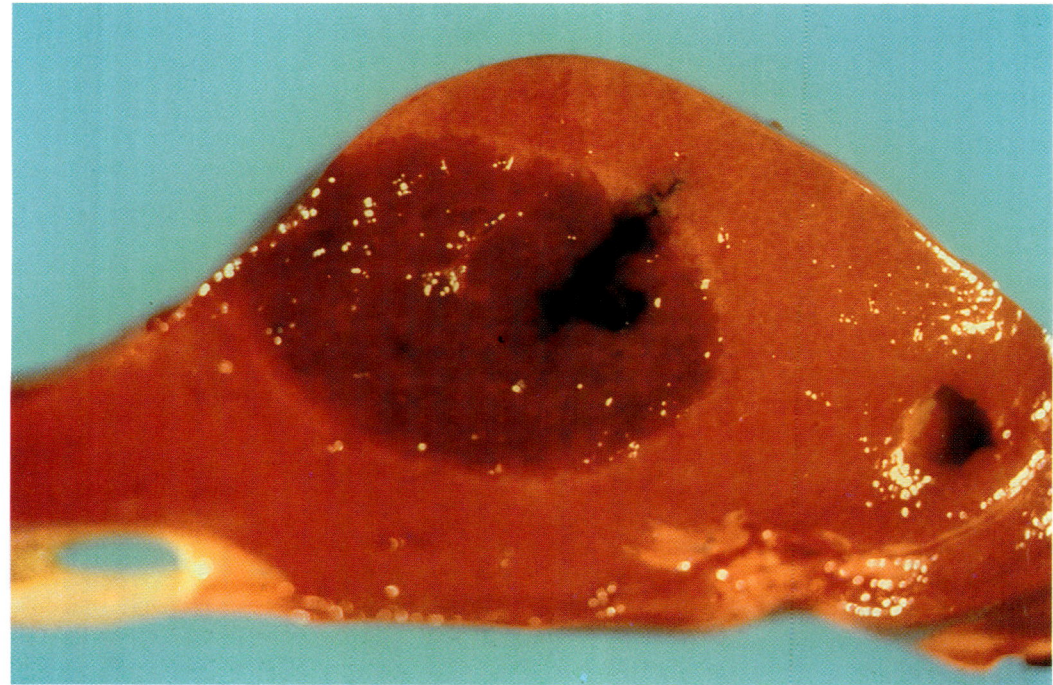

Fig. 9.2.2[2]. An enlarged photograph of a pig liver following laparoscopic hepatic cryosurgery. The black area in the picture is a lesion created by injecting saline and India ink into the liver prior to laparoscopic cryosurgery. This was done by a separate team, so that the team performing the cryosurgery had a target lesion which was visible via ultrasound due to the saline which was injected; this lesion was targeted using laparoscopic ultrasound in order to assess

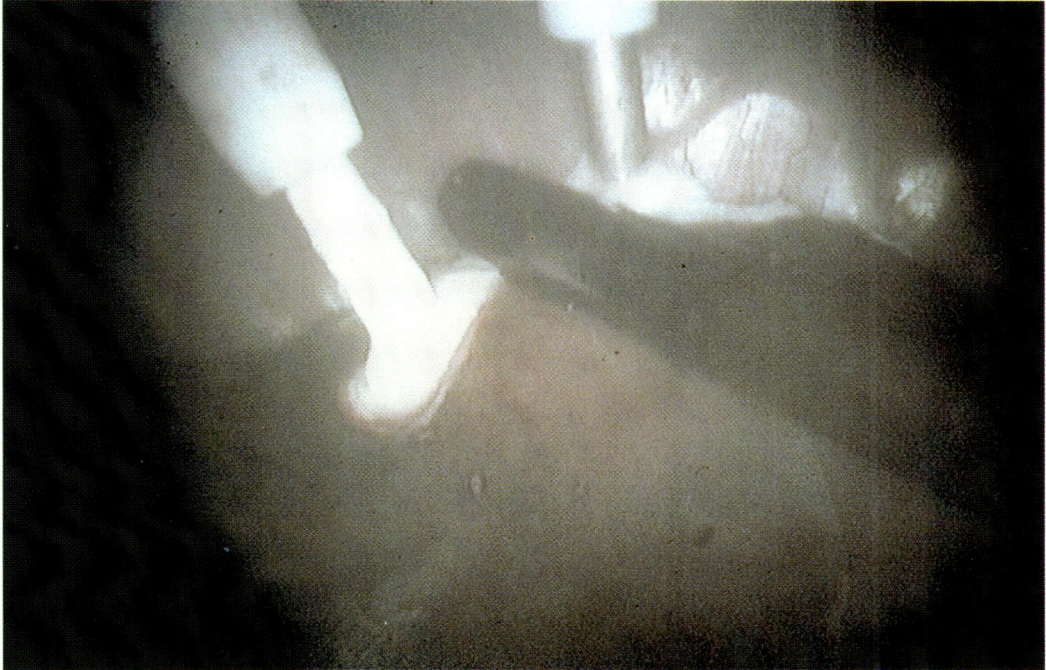

Fig. 9.2.3[2]. Photograph made during laparoscopic cryosurgery on a pig liver; 2 cryoprobes and a laparoscopic ultrasound probe are used

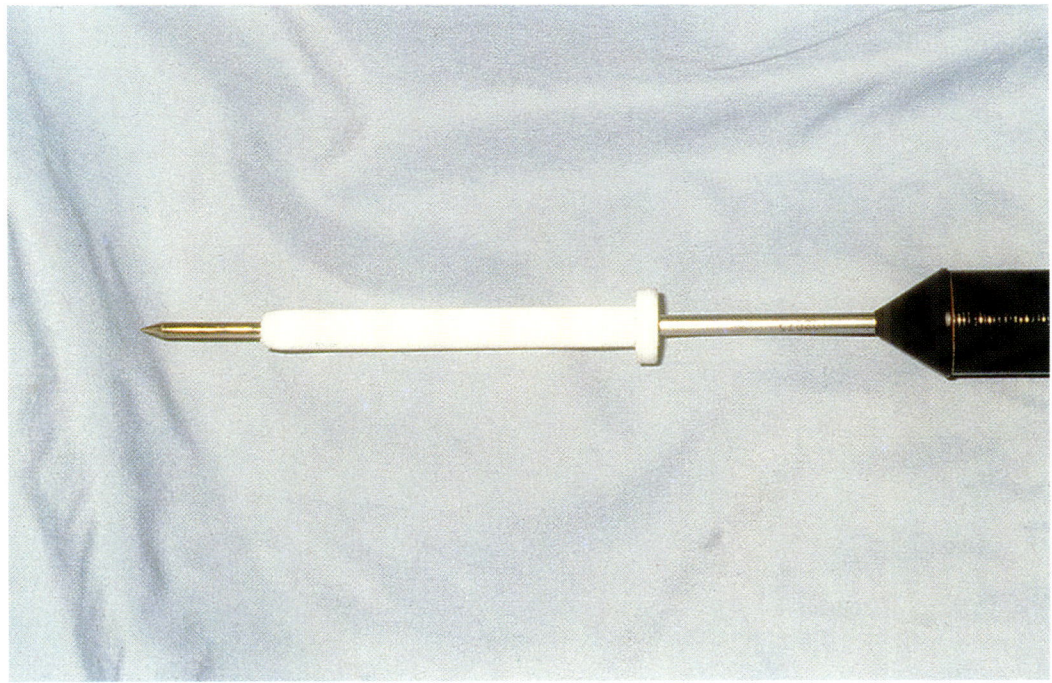

Fig. 9.2.4[2]. Photograph of the standard cryosurgical probe and the sheath, made of Teflon®, which we developed, to act as a laparoscopic trocar and to provide an adequate seal to allow laparoscopic surgery

Chapter 9 Animal Experiment

9.3. Ultrastructural Changes in Liver Tissue

Fig. 9.3.1[1]. In the animal model, we found that it is possible to safely identify, target, and cryoablate specific lesions in the liver. **a** and **b** show the appearance of a dog liver before cryosurgery which was followed by gradual freezing with liquid nitrogen (i.e., −196°C)

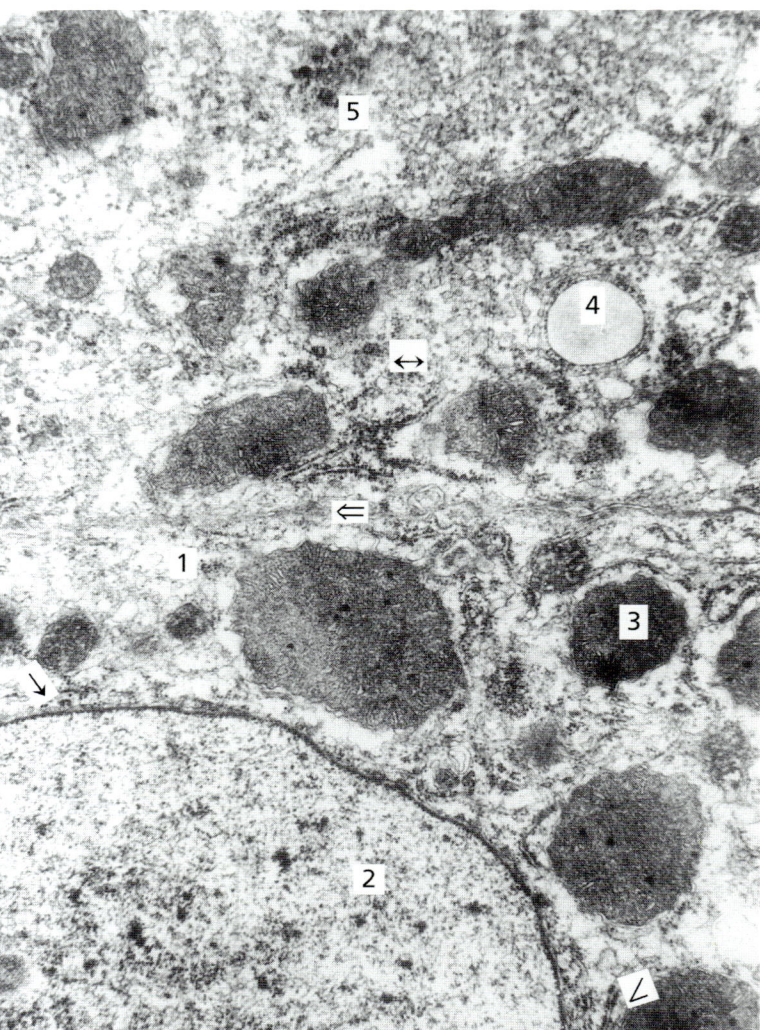

a Electron micrograph showing hepatic cell (1) with nucleus (2), lipid (4) and glycogen (5) inclusions before the cryosurgical exposure. Mitochondrion with matrix (3) as well as plasmatic (⇐) and nuclear (↑) membrane, polysome (→) and endoplasmic canaliculi (∠). Magnification × 18,000

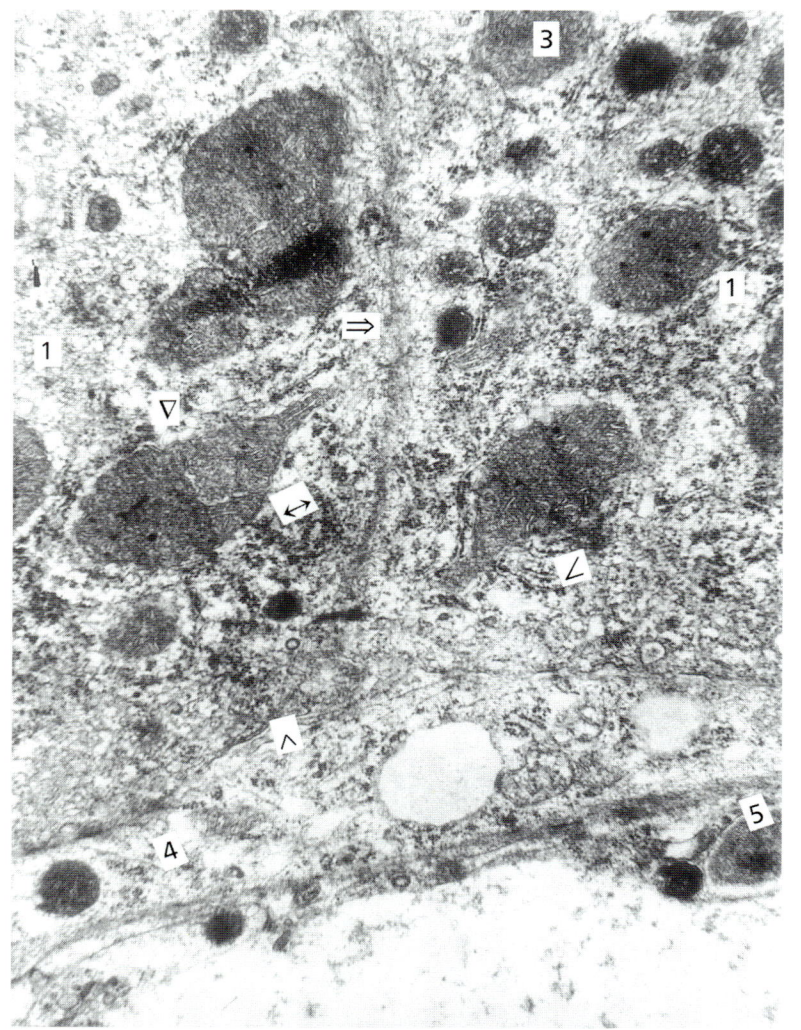

b Electron micrograph shows hepatic cell (1) with plasmatic membrane (⇑), mitochondrion (3), adinocyte (4), and endotheliocyte (5) before the cryosurgical exposure. Sinusoidal surface of the hepatocyte (∧), canaliculi of the endoplasmic granular (∠) and agranular (∇) reticulum, polysome (→). Magnification × 18,000

Section E Experimental Aspects

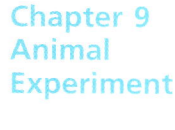

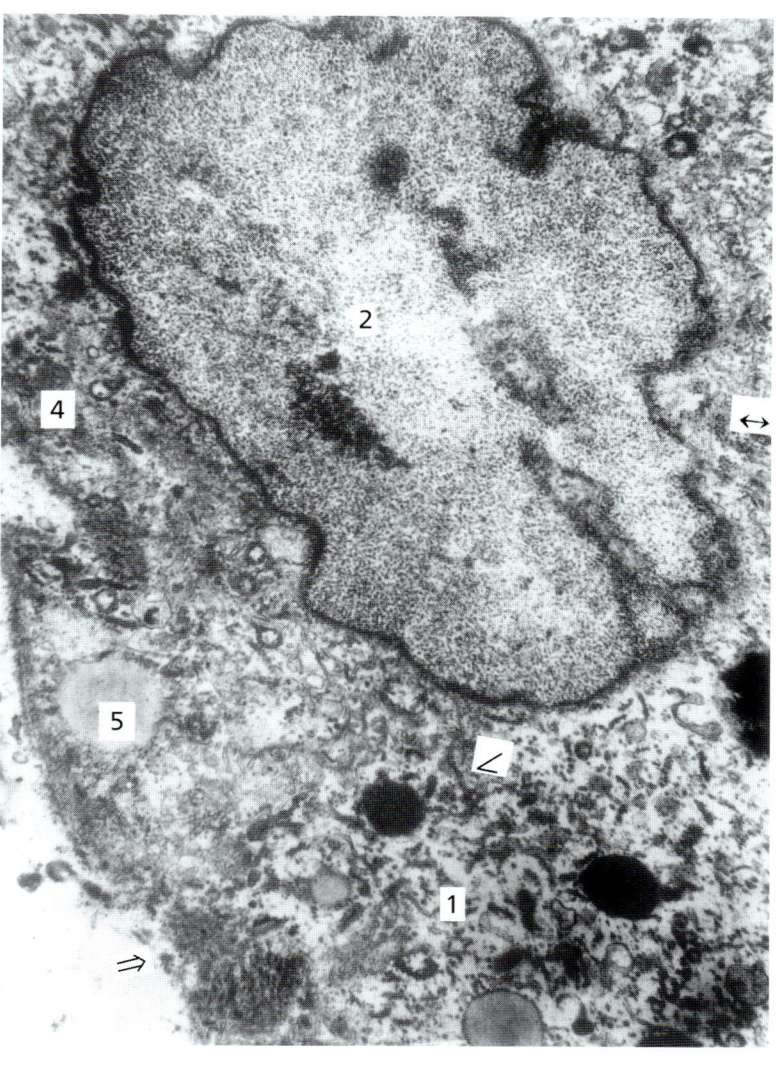

Fig. 9.3.3[1]. Electron micrograph shows hepatic cell with cytolysis (1) *immediately* after the cryosurgical session at a temperature of −180°C. Liver tissue from the cryogenic center zone. The canaliculi are fragmented (▽). Plasmatic membrane is partly intact (↑) and partly amorphous (⇑). Mitochondrion with matrix (3), lipid inclusions (5), dilated canaliculi of the endoplasmic granular reticulum (∠), ribosome and polysome (↔), granulata of glycogen (∧). Magnification × 17,000

Fig. 9.3.2[1]. Electron micrograph showing hepatic cell with cytoplasm (1) *immediately* after the cryosurgical session at a temperature of −180°C. Liver tissue from the cryogenic center zone. Plasmatic membrane (⇑) is lysed. The canaliculi of the endoplasmic granular reticulum (∠) are fragmented. Nucleus of the hepatocyte (2), mitochondrion with matrix (4), lipid inclusions (5), ribosome and polysome (↔). Magnification × 15,000

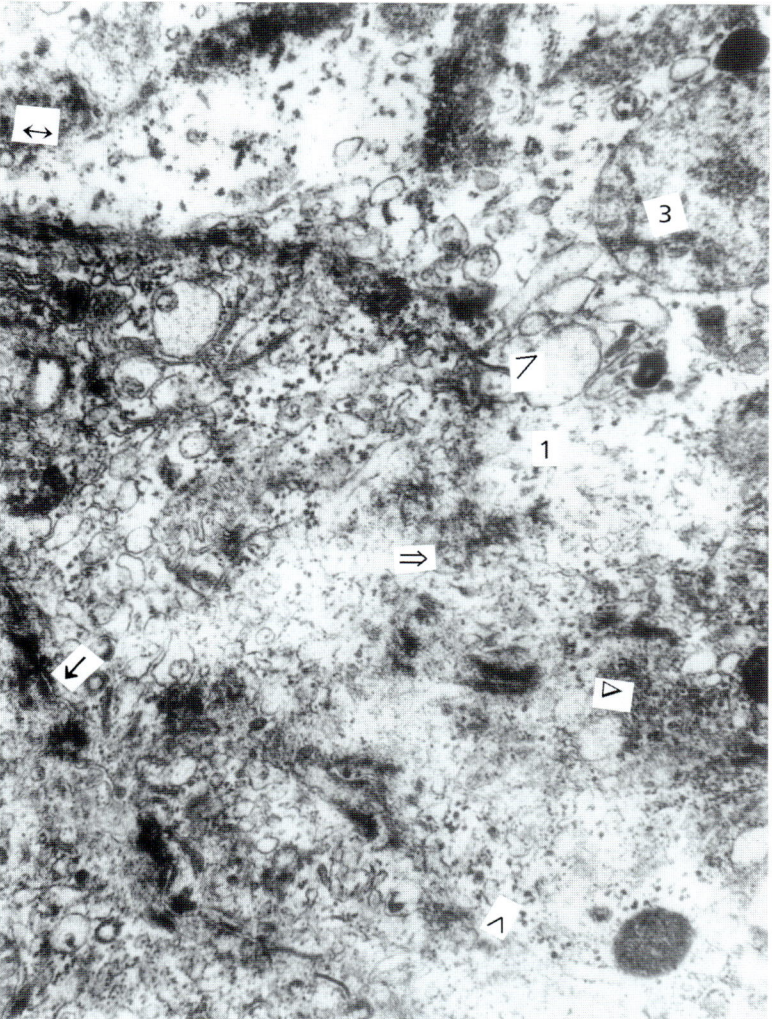

Chapter 9
Animal
Experiment

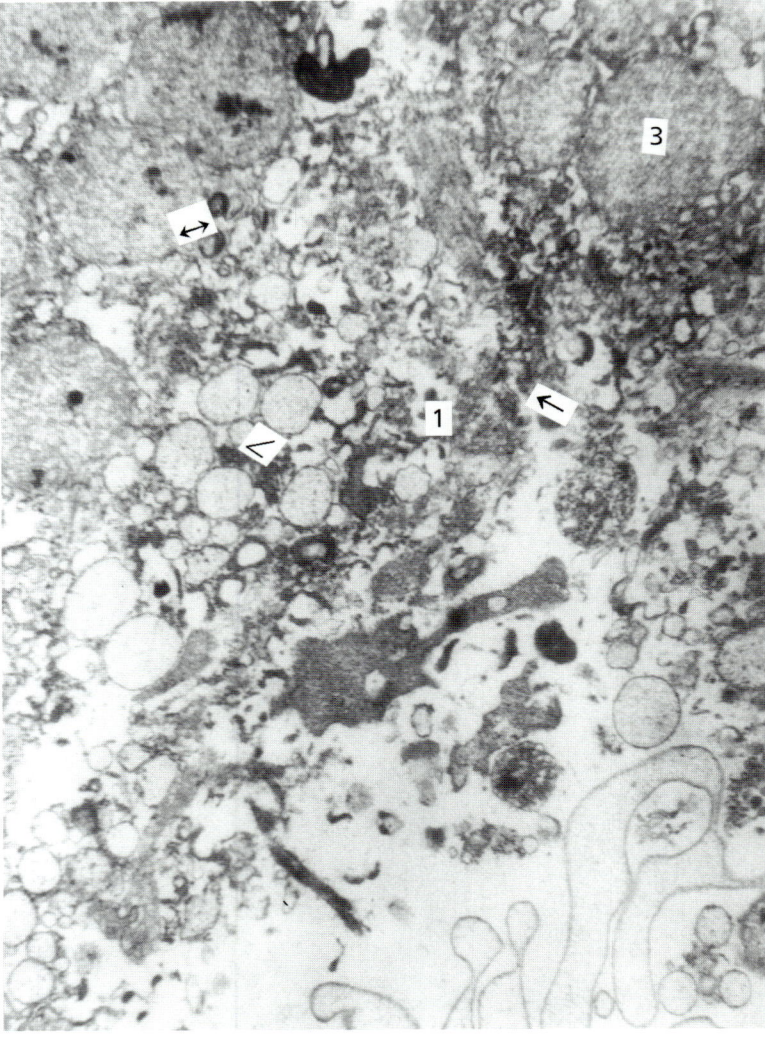

Fig. 9.3.4[1]. Electron micrograph showing hepatic cell (1) 1 h after a cryosurgical session at a temperature of −180°C. Liver tissue from the cryogenic center zone. The plasmatic membrane (↑) is totally lysed. Mitochondrion with matrix (3), dilated canaliculi of the endoplasmic reticulum (∠), cytoplasmic hepatocyte with myelin-like structures (→). Magnification × 12,000

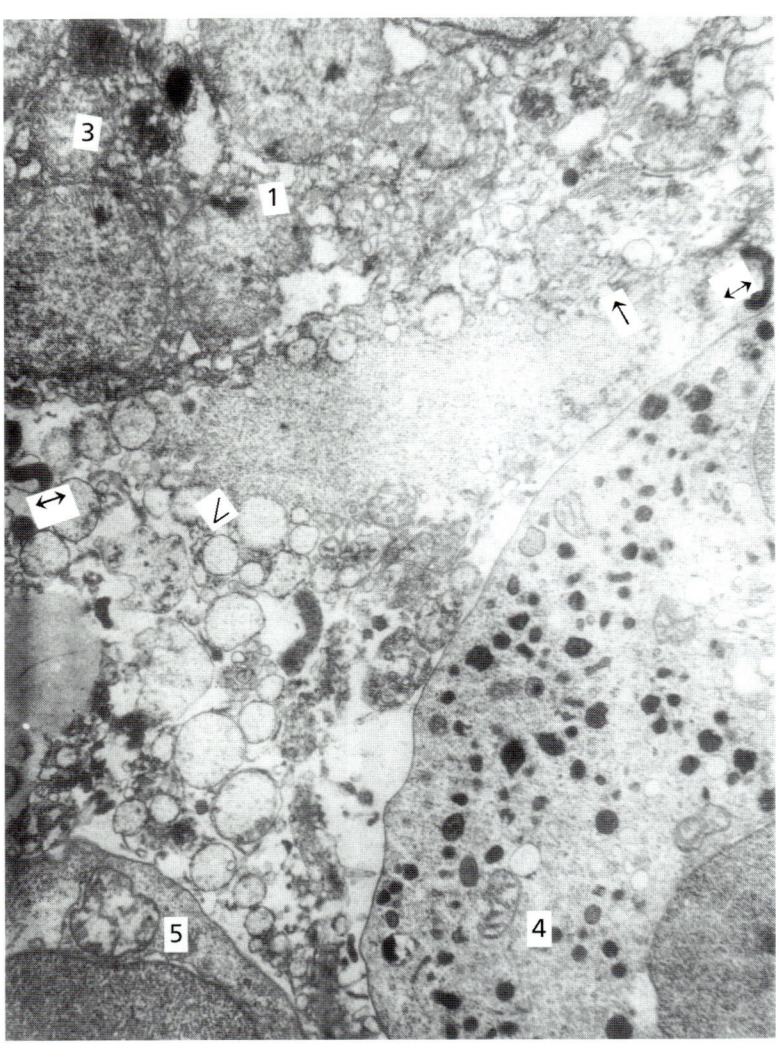

Fig. 9.3.5[1]. Electron micrograph shows hepatic cell (1) 1 h after a cryosurgical session at a temperature of −180°C. Liver tissue from the cryogenic center zone. Mitochondrion (3) after the plasmatic membrane has been totally destroyed (↑). Neutrophil (4) and lymphocyte (5) in the area of sinusoids, myelin-like structures in the cytoplasmic hepatocyte (→), dilated canaliculi of the endoplasmic reticulum (∠). Magnification × 18,000

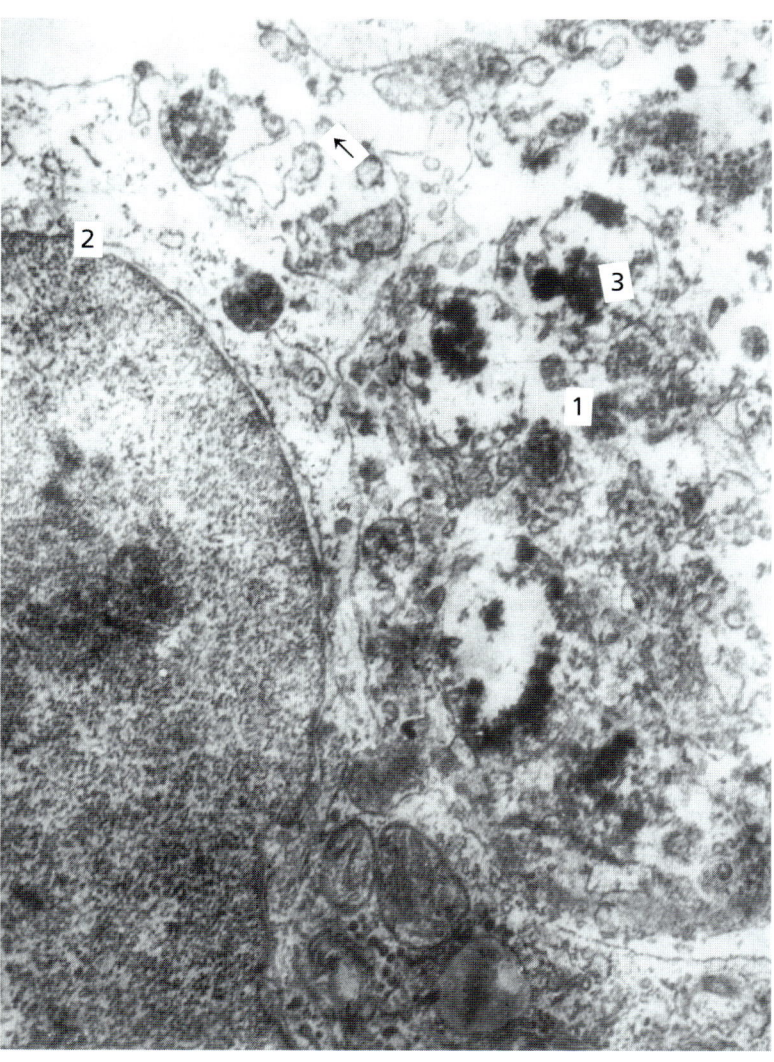

Fig. 9.3.6¹. 24 h after a cryosurgical session at a temperature of −180°C. Liver tissue from the cryogenic center zone. Electron micrograph showing hepatic cell (1) with macrophages (2). The plasmatic membrane of hepatocyte (↑) is fully lysed. Mitochondrion with lysed matrix (3). Magnification × 20,000

Fig. 9.3.7¹. 24 h after a cryosurgical session at −180°C. Liver tissue from the cryogenic center zone. Electron micrograph shows the deglutition of cell detritus (1) by macrophage (2). Magnification × 20,000

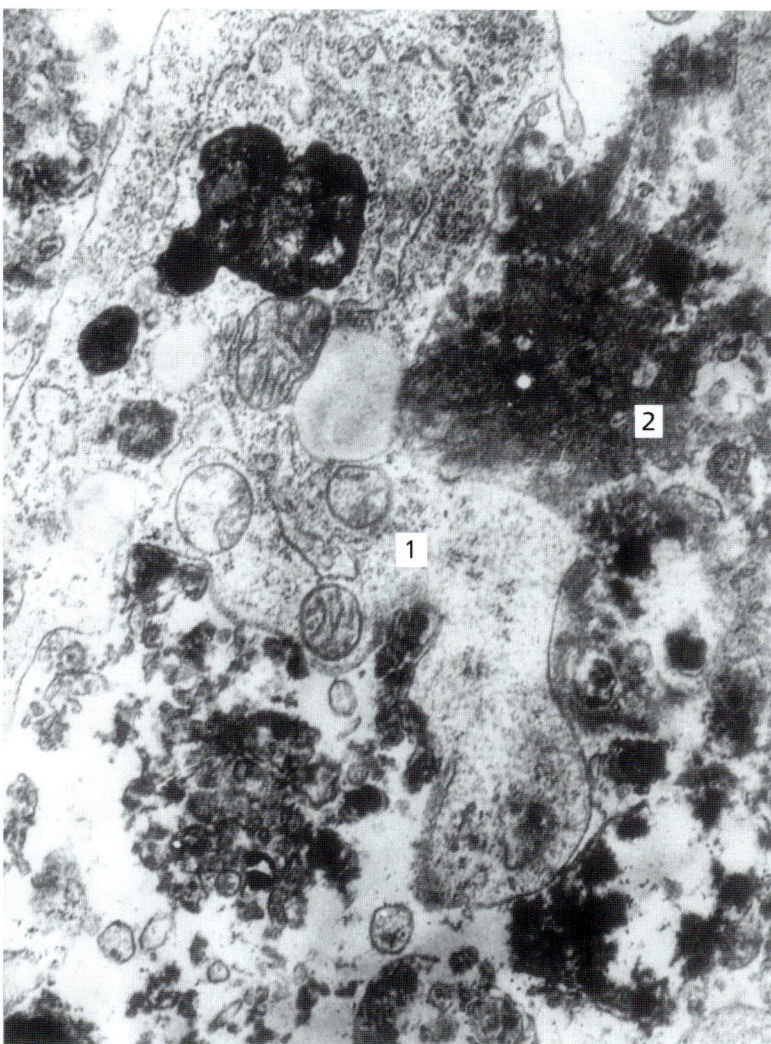

Chapter 9 Animal Experiment

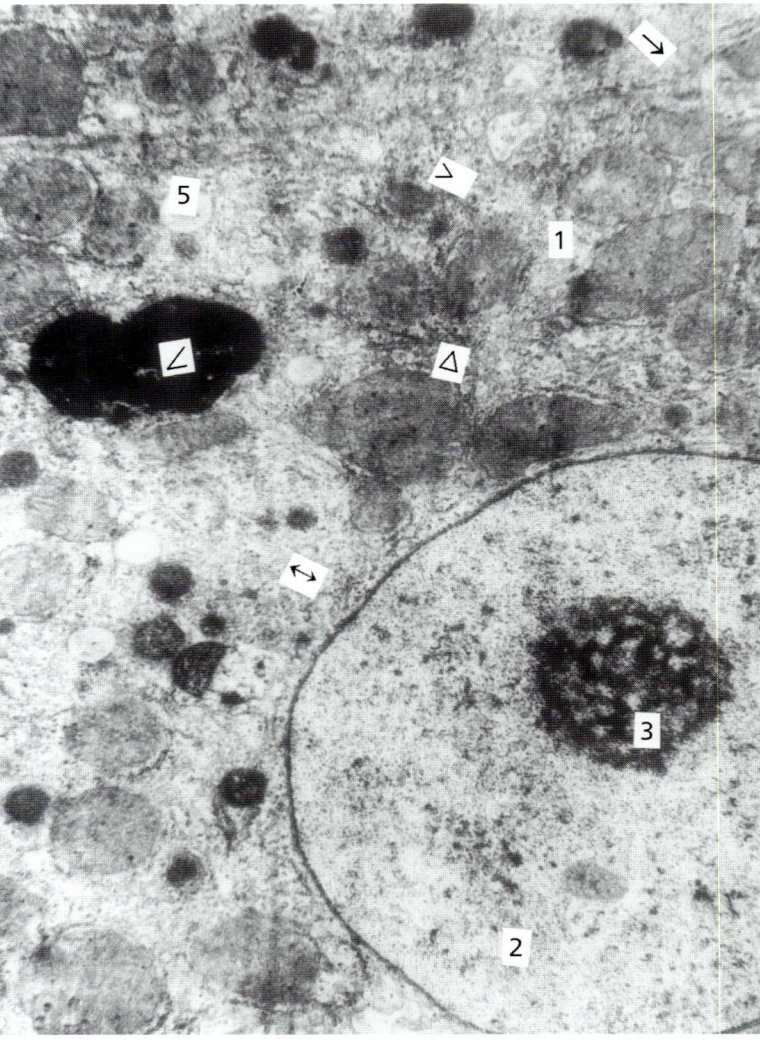

Fig. 9.3.8¹. Cryosurgical session at −180°C. Liver tissue in the border between the cryozone and the non-destroyed liver parenchyma *immediately* after thawing. Electron micrograph showing hepatic cell (1) with nucleus (2) and nucleolus (3) without unequivocal structural changes. The canaliculi of endoplasmic reticulum (∇) are not dilated. The lipid inclusions (5) of lysosome (∠) are evident. Further, the ribosome and polysome (→), and granulata of glycogen (∧) are seen. Magnification × 12,000

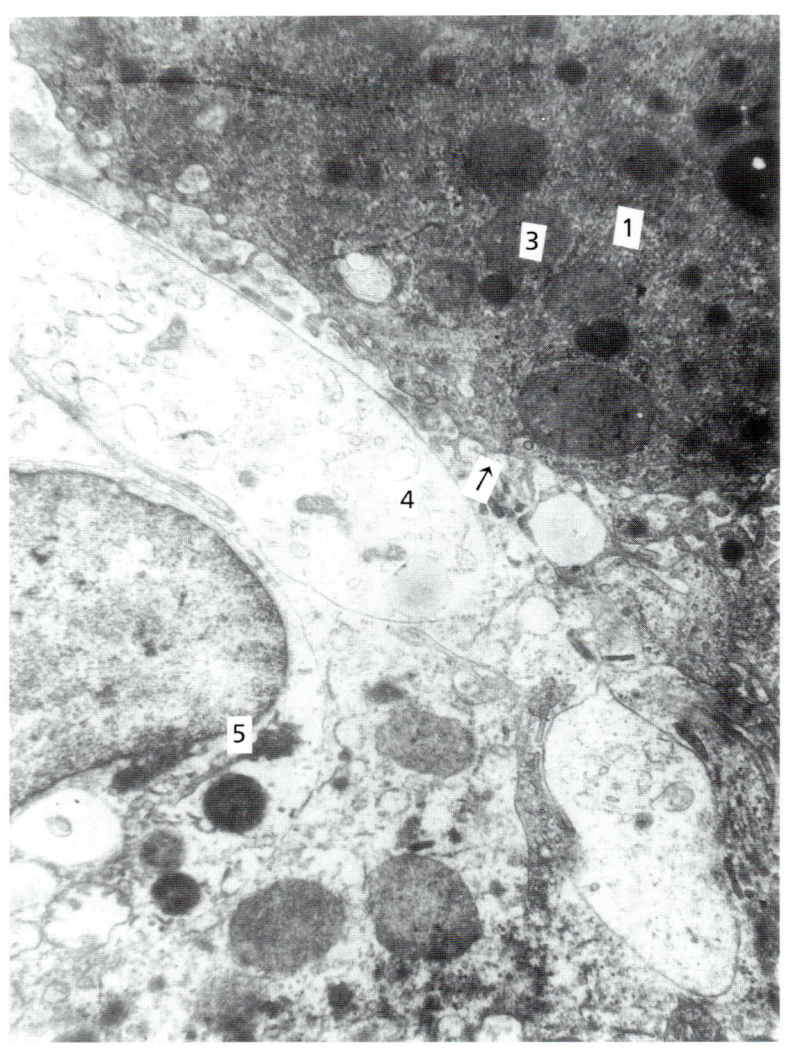

Fig. 9.3.9¹. Cryosurgical session at −180°C. Liver tissue in the border between the cryozone and the non-destroyed liver parenchyma *immediately* after thawing. Electron micrograph showing hepatic cell (1) with well-preserved plasmatic membrane (↑). Mitochondrion with matrix (3), swollen endothelial cells (4), Kupffer's cells (5). Magnification × 12,000

Section E Experimental Aspects

Chapter 9
Animal
Experiment

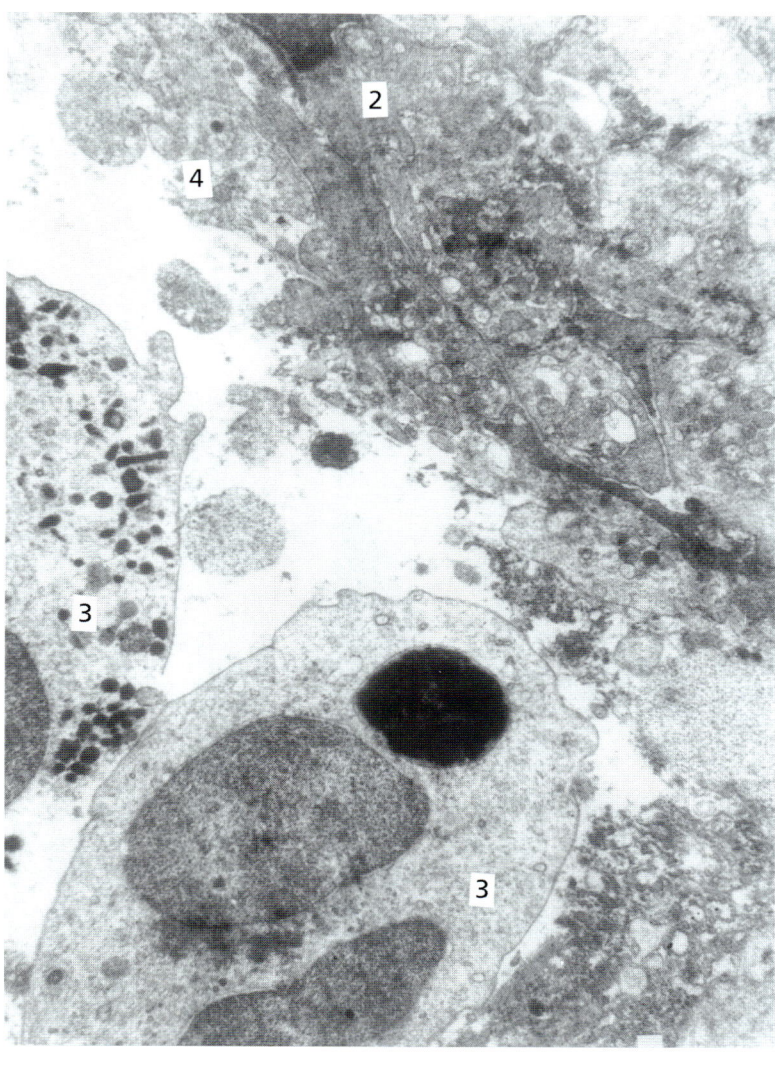

Fig. 9.3.10[1]. Cryosurgical session at −180°C. 1 h after thawing of liver tissue in the border between the cryozone and the non-destroyed liver parenchyma. Electron micrograph showing hepatic cell with lysis: Endothelial cells (2), leukocyte (3) and cell detritus (4). Magnification × 12,000

Fig. 9.3.11[1]. Cryosurgical session at −180°C. 1 h after thawing of liver tissue in the border between the cryozone and the non-destroyed liver parenchyma. Electron micrograph showing hepatic cell (1) with partially lysed plasmatic membrane (⇑) and partially preserved plasmatic membrane (↑). The canaliculi of endoplasmic granular reticulum are fragmented but they are not dilated (▽). Nucleus (2), mitochondrion with matrix (3). Magnification × 12,000

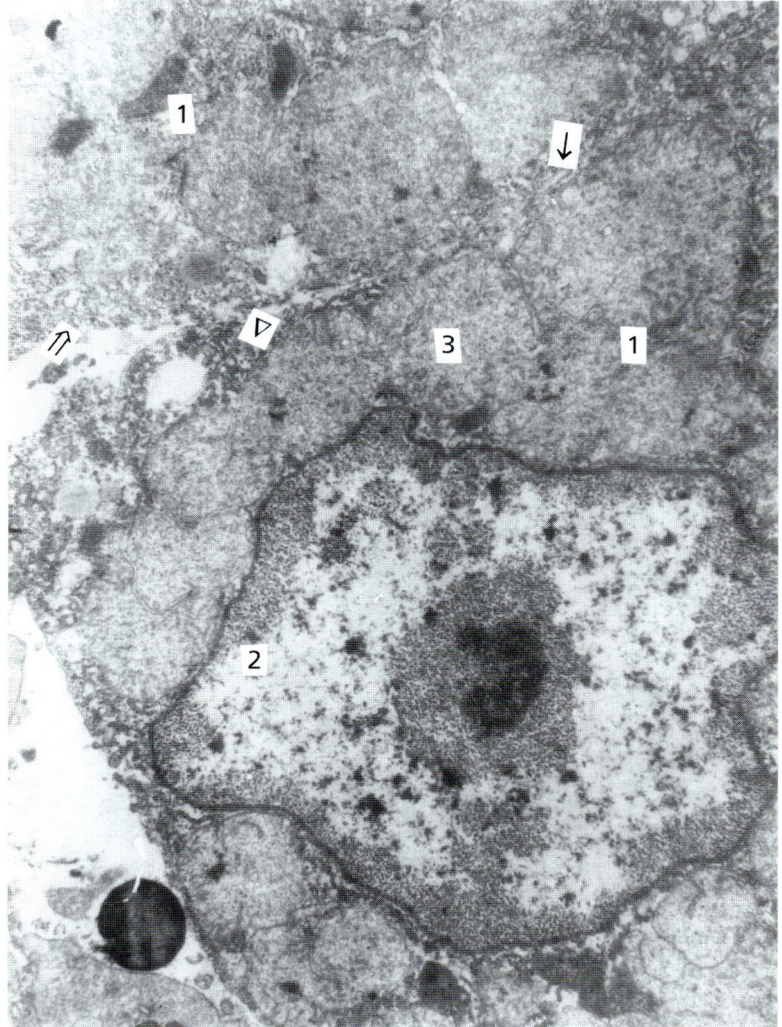

**Chapter 9
Animal
Experiment**

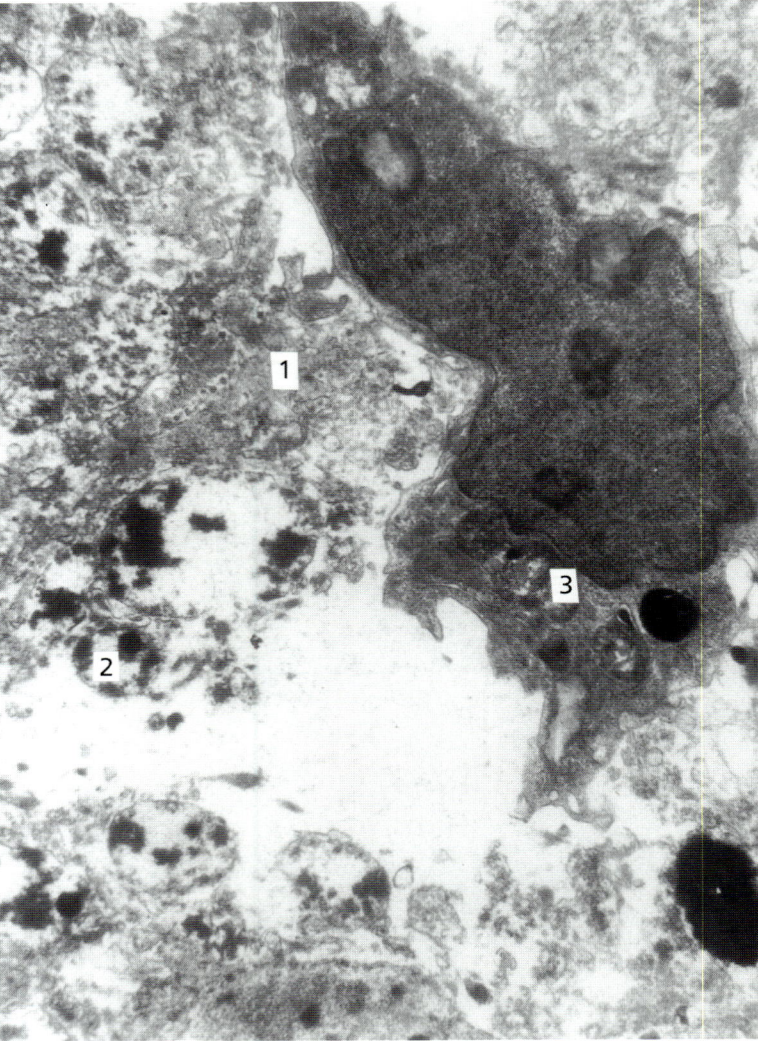

Fig. 9.3.12[1]. 24 h after cryosurgical exposure at −180°C. Liver tissue in the border between the cryozone and the non-destroyed liver parenchyma. Electron micrograph showing the remaining hepatic cell with totally destroyed plasmatic membrane and non-structural matrix (1). Mitochondrion (2), active functional macrophage (3). Magnification × 12,000

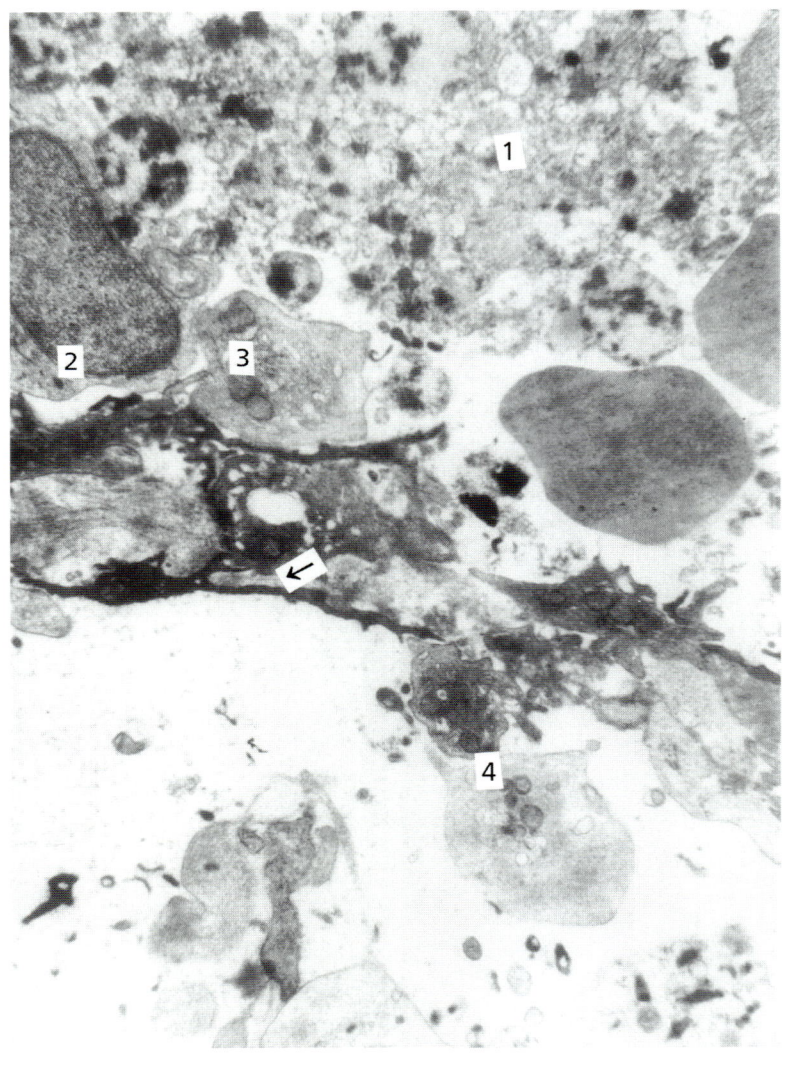

Fig. 9.3.13[1]. 24 h after cryosurgical exposure at −180°C. Liver tissue in the border between the cryozone and the non-destroyed liver parenchyma. Electron micrograph shows the remaining hepatic cell with totally destroyed plasmatic membrane and non-structural matrix (1). Erythrocyte (2) and macrophage (3) in the perisinusoidal Disse space. Further, thrombocyte (4) in the sinusoidal space - beginning of thrombus formation. Endothelial cell and Kupffer's cells (↑). Magnification × 12,000

Chapter 9
Animal Experiment

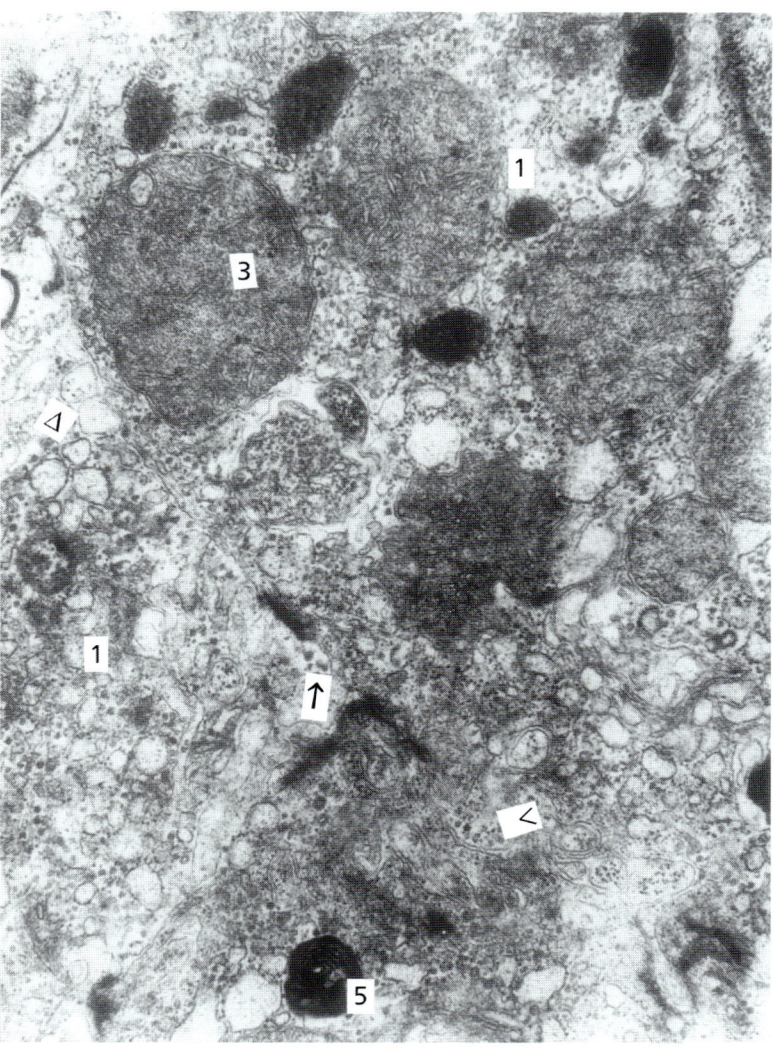

Fig. 9.3.14[1]. *Immediately* after cryosurgical exposure at a temperature of −60°C. Liver tissue in the cryogenic centre zone. Electron micrograph showing hepatic cell (1) with the well-preserved plasmatic membrane (↑) which is lysed. The canaliculi of endoplasmic reticulum (∇) are dilated. Mitochondrion with matrix (3), myelin-like structures (5), ribosome and polysome (↔), granulata of glycogen (∧). Magnification × 15,000

Fig. 9.3.15[1]. *Immediately* after cryosurgical exposure at a temperature of −60°C. Liver tissue in the cryogenic centre zone. The electron micrograph shows the accumulation of collagenous fibres (↑) in the dilated Disse space (1). The erythrocyte is partially hemolysed (3). Magnification × 18,000

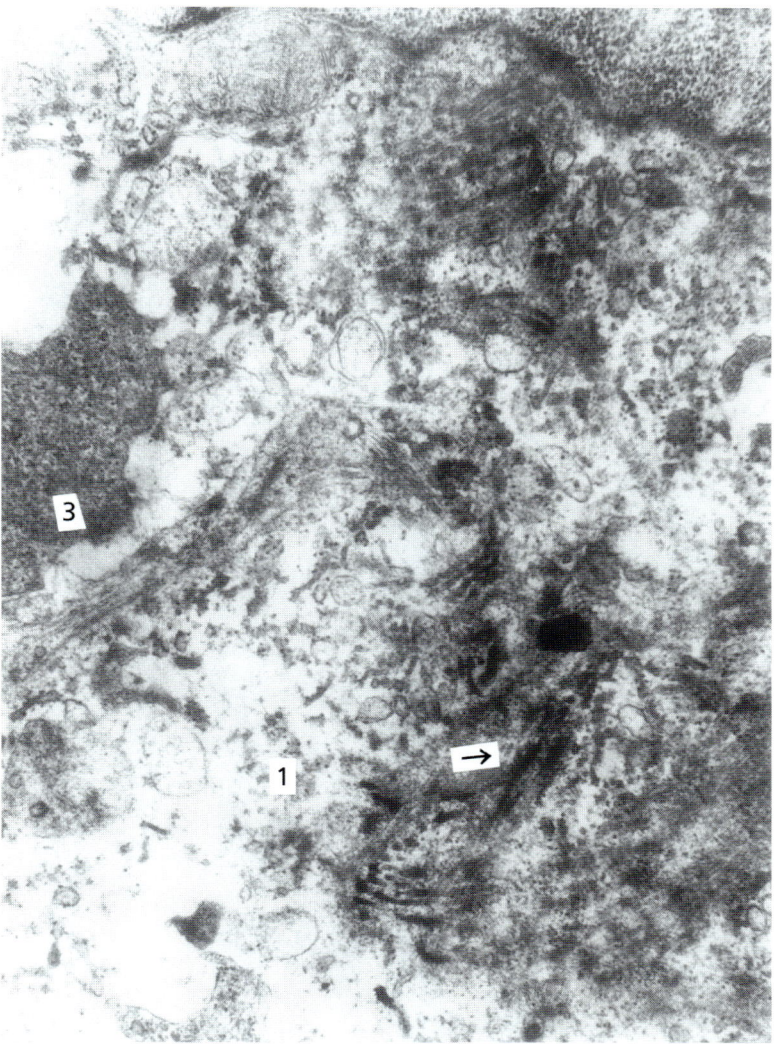

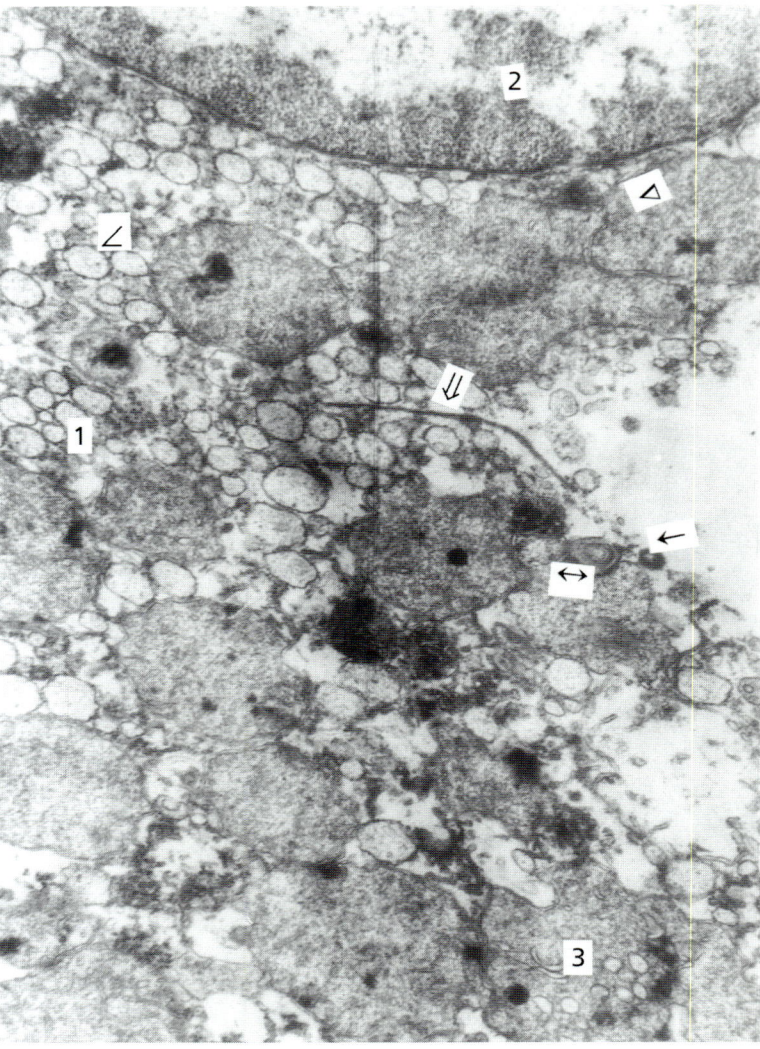

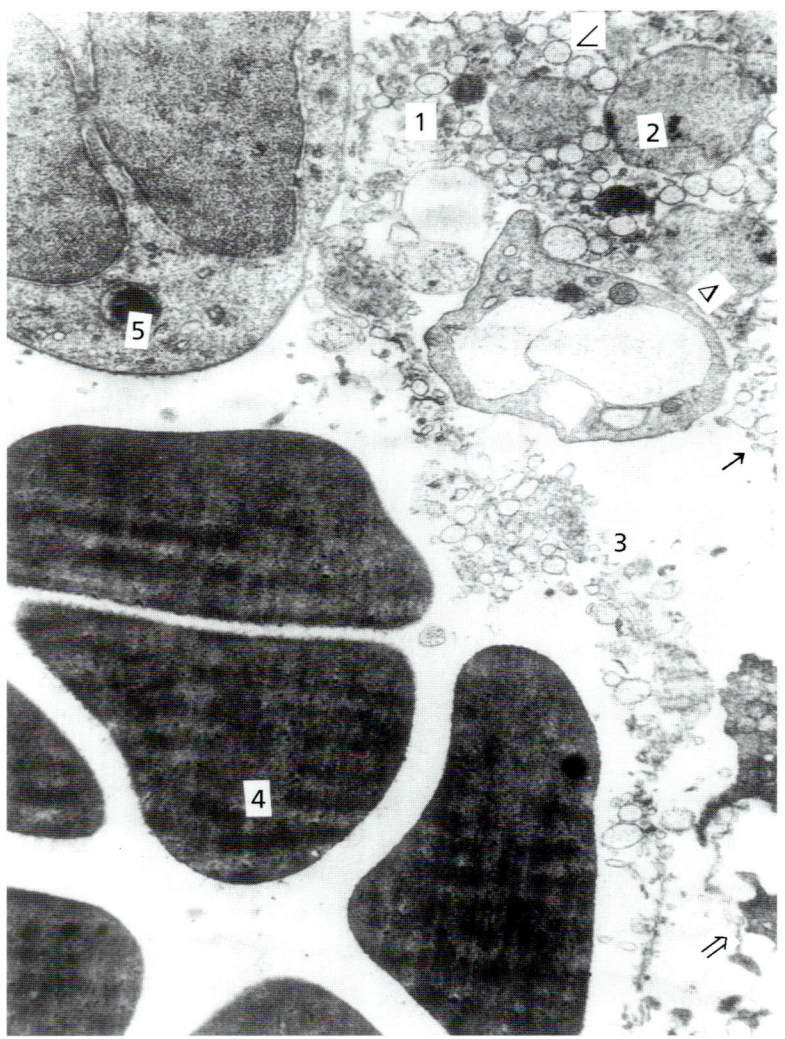

Fig. 9.3.17[1]. Liver tissue sample taken 1 h after cryosurgical exposure at −60°C. Hepatocytes (1). Plasmatic membrane on the sinusoidal surface (↑) of the hepatocytes is completely absent. Mitochondria with electron translucent matrix and partly destroyed external and internal membranes (∇) with coagulated protein components (2). One part of them contains dense inclusions of coagulated protein components (3), fragmental and slightly dilated canaliculi of the rough endoplasmic reticulum (∠). Space of Disse (3). The remainder of the sinusoids' endothelial cells (⇑). Erythrocytes (4) and monocyte (5) in the sinusoidal space. Magnification × 12,000

Fig. 9.3.16[1]. 1 h after cryosurgical exposure at −60°C. Tissue sample taken *immediately* after thawing. Hepatocytes (1). Plasmatic membrane on the sinusoidal surface (↑) of the hepatocytes is almost completely absent, and on the lateral surface partially preserved (⇑). Nucleus (2) with the translucent nuclear matrix and marginally situated heterochromatin. Mitochondria with electron translucent matrix and partly destroyed external and internal membranes (∇). One part of them contains dense inclusions of coagulated protein components (3), fragmental and slightly dilated canaliculi of the rough endoplasmic reticulum (∠). Single myelin-like structures (↔) in the cytoplasm of the hepatocytes. Magnification × 15,000

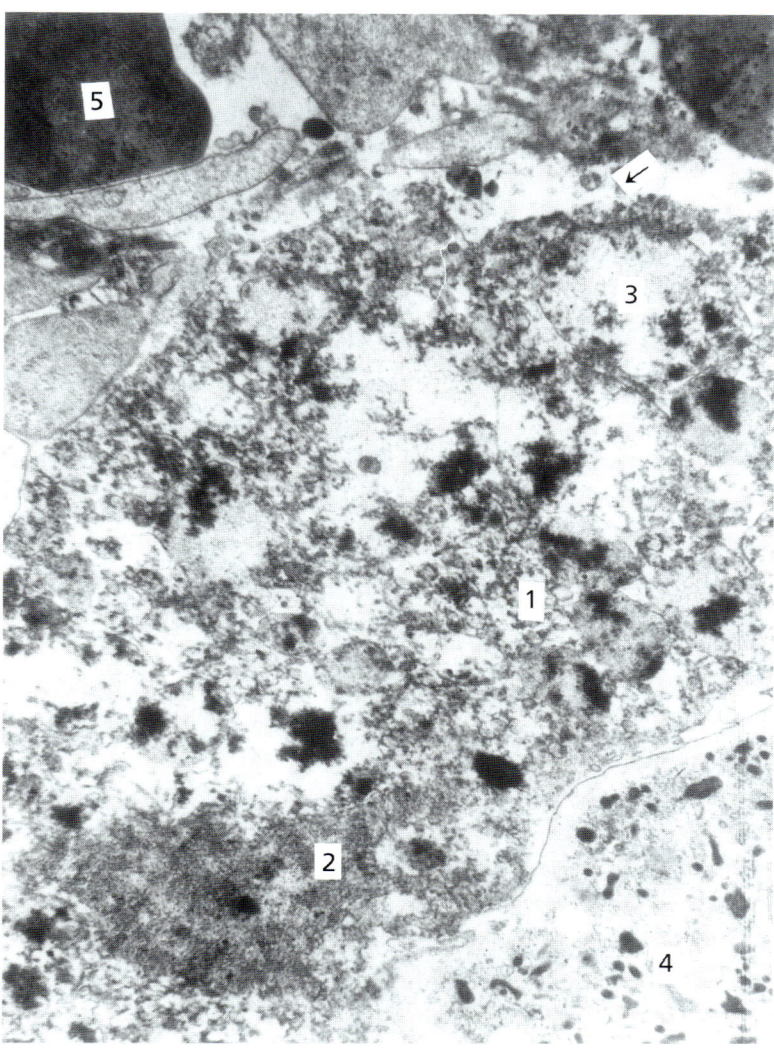

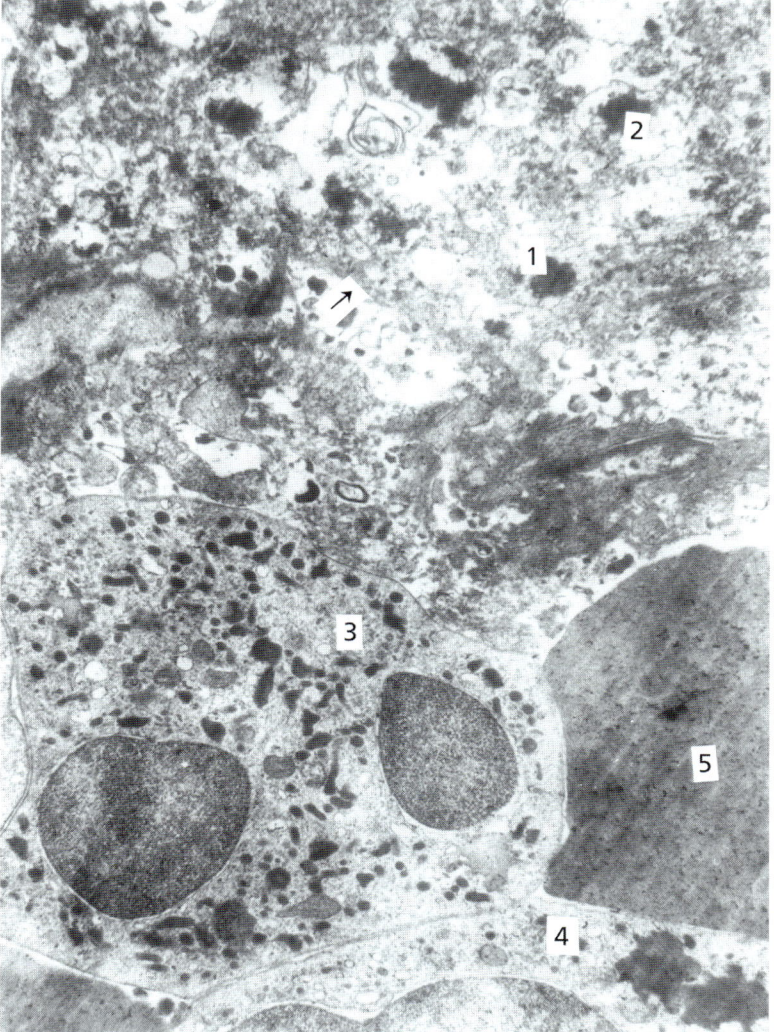

Fig. 9.3.19[1]. Liver tissue sample taken 24 h after cryosurgical exposure at −60°C. Destructively altered hepatocyte (1). Full lysis of plasmatic membrane (↑). Mitochondria with lysed matrix and destroyed external and internal membranes as well as inclusions of coagulated protein components (2). The space of the former sinusoidal capillary is filled with cell detritis and blood cells - neutrophil (3), macrophage (4) and erythrocyte (5). Magnification × 12,000

Fig. 9.3.18[1]. Liver tissue sample taken 24 h after cryosurgical exposure at −60°C. Destructively changed hepatocyte (1). Full lysis of plasmatic membrane (↑). Pyknotically transformed nucleus (2). Mitochondria with lysed matrix and destroyed external and internal membranes as well as inclusions of coagulated protein components (3), neutrophil (4), erythrocytes (5). Magnification × 12,000

Fig. 9.3.21[1]. After cryosurgical exposure at −60°C. Liver tissue sample taken *immediately* from the border between the cryozone and the undamaged liver parenchyma. Dilated Disse space, which is full of collagen fibres (1), and fragments of the ultrastructure of the hepatocytes (⇑), which have exited the cell as a result of plasmalemma lysis. Magnification × 15,000

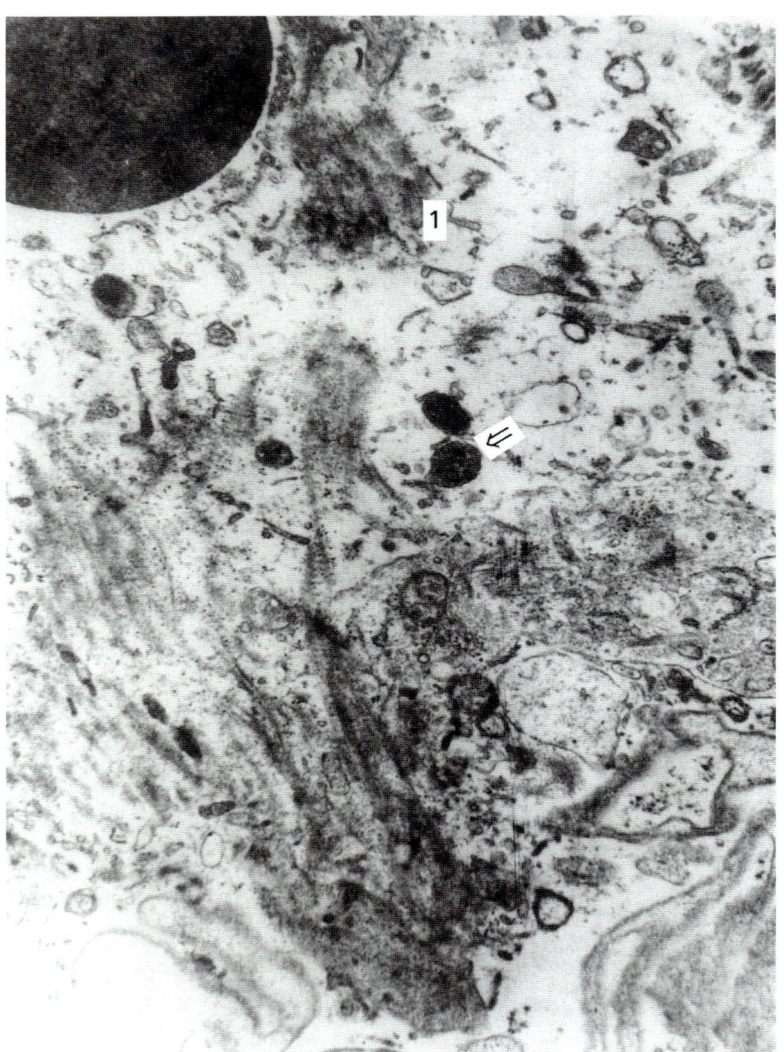

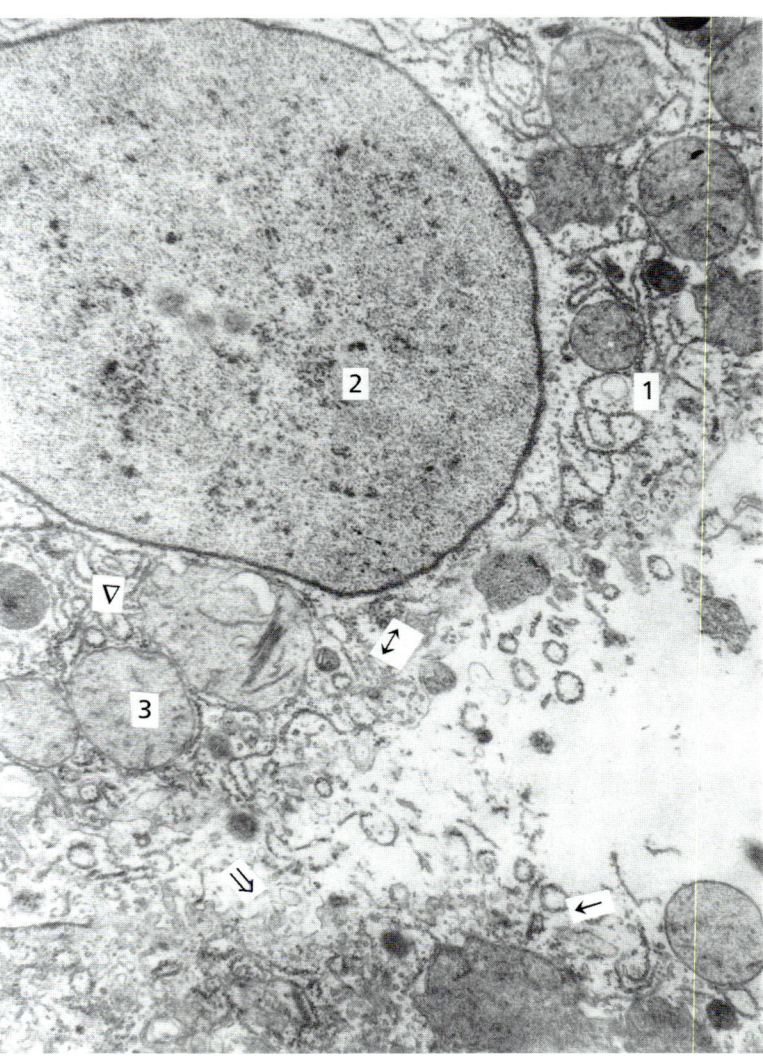

Fig. 9.3.20[1]. After cryosurgical exposure at −60°C. Liver tissue sample taken *immediately* from the border between the cryozone and the undamaged liver parenchyma. Hepatocytes (1). Plasmatic membrane in one area of the sinusoidal surface (↑) of the hepatocytes has been destroyed but partially preserved in other areas (⇑). Nucleus (2) of the hepatocyte is without significant changes. Mitochondria mostly contain clear structured external and internal membranes and electron translucent matrix (3). Canaliculi of the rough endoplasmic reticulum are moderately dilated and partly fragmented (∇). Ribosomes and polysomes (↔). Magnification × 12,000

Section E Experimental Aspects

Chapter 9
Animal
Experiment

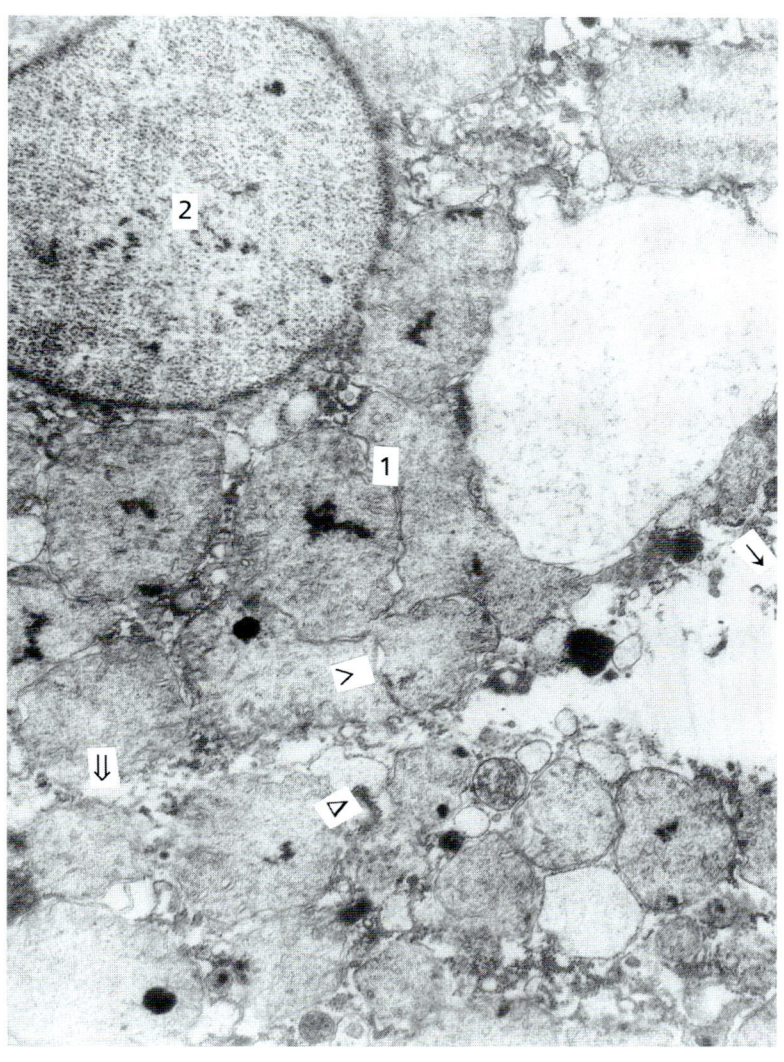

Fig. 9.3.22[1]. Cryosurgical exposure at −60°C. Liver tissue sample taken from the border between the cryozone and the undamaged liver parenchyma 1 h after thawing. Hepatocytes (1). Plasmatic membrane on the sinusoidal (↑) and lateral (⇑) surfaces of the hepatocytes is absent. Nucleus (2) of the hepatocyte with eroded karyolema and equally dilated chromatin in the karyoplasm. Mitochondria contain clearly structured matrix. Local lysis of the external and internal membranes (∧) can be observed. Dilated canaliculi of the rough endoplasmic reticulum (∇). Magnification × 12,000

Fig. 9.3.23[1]. Cryosurgical exposure at a temperature of −60°C. Liver tissue sample taken from the border between the cryozone and the undamaged liver parenchyma 1 h after thawing. Hepatocytes (1). Plasmatic membrane on the sinusoidal surface (↑) of the hepatocytes is absent. Mitochondria (2) contain clearly structured matrix. Local lysis of the external and internal membranes (∧) and dilated canaliculi of the rough endoplasmic reticulum (∇) can be observed in some of them. Neutrophil (3) and hemolytic erythrocyte (4) are situated in the sinusoidal space. Magnification × 12,000

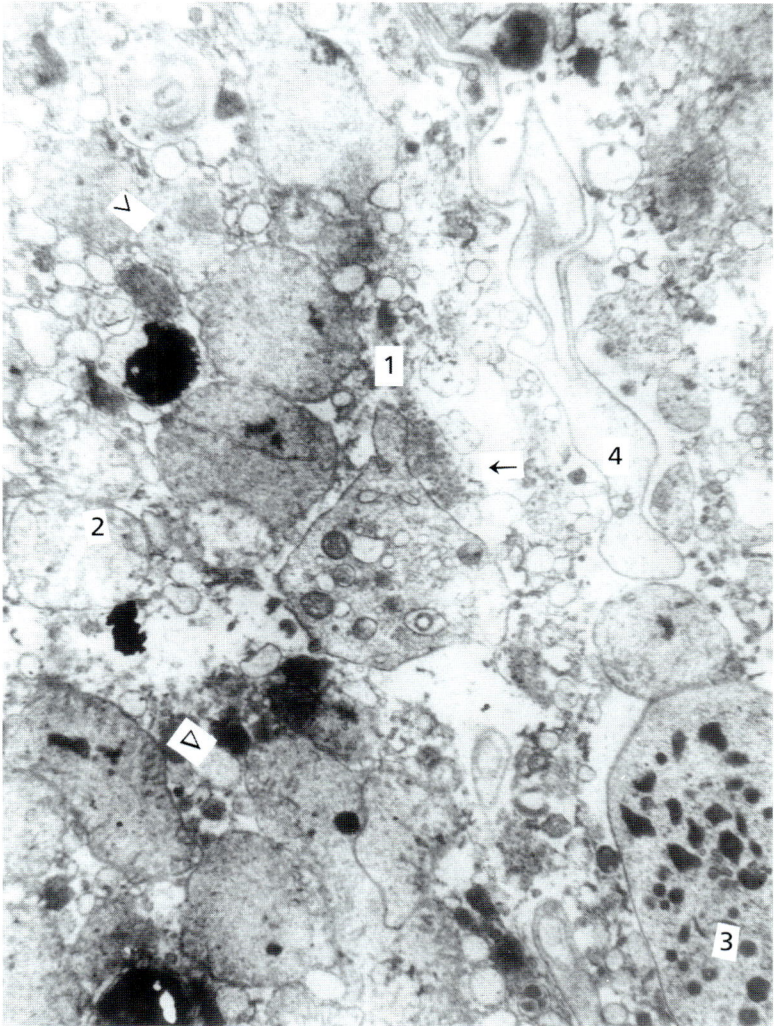

Chapter 9
Animal Experiment

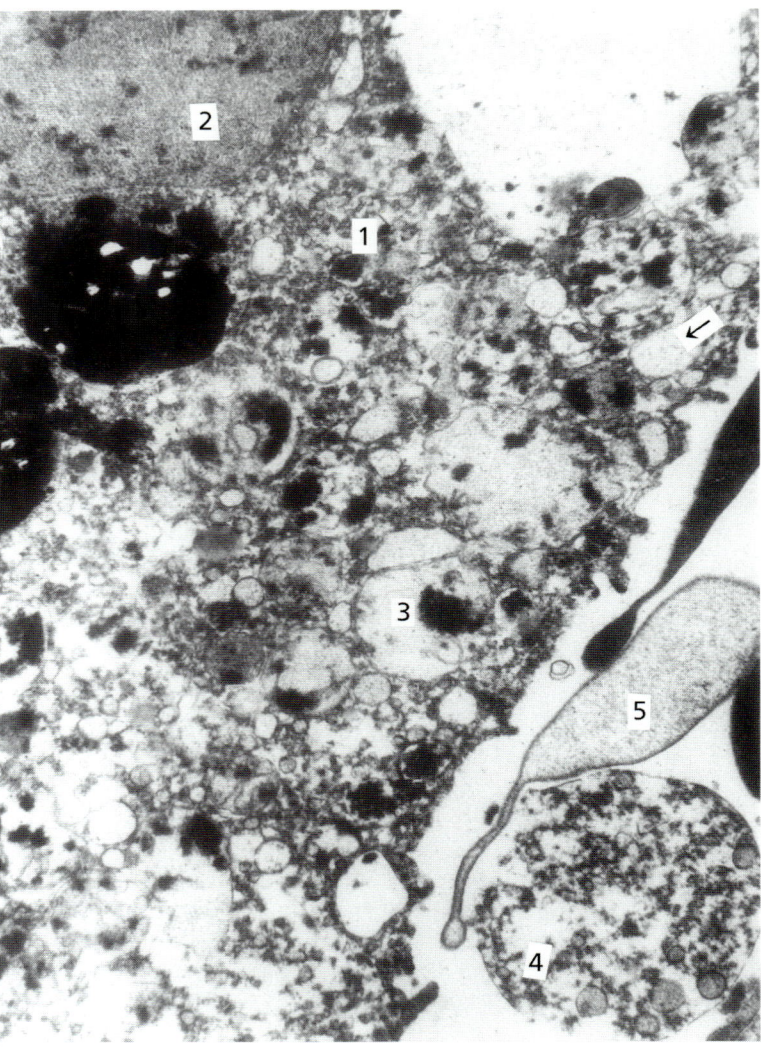

Fig. 9.3.25¹. Cryosurgical exposure at a temperature of −60°C. Liver tissue sample taken from the border between the cryozone and the undamaged liver parenchyma 24 h after thawing. Hepatocyte (1) with unstructured plasmolemma. Nucleus (2) of the hepatocyte with densified karyomatrix (2). Nucleus (2) of the hepatocyte with lysed karyomatrix (3). Mitochondria in the different stages of destructive changes (4). Dilated canaliculi of the rough endoplasmic reticulum (↑). Magnification × 12,000

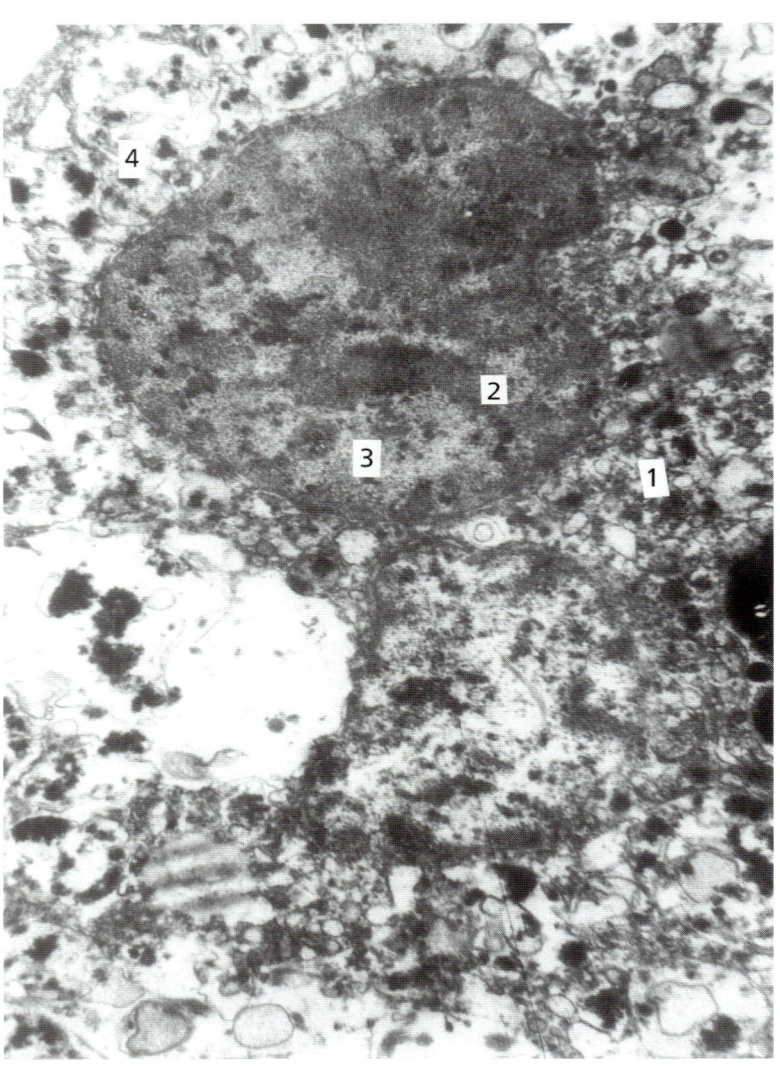

Fig. 9.3.24¹. Cryosurgical exposure at a temperature of −60°C. Liver tissue sample taken from the border between the cryozone and the undamaged liver parenchyma 24 h after thawing. Hepatocyte (1) with destructured plasmolemma. Nucleus (2) of the hepatocyte with eroded nucleus membrane and slightly densified karyomatrix. Mitochondria (2) in the different stages of destructive changes (3). Dilated canaliculi of the rough endoplasmic reticulum (↑). Sequestered part of the hepatocyte (4), hemolytic erythrocyte (5) in the former sinusoidal space. Magnification × 18,000

Section E   Experimental Aspects

9.4. Histological Study of the Liver

Chapter 9
Animal
Experiment

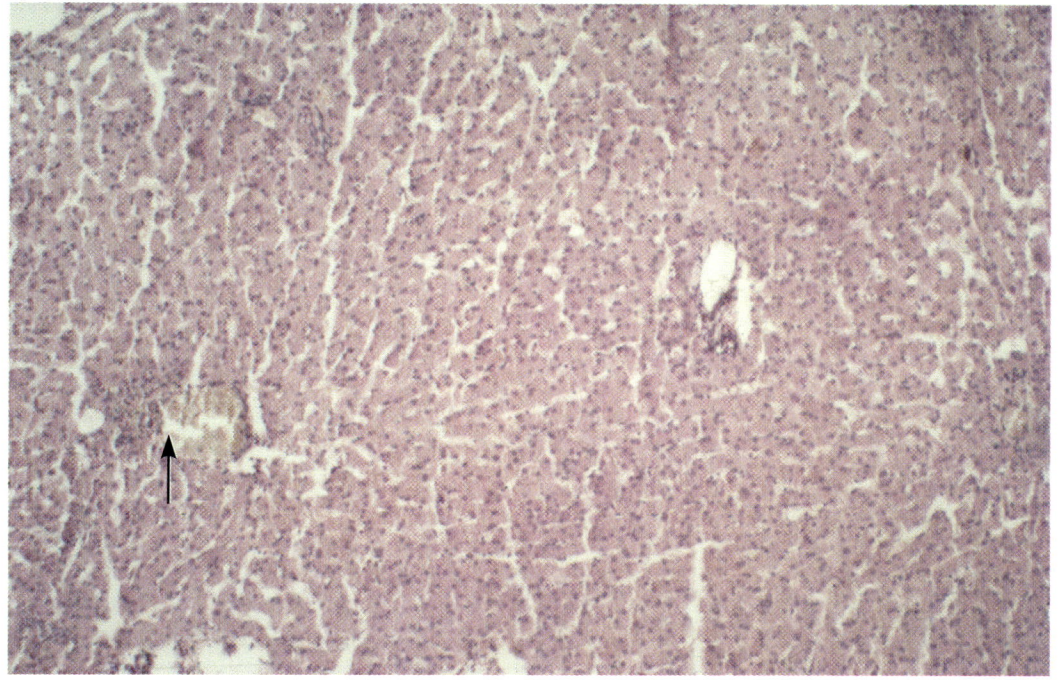

Fig. 9.4.1[1]. *Before* cryosurgical session. Healthy dog liver tissue. Liver tissue with periportal fields (↑). Hematoxylin and eosin staining. Magnification × 100

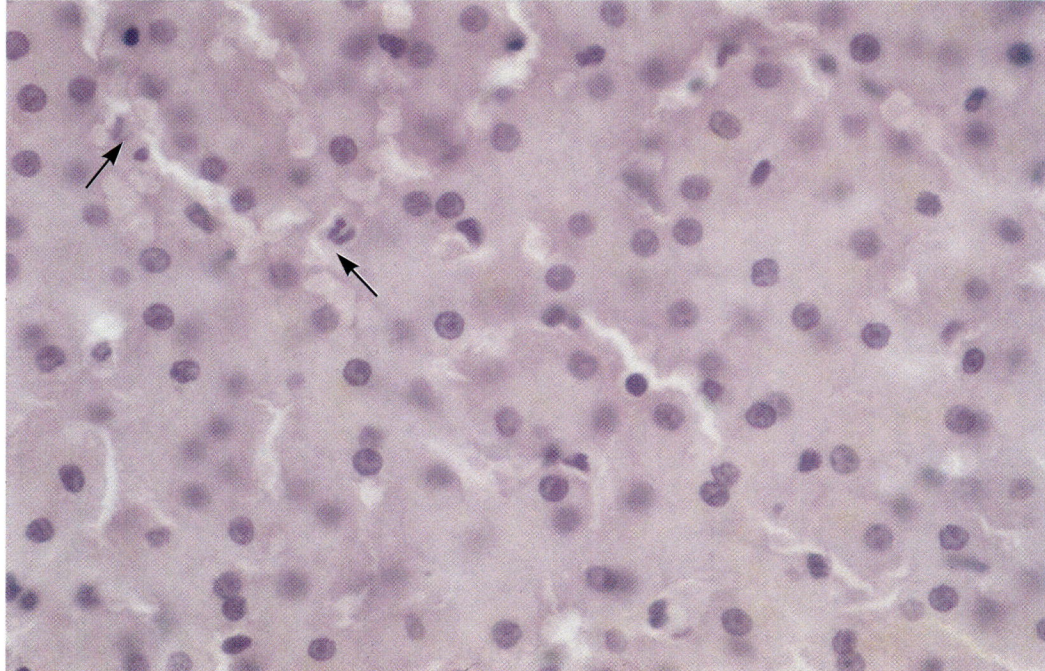

Fig. 9.4.2[1]. 30 min after the single freeze-thaw cycle at a temperature of −180°C. Biopsy from the center of the cryonecrosis. Liver tissue with sinusoids which contain individual inflammation cells (↑). Hematoxylin and eosin staining. Magnification × 600

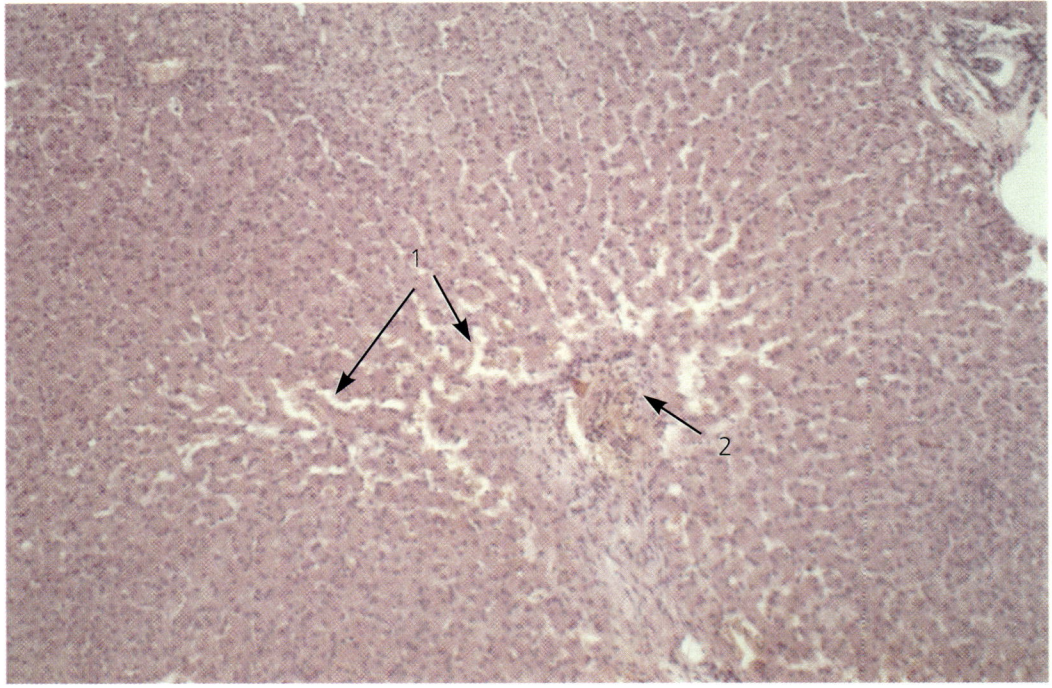

Fig. 9.4.3[1]. 30 min after the single freeze-thaw cycle at a temperature of −180°C. Biopsy from the border between the cryonecrosis and healthy tissue. In the outline still recognizable liver structure with elongated sinusoids (1). Hematoxylin and eosin staining. Magnification × 100

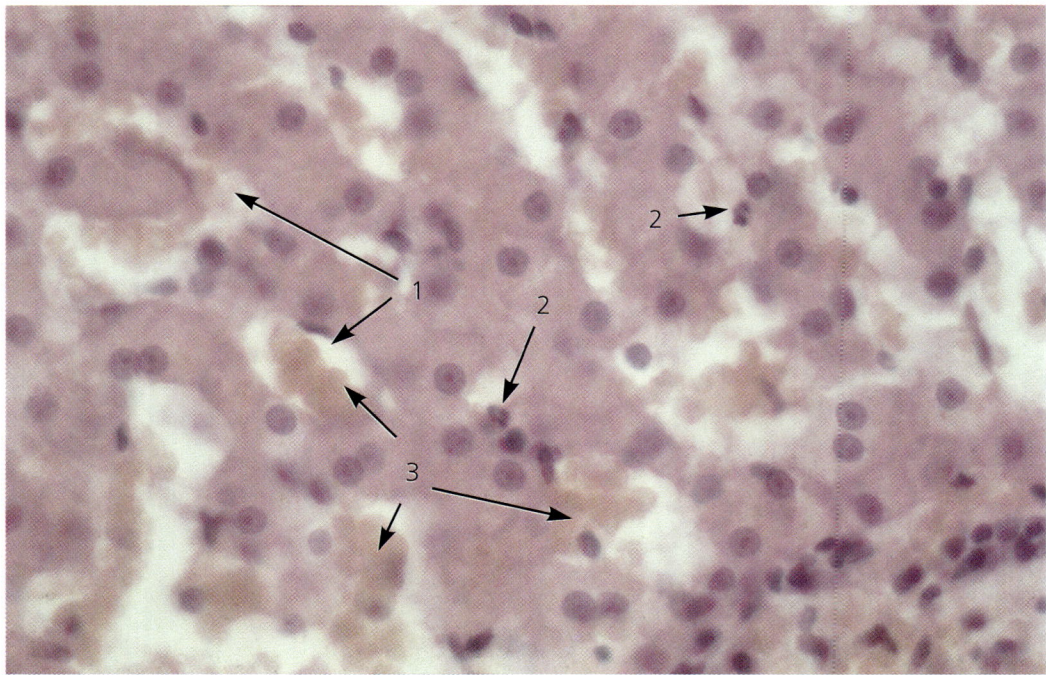

Fig. 9.4.4[1]. 30 min after the single freeze-thaw cycle at a temperature of −180°C. Biopsy from the border between the cryonecrosis and healthy tissue. Wide sinusoids (1) with erythrocytes (3) and view of inflammation cells (2). Hematoxylin and eosin staining. Magnification × 600

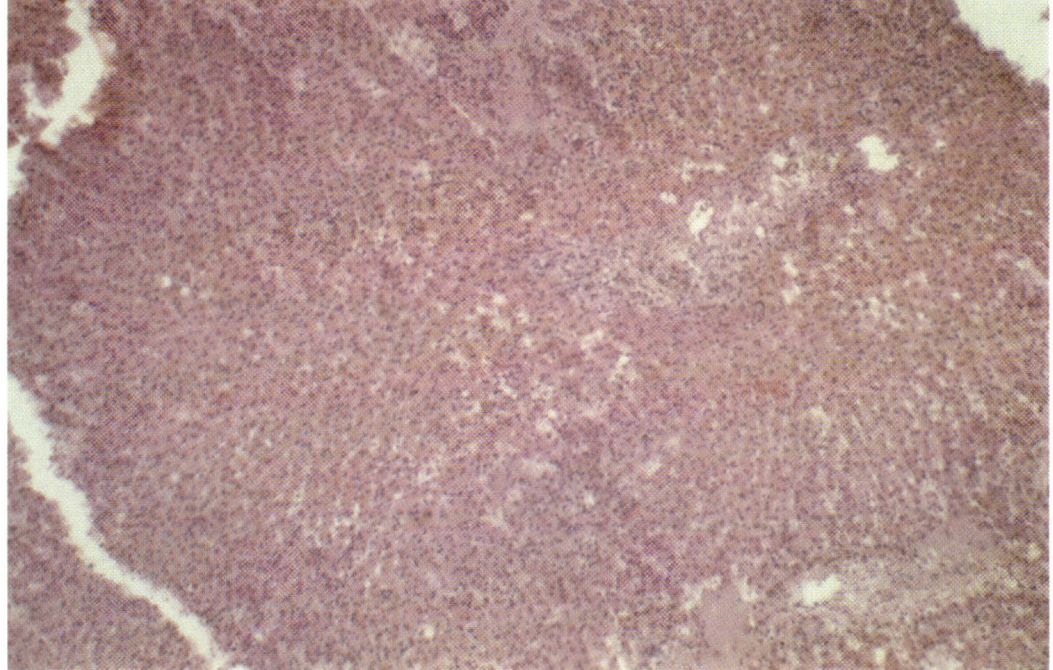

Fig. 9.4.5[1]. 1 h after the single freeze-thaw cycle at a temperature of −180°C. Biopsy from the center of the cryonecrosis. Cryonecrosis with immigration of inflammation cells. Hematoxylin and eosin staining. Magnification × 100

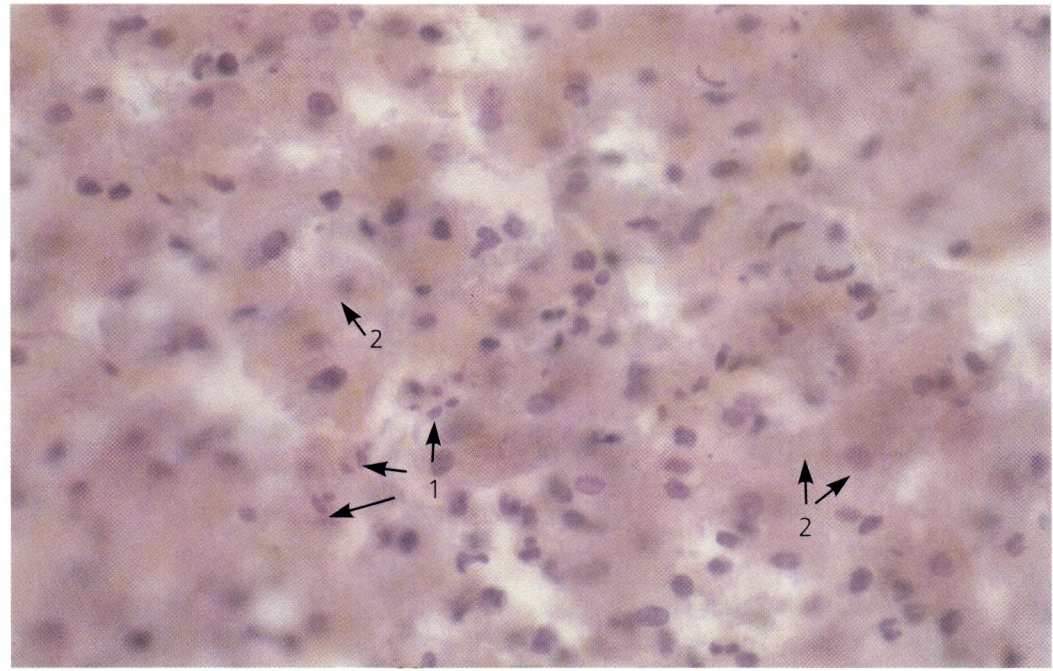

Fig. 9.4.6[1]. 1 h after the single freeze-thaw cycle at a temperature of −180°C. Biopsy from the center of the cryonecrosis. Cryonecrosis with inflammatory cells (1), cell destruction and cell boundaries recognizable in shadows only (2). Hematoxylin and eosin staining. Magnification × 600

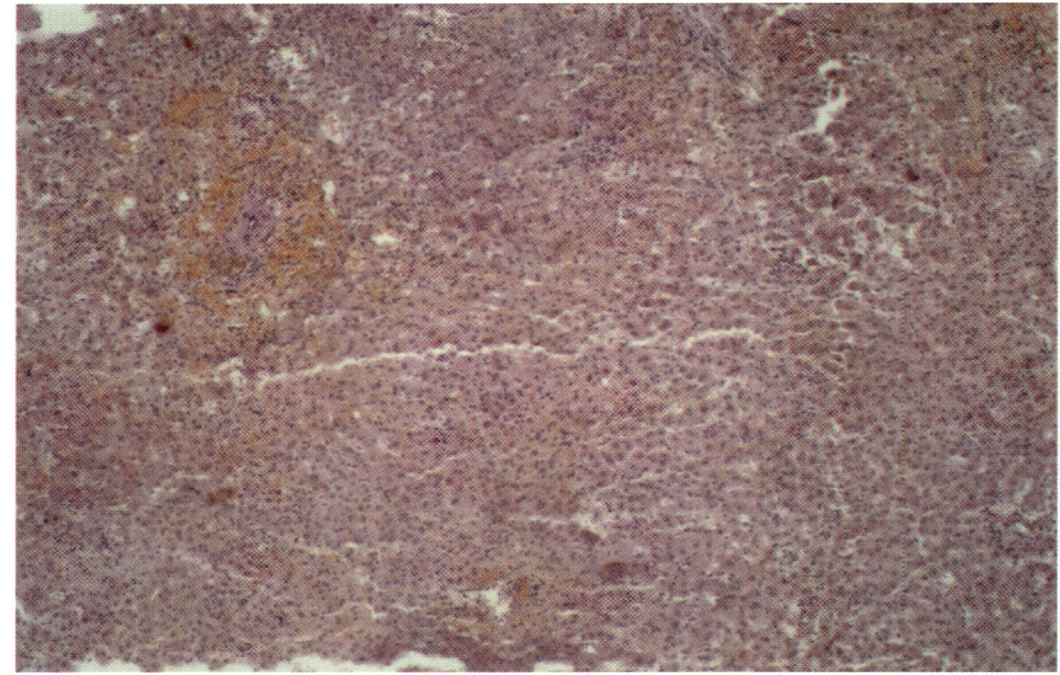

Fig. 9.4.7[1]. 1 h after the single freeze-thaw cycle at a temperature of −180°C. Biopsy from the border between the cryonecrosis and healthy tissue. Transition zone between cryonecrosis (top left) and surviving liver tissue (bottom right). Hematoxylin and eosin staining. Magnification × 100

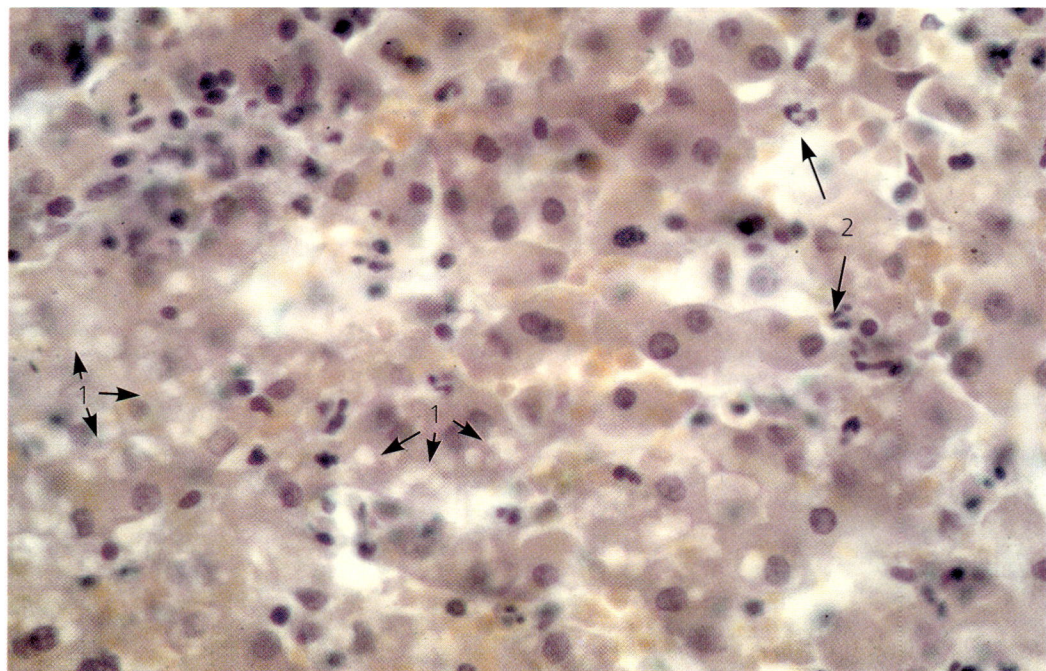

Fig. 9.4.8[1]. 1 h after the single freeze-thaw cycle at a temperature of −180°C. Biopsy from the border between the cryonecrosis and healthy tissue. Foaming vacuolization of the hepatocytes (1), inflammatory infiltration (2). Hematoxylin and eosin staining. Magnification × 600

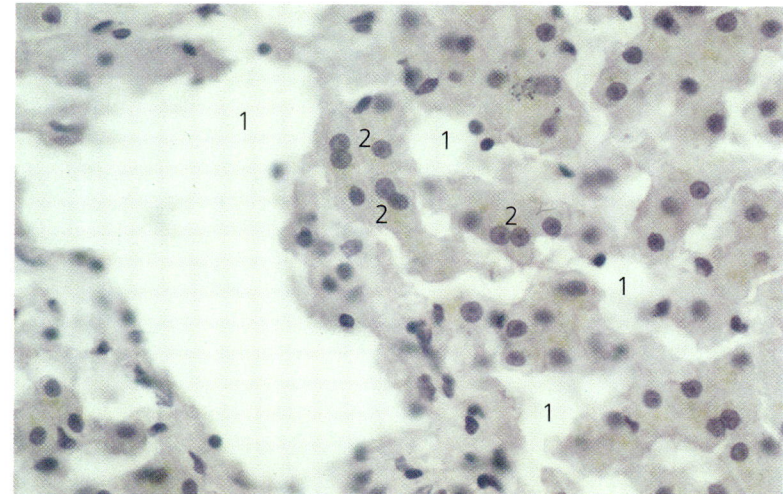

Fig. 9.4.9[1]. 30 min after the single freeze-thaw cycle at a temperature of −60°C. Biopsy from the center of the cryonecrosis. Wide sinusoids (1). Double nucleated hepatocytes (2). Hematoxylin and eosin staining. Magnification × 600

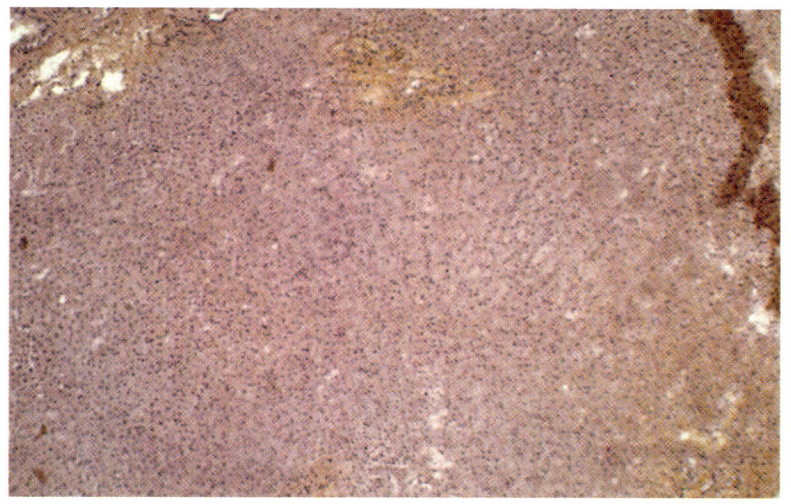

Fig. 9.4.10[1]. 30 min after the single freeze-thaw cycle at a temperature of −60°C. Biopsy from the border between the cryonecrosis and healthy tissue. Transition between cryonecrosis (right) and remaining liver parenchyma (left). Hematoxylin and eosin staining. Magnification × 100

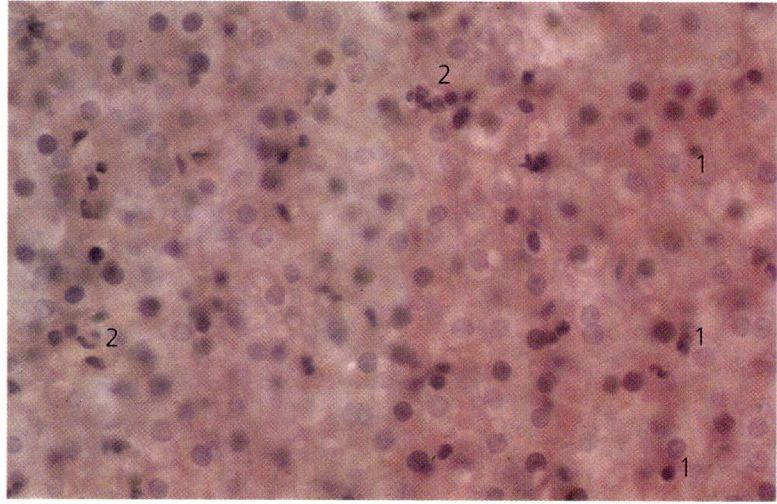

Fig. 9.4.11[1]. 30 min after the single freeze-thaw cycle at a temperature of −60°C. Biopsy from the border between the cryonecrosis and healthy tissue. Individual pyknotic nuclei (1), inflammation cells (2). Hematoxylin and eosin staining. Magnification × 600

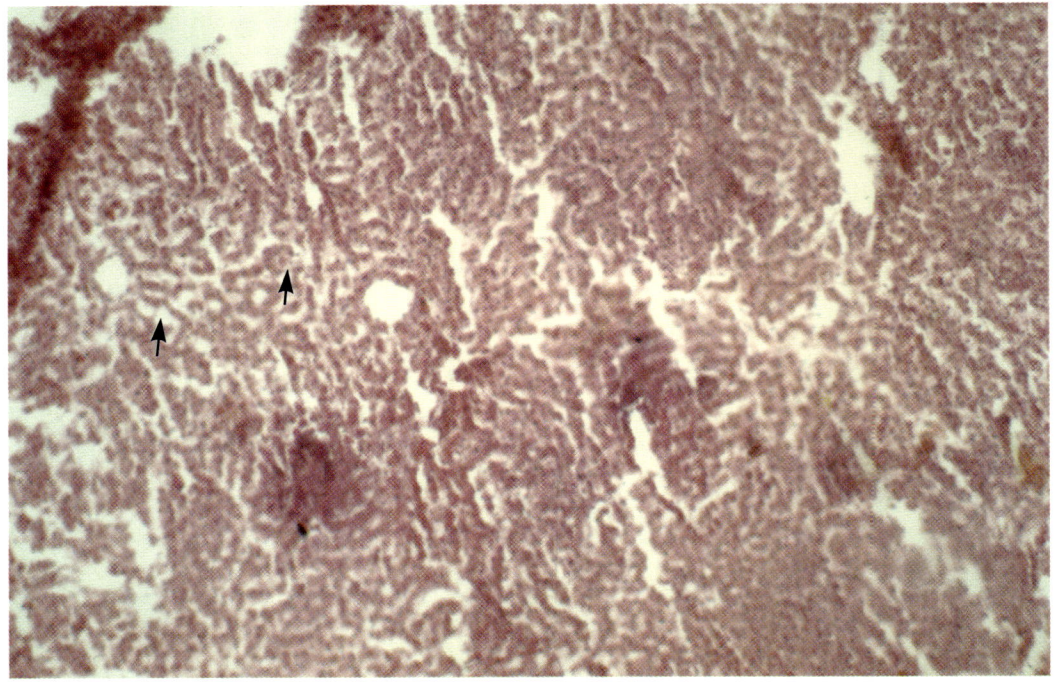

Fig. 9.4.12[1]. 1 h after the single freeze-thaw cycle at a temperature of −60°C. Biopsy from the center of the cryonecrosis. Still recognizable structure with wide sinusoids (↑). Hematoxylin and eosin staining. Magnification × 100

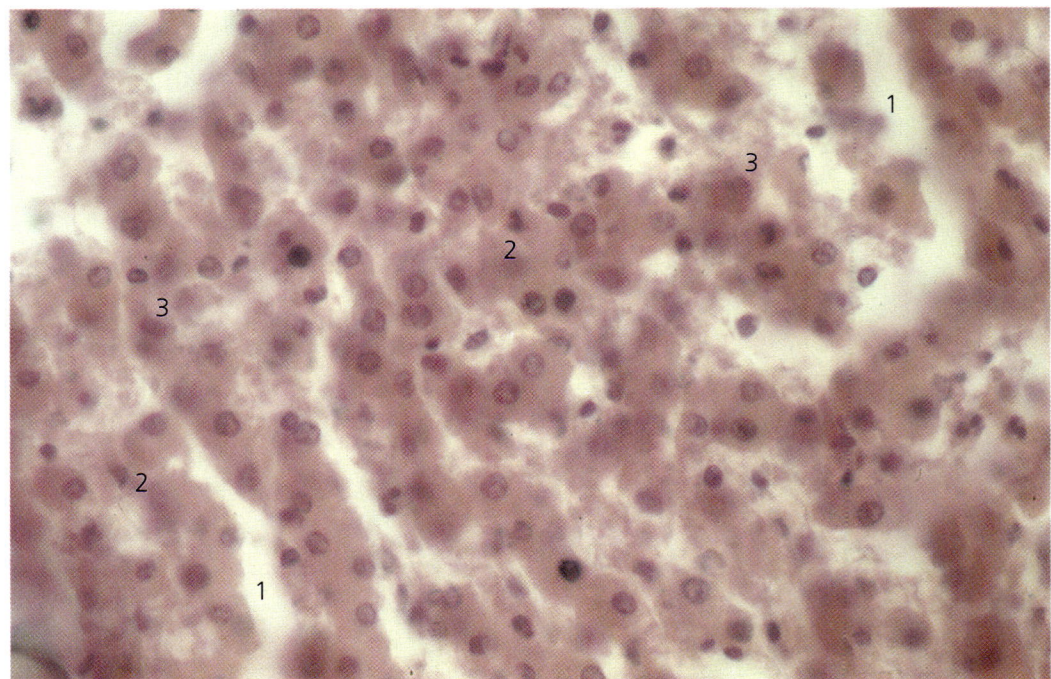

Fig. 9.4.13[1]. 1 h after the single freeze-thaw cycle at a temperature of −60°C. Biopsy from the center of the cryonecrosis. Wide sinus (1), pyknosis (2) of nucleus and individual cell destruction (3). Hematoxylin and eosin staining. Magnification × 600

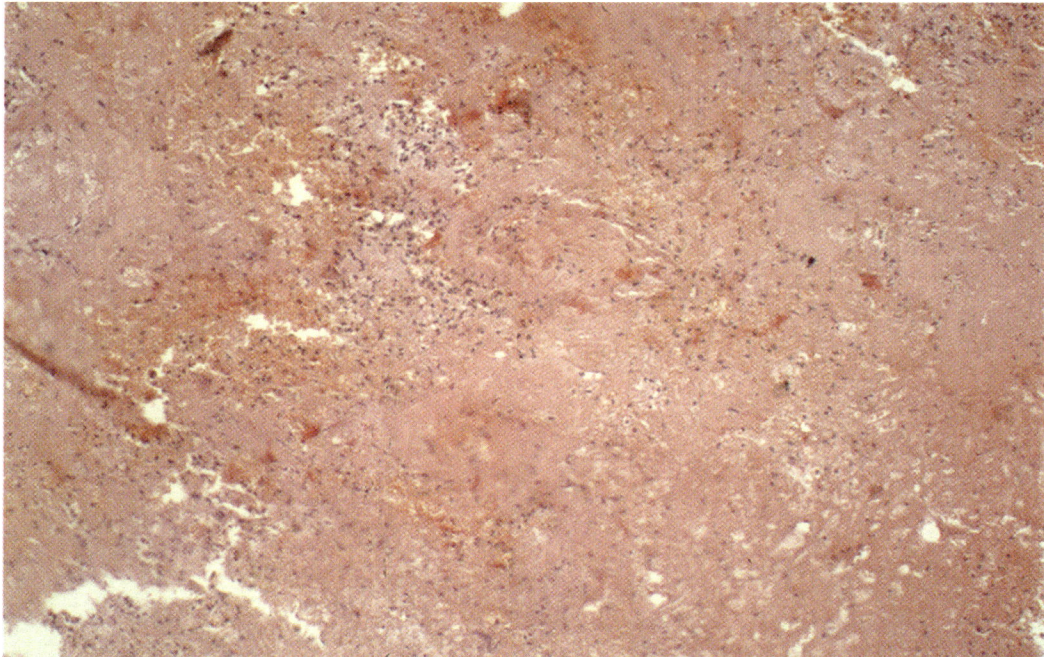

Fig. 9.4.14[1]. 1 h after the single freeze-thaw cycle at a temperature of −60°C. Biopsy from the border between the cryonecrosis and healthy tissue. Total necrosis. Hematoxylin and eosin staining. Magnification × 100

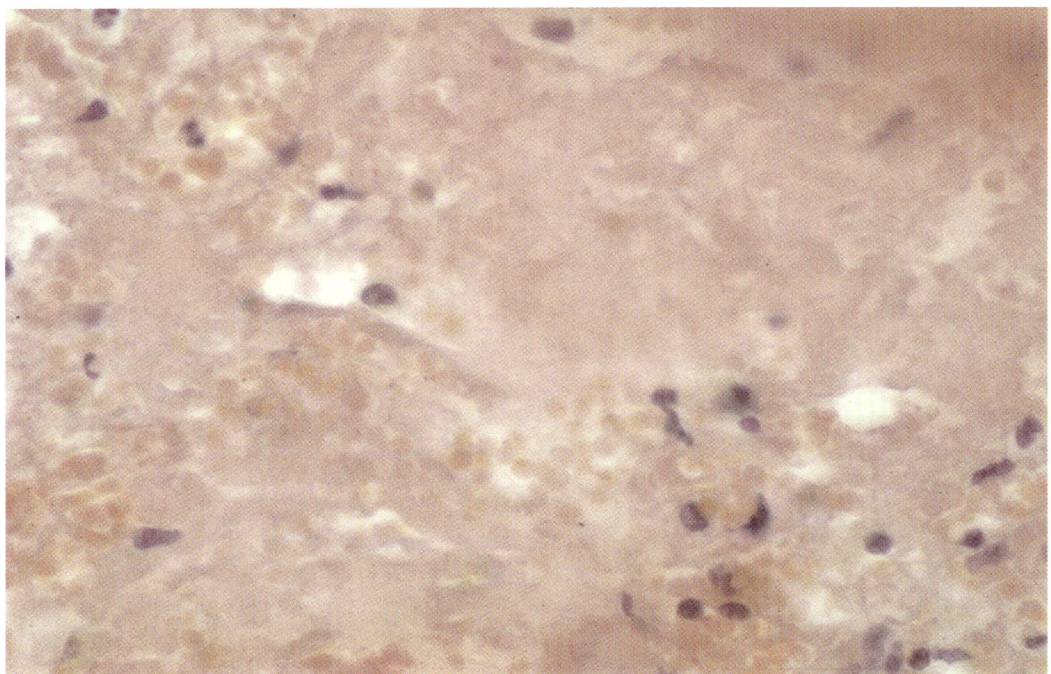

Fig. 9.4.15[1]. 1 h after the single freeze-thaw cycle at a temperature of −60°C. Biopsy from the border between the cryonecrosis and healthy tissue. The cellular reaction is weak. Hematoxylin and eosin staining. Magnification × 600

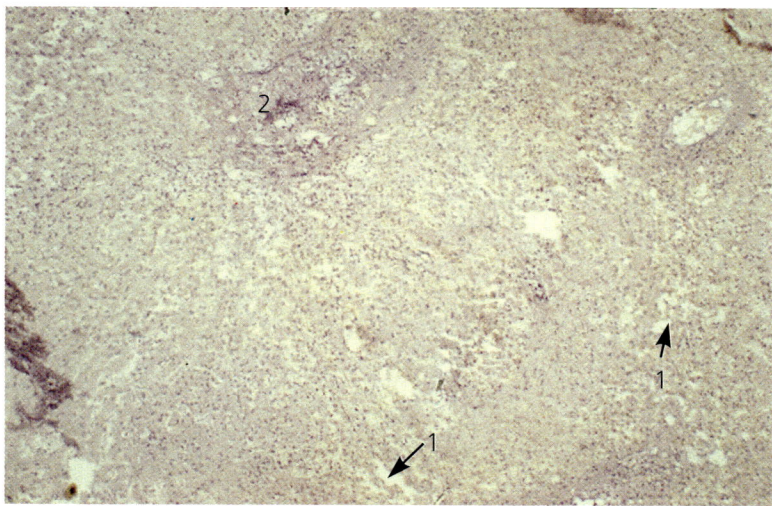

Fig. 9.4.16[1]. 24 h after the single freeze-thaw cycle at a temperature of −180°C. Biopsy from the border between the cryonecrosis and healthy tissue. Cryonecrosis with structure that is recognizable in shadow only, wide sinus (1) and periportal fields (2) without any recognizable individual structures. Hematoxylin and eosin staining. Magnification × 100

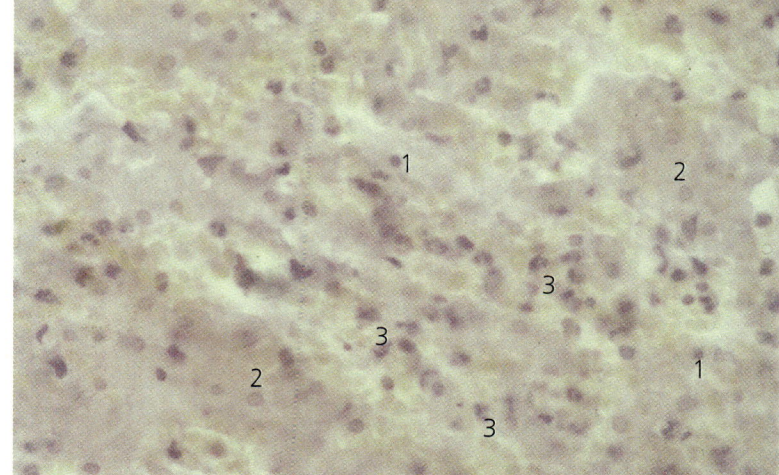

Fig. 9.4.17[1]. 24 h after the single freeze-thaw cycle at a temperature of −180°C. Biopsy from the border between the cryonecrosis and healthy tissue. Cryonecrosis with nuclear pyknosis (1), loss of cellular boundaries (2) and inflammatory infiltration (3). Hematoxylin and eosin staining. Magnification × 600

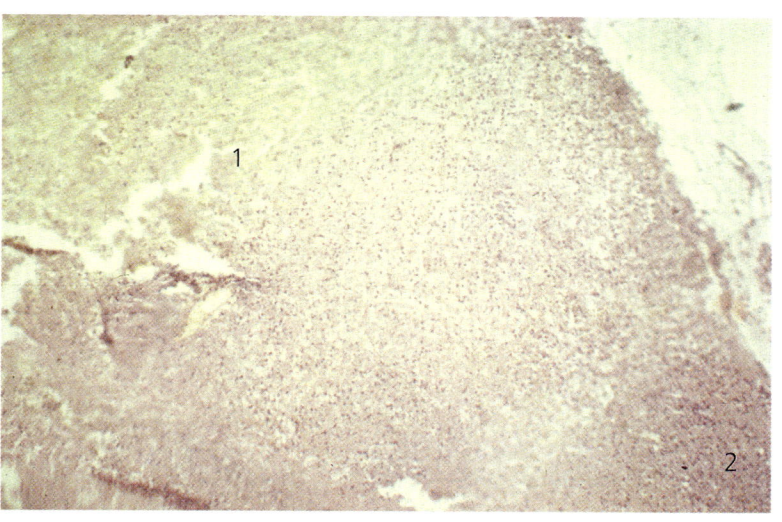

Fig. 9.4.18[1]. 24 h after the single freeze-thaw cycle at a temperature of −60°C. Biopsy from the board between the cryonecrosis and healthy tissue. Coagulation necrosis with extravasions of erythrocytes (1) and transition in still recognizable liver tissue (2) (bottom right). Partial destruction as a result of coagulation necrosis. Hematoxylin and eosin staining. Magnification × 100

Pancreas Cryosurgery. An Animal Experiment

*Nikolai N. Korpan
with contributions by
Iwan S. Tchekman, Jaroslav V. Zharkov
and Franz Beer*

10.0 Introduction

In recent years, the application of cryogenic techniques for the resection of parenchymal organs and *in situ* ablation of tumors using sub-zero temperatures has been studied. The process of freezing in healthy livers and human liver tumors has also been examined.

The renaissance of cryosurgery in the 1990s has also stimulated experimental and clinical cryosurgical research in different medical fields. The advances in cryosurgical technology have encouraged interest in applying cryosurgery in the treatment of pancreatic diseases, particularly pancreatic malignancies.

It has been suggested that cryoablation should be carried out for a pancreatic tumor deemed unresectable. Cryosurgery might become a significant adjunct in the treatment of inoperable pancreatic neoplasms, especially since analgesia results directly from the freezing process. To date there have been no morphological studies on the response of normal and pathological pancreatic tissue to cryosurgical exposure. In the literature to date there is no definition of the *in vivo* sensitivities of pancreatic parenchyma to different cryosurgical exposures, and the minimum temperature required to cause adequate cryodestruction and thus prevent tumor recurrence has not yet been defined.

The experimental basis for pancreatic cryosurgery has not yet been sufficiently discussed.

The existing inadequacy in the treatment of pancreatic malignancies prompted this investigation of the pathohistological consequences of freezing animal pancreata.
The effect of temperature application in the freeze-thawing process and the cryosurgical response in normal pancreatic tissue in animal experiments are presented in this chapter as a basis for evaluating the cryosurgical technique as a treatment option in pancreatic diseases, particularly pancreatic tumors.

This is the first time ever that the phenomenon described in the following, which we have called 'lunar eclipse', has been observed macroscopically. Immediately after freezing, during the thawing process, the snow-white pancreas parenchyma, frozen hard to an ice-block, and resembling a full moon with a sharp demarcation line, gradually took on a ruby-red shade and hemispherical shape as it grew in size in the direction of blood flow. This snow-white cryogenic lesion dissolved in the same way in all of the animals.

Chapter 10 Pancreas Cryosurgery

10.1 Pancreatic Cryosurgery: Experimental Basis

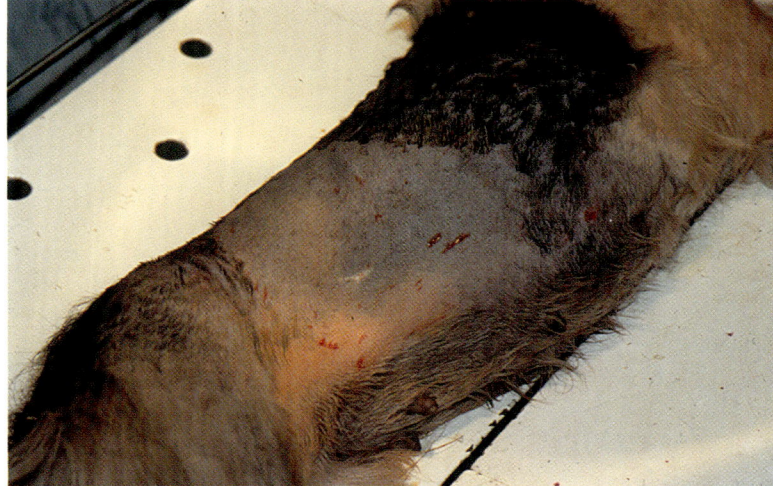

Fig. 10.1.1. Experimental freezing of a dog pancreas. Preparation for access to operating area on pancreas (**A, B**)

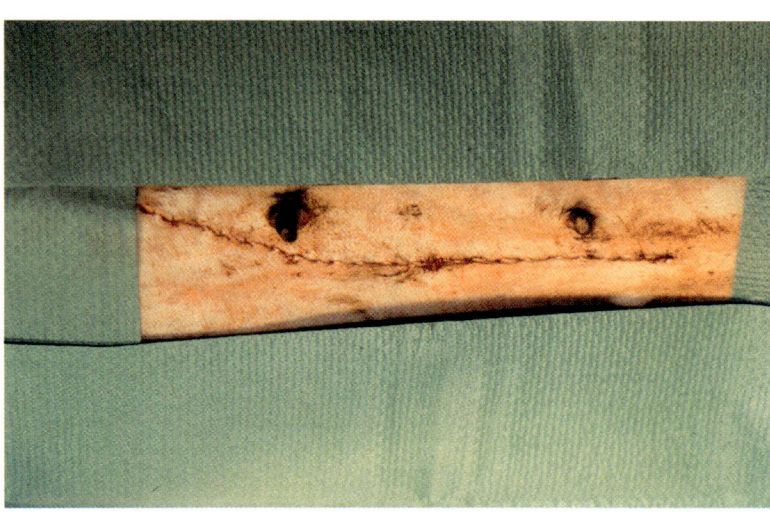

Fig. 10.1.2. Laparotomy with oblique abdominal section using an incision curved like a hockey-stick in the direction of the left costal arch

Section E   Experimental Aspects

Chapter 10
Pancreas
Cryosurgery

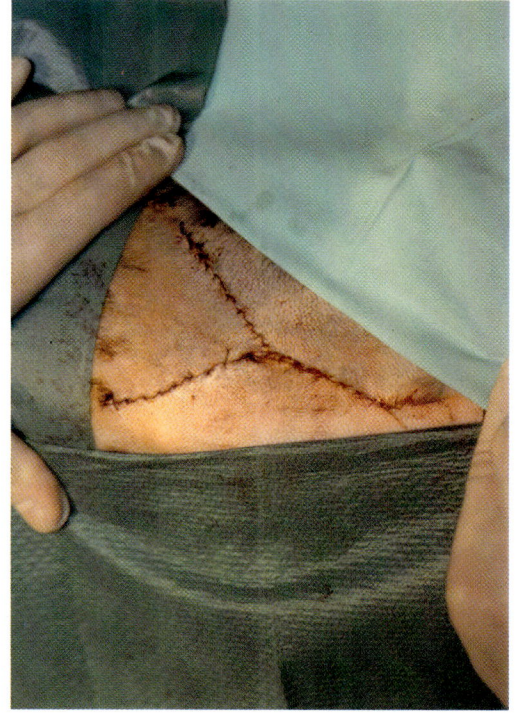

Fig. 10.1.3. Laparotomy with oblique abdominal section using a fork-shaped incision to both costal arches

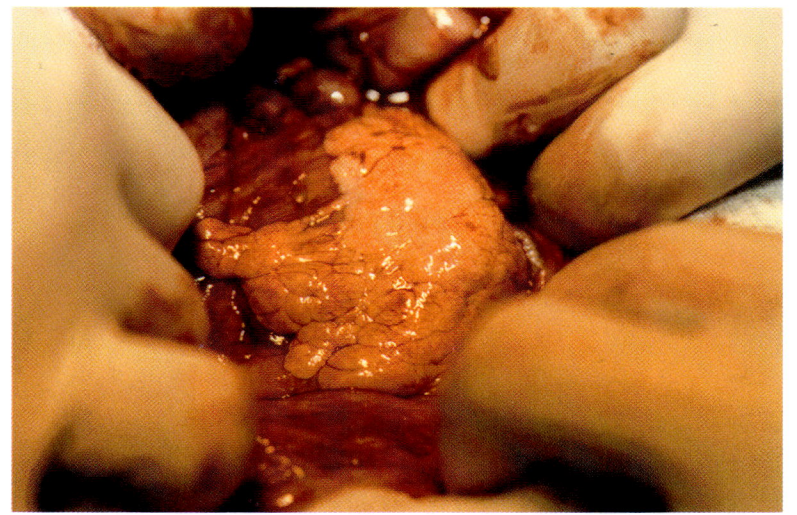

Fig. 10.1.4. Appearance of a dog pancreas before cryosurgery

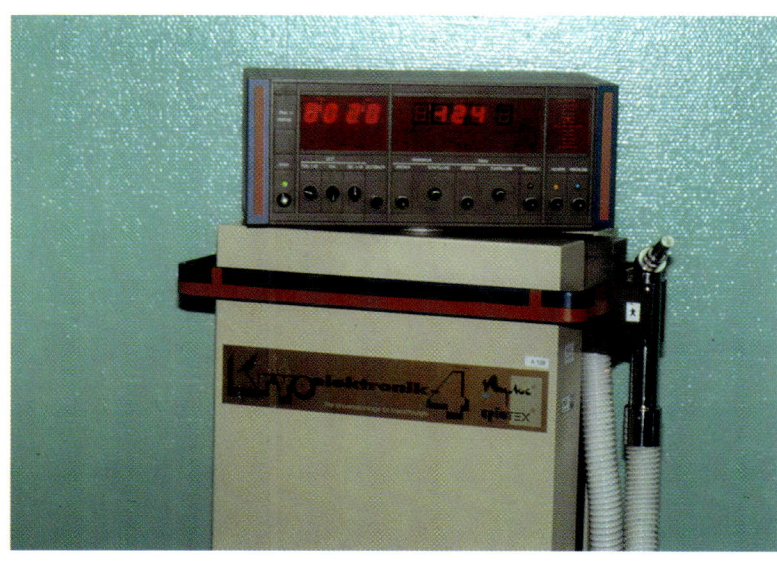

Fig. 10.1.5. The technique of cryosurgery. The cryosurgical unit is a liquid nitrogen-based universal system (Cryotechnological Research Company "Pulse", Kiev, Ukraine)

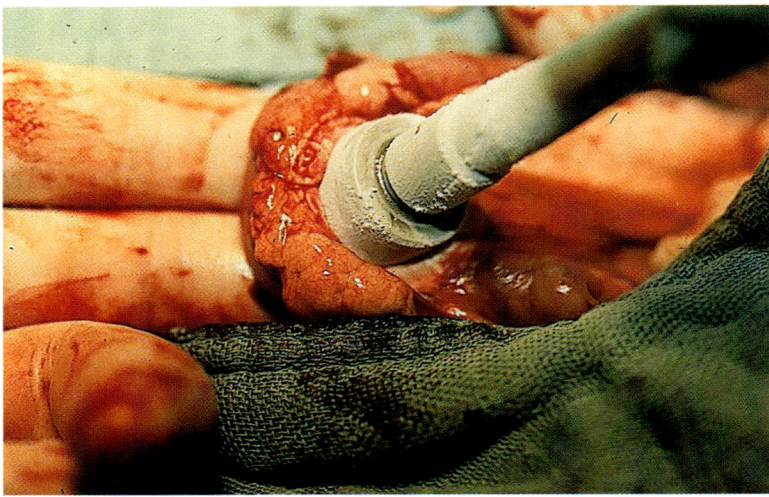

Fig. 10.1.6. Cryosurgical application. The technique of cryosurgery, showing a disc probe with a diameter of 15 mm which is placed on the pancreas at a temperature of −180°C for 9 min using a single freeze-thaw cycle to induce aseptic cryonecrosis (tissue destruction)

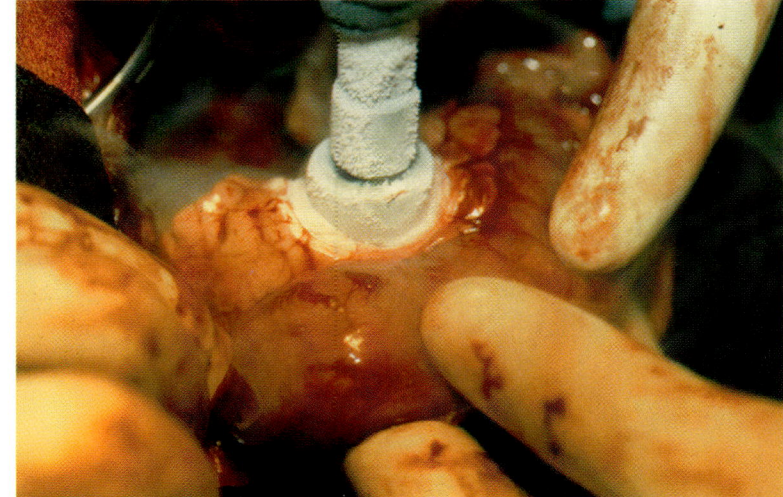

Fig. 10.1.7. Formation of an ice ball with the cryozone line of demarcation around the cryoprobe

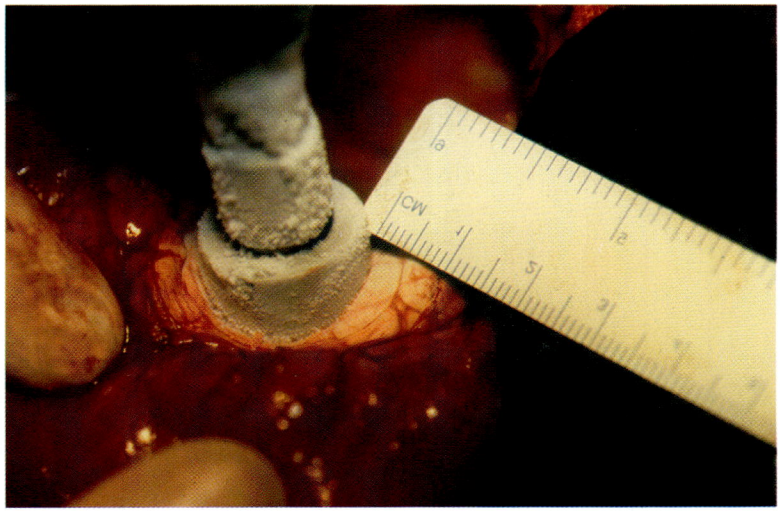

Fig. 10.1.8. The cryozone including a 12 mm margin to the surrounding, normal-looking pancreas parenchyma

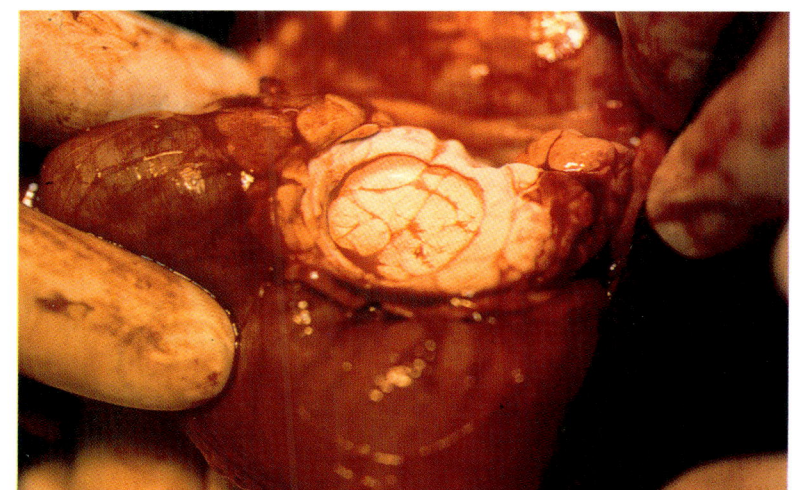

Fig. 10.1.9. Appearance of a cryozone *immediately* after cryosurgical session with the ice crater in the middle and the ice margin with the line of demarcation

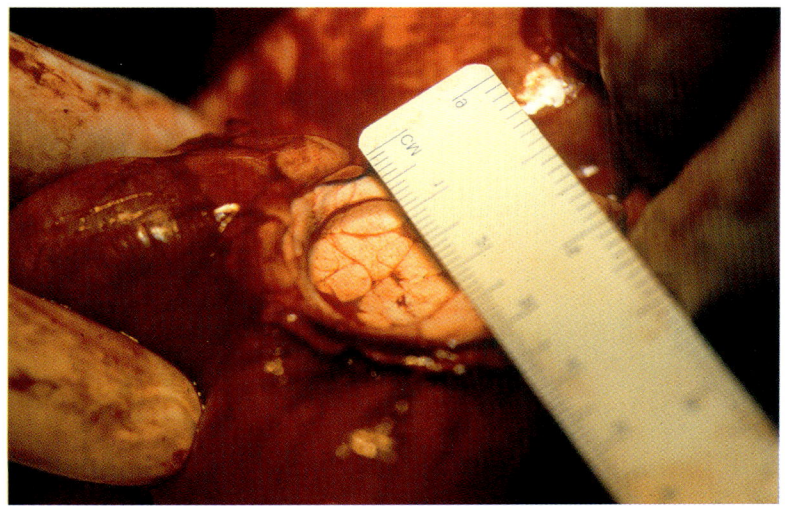

Fig. 10.1.10. The cryozone measures 39 mm in diameter after a single freeze-thaw cycle with a cryoprobe 15 mm in diameter at a temperature of −180°C for 9 min

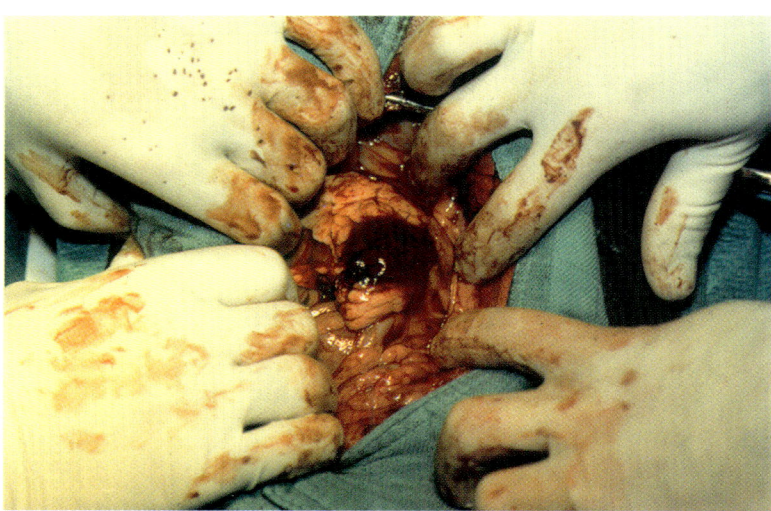

Fig. 10.1.11. Post-cryosurgical view. *Immediately* after the full thawing of a pancreas parenchyma cryozone

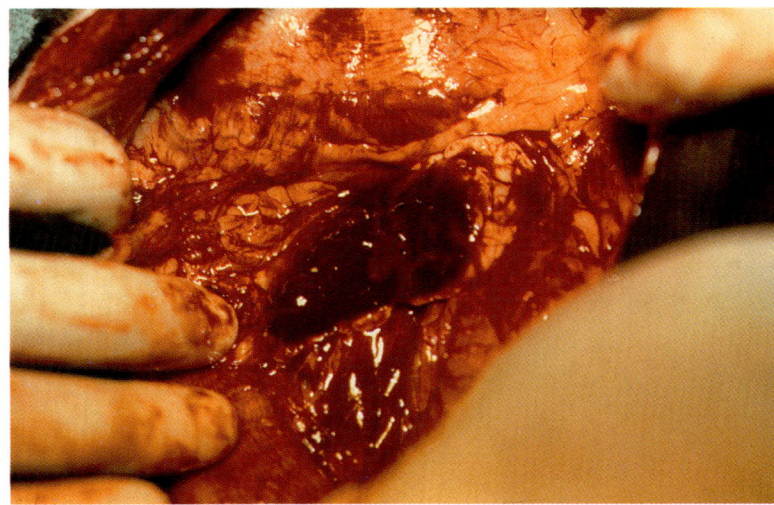

Fig. 10.1.12. Appearance of a cryosurgical necrosis *immediately* after the multiple biopsies from the margin between the frozen and normal pancreas parenchyma and from the middle of the cryonecrosis *immediately* after the biopsy

Fig. 10.1.13. Intraoperative monitoring of pancreas cryosurgery. Intraoperative ultrasound of the pancreas: before (**A**), during and after (**B**) cryosurgical session

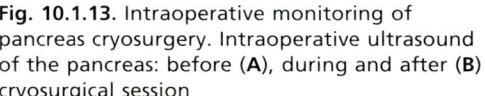

A

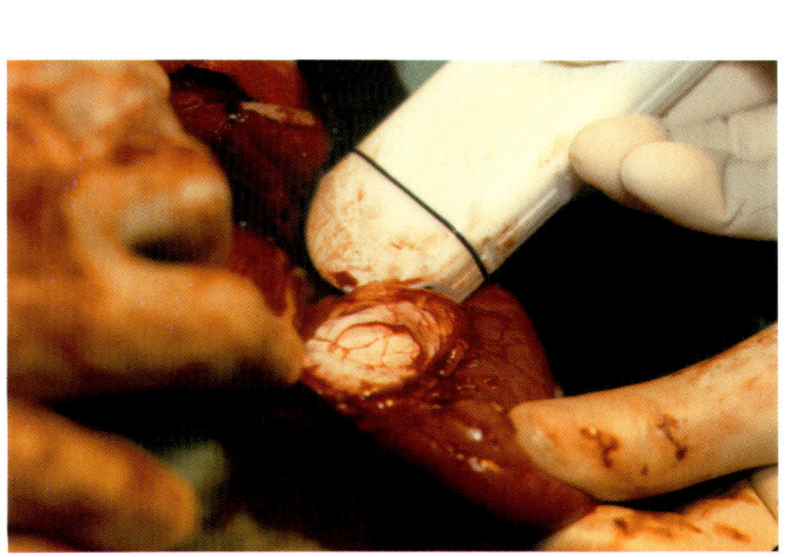

B

Section E   Experimental Aspects   143

Chapter 10
Pancreas
Cryosurgery

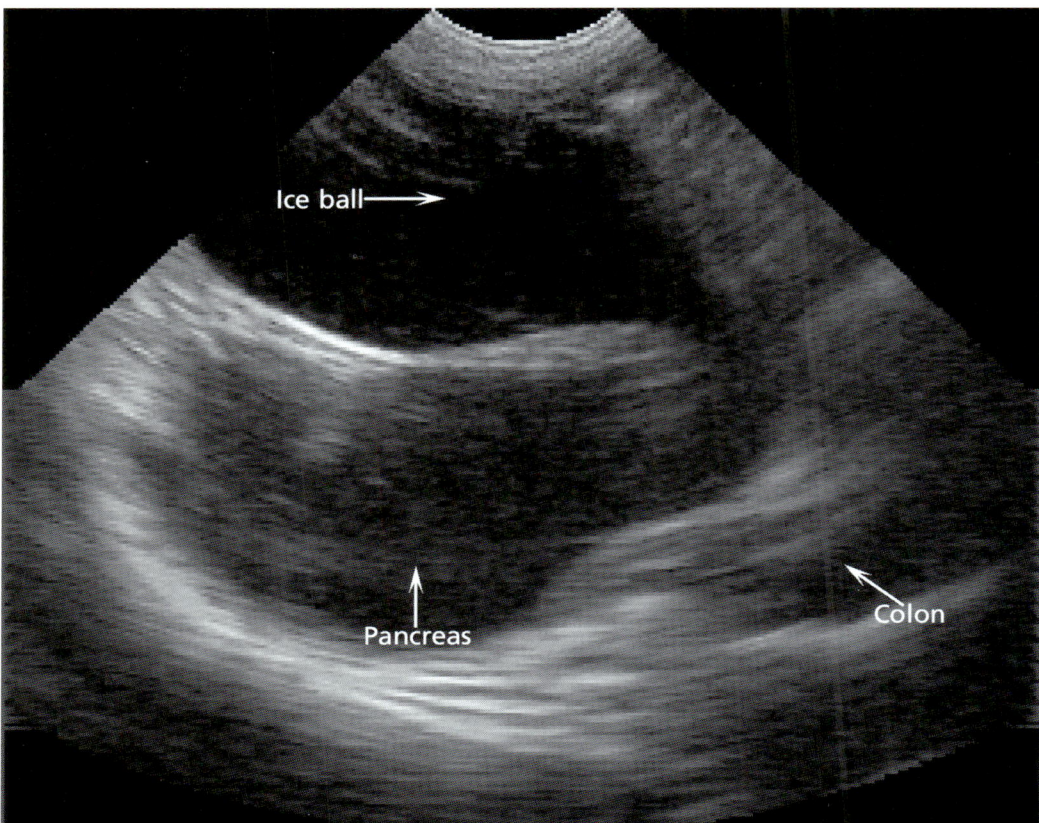

Fig. 10.1.14. Intraoperative ultrasound monitoring of pancreas cryosurgery. The hyperechoic rim of the frozen front and postacoustic shadowing are evident. The cryosurgical area measures 30.7 mm × 60 mm after application of a cryoprobe 15 mm in diameter at a temperature of −180°C for 5 min

Chapter 10 Pancreas Cryosurgery

10.2 The 'Lunar Eclipse' Phenomenon

The phenomenon of the lunar eclipse is a rare feature in nature. To be able to watch it with your own eyes certainly belongs to the most astonishing experiences in life. Thus, it was remarkable and indeed unique to observe something like a lunar eclipse in real life but 'transferred' into the field of medicine. For the first time in medical history, this phenomenon was observed by the author during the course of experimental cryosurgery on an animal pancreas. The scientific data which are presented in this book may be not only of interest to specialists in different fields of science (experimental and practical medicine, cryomedicine, including cryosurgery, cryobiology, physics, particularly the physics of low temperatures, and cryogenic technology) but also to the general public.

A recent study of the freezing process in healthy livers and in human liver tumors has shown that when liquid nitrogen was used as the freezing liquid, it was possible to destroy local parenchyma. This study shows the effect of different temperature applications on the freeze-thawing process, and the response of normal pancreas tissue in animal experiments to cryosurgical exposure, with the objective of evaluating the cryosurgical technique as an optional treatment of diseases of the pancreas, primarily of pancreas tumors.

This is the first time that the effect of freeze-thawing processes with different temperature applications on animal pancreatic parenchyma has been investigated. Presented here is the latest experimental study in the field of pancreas cryosurgery, in which a new phenomenon, the 'lunar eclipse' after cryosurgery on the animal pancreas, is shown.

Section E   Experimental Aspects   145

Chapter 10
Pancreas
Cryosurgery

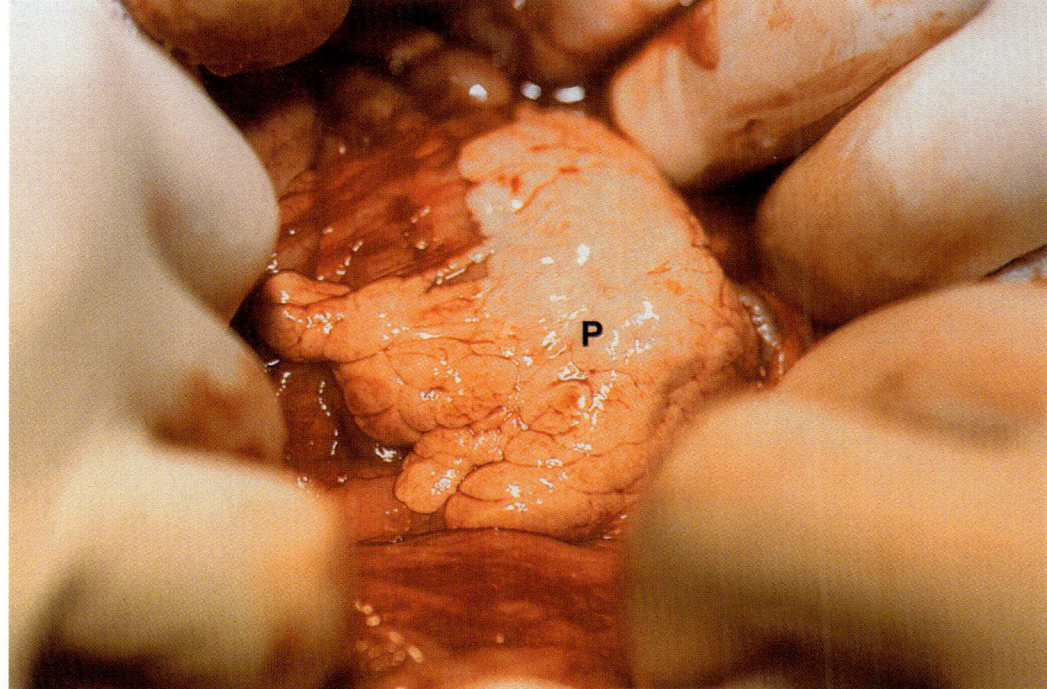

P Pancreas

Fig. 10.2.1. Animal pancreas. View of a dog pancreas before cryosurgery

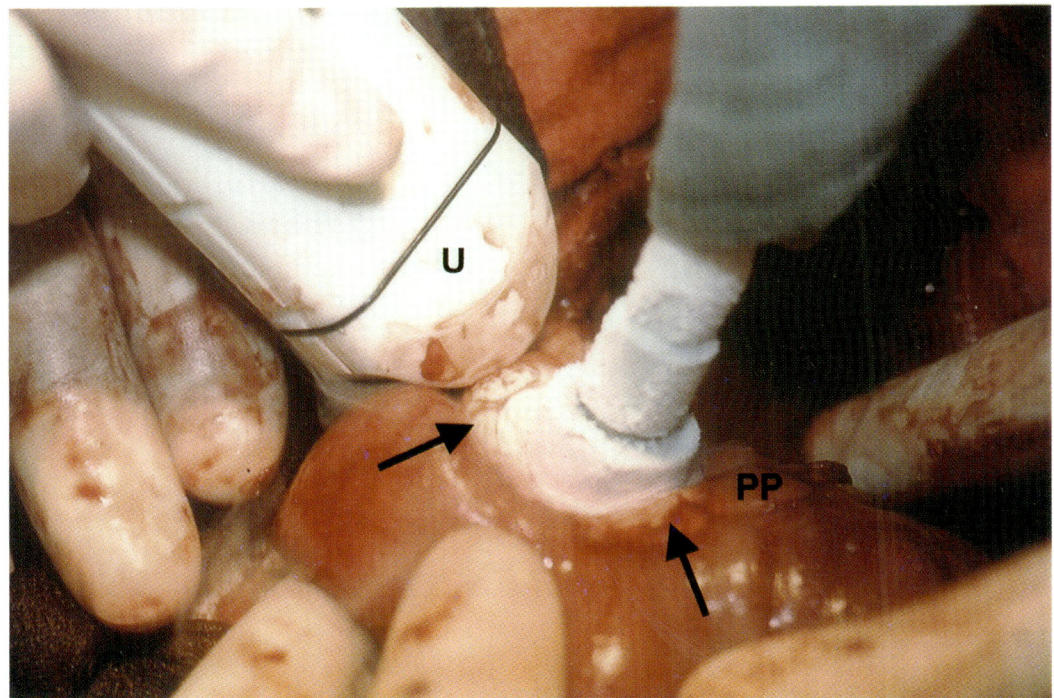

PP Pancreas parenchyma, *U* ultrasound, ← ice-margin

Fig. 10.2.2. Cryosurgical application. The technique of cryosurgery, showing a disc probe with a diameter of 20 mm which is placed on the pancreas at a temperature of −196°C for 9 min in a single freeze-thaw cycle

Chapter 10
Pancreas Cryosurgery

PP Pancreas parenchyma, *CZ* cryozone, *CN* cryonecrosis, 1 ← cryozone demarcation line which corresponds exactly to the diameter of the cryoprobe (inner ring of the cryozone), 2 ← demarcation line between the cryonecrosis and the undamaged pancreas parenchyma (outer ring of the cryozone), a - ice margin between the inner and outer rings of the cryozone

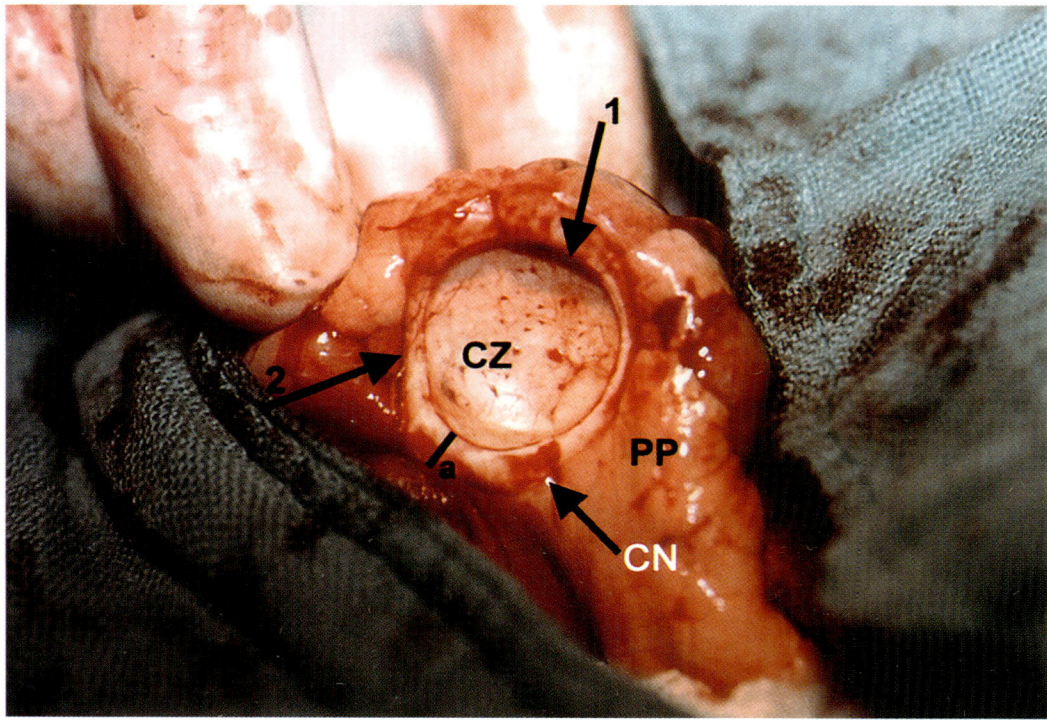

Fig. 10.2.3. Ice ball. View of a cryozone with the ice crater in the middle, and of the ice margin with the line of demarcation around the cryoprobe, *immediately* after the cryosurgical session. The cryozone includes a margin of 7 mm which surrounds the normal-looking pancreas parenchyma

PP Pancreas parenchyma, *CN* cryonecrosis, *CZ* cryozone, 1 ← line of the gradual "coming" the eclipse, 2 ← line of demarcation between the cryonecrosis and the undamaged pancreas parenchyma

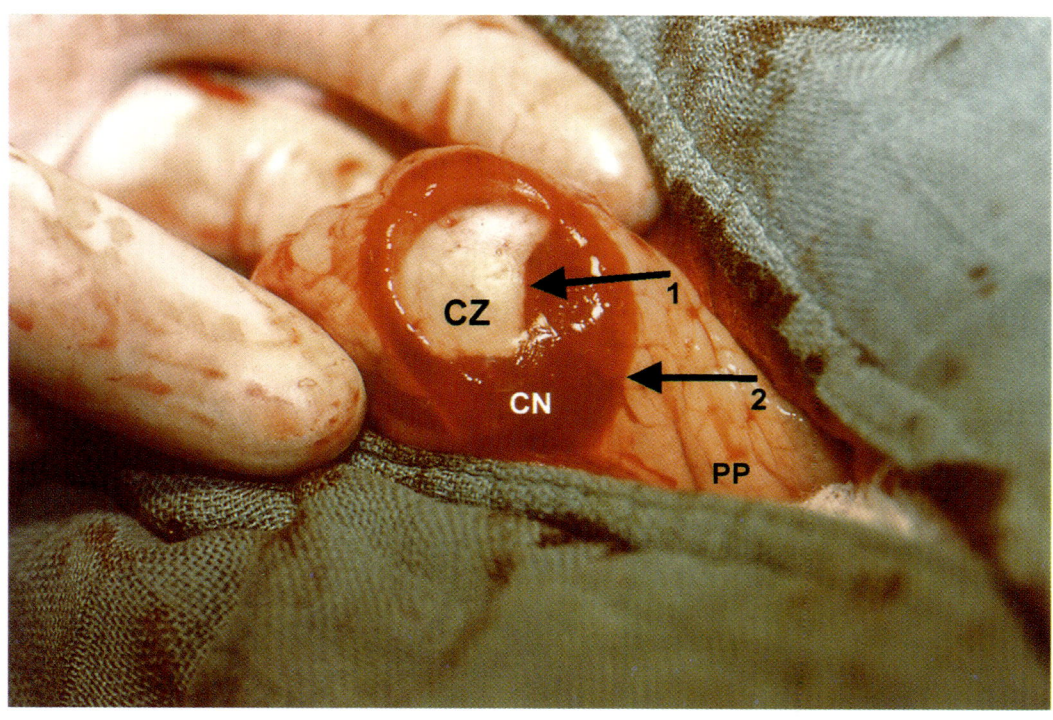

A

Fig. 10.2.4. (A–D). 'Lunar eclipse'. The ice block *immediately* after cryosurgery. Beginning of the 'lunar eclipse'. The set of photographs (A–D) shows the frozen-hard, snow-white ice block of the pancreas parenchyma which resembles a full moon with a sharp demarcation line. It gradually assumes a ruby-red shade and hemispherical shape, increasing in size in the direction of blood flow. This is when the form of the 'lunar eclipse' first appears. **A** Beginning of the 'eclipse'; **B** two-thirds of the cryozone has been taken over by the 'lunar eclipse'; **C** cryonecrosis increases until it covers three-quarters of the cryozone; **D** hardly any imprints are left on the cryozone, - only a pea-shaped area remains

Section E   Experimental Aspects   **147**

Chapter 10
Pancreas
Cryosurgery

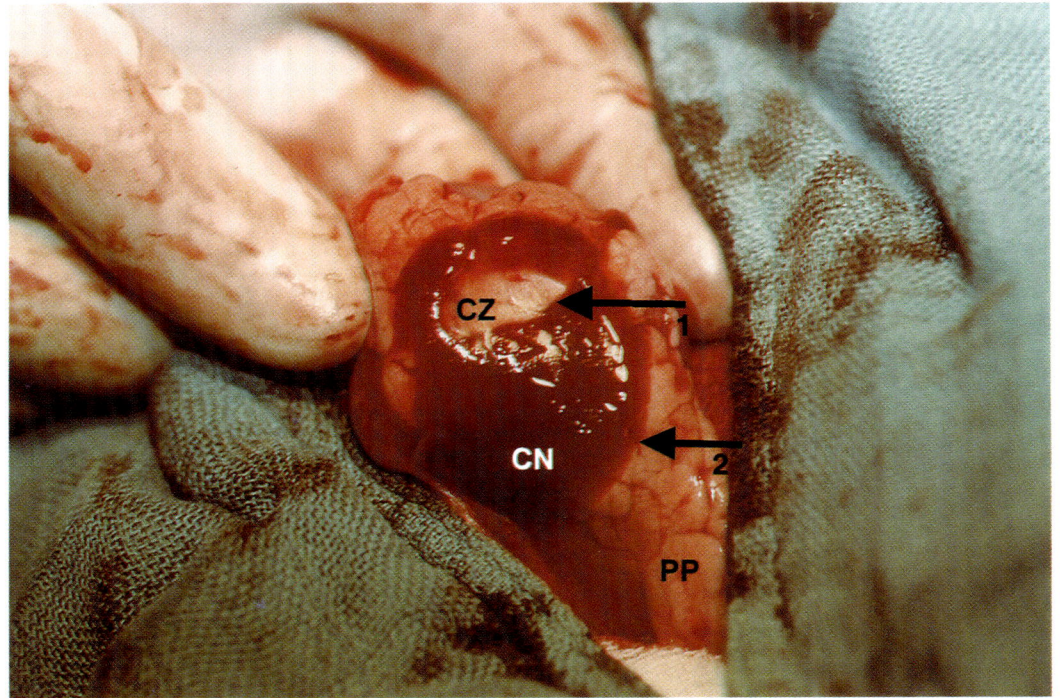

B

Fig. 10.2.4 (*continued*)

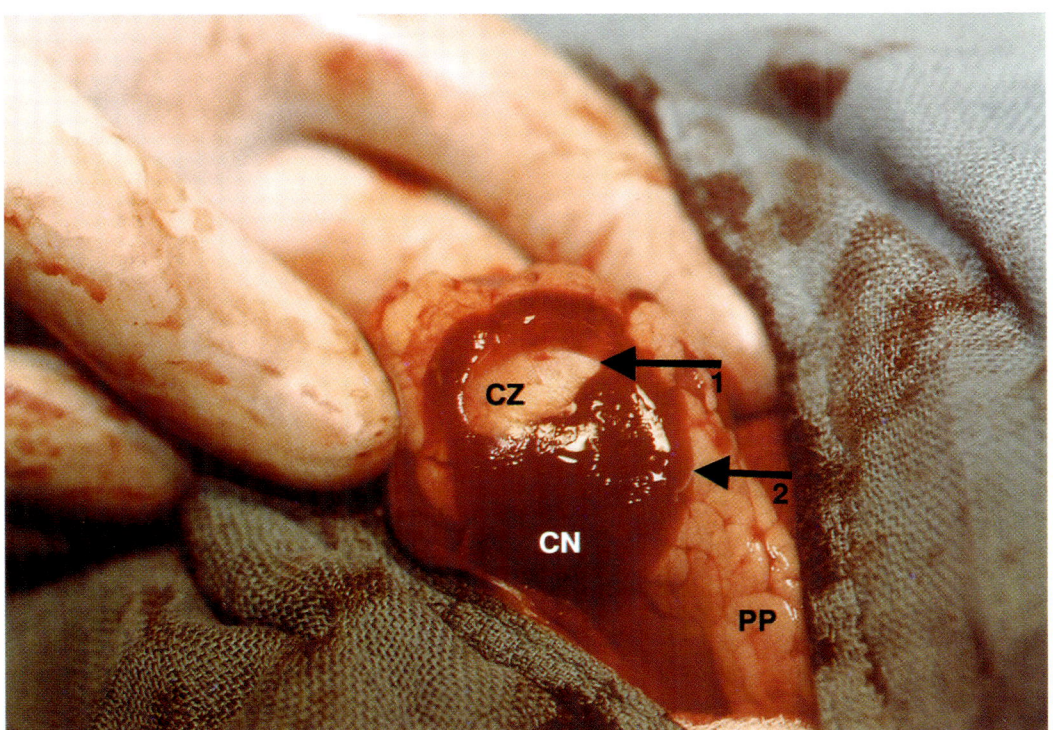

C

PP Pancreas parenchyma, *CN* cryonecrosis, *CZ* cryozone, $_1 \leftarrow$ line of the gradual "coming" the eclipse, $_2 \leftarrow$ line of demarcation between the cryonecrosis and the undamaged pancreas parenchyma

Chapter 10
Pancreas
Cryosurgery

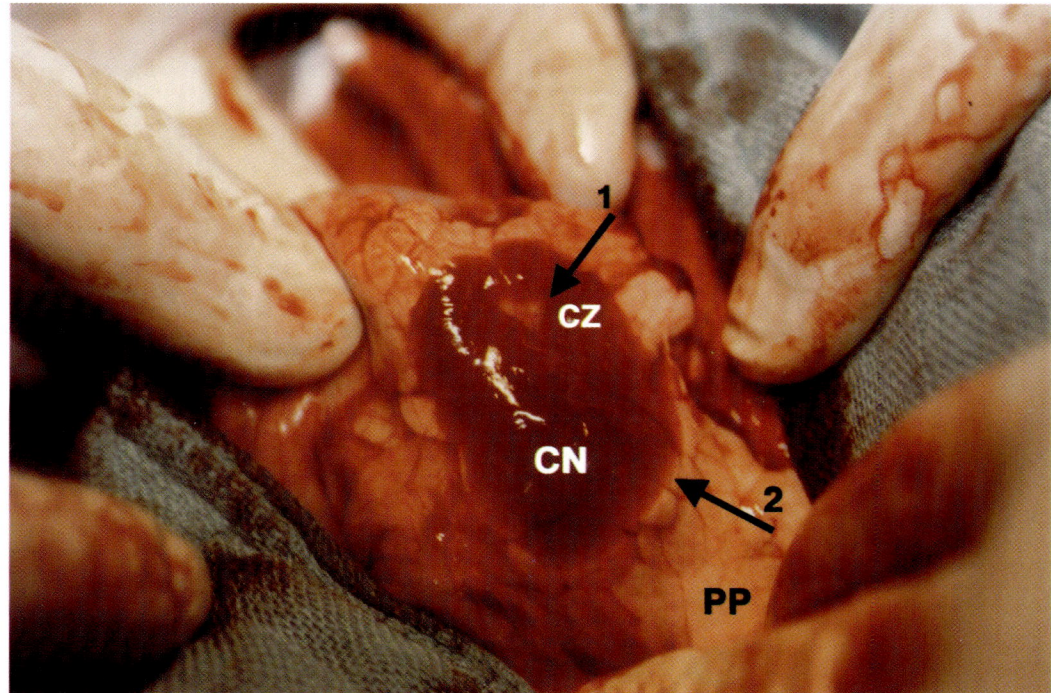

D

Fig. 10.2.4 (continued)

PP Pancreas parenchyma, *CN* cryonecrosis, ← line of demarcation between the cryonecrosis and the undamaged pancreas parenchyma

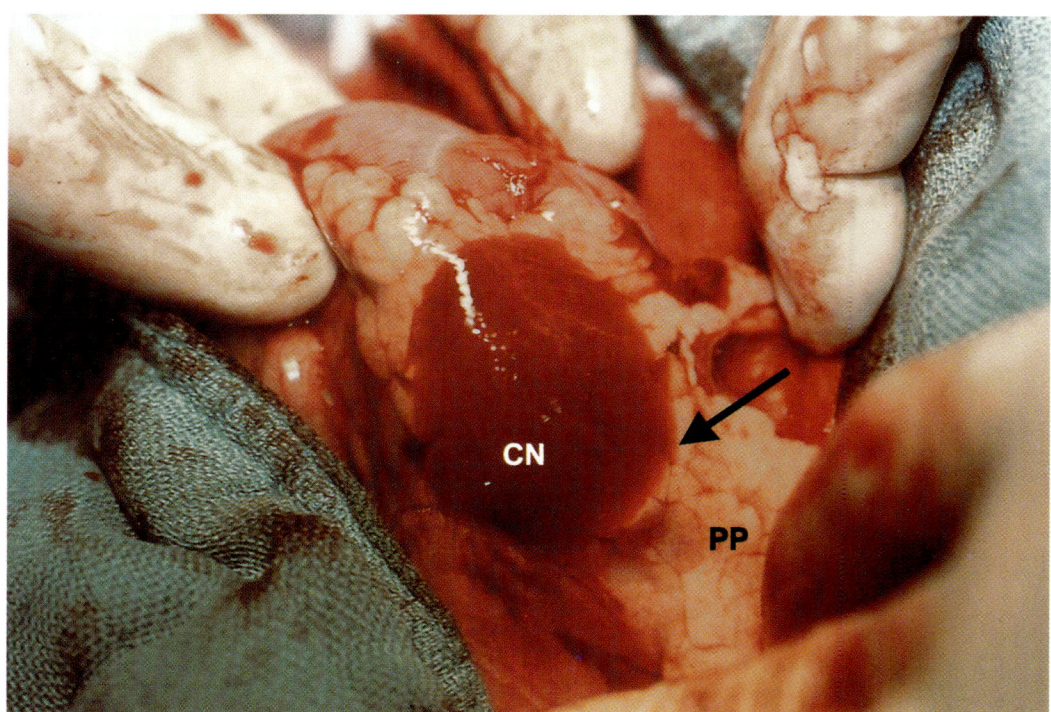

Fig. 10.2.5. Post-cryosurgical view. Immediately after the full thawing of the pancreas parenchyma cryozone. Intense ruby-red shade. The 'lunar eclipse' is complete

Section E Experimental Aspects

10.3 Ultrastructural Changes in Pancreas Tissue

Chapter 10
Pancreas
Cryosurgery

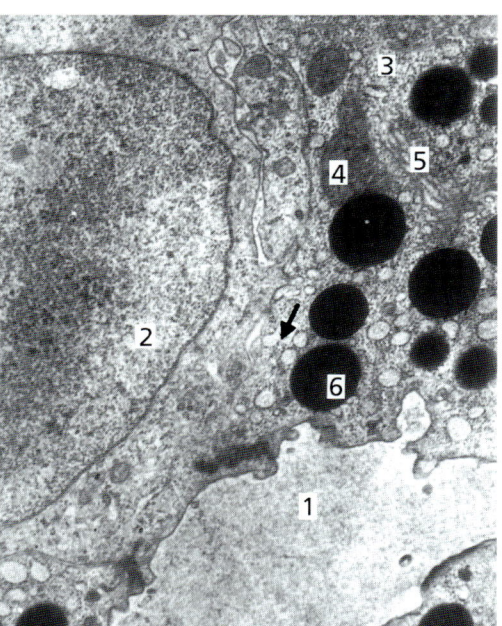

Fig. 10.3.1.a Electron micrograph showing the pancreatic cell with pancreatic acini (1), centro-acinar cell with nucleus (2), exocrine pancreatic cells (3) which have mitochondria (4), Golgi body (5), canaliculi of the rough endoplasmic reticulum (←), zymogen granules (6)

Fig. 10.3.1. (a-d) Dog pancreas cells before cryosurgery which was followed by gradual freezing using liquid nitrogen (at a temperature of −196°C)

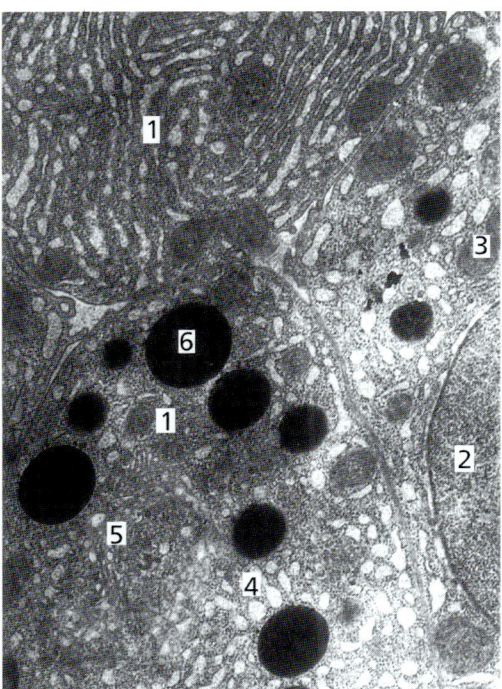

Fig. 10.3.1.b Exocrine pancreatic cells (1). Nucleus with evenly distributed chromatin (2). Mitochondria with a dense electron matrix, and a small number of cristae (3), canaliculi of the rough endoplasmic reticulum (4), Golgi body (5), zymogen granules (6)

Chapter 10
Pancreas Cryosurgery

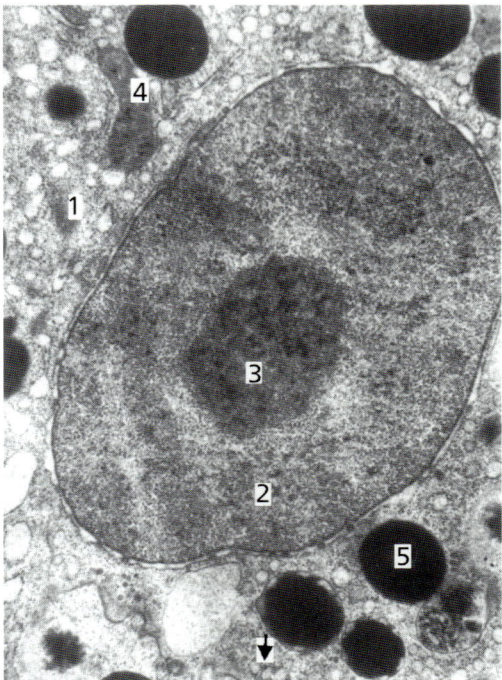

Fig. 10.3.1.c The exocrine pancreatic cell (1). Nucleus (2) with evenly distributed chromatin and nucleolus (3). Mitochondria (4), canaliculi of the rough endoplasmic reticulum (—), zymogen granules (5)

Fig. 10.3.1 (a-d) Dog pancreas cells before cryosurgery which was followed by gradual freezing using liquid nitrogen (at a temperature of −196°C)

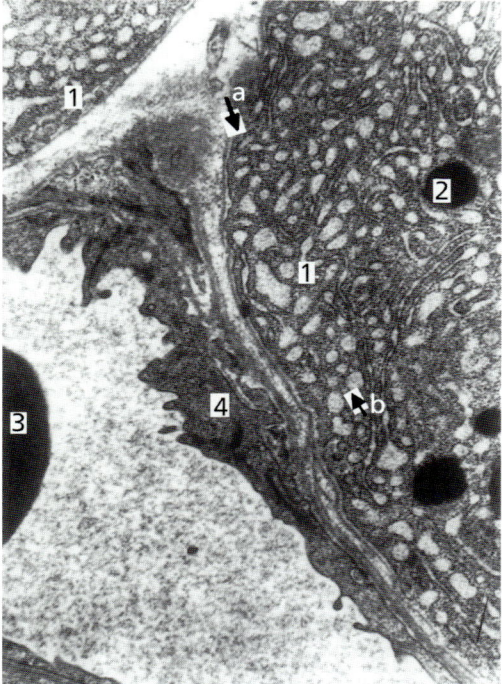

Fig. 10.3.1.d Exocrine pancreatic cells (1). The plasmatic membrane and basement membrane of these cells from the side of the basement surface (← a). Canaliculi of the rough endoplasmic reticulum (← b), zymogen granules (2). Erythrocytes (3) in the vascular capillary space. Endothelium cells (4) covering the hemomicrovessel

Section E Experimental Aspects

Chapter 10
Pancreas
Cryosurgery

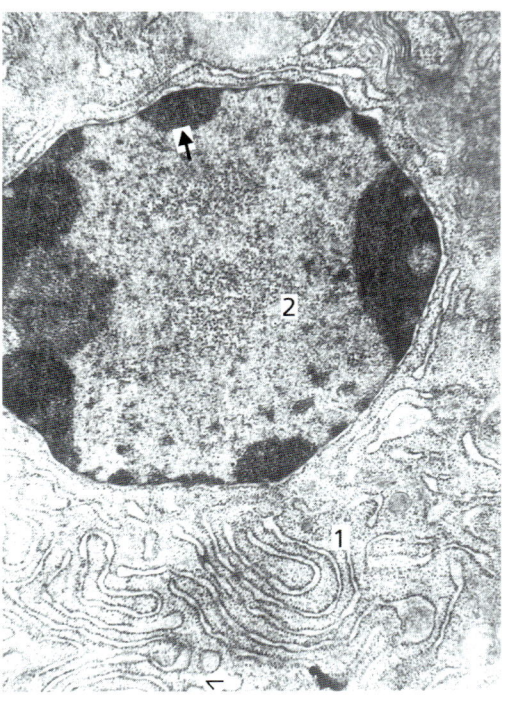

Fig. 10.3.2. The freeze-thaw cycle at a temperature of −180°C. Exocrine pancreatic cell (1). Nucleus (2), with a well-preserved nuclear envelope (membrane), the perinuclear space insignificantly dilated throughout, margination of the chromatin into large aggregates (—). The canaliculi of the rough endoplasmic reticulum are slightly dilated and partly fragmented (∠). The zymogen granules are absent

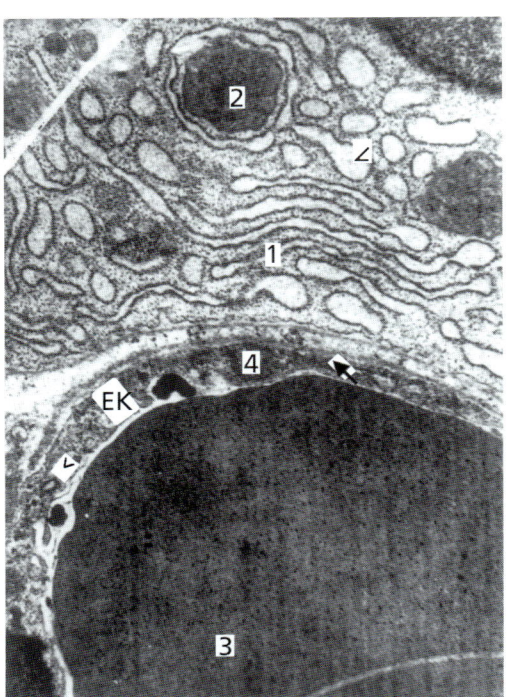

Fig. 10.3.3. The basement area of the pancreatic exocrine cell (1) Mitochondria with a dense electron matrix and a small number of cristae (2). The canaliculi of the rough endoplasmic reticulum are slightly dilated and partly fragmented (∠). Erythrocytes (3) in the vascular capillary space. An endothelium cell (EK), which has electron-dense mitochondria (4), canaliculi of the endoplasmic reticulum (^), ribosomes. The basement membrane (—) of the endothelium cell is powdery

Chapter 10
Pancreas
Cryosurgery

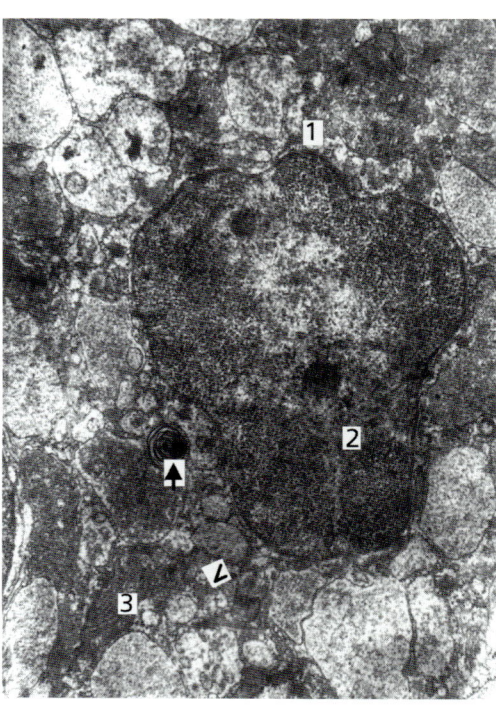

Fig. 10.3.4. Pancreatic exocrine cell (1). Nucleus (2) with dense chromatin. Mitochondria with an electron-dense matrix and a small number of cristae (3). Dilated canaliculi of endoplasmic reticulum which are full of an amorphous, flake-like substance (∠). There are no ribosomes on their membranes. The number of ribosomes in the cytoplasm suddenly decreased as a result of cryosurgical exposure. The appearance of myelin-like structures (←) in the cytoplasm confirms the increase of free radicals

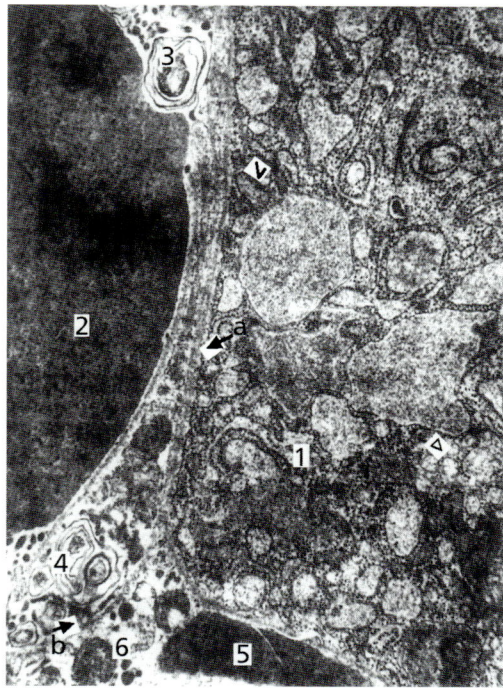

Fig. 10.3.5. Pancreatic exocrine cell (1). The plasmatic membrane on the basement surface is not clearly structured. The canaliculi of the endoplasmic reticulum (∠) have fragmented. Extended edema and loose ribosomes can be observed. Erythrocyte (2) and myelin-like structure (3) in the vascular capillary space where the endothelial structure is locally damaged (←). Myelin-like structure in the endothelial cell (4) and the remains of the cell organelles (6) in the interstitial space

Section E Experimental Aspects

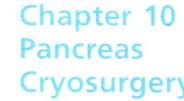

Chapter 10
Pancreas
Cryosurgery

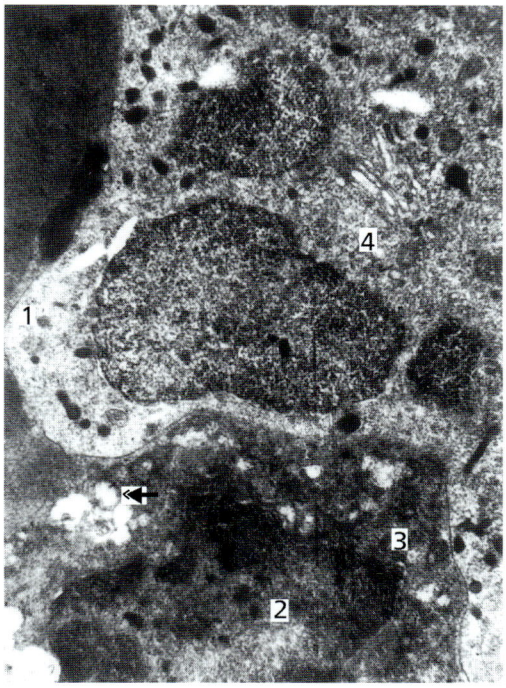

Fig. 10.3.6. The exocrine pancreatic cell (1) has a pyknotically transformed nucleus (2). The cytoplasm is filled with electron-dense homogeneous contents (3) and the remains of the canaliculi of the endoplasmic reticulum (↑). Segmented neutrophil (4) in the center of the inflammation

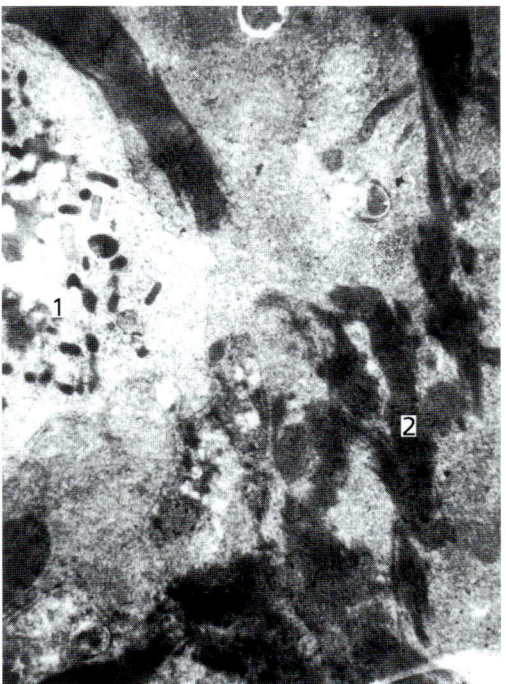

Fig. 10.3.7. Cell detritus (1) and fibrin fibers (2)

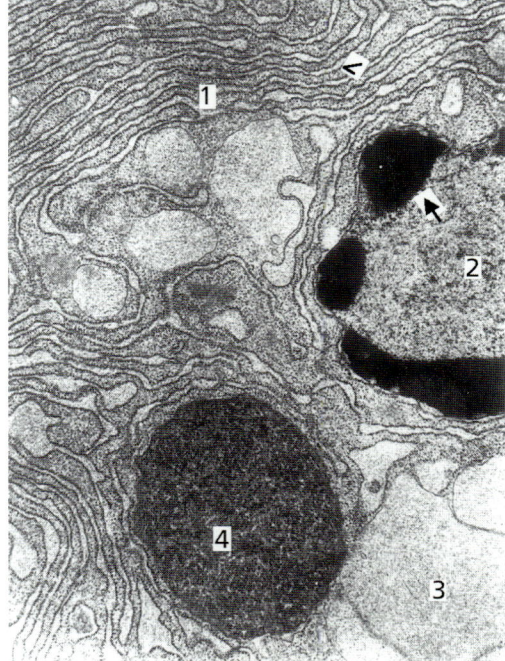

Fig. 10.3.8. The freeze-thaw cycle at a temperature of −60°C. Exocrine pancreatic cell (1). Nucleus (2) with the chromatin and sharply outlined with the creation of aggregates (←). Undilated canaliculi of the rough endoplasmic reticulum (△), dilated canaliculi of the rough endoplasmic reticulum, with loose ribisomes (3). Zymogen granules are absent. A drop of the electron-dense homogeneous substance can be seen (4)

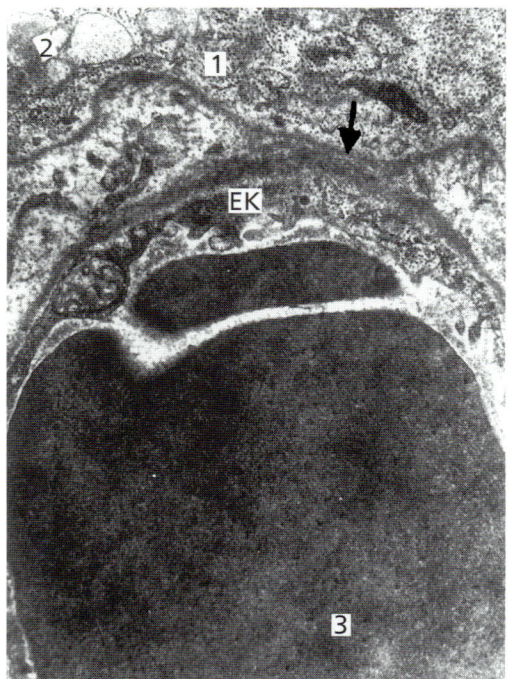

Fig. 10.3.9. Exocrine pancreatic cell (1). Plasmatic and basement membranes (←) of the cells from the side of the basement surface have been preserved. There are countless ribosomes and insignificantly dilated canaliculi of the endoplasmic reticulum (2). Erythrocytes (3) in the vascular capillary space, endothelial cells (EK) of the vascular capillary have mostly been preserved

Section E　　Experimental Aspects

Chapter 10
Pancreas
Cryosurgery

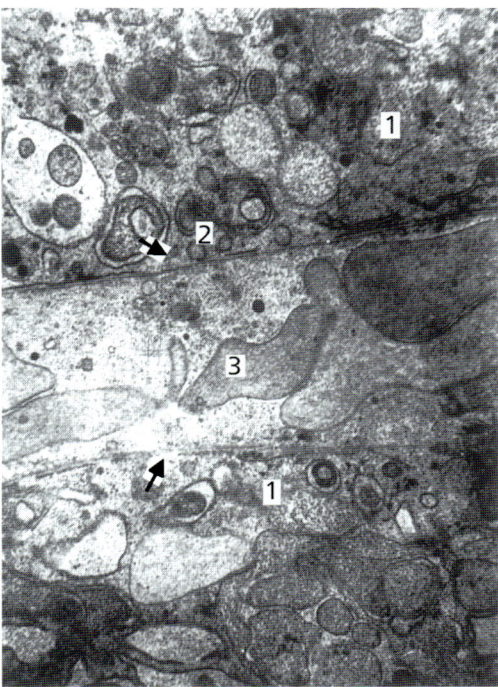

Fig. 10.3.10. Exocrine pancreatic cell (1). Plasmatic membrane (—) of cells on the basement surface is locally lysed. Canaliculi of the rough endoplasmic reticulum (2) are filled with an amorphous, flake-like material of varying electron density. Empty erythrocytes (3) in the interstitial space

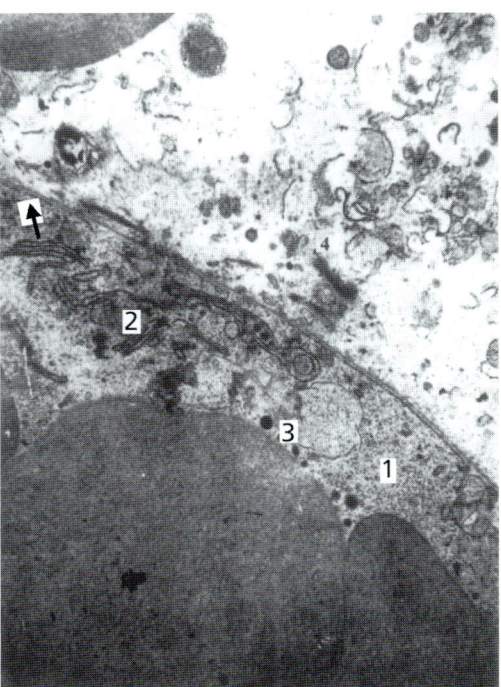

Fig. 10.3.11. Exocrine pancreatic cell (1). Plasmatic membrane (—) is locally lysed. Canaliculi of the rough endoplasmic reticulum (2). Drops of an electron-dense homogeneous substance are present (3). Cell detritus (4) in the interstitial space

Chapter 10
Pancreas Cryosurgery

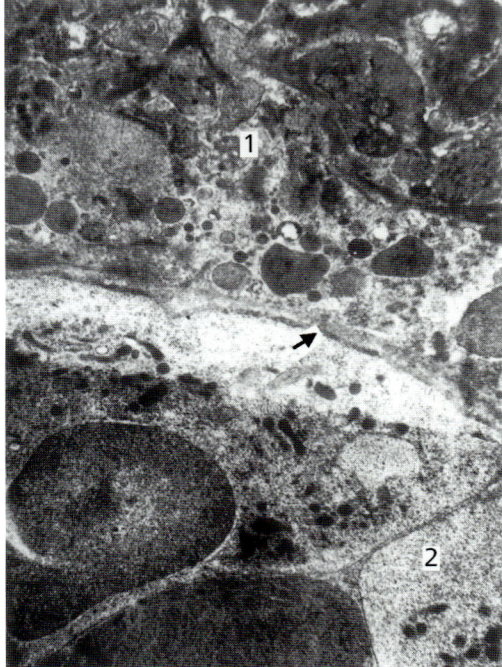

Fig. 10.3.12. Cell detritus (1) has formed from the exocrine pancreatic cells. The damaged blood cells (2) are found in the vascular space, the endothelium covering is fully desquamated, the basement membrane is powdery (→)

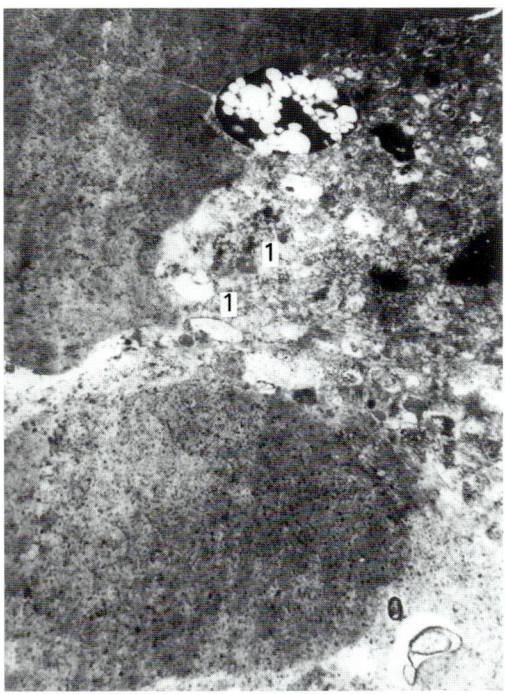

Fig. 10.3.13. 24 h after thawing. The central part of the cryozone in the dog's pancreas. The damaged exocrine cells (1)

Section E   Experimental Aspects

10.4 Morphological Study of the Pancreas

Chapter 10
Pancreas
Cryosurgery

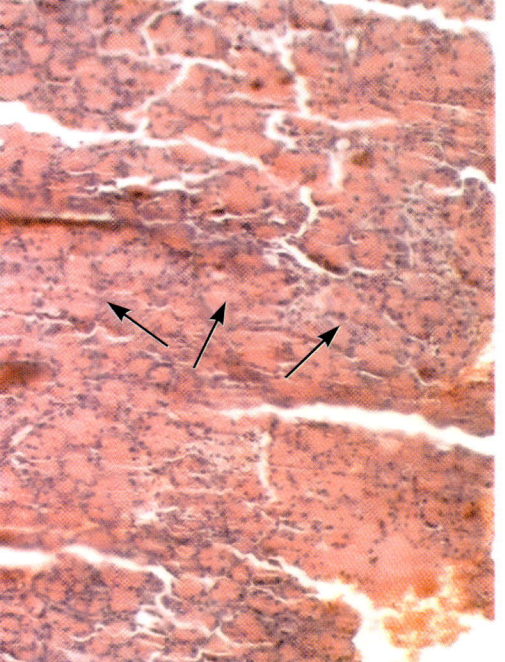

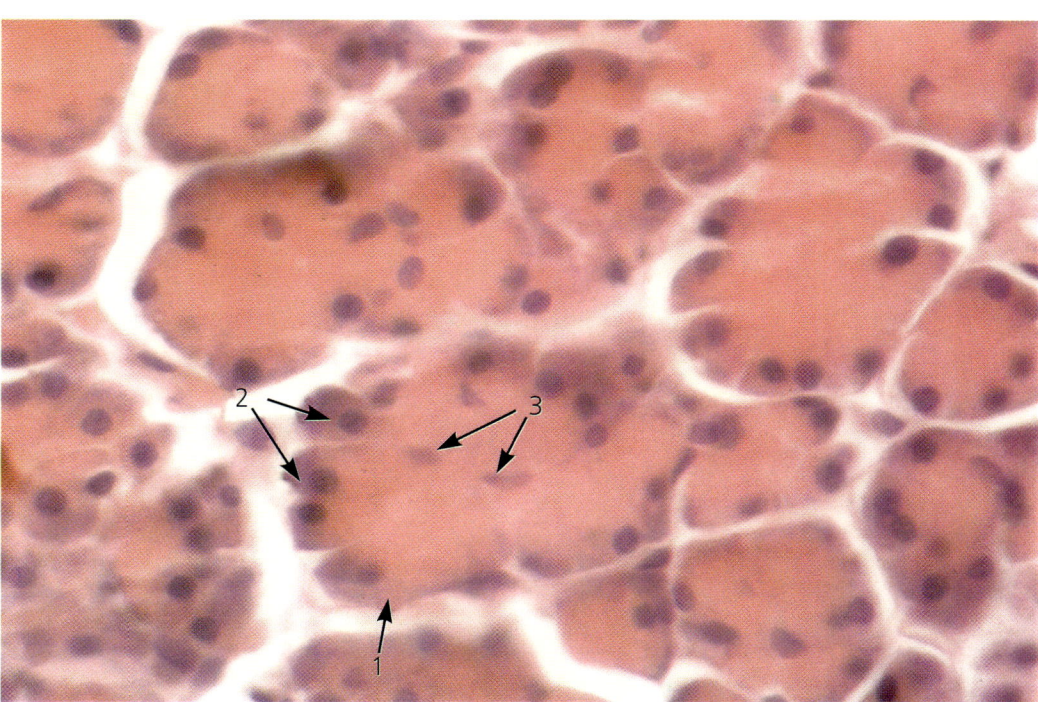

Fig. 10.4.1 a,b. *Before* cryosurgical session. Healthy dog pancreas tissue. Exocrine pancreatic tissue - acinus with secretory glands (—) (**a**). Acinus with basal membrane (1), acinic cells (2) with cytogenic granula and centroacinic cells (3) (**b**). Hematoxylin and eosin staining. Magnification: **a** ×100; **b** ×600

Chapter 10
Pancreas
Cryosurgery

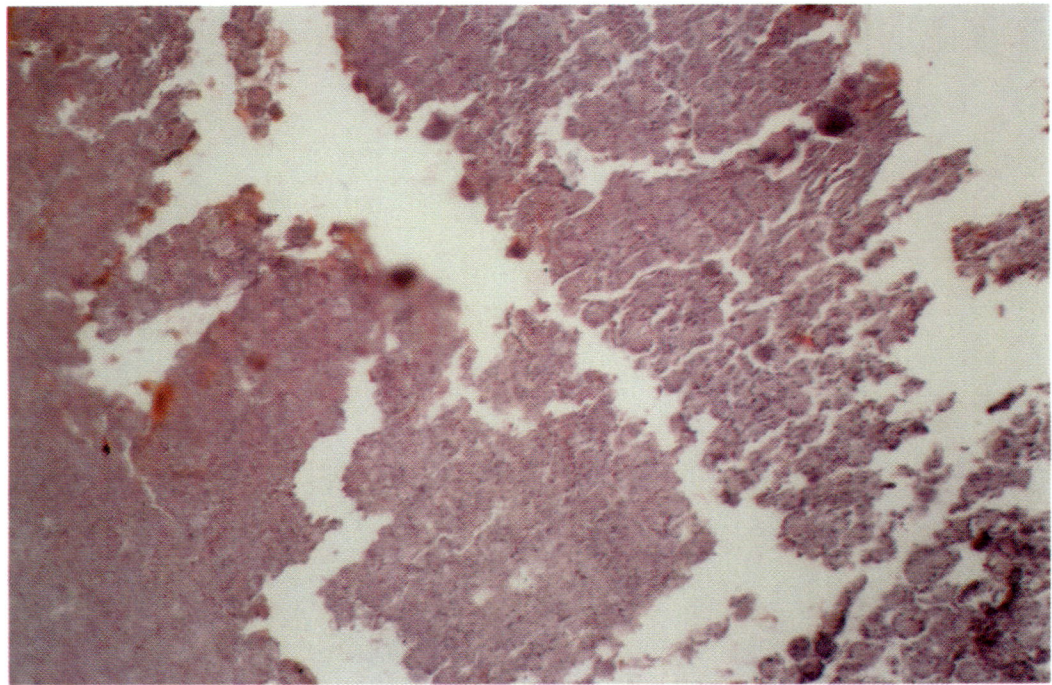

Fig. 10.4.2. *Immediately* after the single freeze-thaw cycle at a temperature of −180°C. Biopsy from the center of the cryonecrosis. Cryonecrosis with acinus in shadow only. Hematoxylin and eosin staining. Magnification × 100

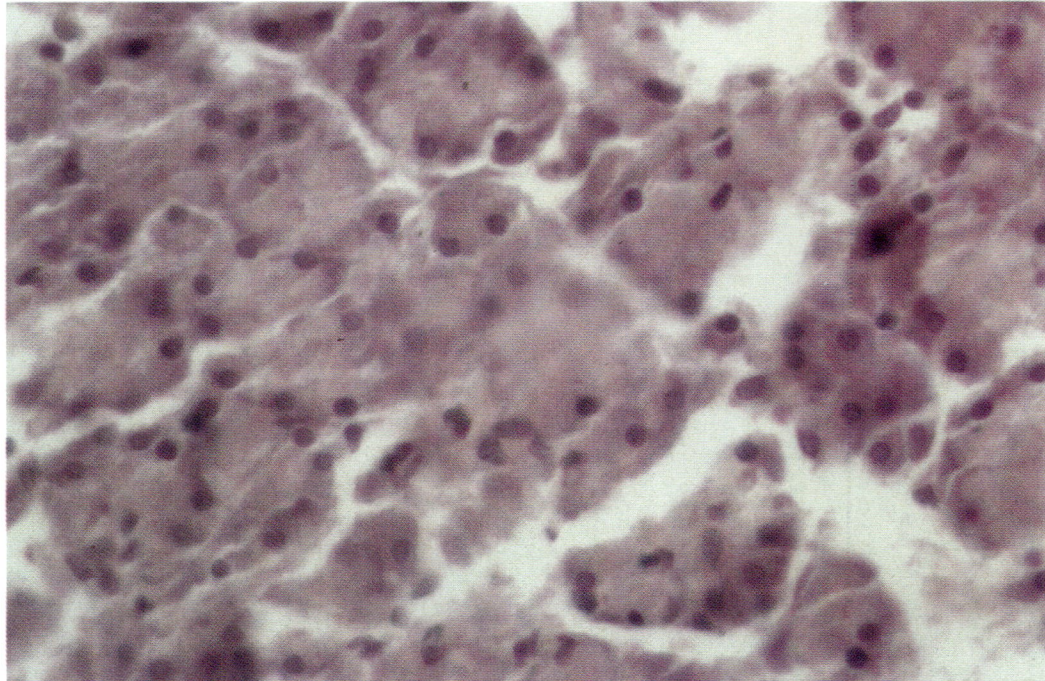

Fig. 10.4.3. *Immediately* after the single freeze-thaw cycle at a temperature of −180°C. Biopsy from the center of the cryonecrosis. Beginning necrosis with faded cell boundaries and individual cell destruction. Hematoxylin and eosin staining. Magnification × 100

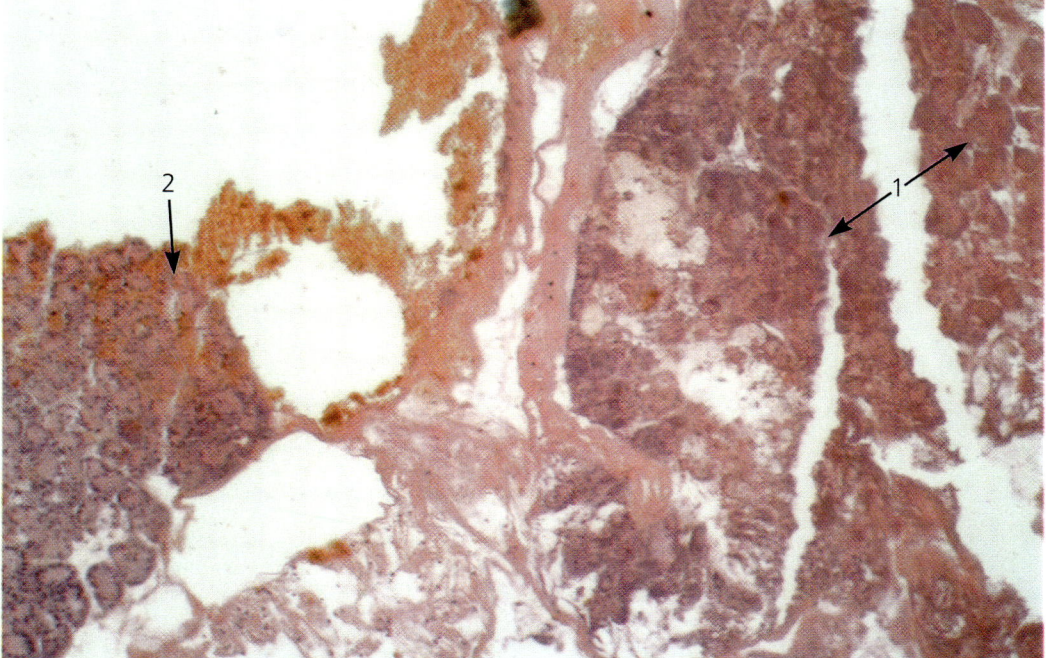

Fig. 10.4.4. 1 h after the single freeze-thaw cycle at a temperature of −180°C. Biopsy from the center of the cryonecrosis. Necrotic pancreatic tissue (1) with focal bleeding (2). Hematoxylin and eosin staining. Magnification × 100

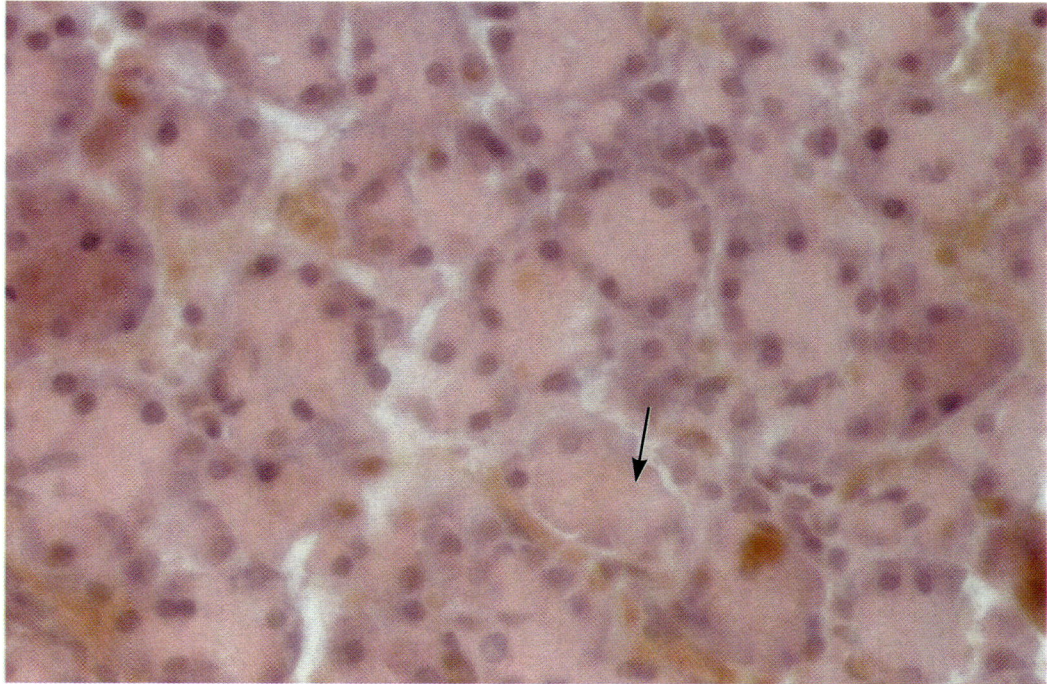

Fig. 10.4.5. 1 h after the single freeze-thaw cycle at a temperature of −180°C. Biopsy from the center of the cryonecrosis. Cryonecrosis with faded cell boundaries (←). Hematoxylin and eosin staining. Magnification × 600

Chapter 10
Pancreas Cryosurgery

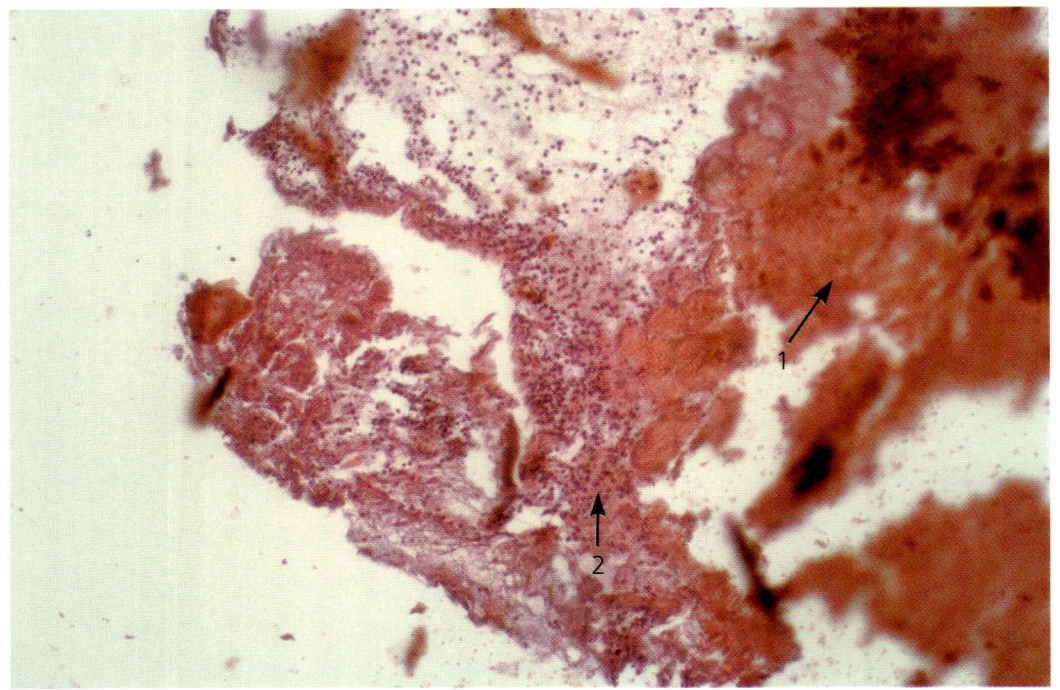

Fig. 10.4.6. 24 h after the single freeze-thaw cycle at a temperature of −180°C. Biopsy from the center of the cryonecrosis. Cryonecrosis (1) with demarcations of inflammatory cells (2). Hematoxylin and eosin staining. Magnification × 100

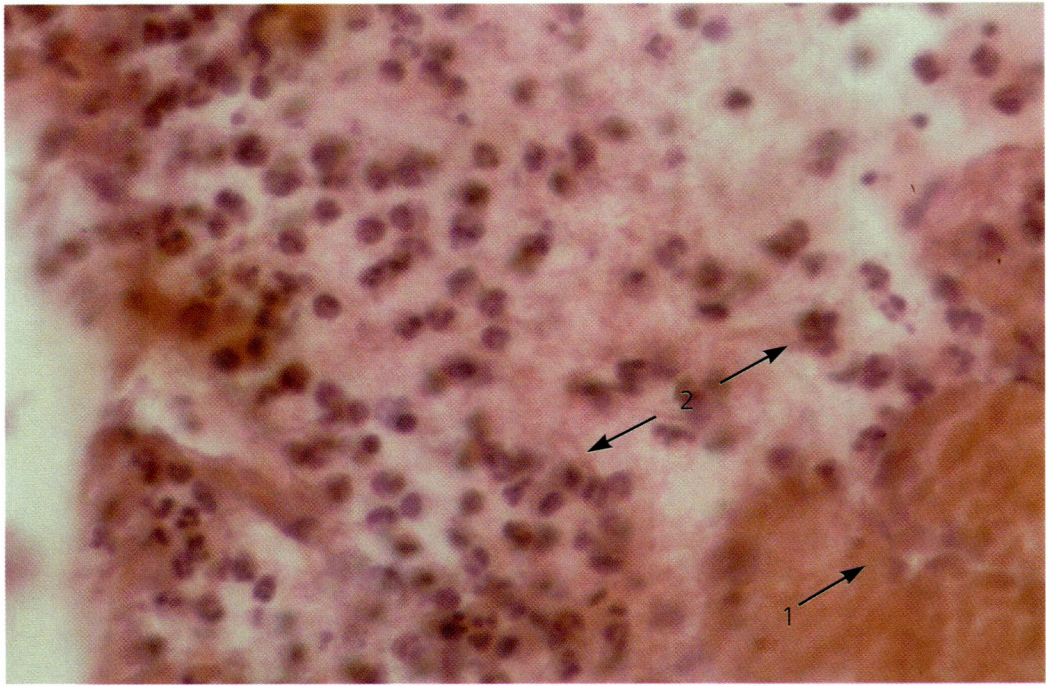

Fig. 10.4.7. 24 h after the single freeze-thaw cycle at a temperature of −180°C. Biopsy from the center of the cryonecrosis. Necrotic pancreatic tissue (1) with demarcation of inflammatory cells (2). Hematoxylin and eosin staining. Magnification × 600

Section E   Experimental Aspects   **161**

Chapter 10
Pancreas
Cryosurgery

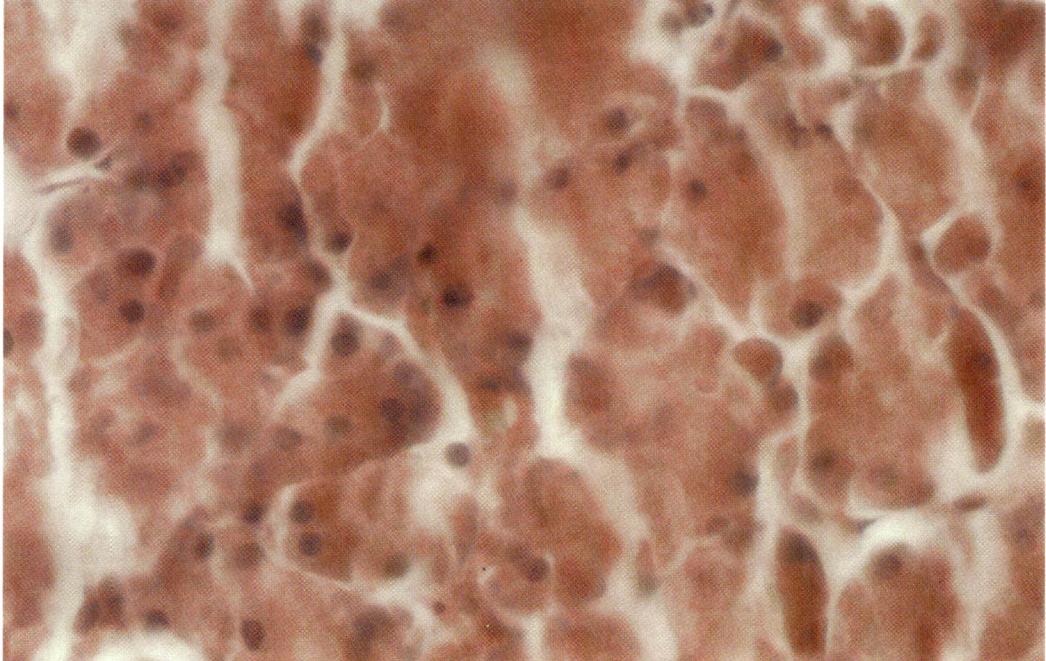

Fig. 10.4.8. Pancreas. *Immediately* after the single freeze-thaw cycle at a temperature of −60°C. Biopsy from the center of the cryonecrosis. Pancreatic tissue with mostly still recognizable cell boundaries and remaining acinar structure. Hematoxylin and eosin staining. Magnification × 600

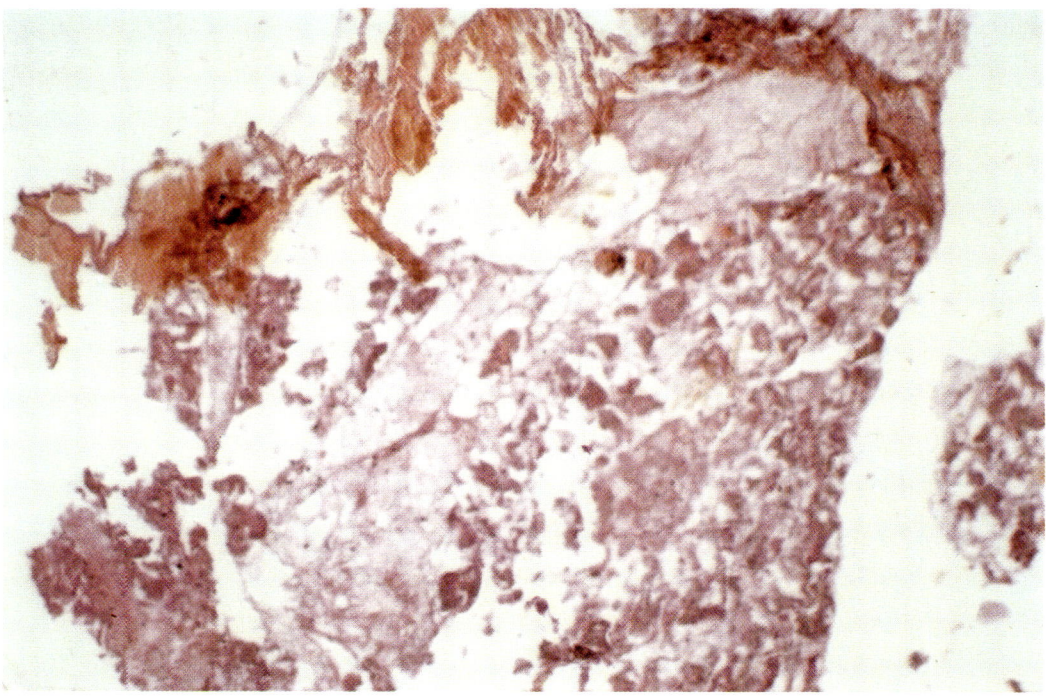

Fig. 10.4.9. 24 h after the single freeze-thaw cycle at a temperature of −60°C. Biopsy from the center of the cryonecrosis. Cryonecrosis with complete loss of architecture but with weak intensity. Hematoxylin and eosin staining. Magnification × 100

Chapter 10
Pancreas Cryosurgery

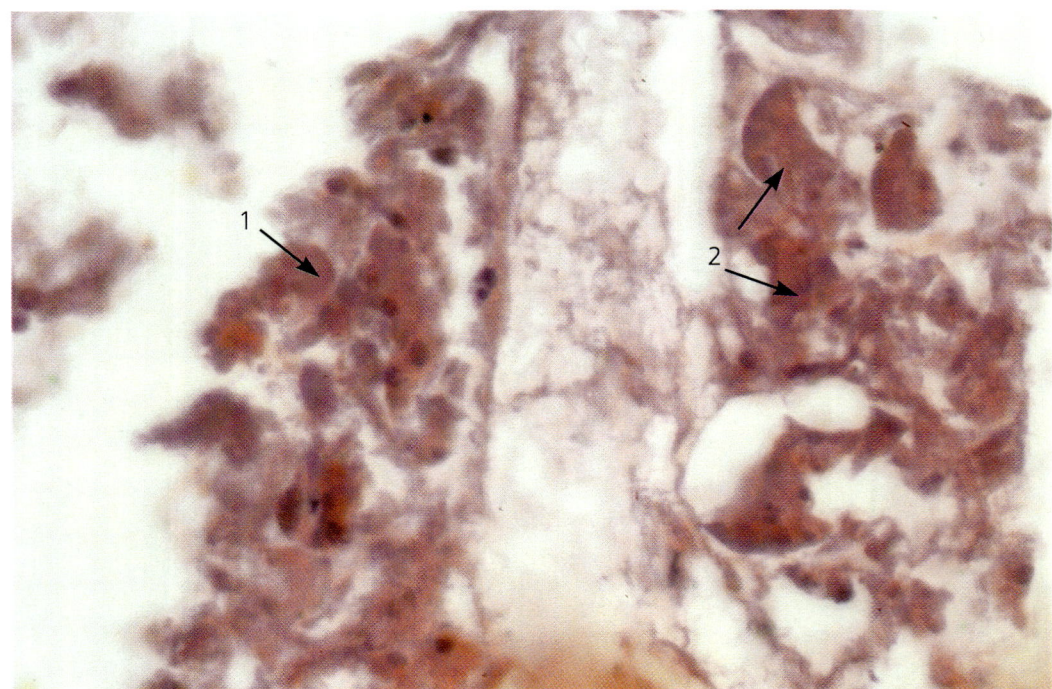

Fig. 10.4.10. 24 h after the single freeze-thaw cycle at a temperature of −60°C. Biopsy from the center of the cryonecrosis. Loss of cell coherence (1), fragments of acinus (2) but with weak intensity. Hematoxylin and eosin staining. Magnification × 600

Section F

Clinical Aspects

Cryosurgical Dermatology

Nikolai N. Korpan[1] with contributions by Joao A. Amaro[2], Jose Carlos Almeida Gonçalves[3], Giuseppe Monfrecola[4], Peter Nordin[5], Patrick J.M. Le Pivert[6], Massimiliano Scalvenzi[4] and Rodney Sinclair[7]

11.0 Introduction

Skin cryosurgery has always been an integral part of dermatology and is widely used in the treatment of cutaneous lesions. Cryosurgery is an excellent and one of the most commonly performed techniques to treat benign, premalignant and malignant lesions of the skin. It has become routine practice in many centers to use freeze-thaw cycles in the treatment of the common types of benign skin tumors. Over the past two decades it has also begun to be more frequently used for the treatment of malignant skin tumors. Because benign lesions require a shorter duration and less deep application of sub-zero temperatures than malignant lesions, it is possible to achieve good to excellent cosmetic results.

Eradication of simple cutaneous lesions by freezing was already attempted at the turn of the twentieth century. Liquid air was applied with a cotton swab or solidified carbon dioxide was placed on the lesion, but destruction was limited. When liquid nitrogen became available it was initially applied with a cotton swab, but in the 1960s new techniques and equipment were developed that permitted deeper destruction. Thus, malignant as well as benign lesions became amenable to cryosurgical management.

Cryosurgery is used alone, in combination with an intralesional steroid injection, or combined with conventional surgery to treat keloids and hypertrophic scars, which are uncommon complications of superficial wounds but are not uncommon in full-thickness wounds.

The standard cryosurgical procedure is carried out for the treatment of such scars. As a rule, the freeze time ranges between 10 and 30 seconds, but large keloids require a longer freeze duration. A single or double freeze-thaw cycle is performed, and more than one treatment session is usually needed. Complete flattening can be achieved. This procedure can be repeated if necessary.

The cryosurgical shaving of scars has had excellent clinical and cosmetic results. This procedure is not difficult. Shaving cryosurgery is therefore an effective new technique to treat hypertrophic scars and keloids.

The incidence of complications after dermatologic cryosurgery is minimal. The cure rates are high, and the cosmetic results are excellent. Some advantages of cryosurgery include simplicity, low cost, ability to treat multiple lesions, minimal or no scarring, no age limitations, safety during pregnancy, and the ability to treat any area of the body. The use of local anesthesia is usually not necessary. Overfreezing should be avoided, as repeated treatment is likely.

Some treatment techniques have become established. The minimal temperature reached by the targeted tissue is important. For maximum destruction, −60°C or lower should be obtained. Of all the cryogens available today, including fluorocarbon sprays, carbon dioxide, and nitrous oxide, liquid nitrogen is the coldest and most versatile, and therefore the freezing agent of choice. The choice of agent depends

Chapter 11
Cryosurgical Dermatology

on the type of lesion and the operator's personal preference. The process of freezing with modern cryosurgical equipment using liquid nitrogen, for example, can be controlled by the duration of freezing (freeze time), the thawing of the lesion (thaw time), and the measurement of the ice ball beyond the target area (lateral spread of freeze).

The cryoprobe technique - contact cryosurgery – involves the use of a metal probe that is cooled internally by a circulating flow of liquid nitrogen. The probe is firmly applied to the lesion until a rim of frozen tissue is observed. The freeze time here is two or three times longer than if the spray technique, for example, is used. Lesions that are suitable for treatment include hemangioma, condyloma, dermatofibroma, etc. A single freeze-thaw cycle administered once is satisfactory for several of these conditions, but repeated treatment at 4- to 6-week intervals may be needed for hemangiomas or condylomata until the desired resolution of the lesion is achieved.

Vascular tumors comprise a range of lesions including the frequently occurring hemangiomas. A common hemangioma of infancy is the capillary hemangioma. They may become quite large, occasionally obstructing such vital functions as vision or smell when located in these areas. These hemangiomas undergo a rapid growth phase followed by spontaneous involution over several years.

The cryosurgical method is also very effective in the treatment of other benign lesions. Patients with problems related to pigmented lesion disorders are among those most commonly evaluated for dermatologic surgery. The vast majority of these lesions are benign and are often treated surgically. However, recent data suggest that some of these lesions may be both markers for and precursors to malignant melanoma. It is, therefore, important that patients with pigmented lesions be carefully evaluated and appropriately treated.

Perhaps the most controversial topic in dermatology is the management of patients with dysplastic nevus syndrome. Dysplastic nevi can be both precursors for malignant melanoma and markers for increased risk of melanoma. The difference has important implications for medical or surgical, including cryosurgical, management. If these lesions are true precursors, appropriate management would be complete cryodestruction.

Congenital nevi are much less prevalent than dysplastic nevi, but melanoma can also develop in congenital nevi. In fact, the giant congenital nevus is most likely to undergo malignant change. The incidence of melanoma in large congenital nevi has been estimated as between 5 and 20% in the patient's lifetime.

The management of congenital nevi depends primarily on their size and the perceived risk of developing malignant melanoma. Large congenital nevi, which have the highest risk of developing melanoma, are the most rare and their management is complex.

One of the most common office procedures for the treatment of warts is cryosurgery. The standard cryosurgical procedure is used to treat these benign epidermal skin tumors which occur in both adults and children.

Cryosurgery is medically indicated in cases involving periocular tumors. The cure rate is higher than that of conventional surgery and the cosmetic result is often superior.

Chapter 11
Cryosurgical Dermatology

The first step in the management of the patient with malignant skin tumors is a biopsy of the suspicious lesion as well as clinical evaluation. The precise surgical procedure for a cutaneous malignant lesion varies somewhat from surgeon to surgeon.

The best data we have in the treatment of malignant skin tumors come from cryogenic surgery.

Theoretical, experimental and clinical experience has shown that obtaining an absolutely constant low temperature is the only requirement for total biological necrosis. Accurate temperature levels and a rapid cooling rate are the two essential factors for modern cryosurgery. During the entire operation, therefore, the control and the stability of the selected temperature usually at −170°C− −190°C in the working part of the cryoprobe (cryosound), which is in contact with the organ or tissue to be necrosed, are essential conditions for a successful cryogenic effect.

Chapter 11 Cryosurgical Dermatology

11.1 Standard Cryosurgical Procedures of Cutaneous Lesions

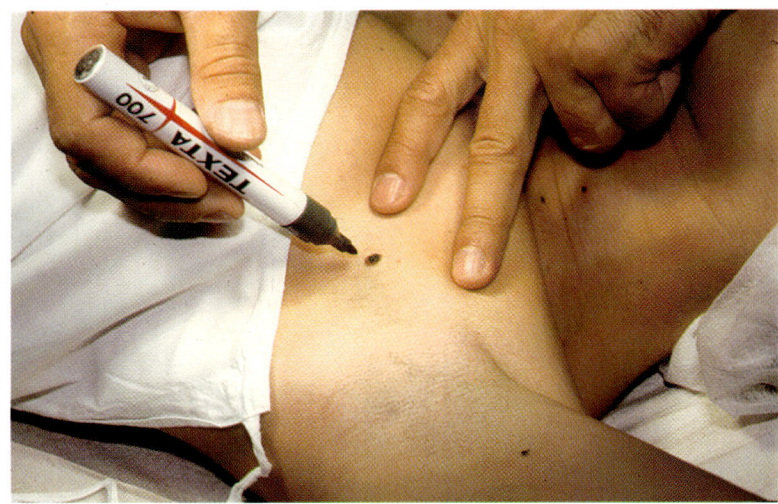

Fig. 11.1.1[1]. *Marking.* The skin lesion is usually marked preoperatively, including the marked surrounding margin of approximately 5–7 mm of normal appearing skin

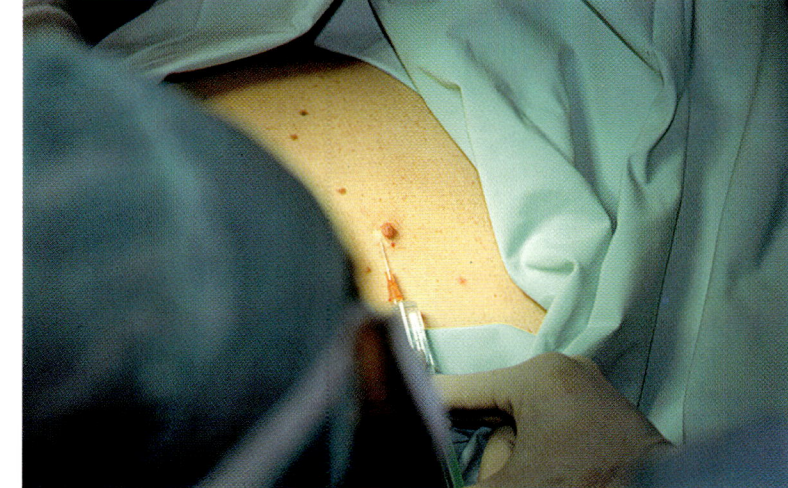

Fig. 11.1.2[1]. *Local anesthesia.* For most small skin lesions, including the small procedures (skin biopsies), local anesthesia is unnecessary. In other cases a variety of local anesthetics may be used (1.0% or 2.0% scandicain, 1.0% or 2.0% xylocain etc.)

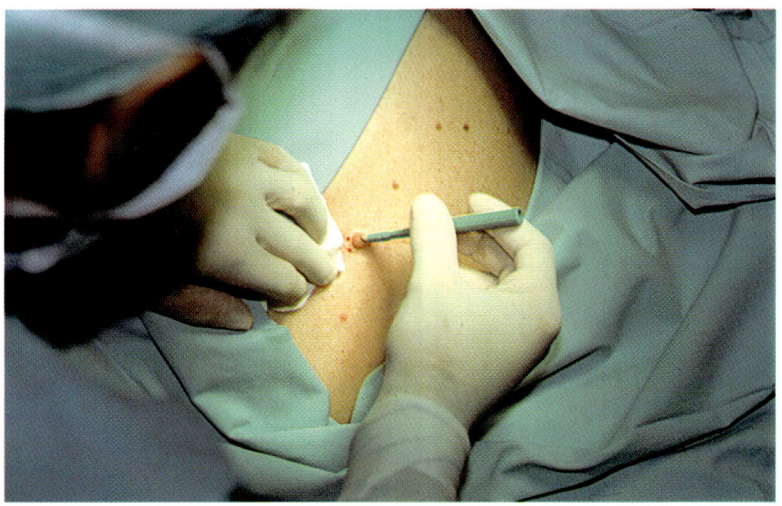

Fig. 11.1.3[1]. *Skin biopsy.* This is a routine diagnostic tool used to evaluate and verify the skin tumor. The standard instrument for skin biopsy is the dermal punch (Keyes' punch)

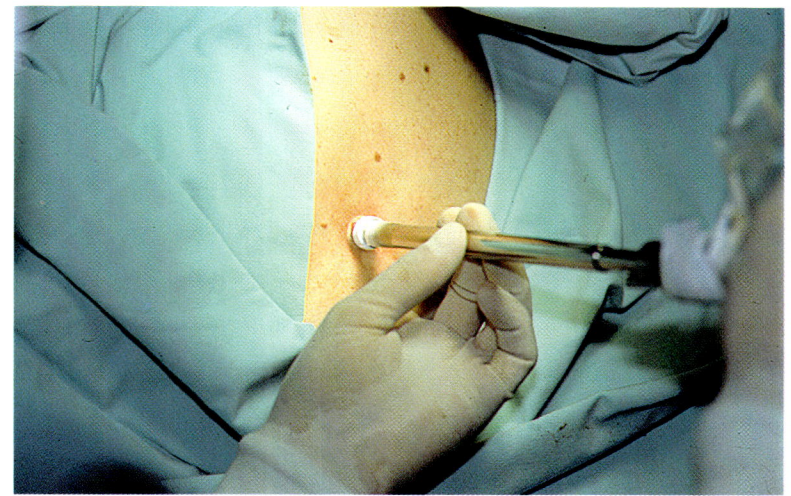

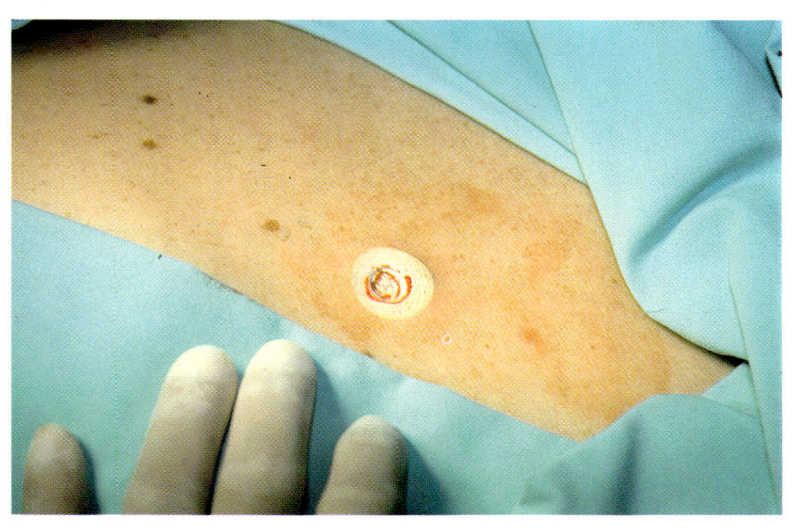

Fig. 11.1.4[1] **a–f.** *Cryosurgical session.* Cryosurgery (**a, c, e**) by means of a cryoprobe. The cryoprobe technique is also known as contact or application cryosurgery. A single freeze-thaw cycle is usually performed. Sometimes two or three freeze-thaw cycles are used for the cryosurgical treatment of cutaneous lesions. Cryozone formation (**b, d, f**) is observed immediately after freezing

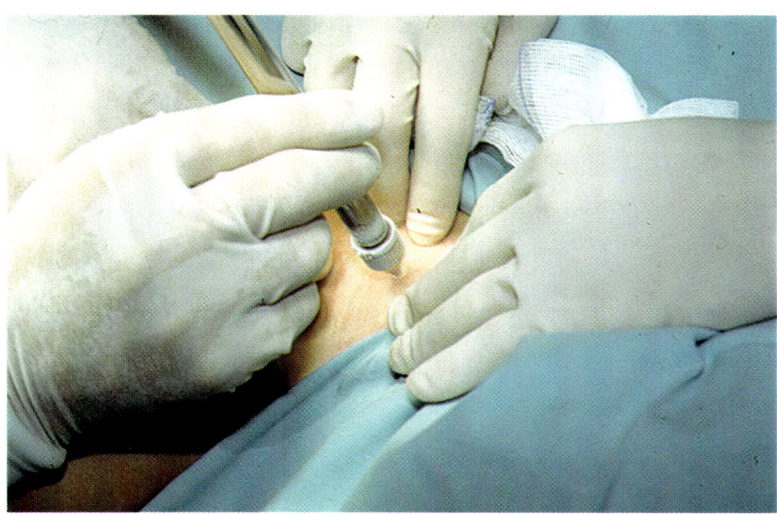

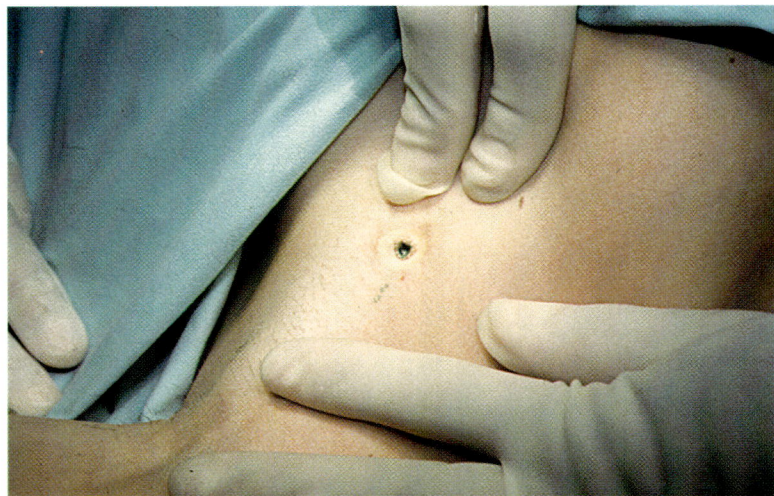

d

e

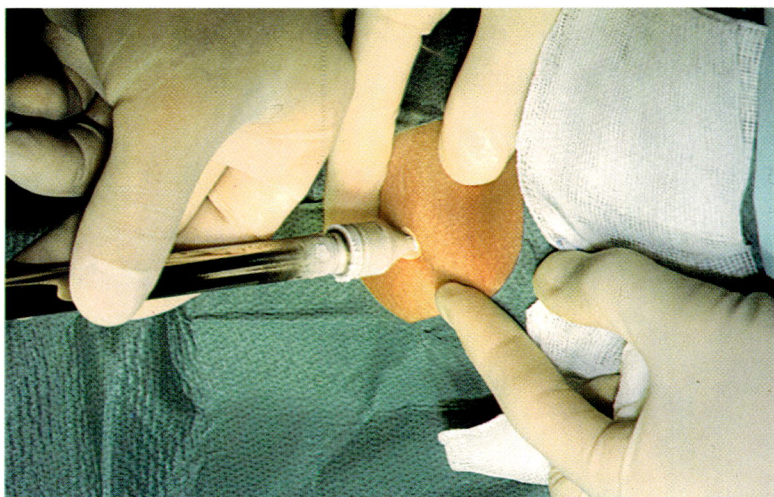

Fig. 11.1.4[1] a–f. *Cryosurgical session.* Cryosurgery (**a, c, e**) by means of a cryoprobe. The cryoprobe technique is also known as contact or application cryosurgery. A single freeze-thaw cycle is usually performed. Sometimes two or three freeze-thaw cycles are used for the cryosurgical treatment of cutaneous lesions. Cryozone formation (**b, d, f**) is observed immediately after freezing

f

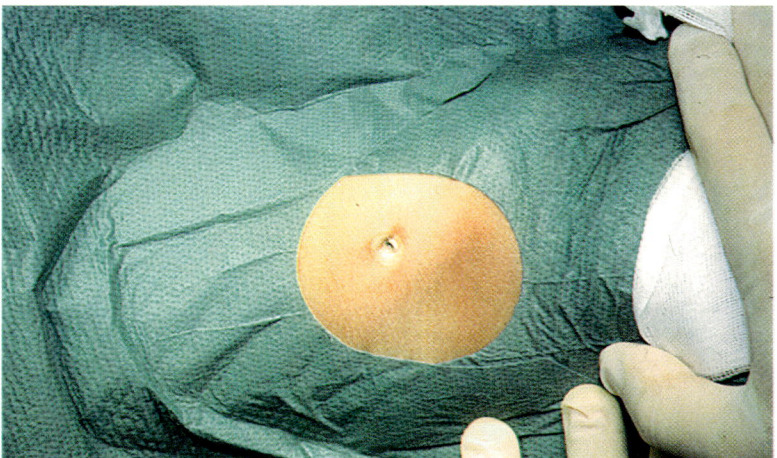

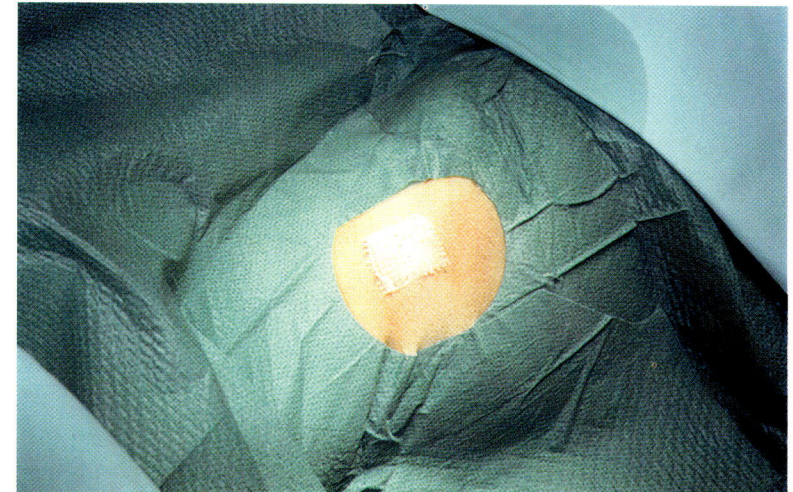

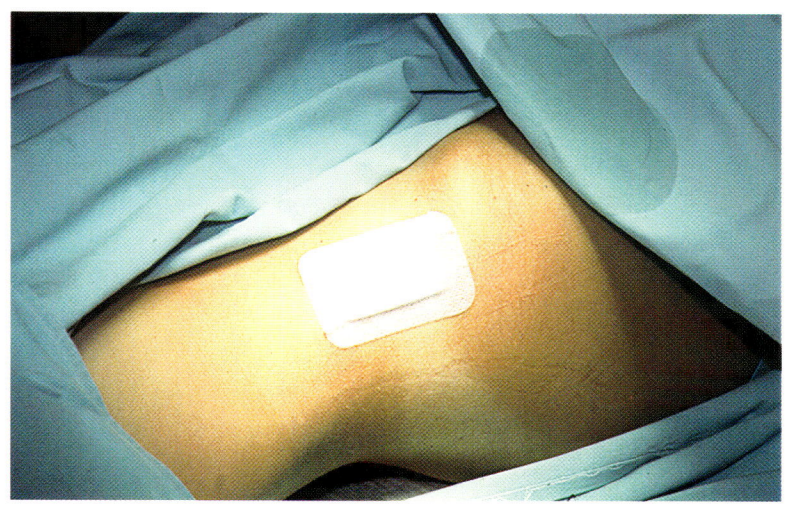

Fig. 11.1.5[1] a, b. *Wound dressing.* A simple wound dressing must serve as a barrier between the wound and the outside environment for the first postoperative days. As a contact layer between the surface of the dressing and the wound a layer of ointment, for example, "Jelonet" or "Sofra-tuell" (**a**) must be applied and covered with an absorbing cotton gauze layer (**b**)

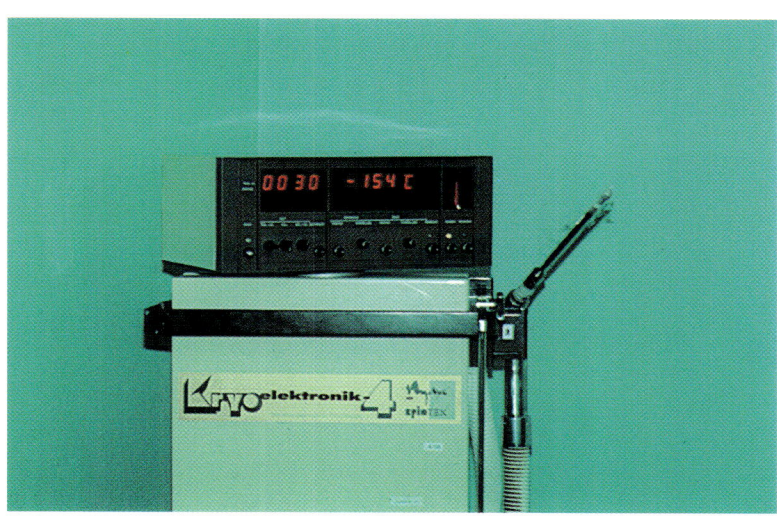

Fig. 11.1.6[1]. *Cryosurgical equipment.* The cryosurgical equipment includes a cryosurgical unit with a set of cryosurgical instruments (cryosurgical universal unit) and cryogenic agents (liquid nitrogen etc.)

11.2 Benign Tumors

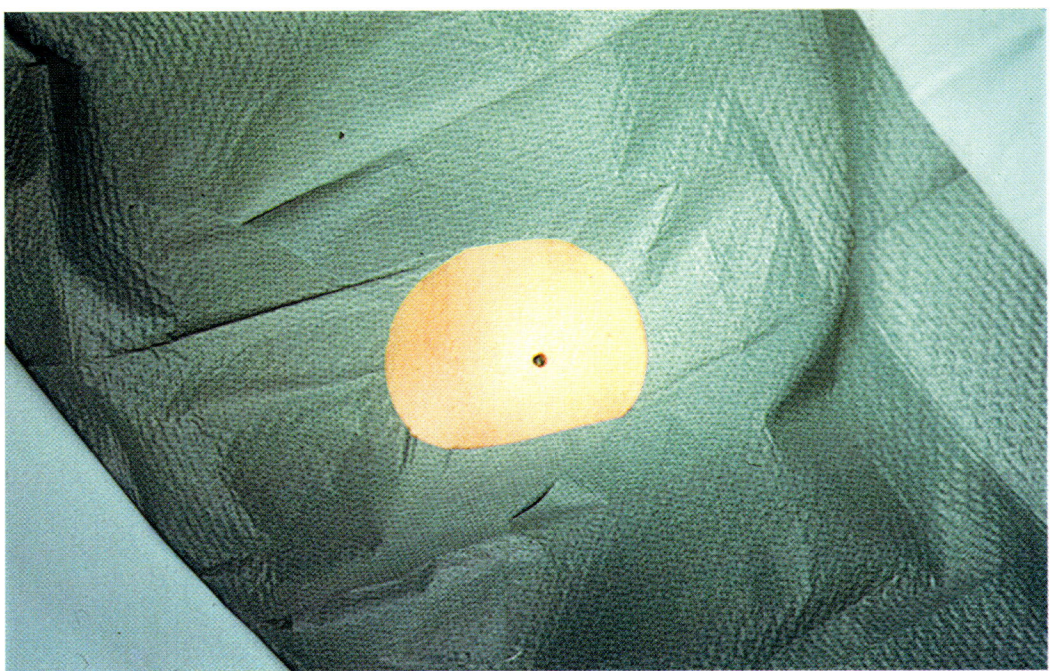

Fig. 11.2.1[1]. Benign pigmented lesion in a 20-year-old girl. Preoperative view

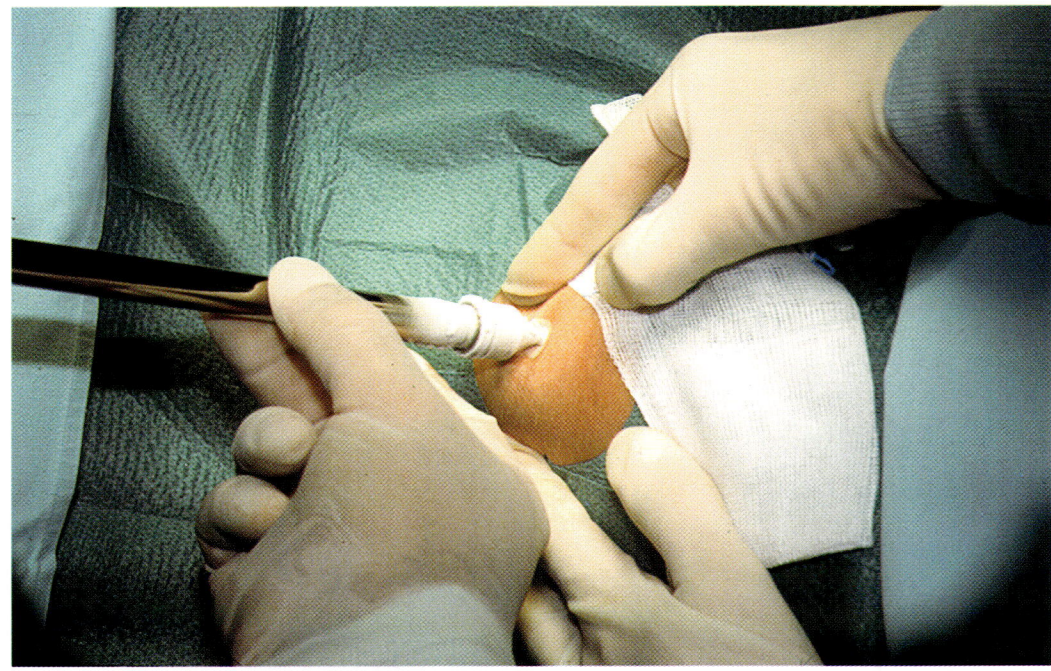

Fig. 11.2.2[1]. The same patient. A simple cryosurgical session using a disc cryoprobe with a diameter of 5 mm which is placed on the skin lesion until a temperature of −180°C is reached. No exposure time. Local anesthesia not necessary

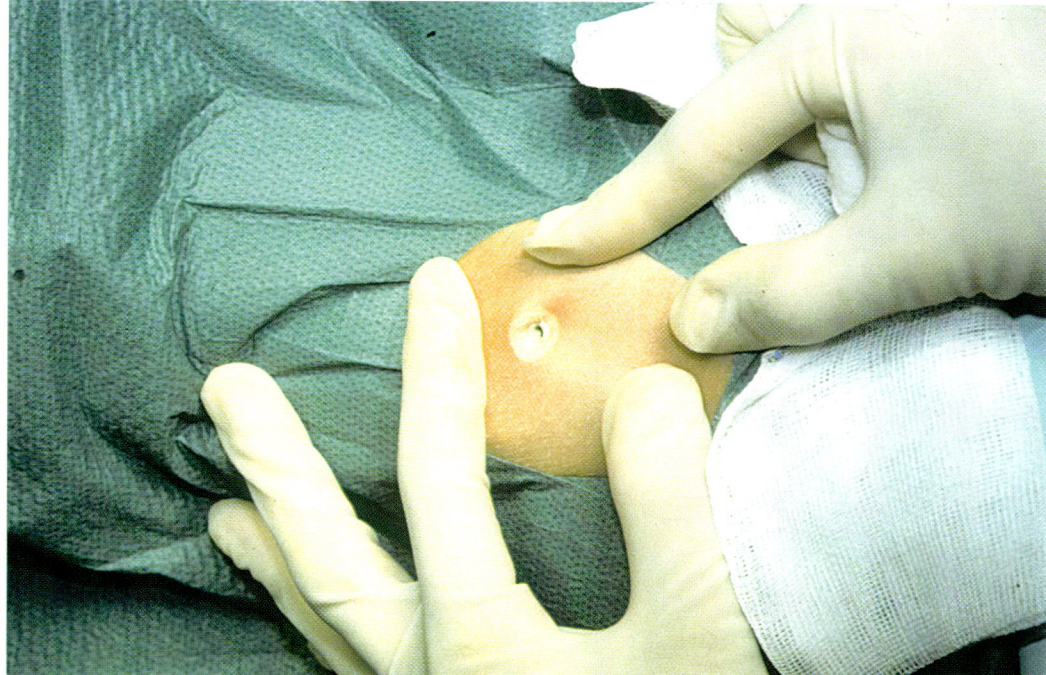

Fig. 11.2.3[1]. The same patient. The skin lesion immediately after cryosurgical debulking

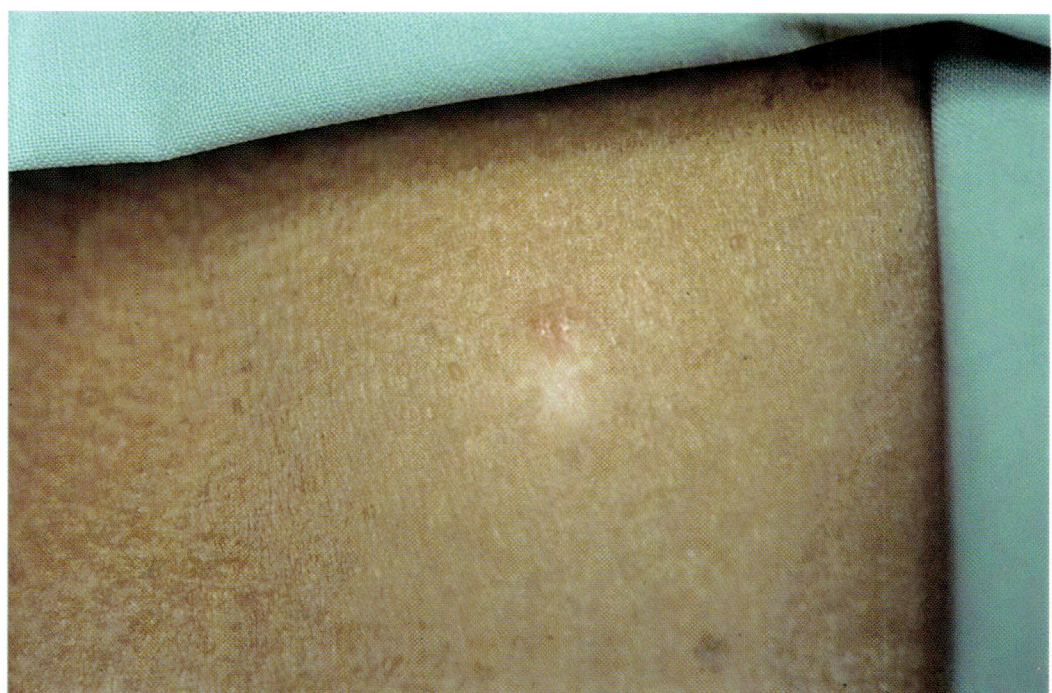

Fig. 11.2.4[1]. Complete healing 5 weeks after cryosurgical treatment in the same patient

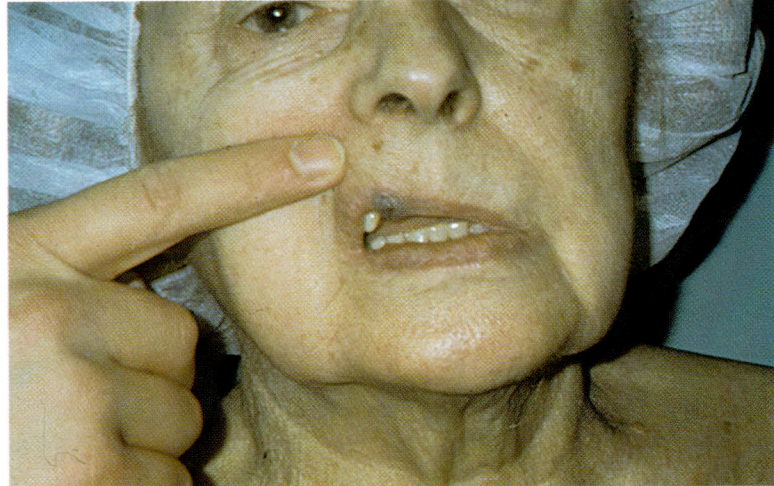

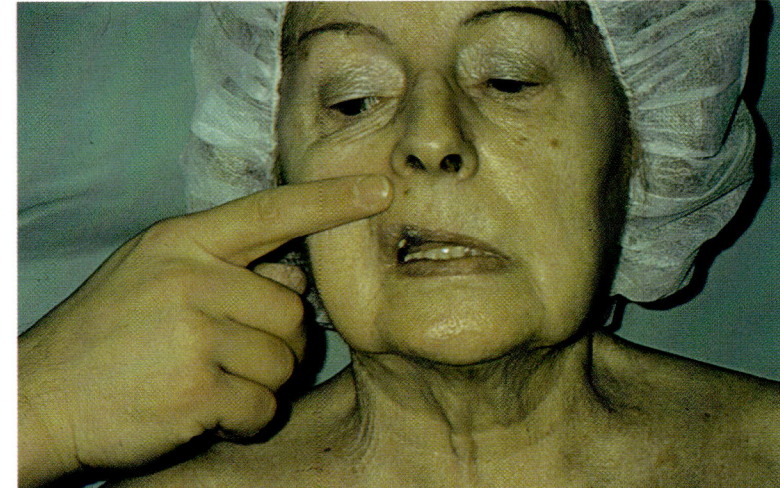

Fig. 11.2.5[1] A, B. Hemangioma simplex on the lip of a 74-year-old woman. Preoperative view

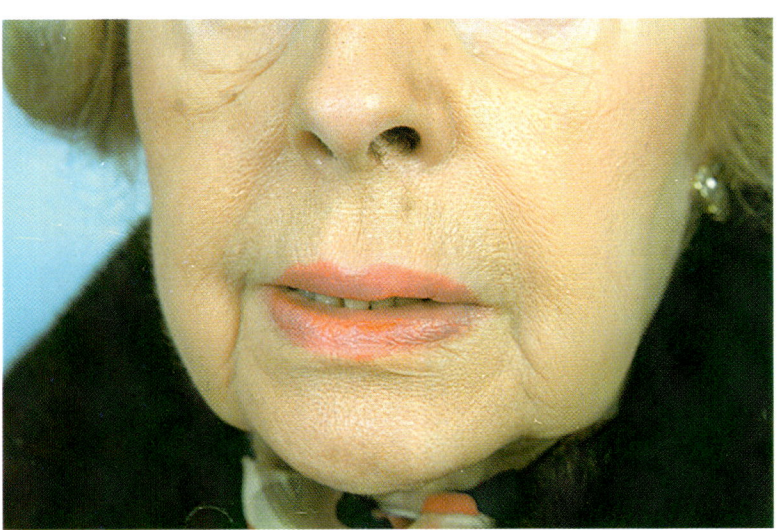

Fig. 11.2.6[1]. Excellent results 8 weeks after cryosurgical treatment. The patient is disease-free

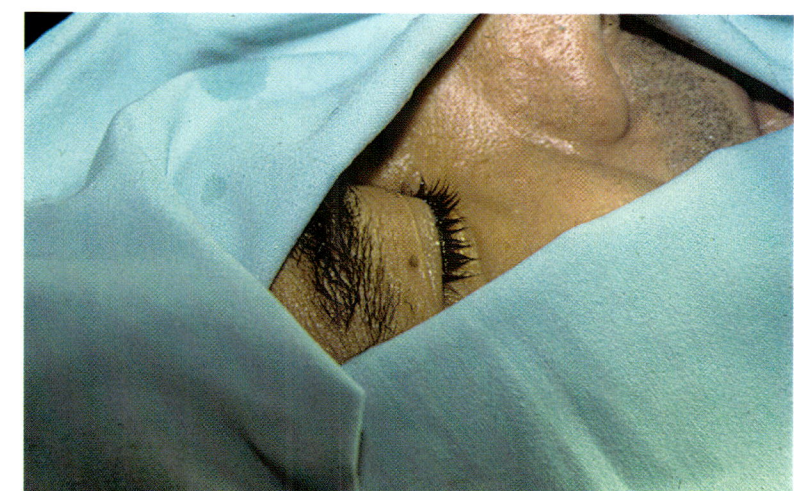

Fig. 11.2.7[1]. Preoperative clinical appearance of a typical nevus of the upper eyelid showing round shape, uniform color, and crisp border demarcation

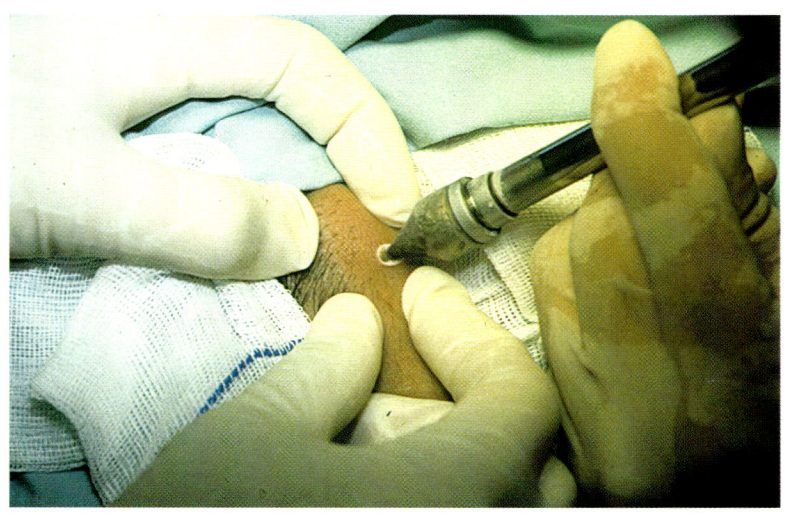

Fig. 11.2.8[1]. Cryosurgical treatment by means of a disc cryoprobe with a diameter of 5 mm which is placed on the skin lesion until a temperature of −170°C is reached. No exposure time. Local anesthesia not necessary

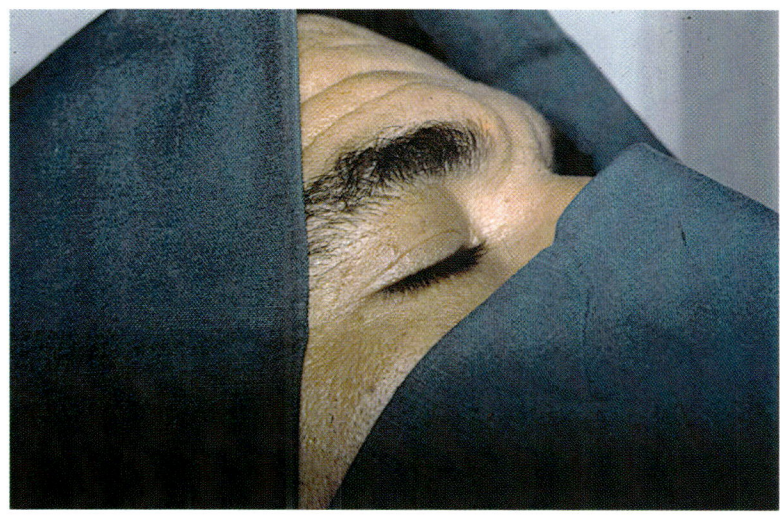

Fig. 11.2.9[1]. Good results 6 weeks after cryosurgical treatment

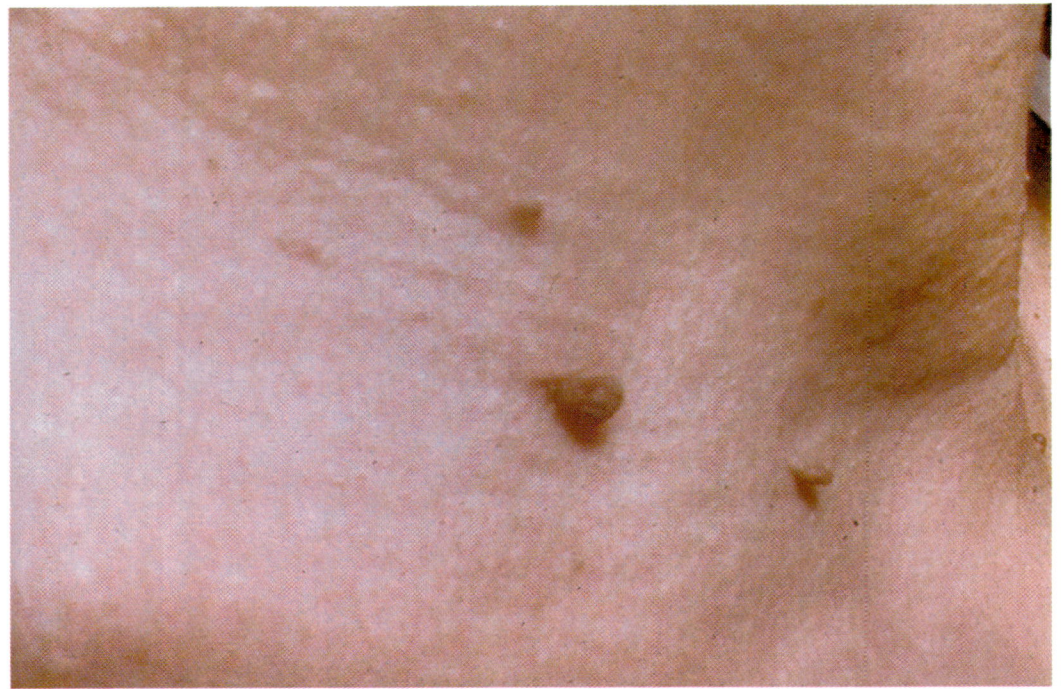

Fig. 11.2.10⁴. The picture shows soft fibromas before cryosurgical treatment

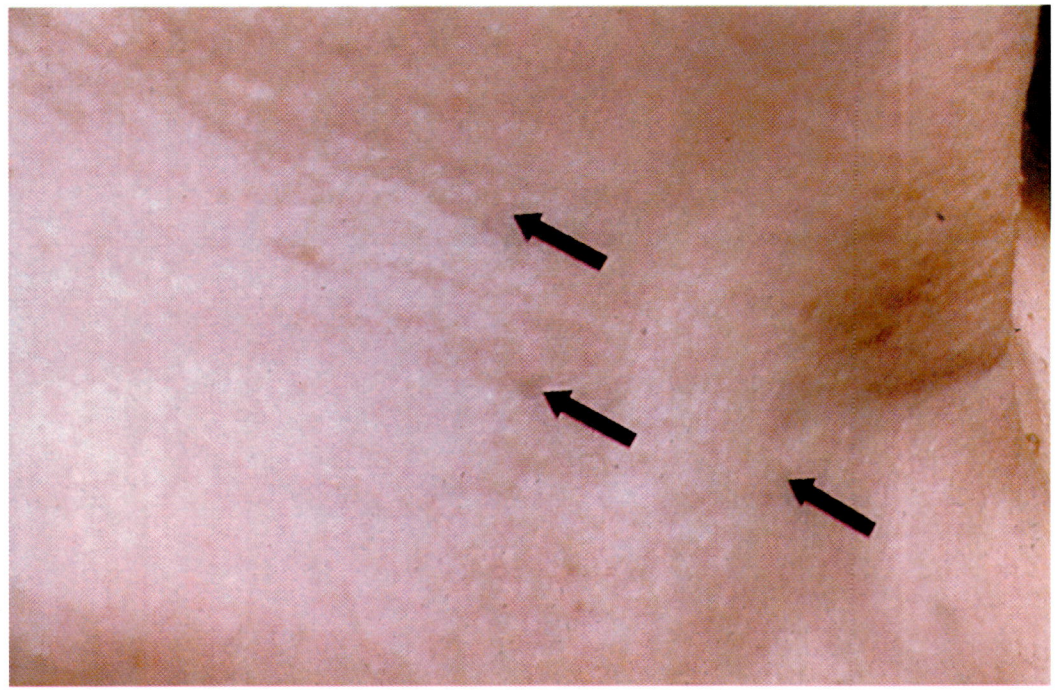

Fig. 11.2.11⁴. The same area 30 days after a single cryosurgical session

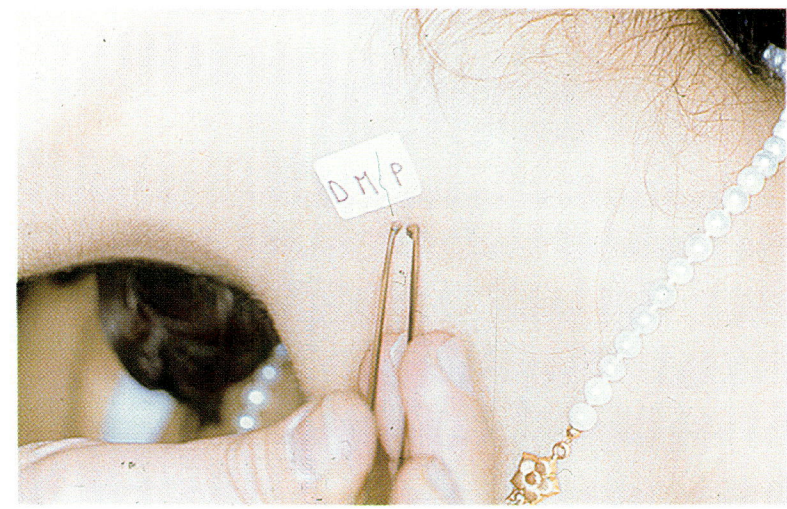

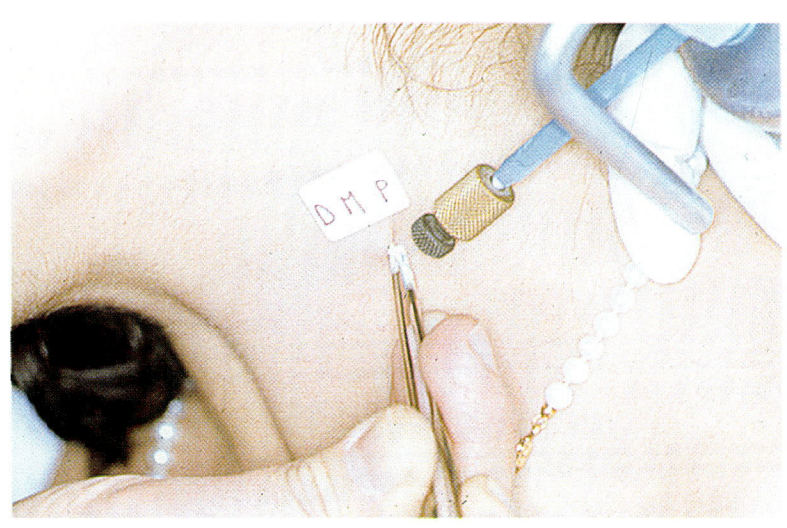

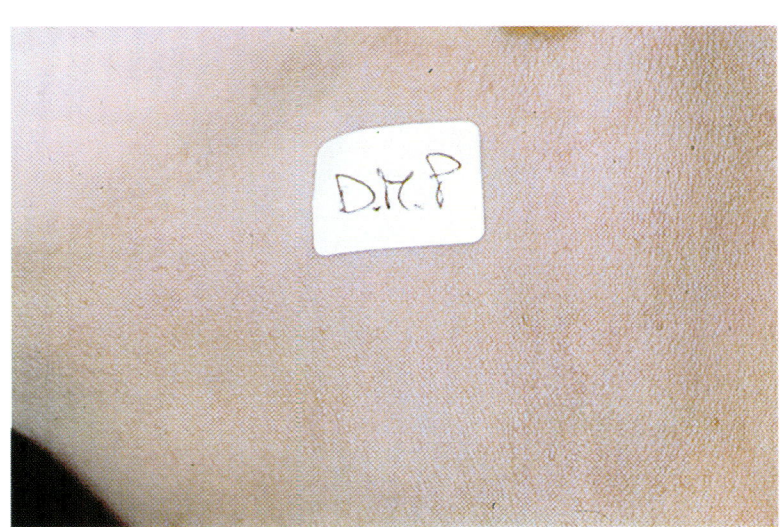

Fig. 11.2.12⁴. The technique employed for the cryosurgical treatment of soft fibromas (**A**): the liquid nitrogen spray is directed towards the distal part of the forceps (**B**) in order to freeze the fibroma, sparing the surrounding tissue. The same area 20 days after a single cryosurgical session (**C**). This technique is only effective for small, soft fibromas less than 5 mm diameter

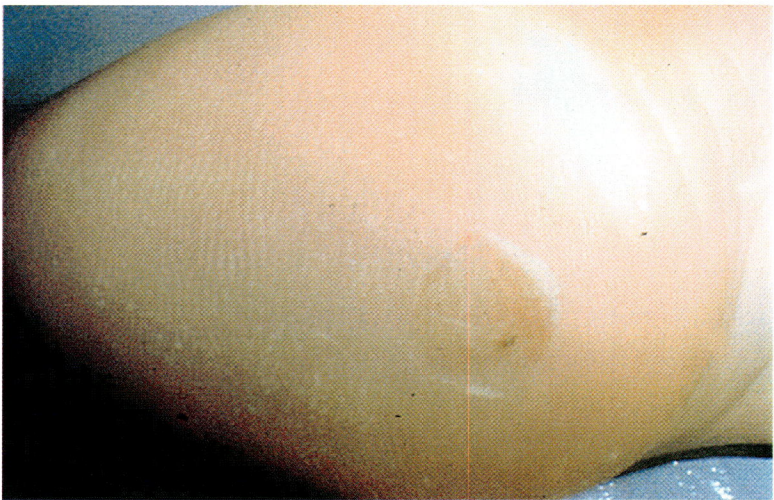

A

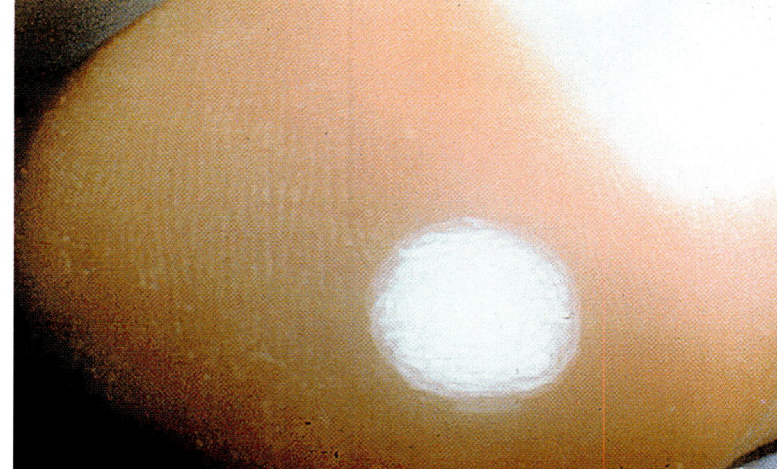

B

Fig. 11.2.13[4]. Plantar wart before (**A**), during the cryosurgical session (**B**) and 5 weeks after cryosurgery (**C**). This kind of lesion can be successfully treated by spray cryogens if it has been pretreated by keratolytic agents (i.e., ointments or plasters containing salicylic acid) in order to remove the hyperkeratotic layers

C

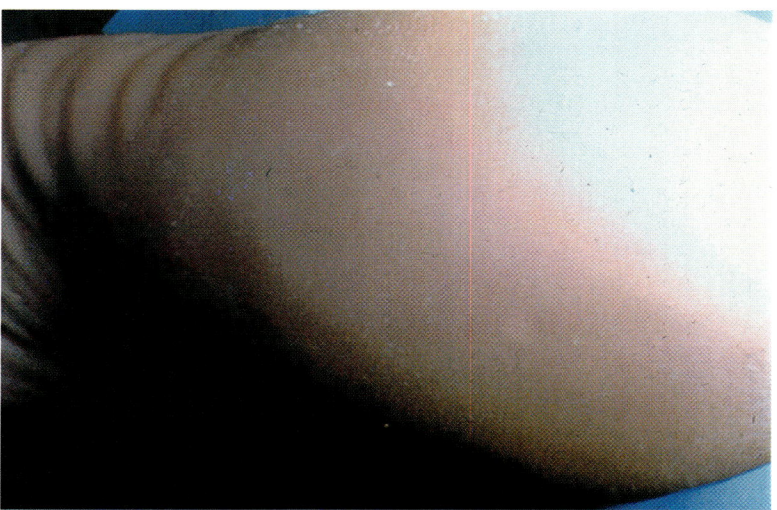

Section F — Clinical Aspects

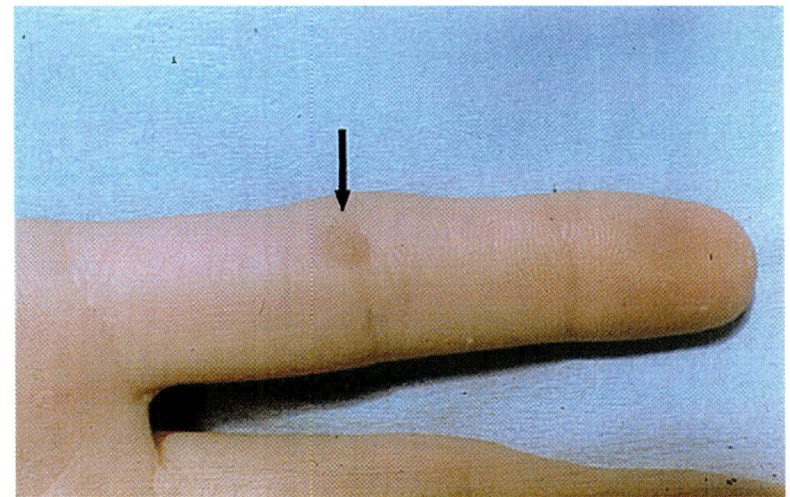

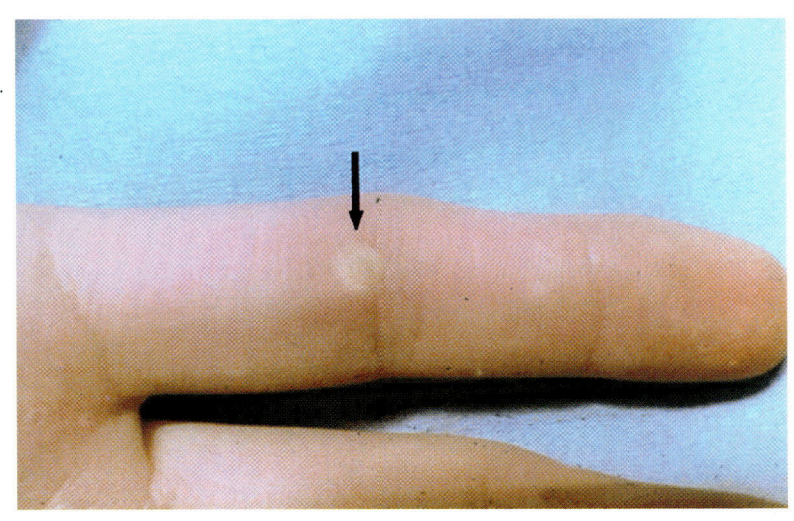

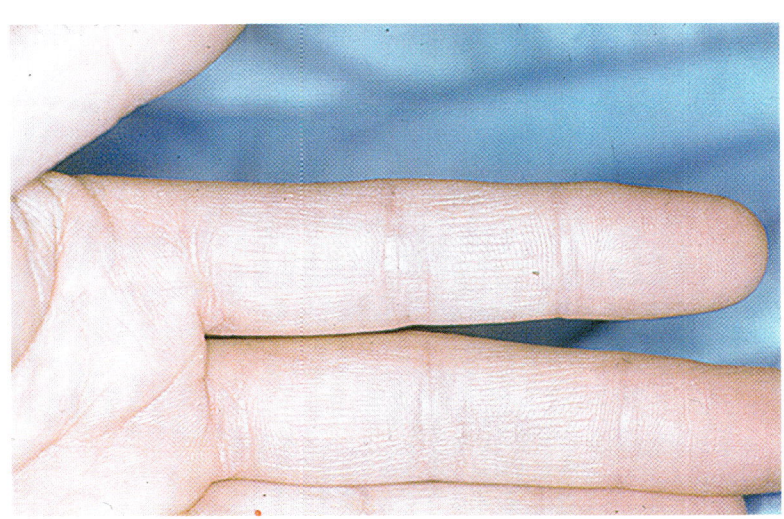

Fig. 11.2.14[4]. Finger wart (**A**), during the cryosurgical session (**B**) and 40 days after cryosurgery (**C**)

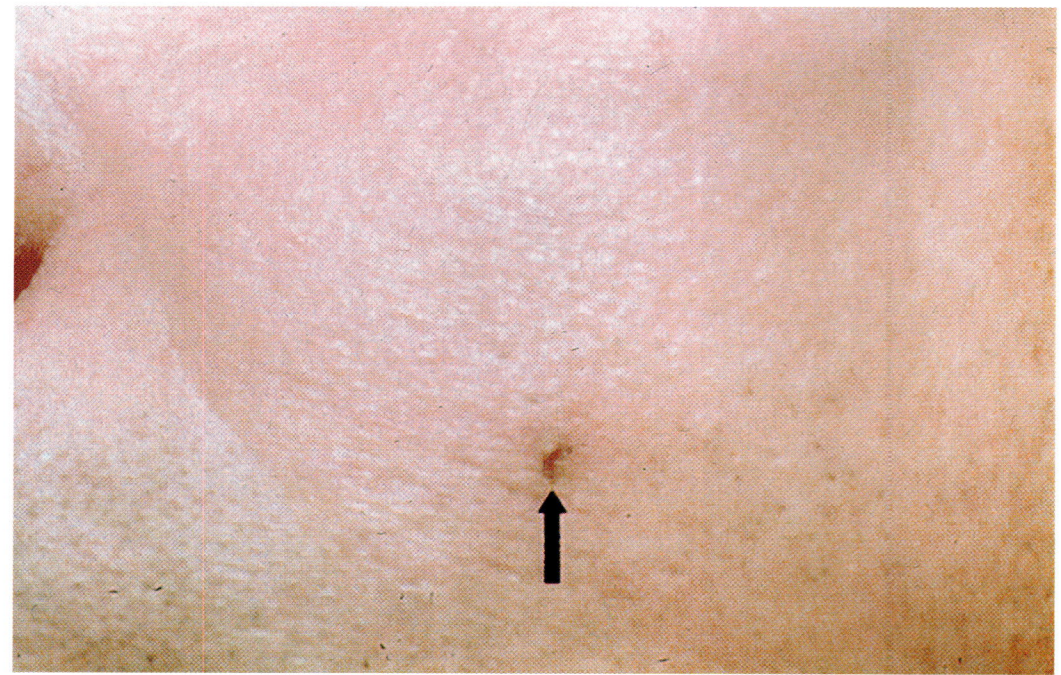

Fig. 11.2.15[4]. Verruca vulgaris of the cheek

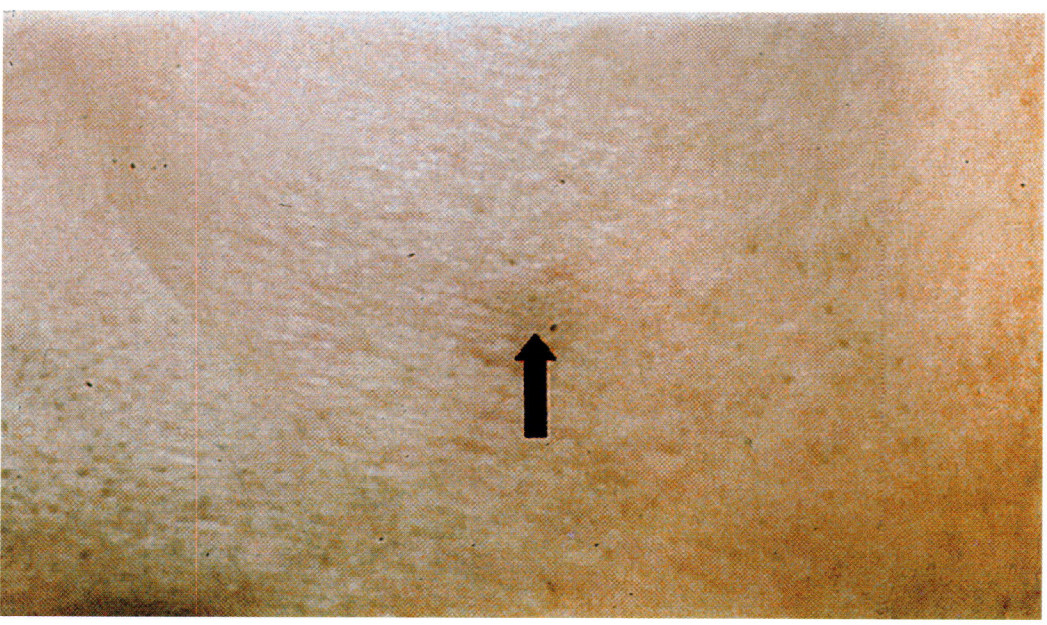

Fig. 11.2.16[4]. Two weeks after cryosurgery (using spray nitrogen)

Section F Clinical Aspects

Chapter 11
Cryosurgical
Dermatology

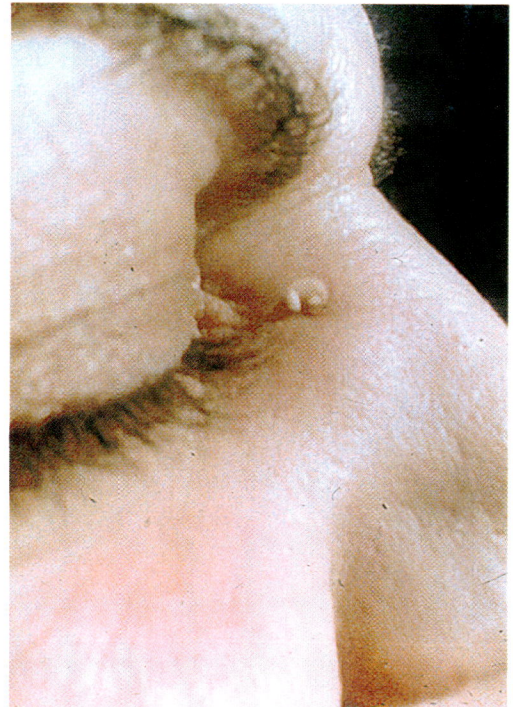

A

Fig. 11.2.17⁴. Filiform verrucae before cryosurgical treatment (**A**) and two weeks after treatment with spray nitrogen (**B**)

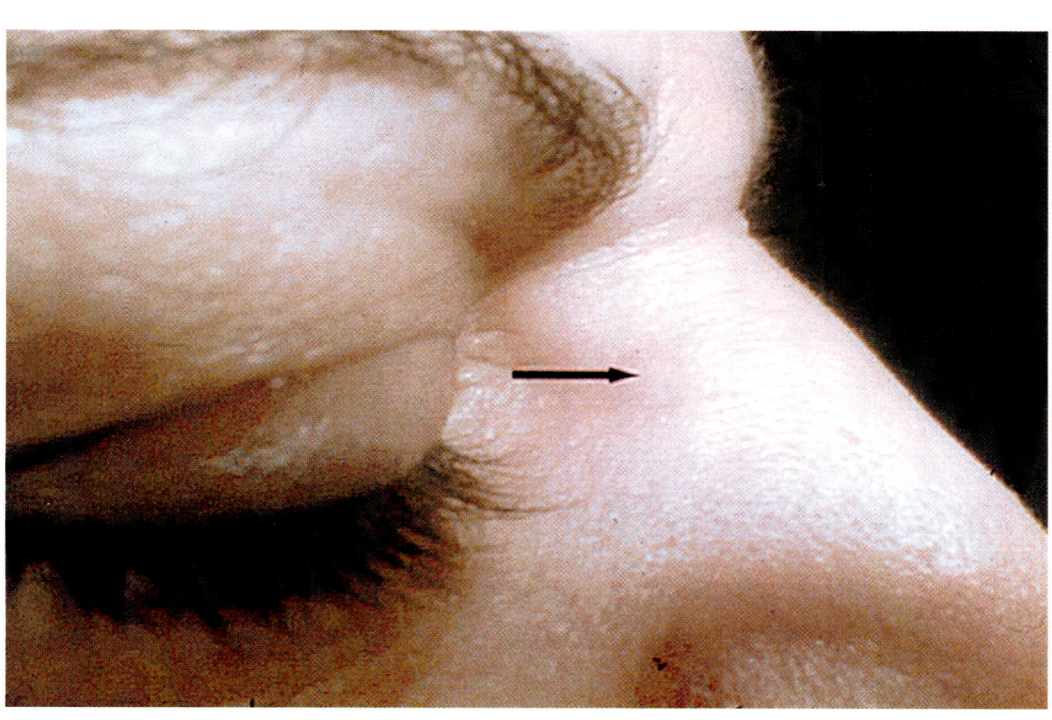

B

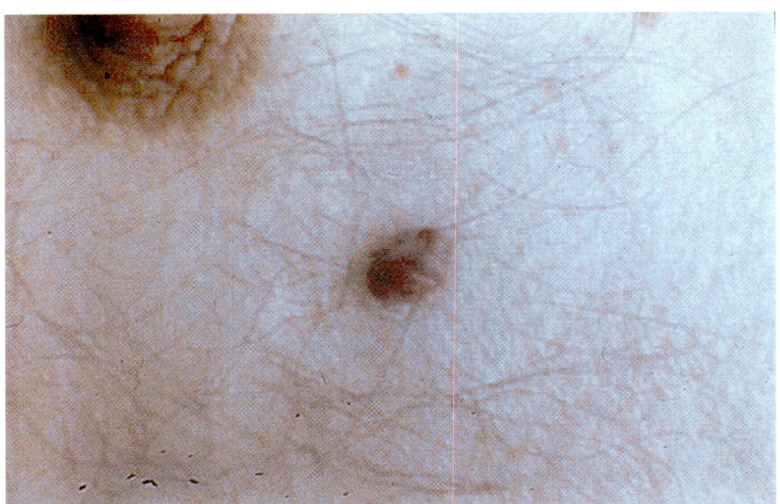

A

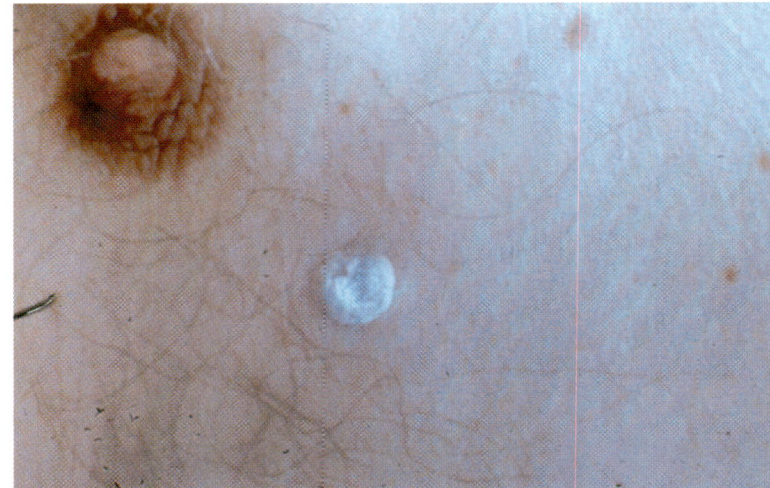

B

Fig. 11.2.18[4]. Senile hemangioma of the chest (**A**), during treatment (**B**) and 3 weeks after cryosurgery (**C**)

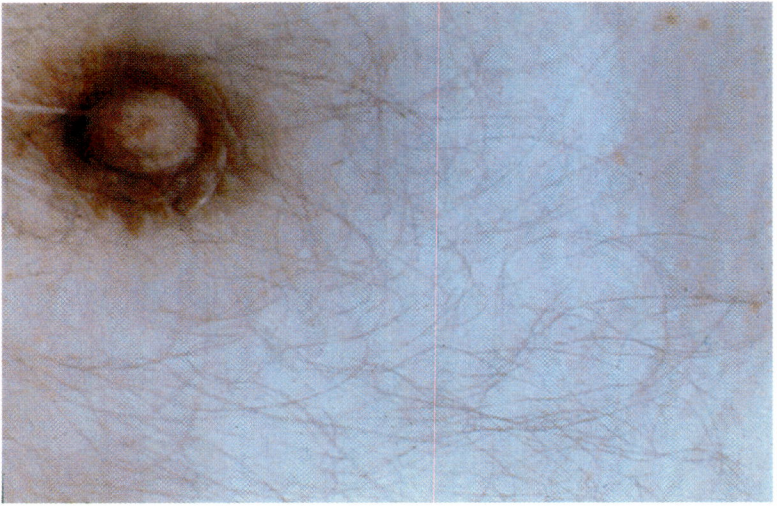

C

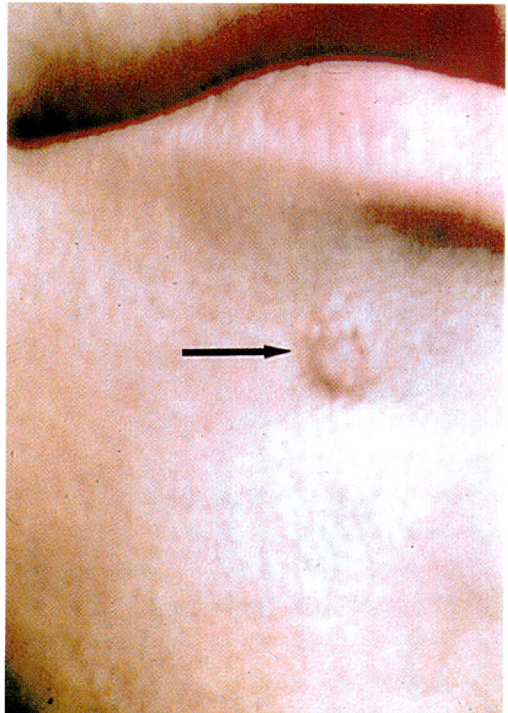

A

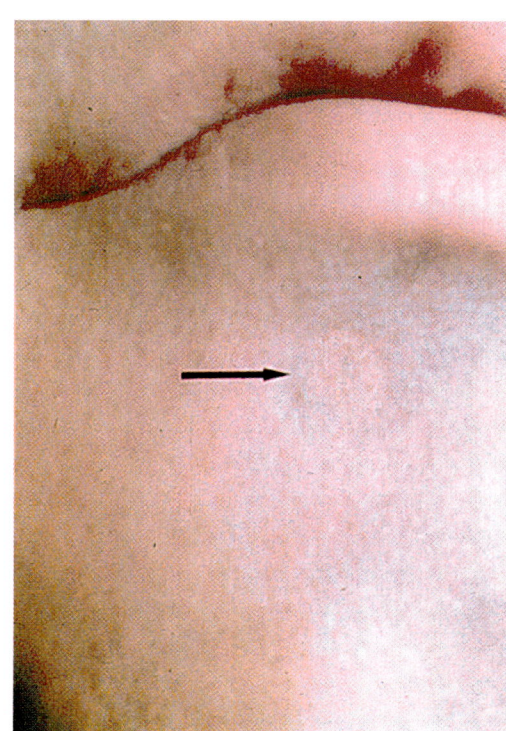

B

Fig. 11.2.19[4]. Chin wart (**A**), 15 days after a single session of cryosurgery (**B**)

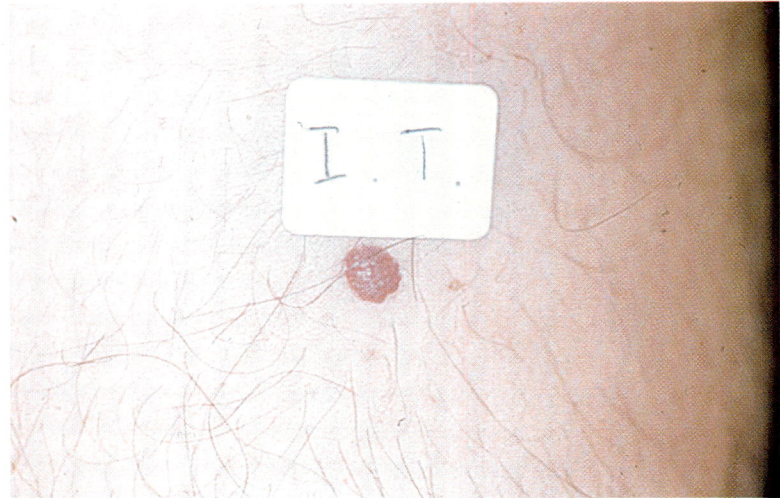

A

B

Fig. 11.2.20⁴. Strawberry hemangioma of the chest (**A**), during cryosurgical treatment (**B**) and one month after a single treatment (**C**)

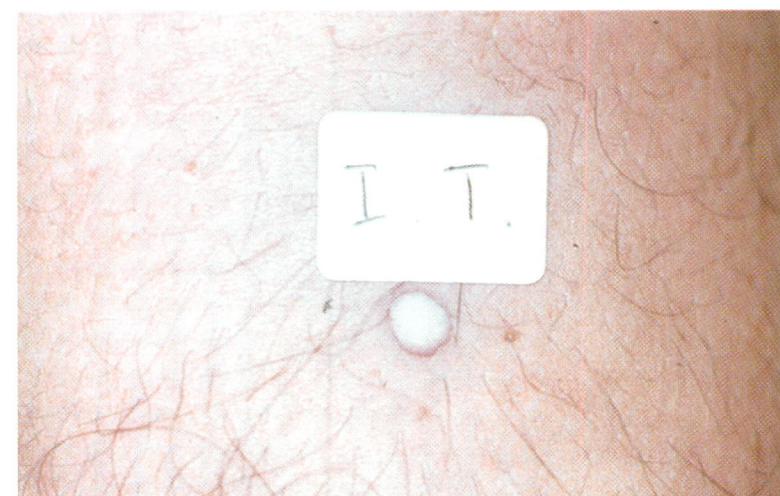

C

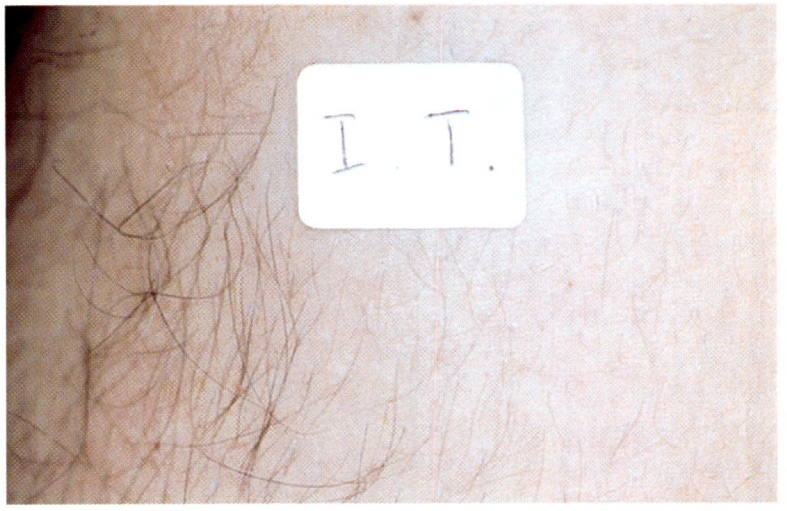

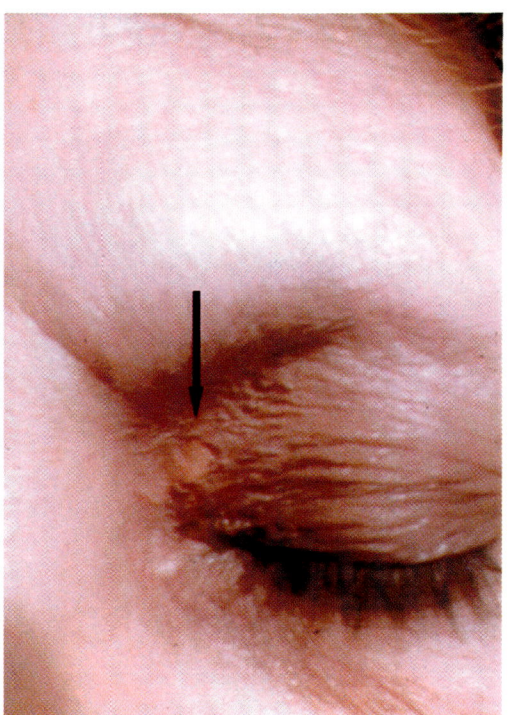

A

Fig. 11.2.21[4]. Xanthelasma before (**A**) and 6 weeks after a single cryosurgical session (**B**)

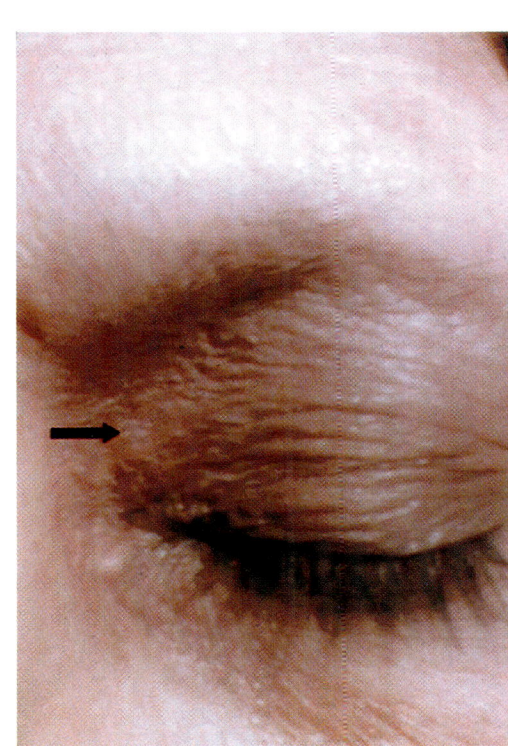

B

Chapter 11
Cryosurgical
Dermatology

11.3 Malignant Tumors

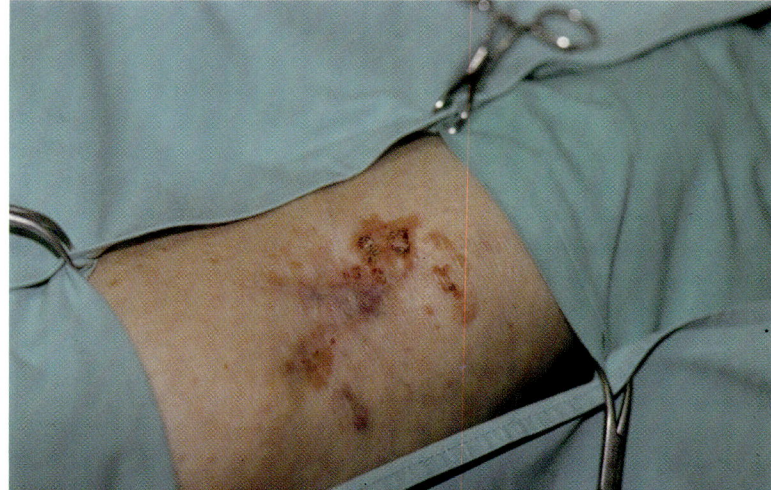

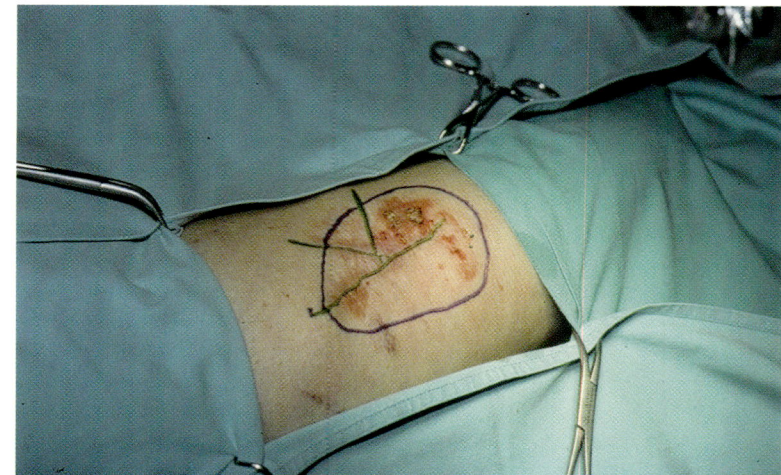

Fig. 11.3.1[1] A, B. Long-standing history of basal cell carcinoma (BCC) on the thigh of a 67-year-old woman (**A**). Patient had undergone five operations with skin grafts. Scars are visible (**B**)

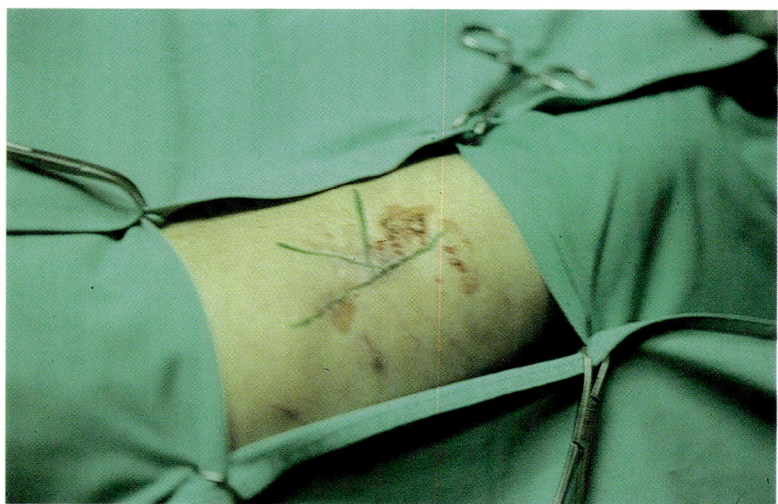

Fig. 11.3.2[1]. Demonstration of the boundary lines of recurrent basal cell carcinoma

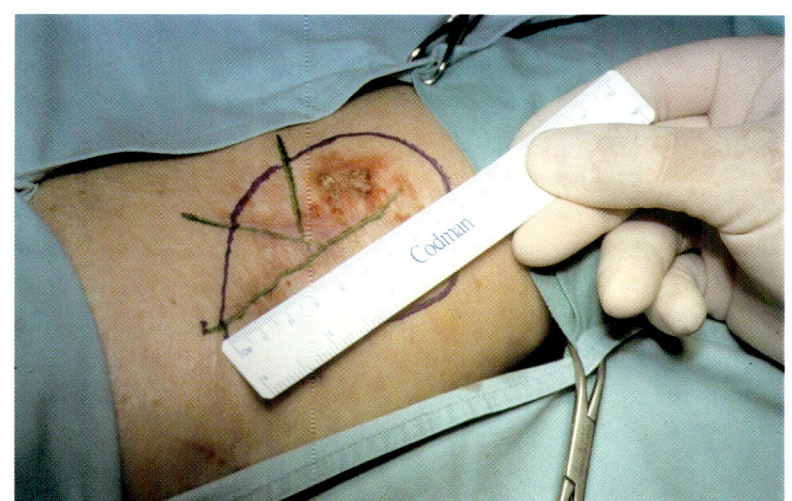

Fig. 11.3.3[1]. The entire area of skin involved measured 90 mm in diameter

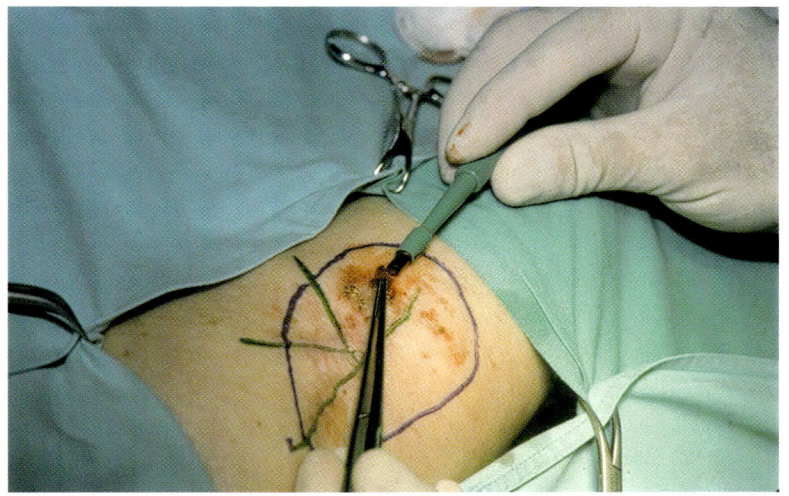

A

B

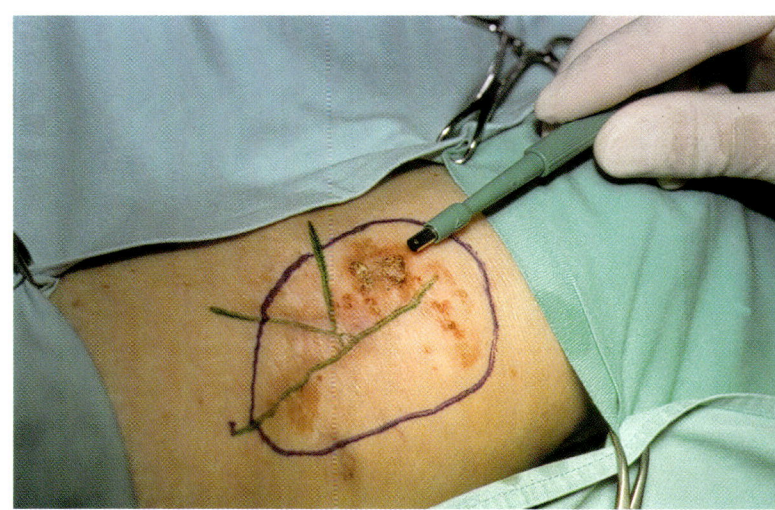

Fig. 11.3.4[1] **A–C.** Preoperative skin biopsy as a routine diagnostic tool used to evaluate and document the extensive skin lesion

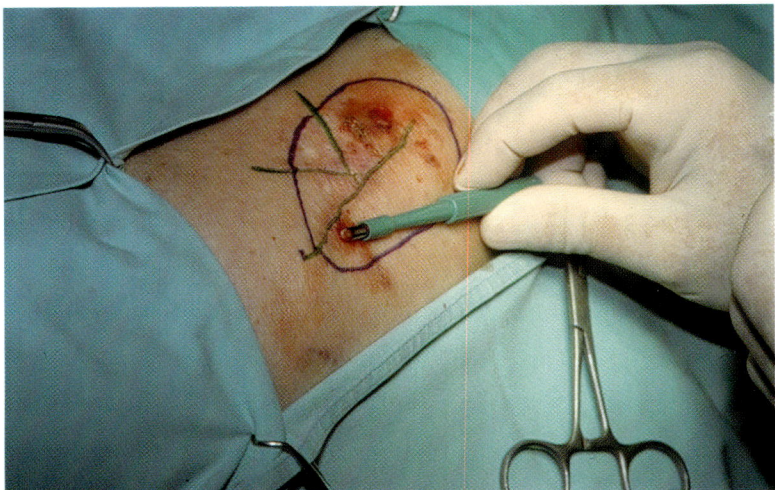

C

Fig. 11.3.4¹ A–C. Preoperative skin biopsy as a routine diagnostic tool used to evaluate and document the extensive skin lesion

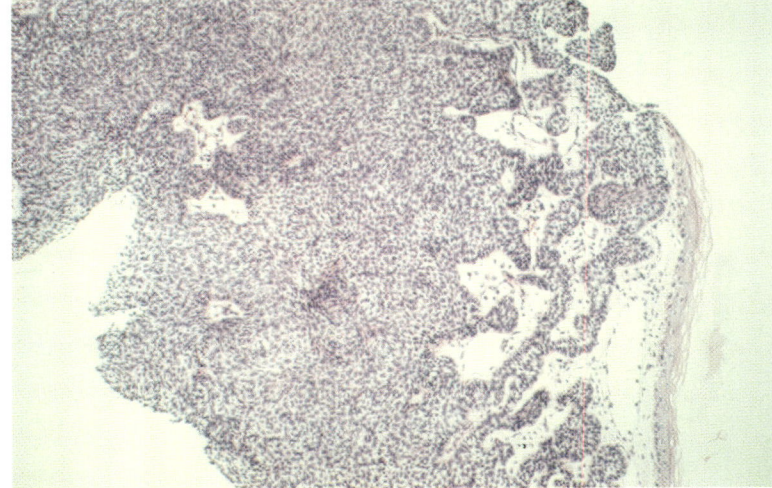

A

B

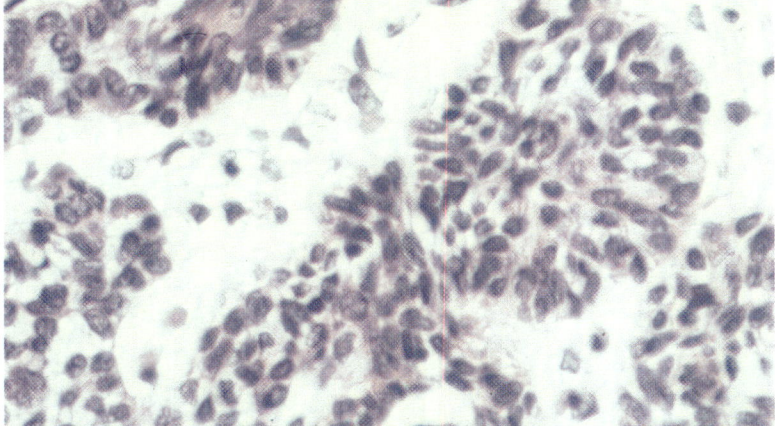

Fig. 11.3.5¹ A, B. Histological report: basal cell carcinoma infiltrate of solid nests of basaloid cells with peripheral palisading, magnified 100 times, (**A**) and solid nests of basaloid cells with palisading and rare mitotic figures, magnified 600 times (**B**)

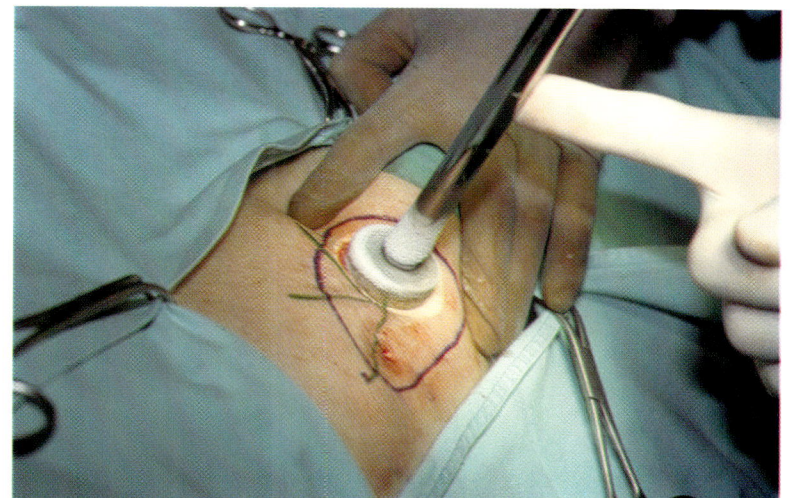

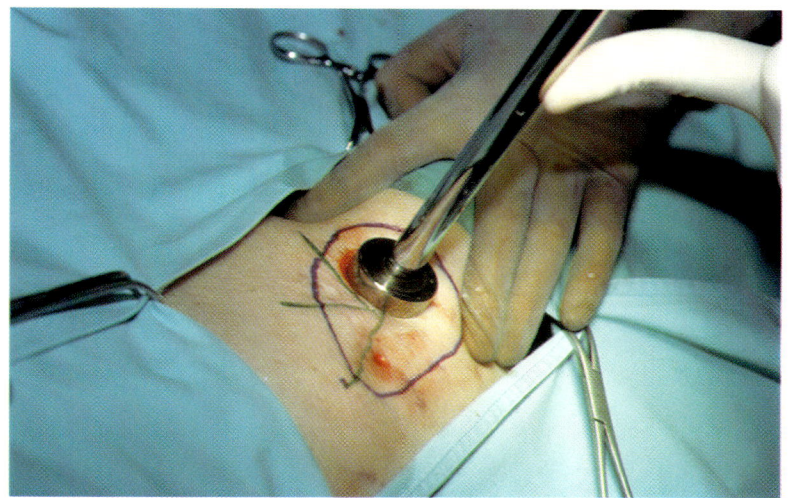

Fig. 11.3.6[1] **A, B.** The cryoprobe is applied to a part of the recurrent skin lesion (**A**) and a single freeze-thaw cycle is started (**B**). One treatment session is usually sufficient

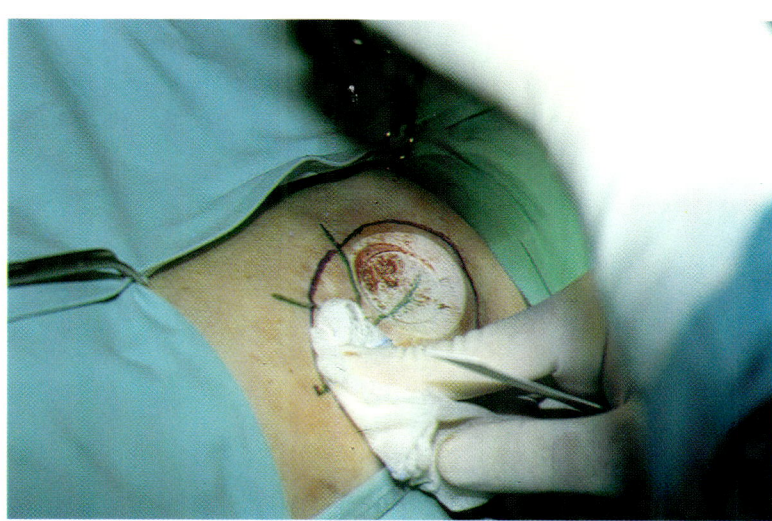

Fig. 11.3.7[1]. View of the cryosurgical zone. The rim of the cryozone clearly demarcates the line between the area cryosurgically destroyed, which was followed by cryogenic necrosis, and the healthy skin

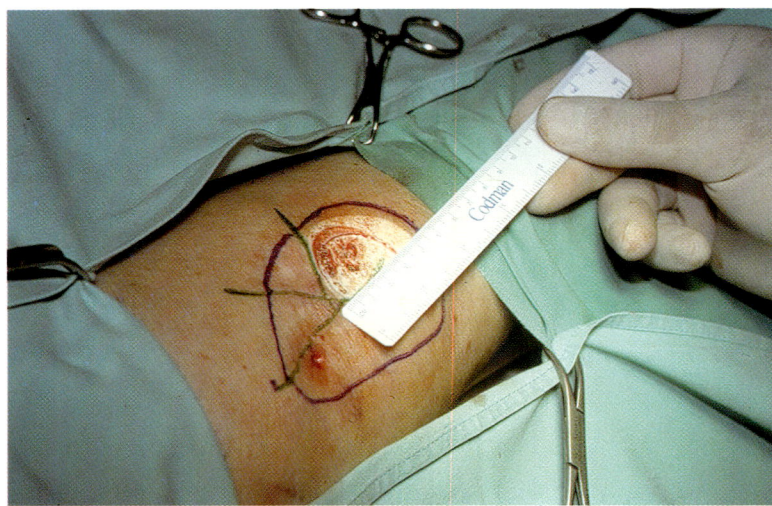

Fig. 11.3.8[1]. Each cryosurgical zone measures 60 mm in diameter

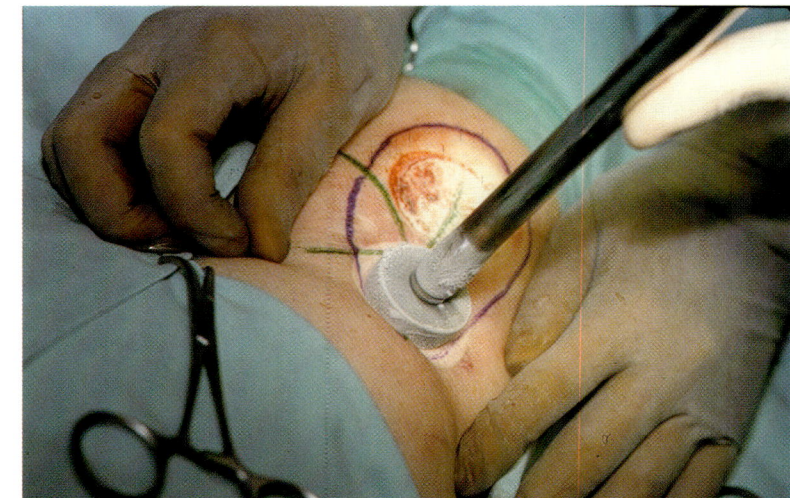

Fig. 11.3.9[1]. The extirpation of the extensive skin lesion is performed in the overlap cryosurgical technique

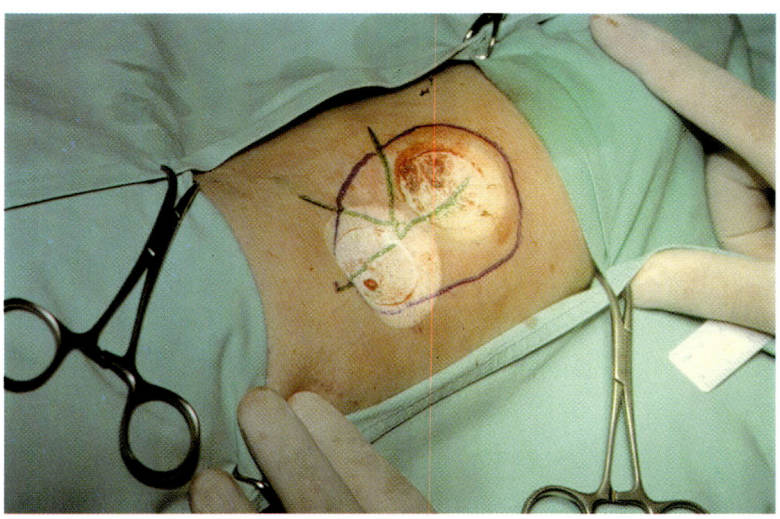

Fig. 11.3.10[1]. View of both cryosurgical zones which cover most of the malignant skin tumor

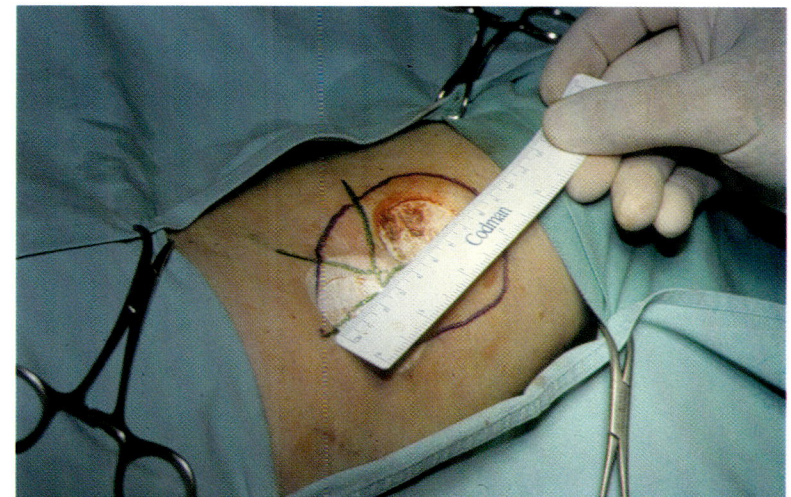

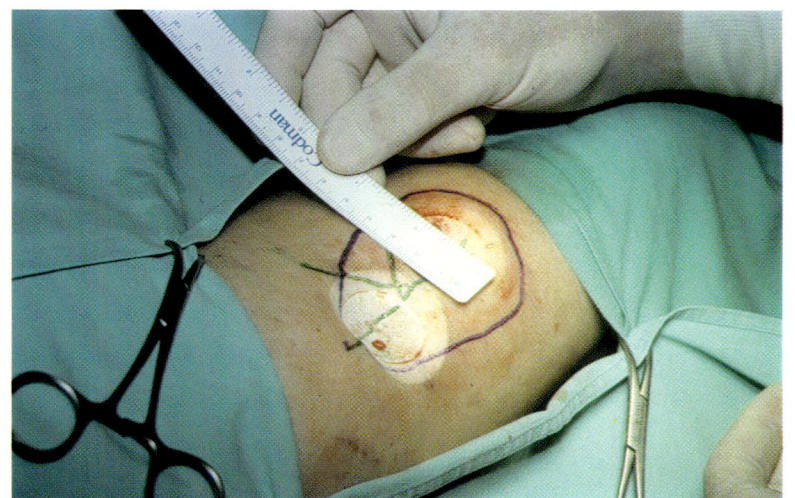

Fig. 11.3.11[1]. After a single freeze-thaw cycle the cryosurgical area measures 104 mm in length (**A**). The cryosurgical bridge measures 26 mm in width between the two cryozones (**B**)

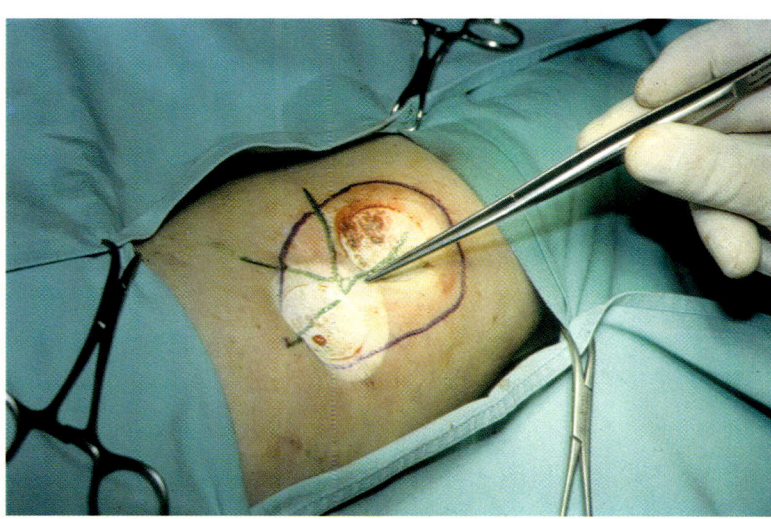

Fig. 11.3.12[1]. The cryosurgical bridge between the two cryozones is clearly visible

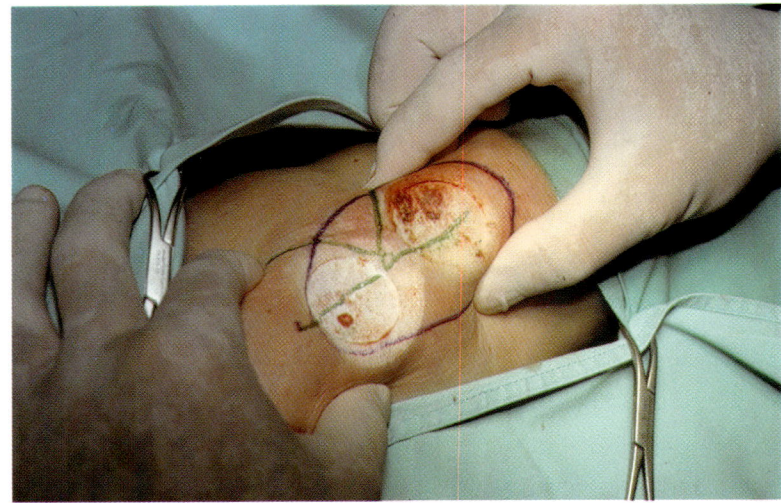

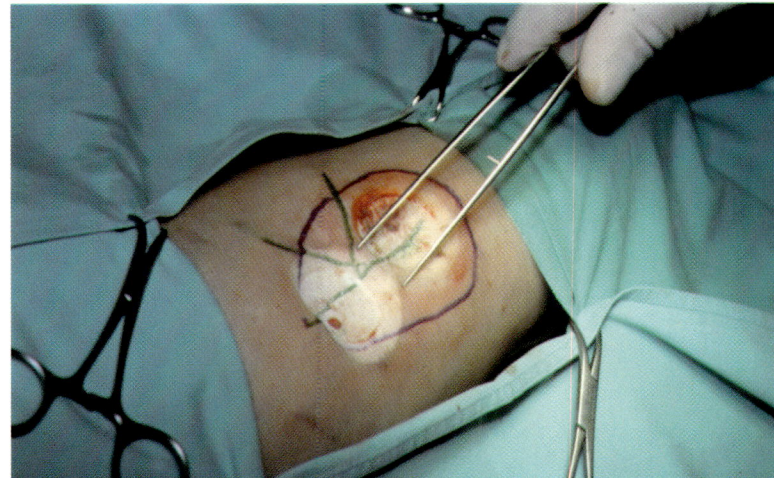

Fig. 11.3.13[1]. The ice block is easily palpable in the area of the cryozone (**A**) as well as clearly visible in the area of the cryosurgical bridge (**B**)

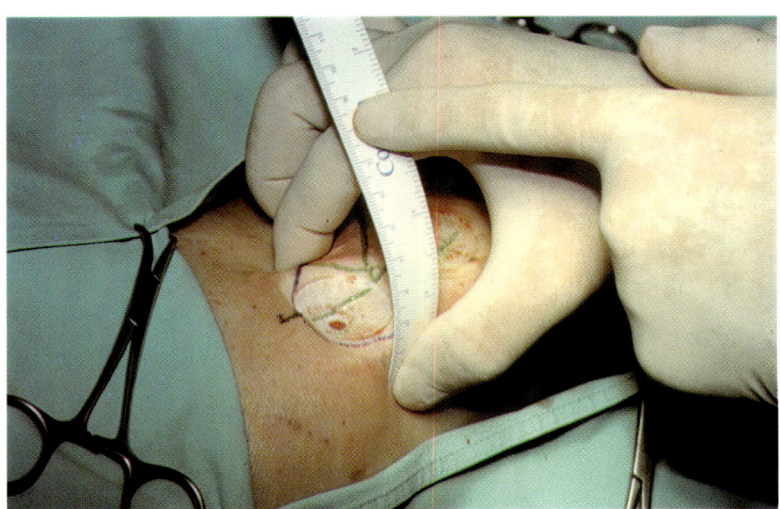

Fig. 11.3.14[1]. Each of the cryozones measures 17 mm in depth immediately after the single freeze-thaw cycle

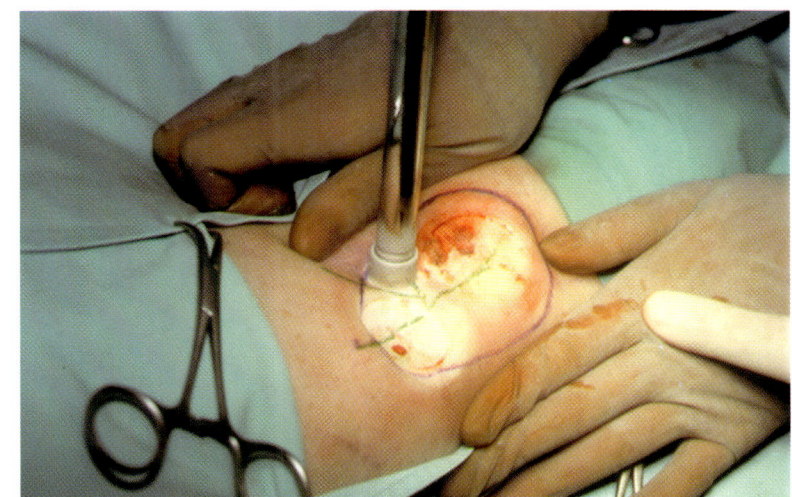

Fig. 11.3.15[1]. Finally, the remaining part of the malignant skin lesion is cryoextirpated using the same cryosurgical overlap technique

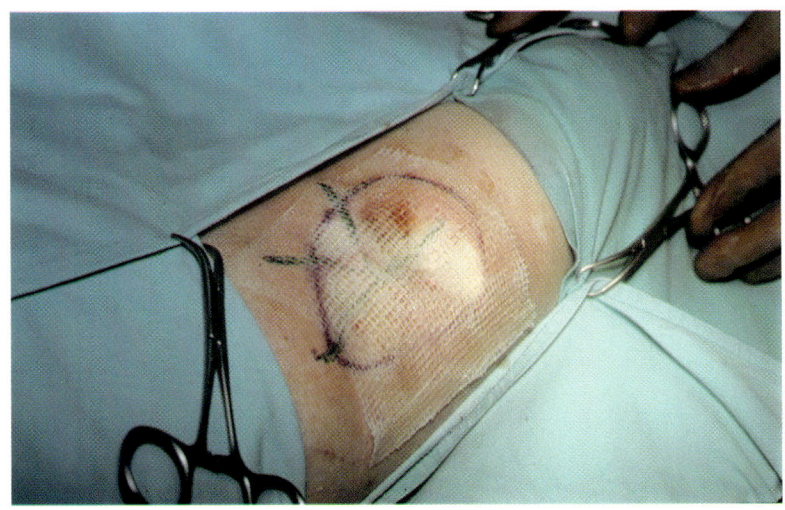

A

B

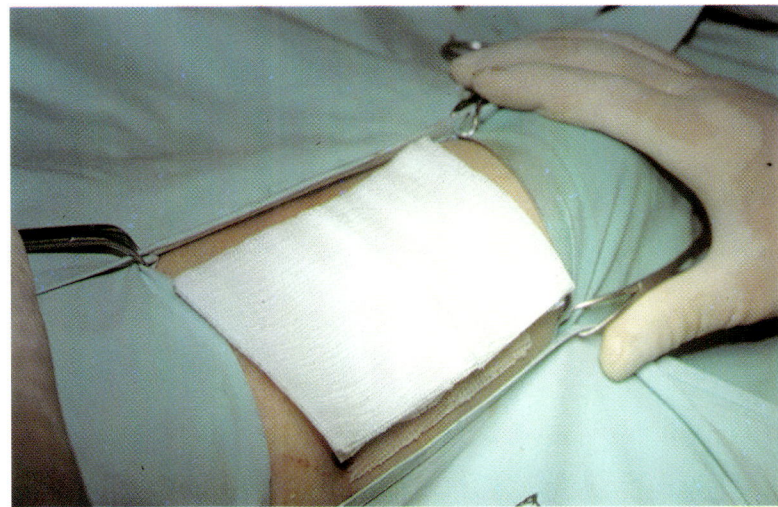

Fig. 11.3.16[1]. Dressing layers. A layer of an ointment (Sofra-tuell) (A) and an absorbent cotton gauze layer (B) is used as a contact layer between the dressing and the wound surface

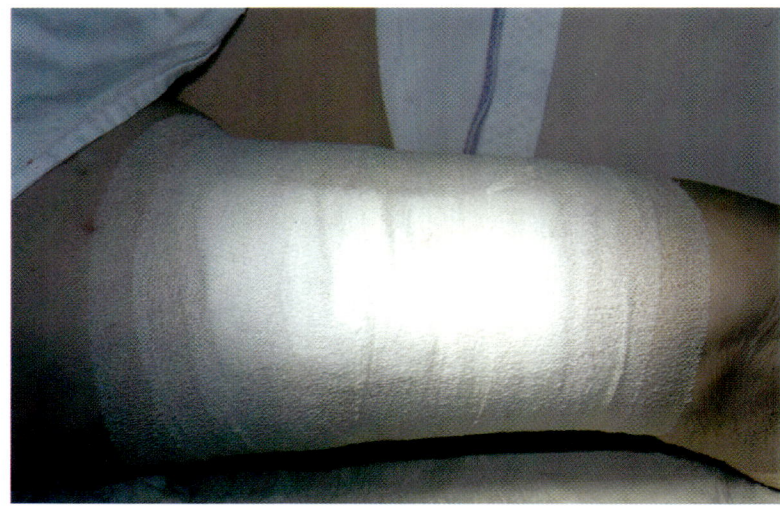

Fig. 11.3.17[1]. View of the wound dressing

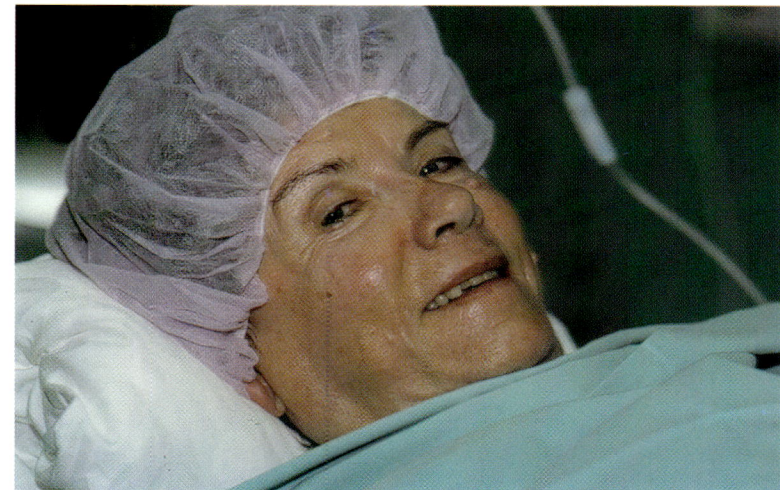

Fig. 11.3.18[1]. Patient smiling happily after the cryosurgical operation

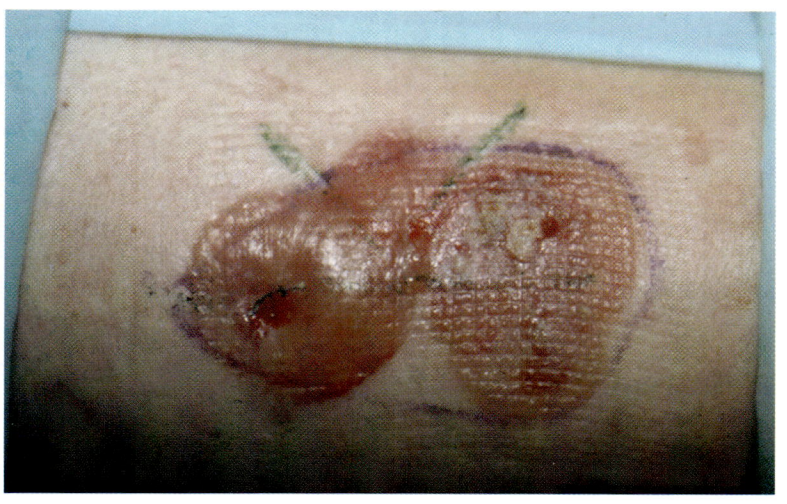

Fig. 11.3.19[1]. Wound healing. 24 h after cryosurgical treatment

Section F Clinical Aspects

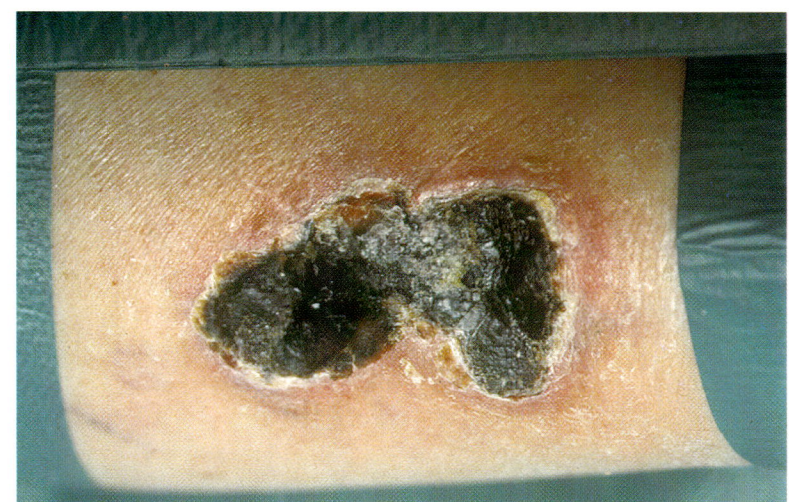

Fig. 11.3.20[1]. Wound healing. 6 weeks after cryosurgical treatment

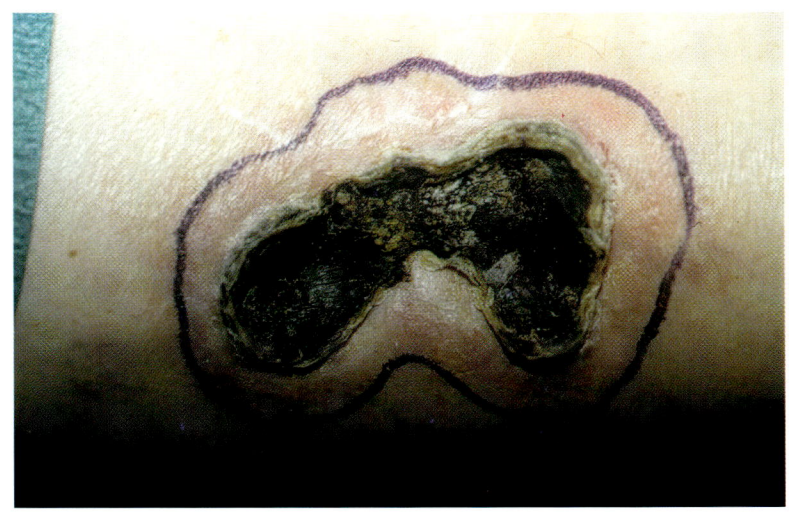

A

B

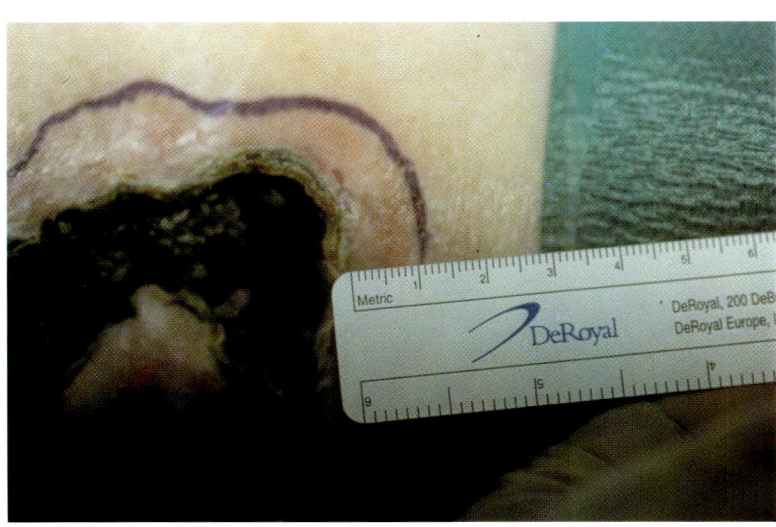

Fig. 11.3.21[1]. Wound healing. 8 weeks after cryosurgical treatment with crust formation (**A**). The crust will slowly be sloughed off and new connective tissue can be seen (**B**). The new tissue measures 12 mm in diameter

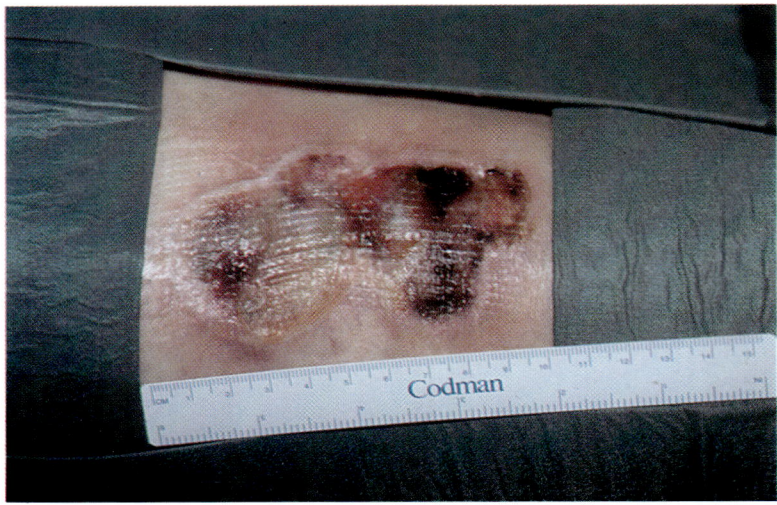

Fig. 11.3.22¹. Wound healing. 10 weeks after cryosurgical treatment showing that the crust has fallen off

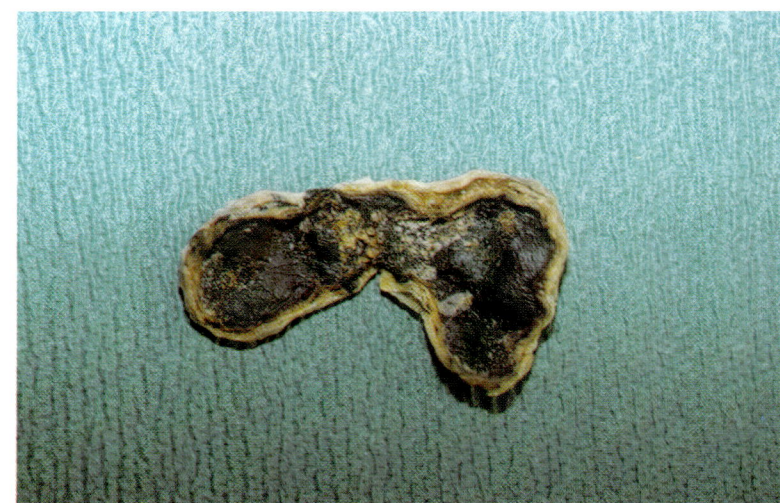

A

B

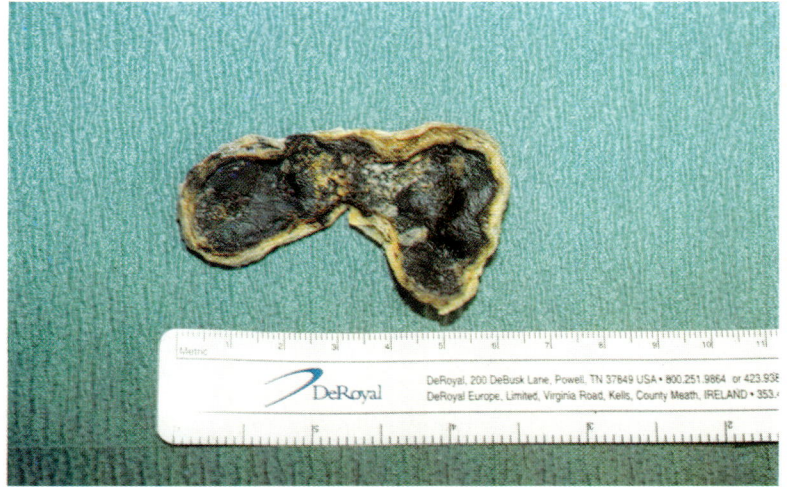

Fig. 11.3.23¹. The sloughed-off crust 10 weeks after cryosurgical treatment of recurrent extensive basal cell carcinoma (**A**) measures a total of 60 mm in diameter (**B**)

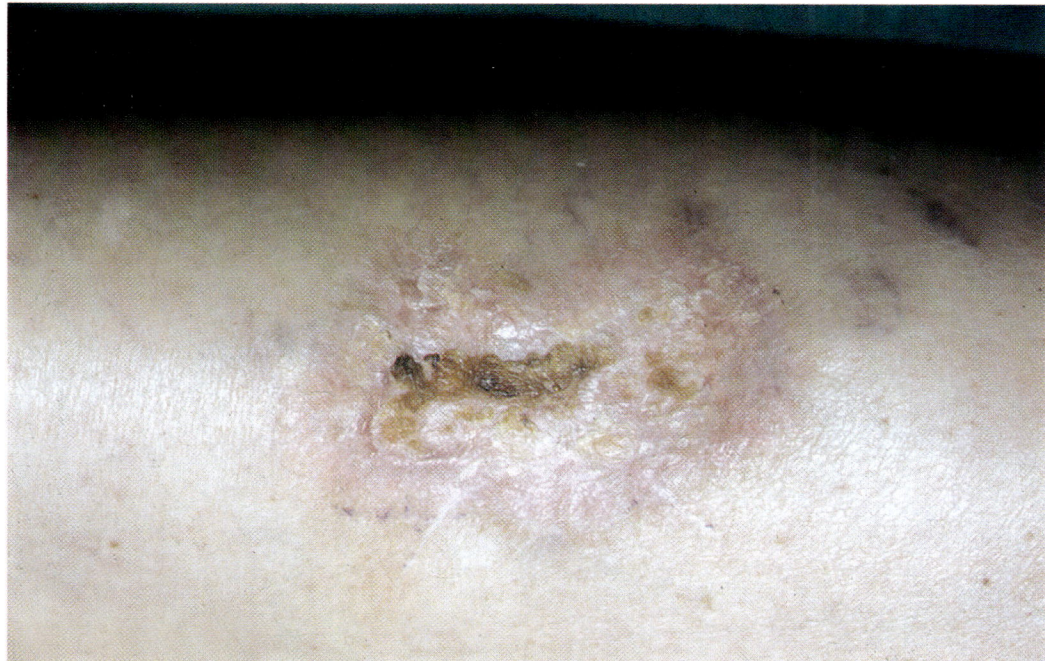

Fig. 11.3.24[1]. Wound healing. Cosmetic result 3 months after cryosurgical treatment

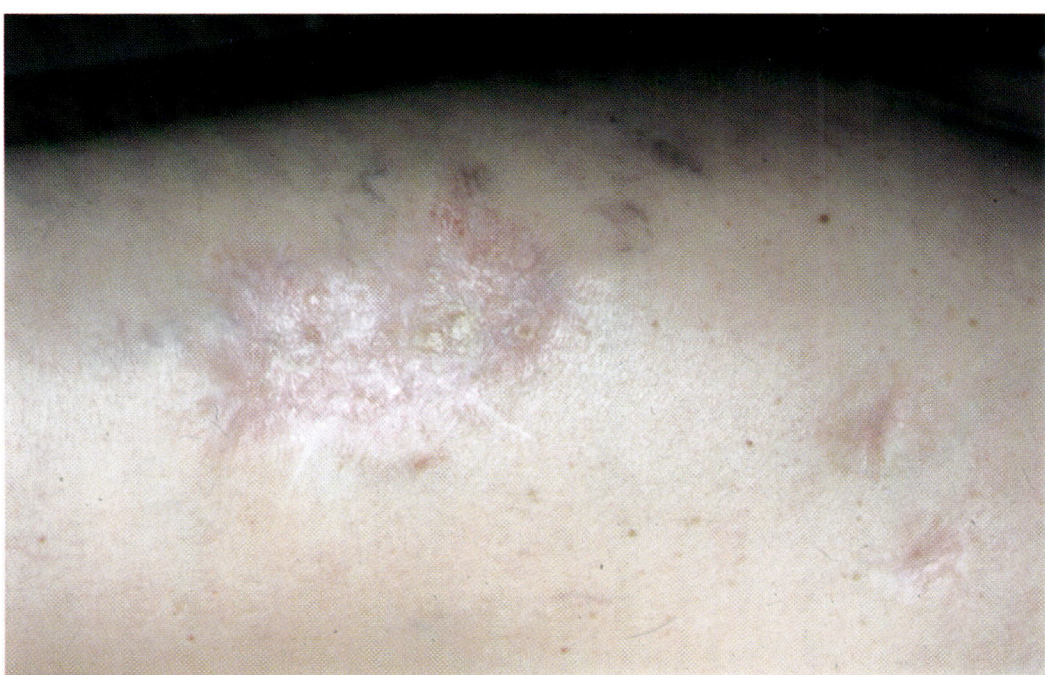

Fig. 11.3.25[1]. Excellent cosmetic result 1 year after cryosurgical treatment. No recurrence. Also, two other small BCCs can be seen on the right side after cryosurgical treatment six months before the picture was taken

Chapter 11
Cryosurgical Dermatology

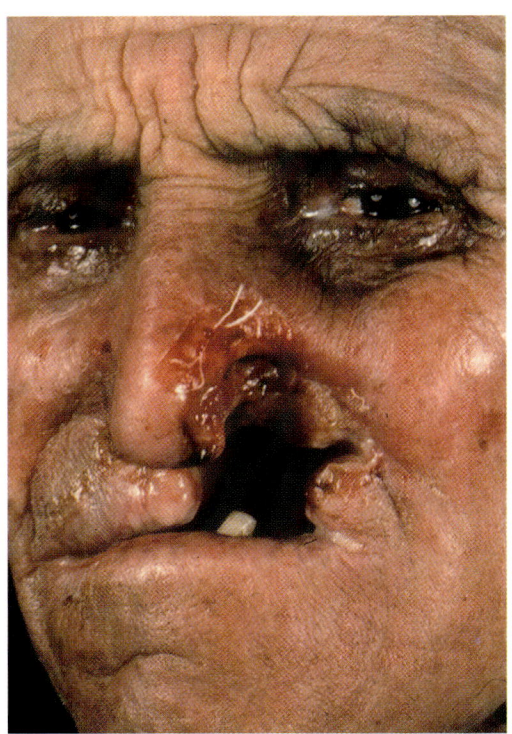

Fig. 11.3.26[2]. "Ulcus rodens" recurrence after radiotherapy (**A**). Clinical cure after cryosurgery (**B**)

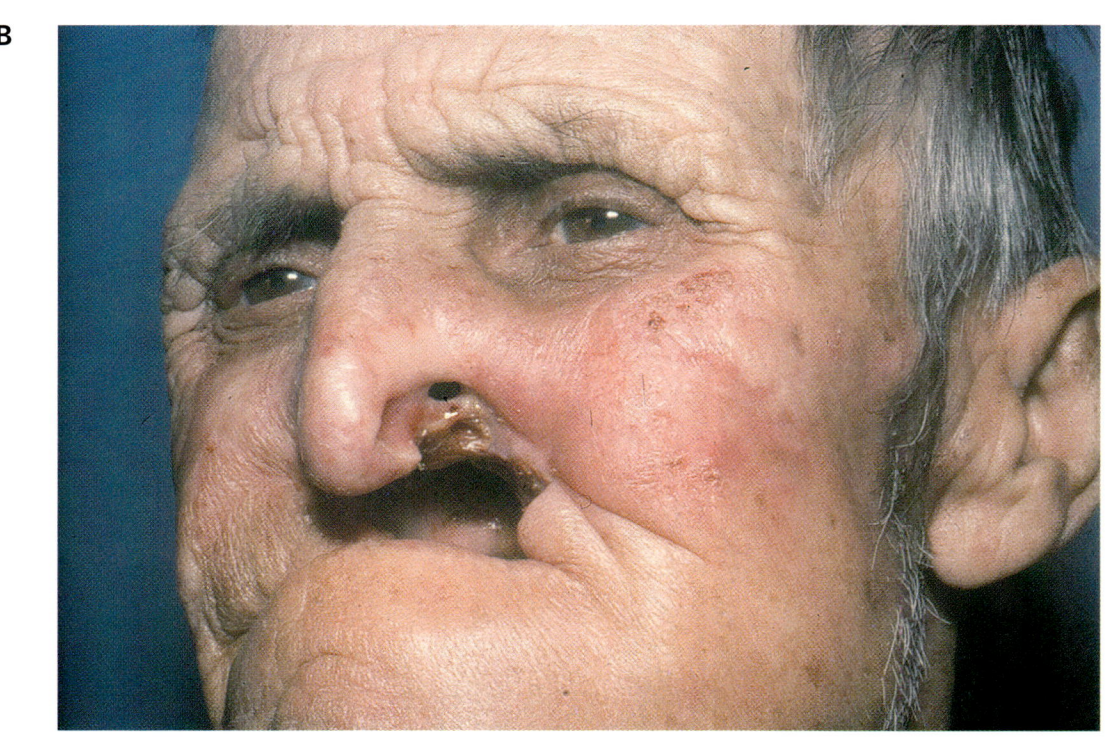

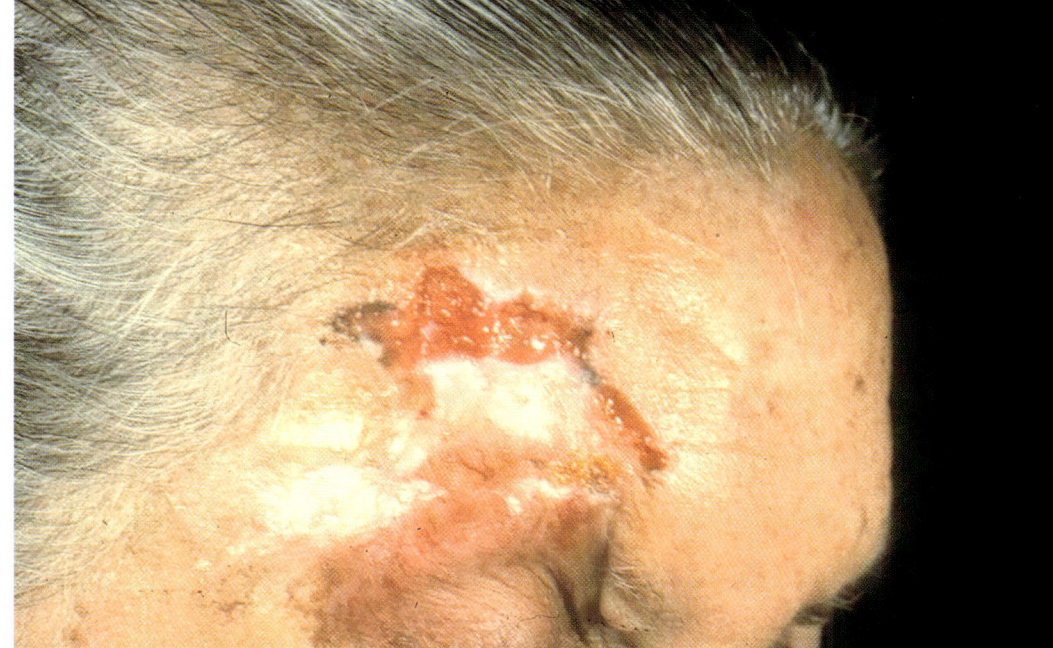

Fig. 11.3.27². Basal cell carcinoma, recurrence after radiotherapy (**A**). After cryosurgery, no recurrence after 5 years (**B**)

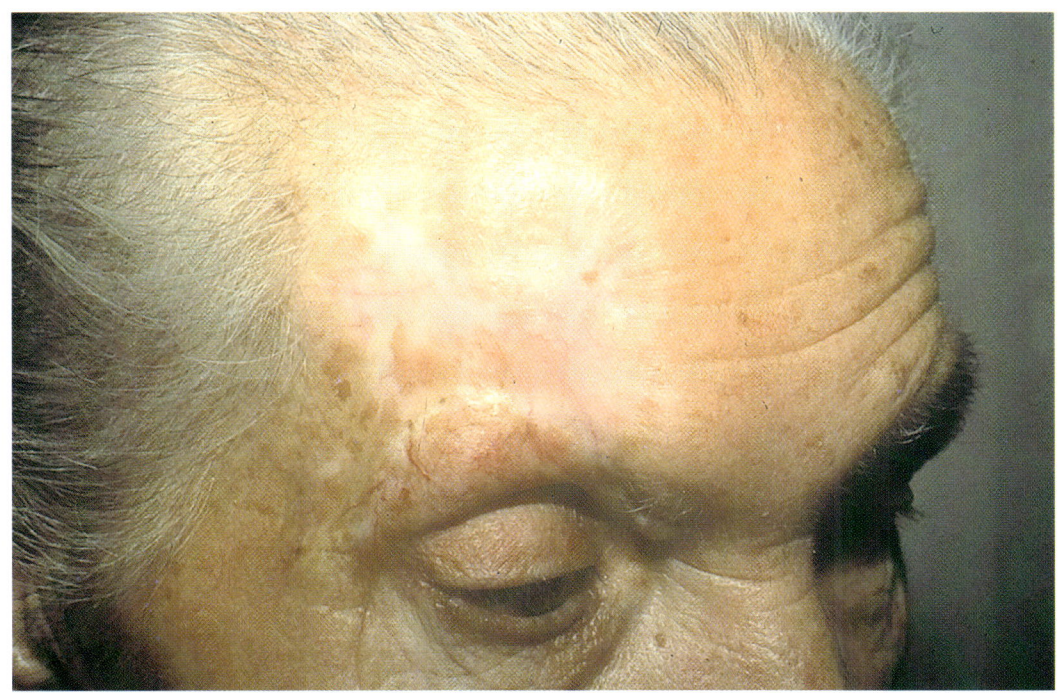

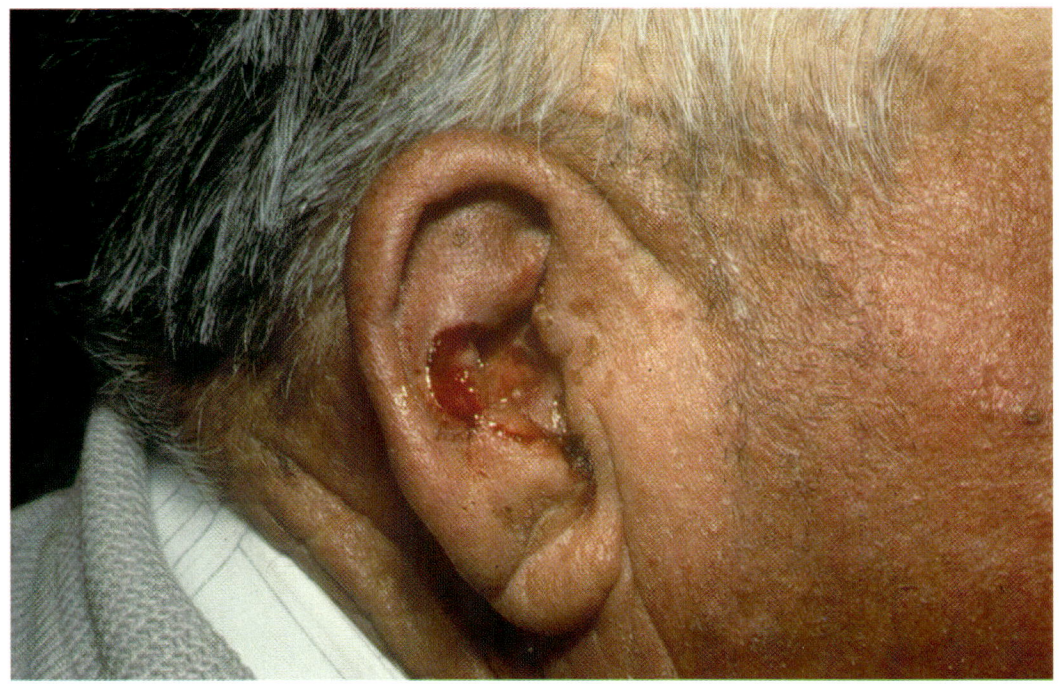

Fig. 11.3.28². Basal cell carcinoma (A). Clinical cure after cryosurgery (B)

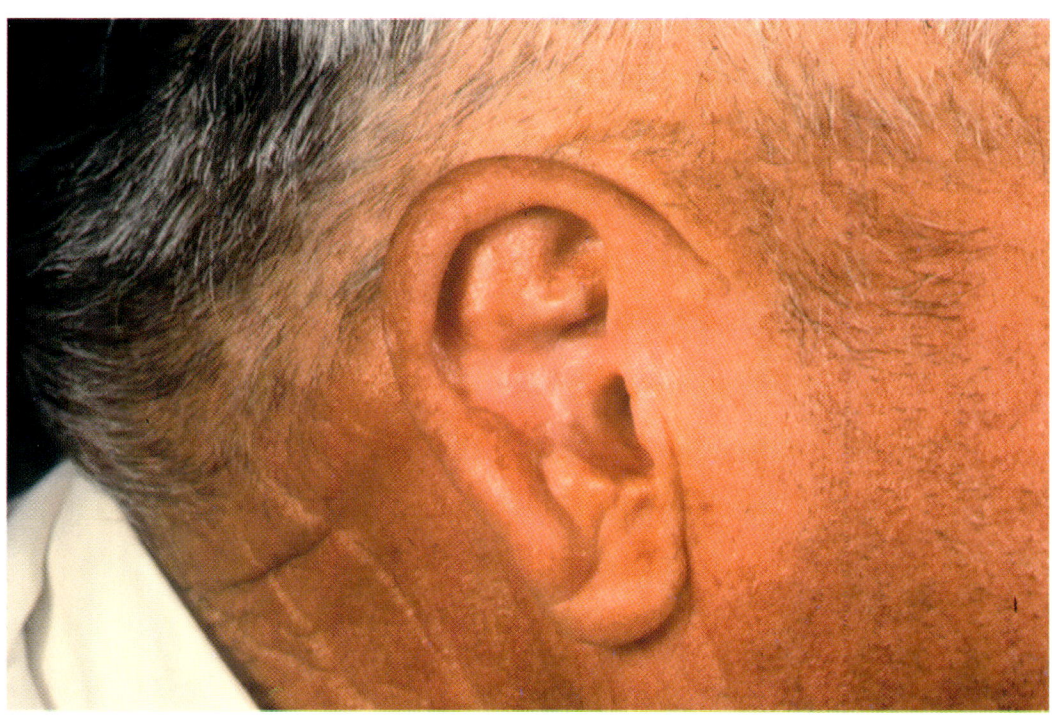

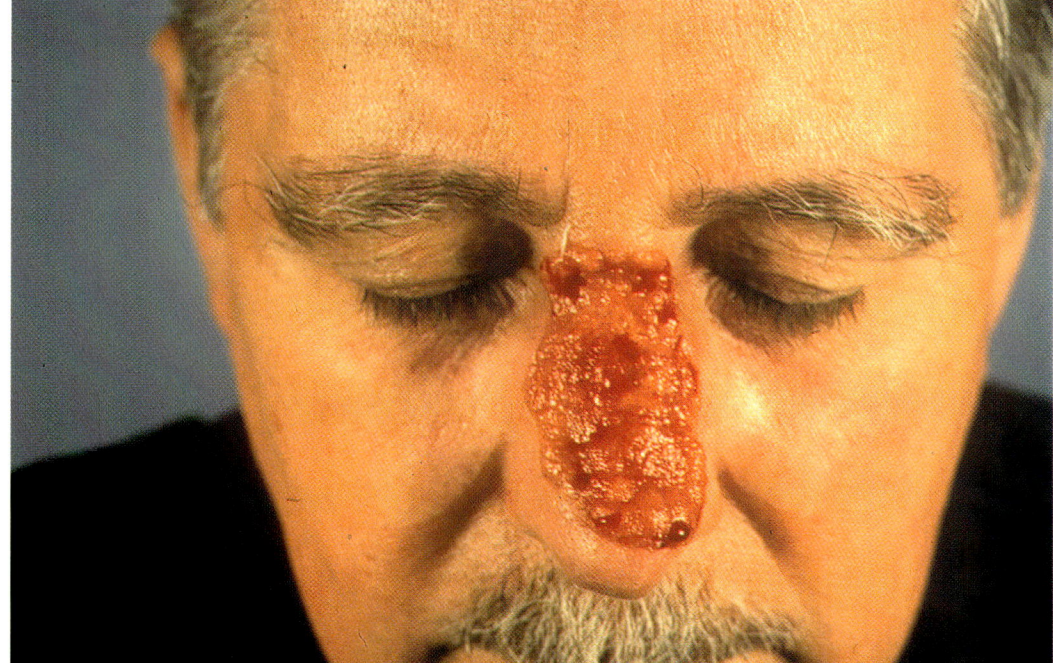

Fig. 11.3.29[2]. Basal cell carcinoma (A). After cryosurgery, no recurrence after 10 years (B)

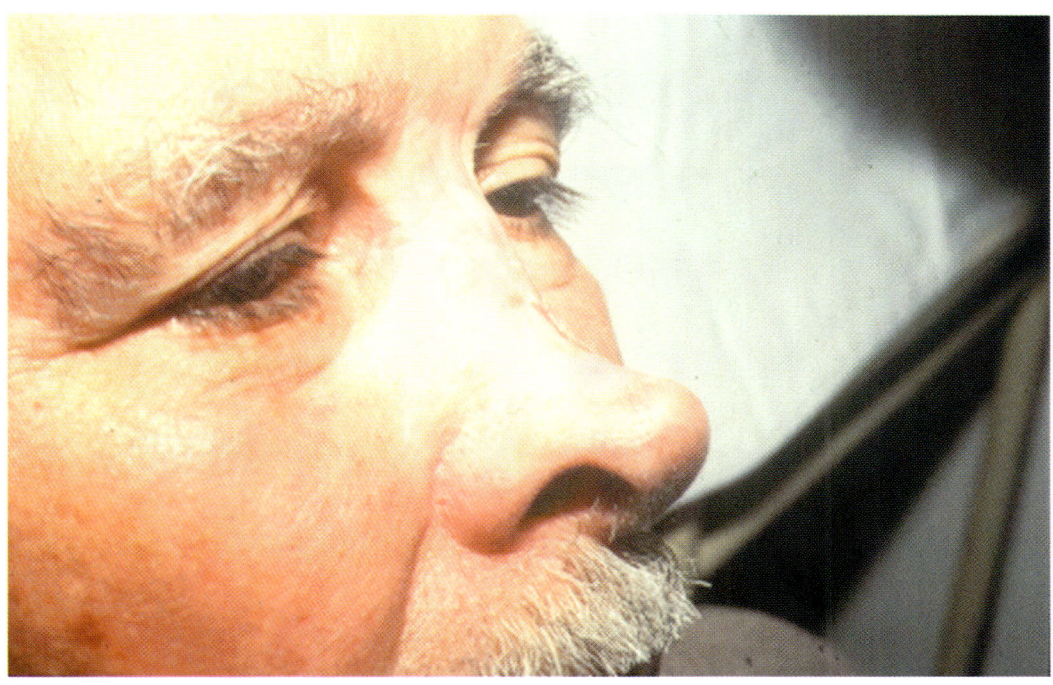

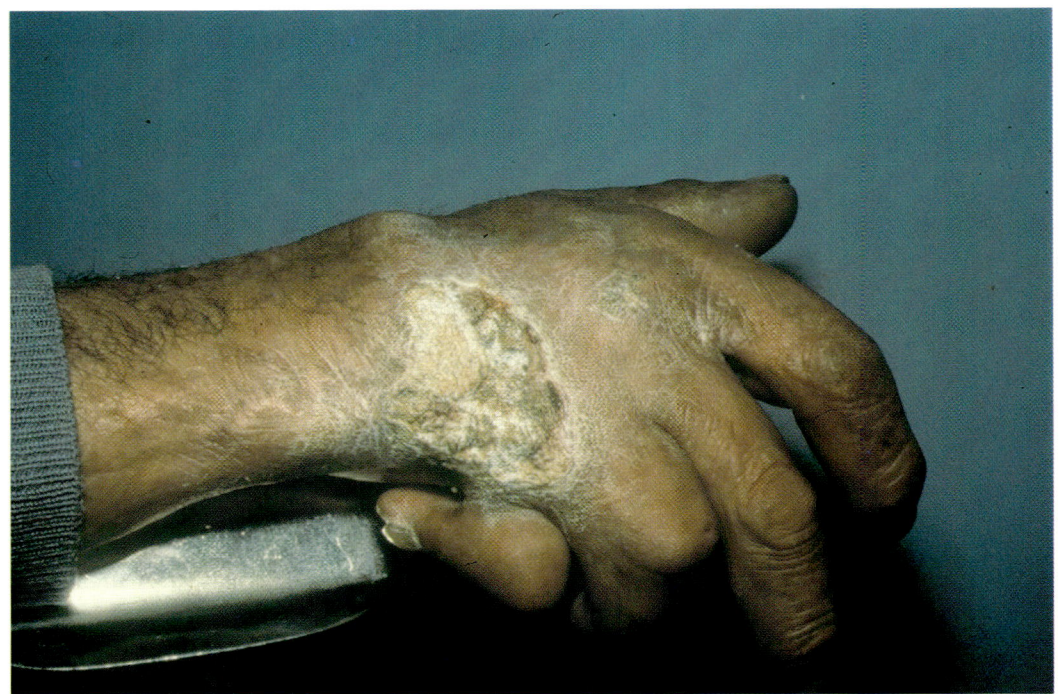

Fig. 11.3.30². A long-existing squamous cell carcinoma which had developed on the scar tissue from a burn. Amputation was proposed (**A**). After cryosurgery, no recurrence after a 5-year observation period (**B**)

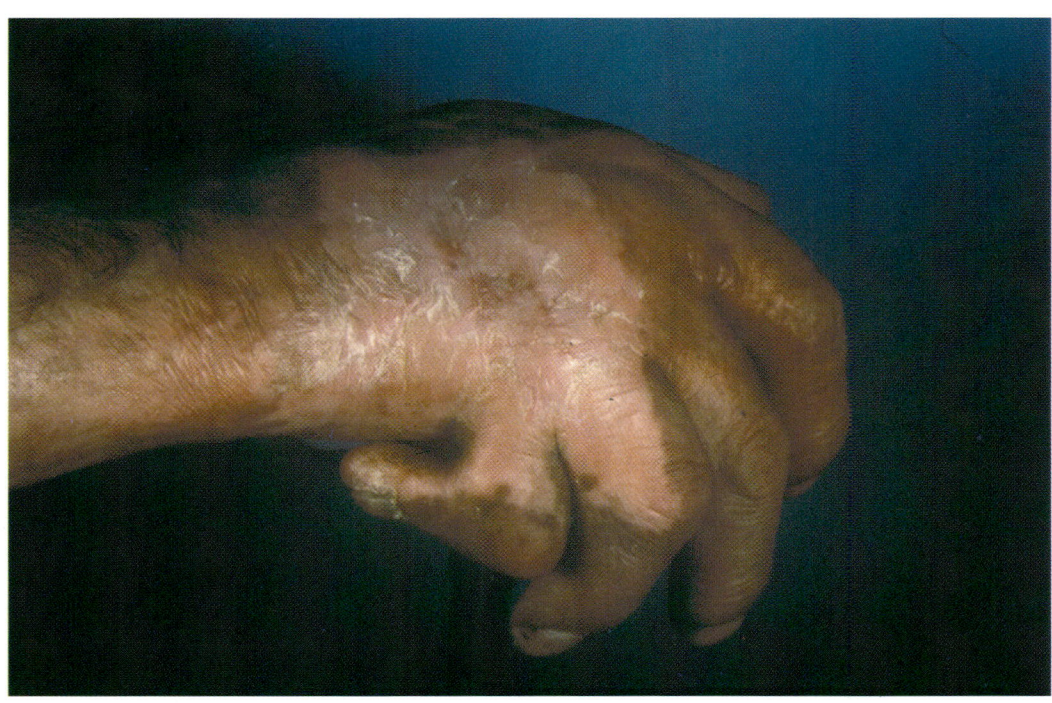

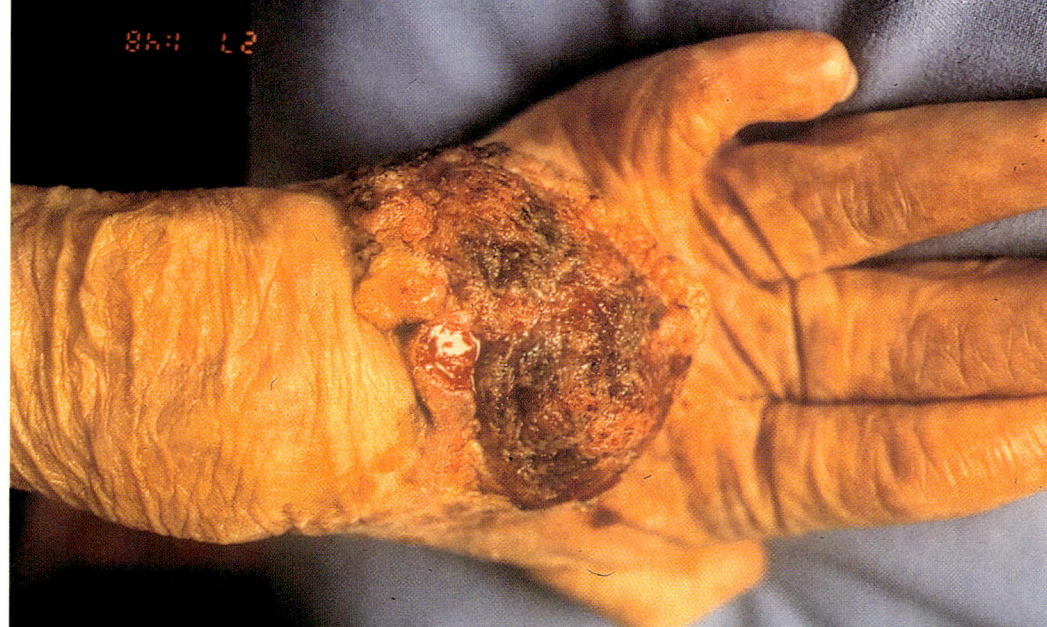

Fig. 11.3.31[2]. A long-existing squamous cell carcinoma which had developed on scar tissue. Amputation was proposed (**A**). After cryosurgery, no recurrence after a 3-year observation period (**B**)

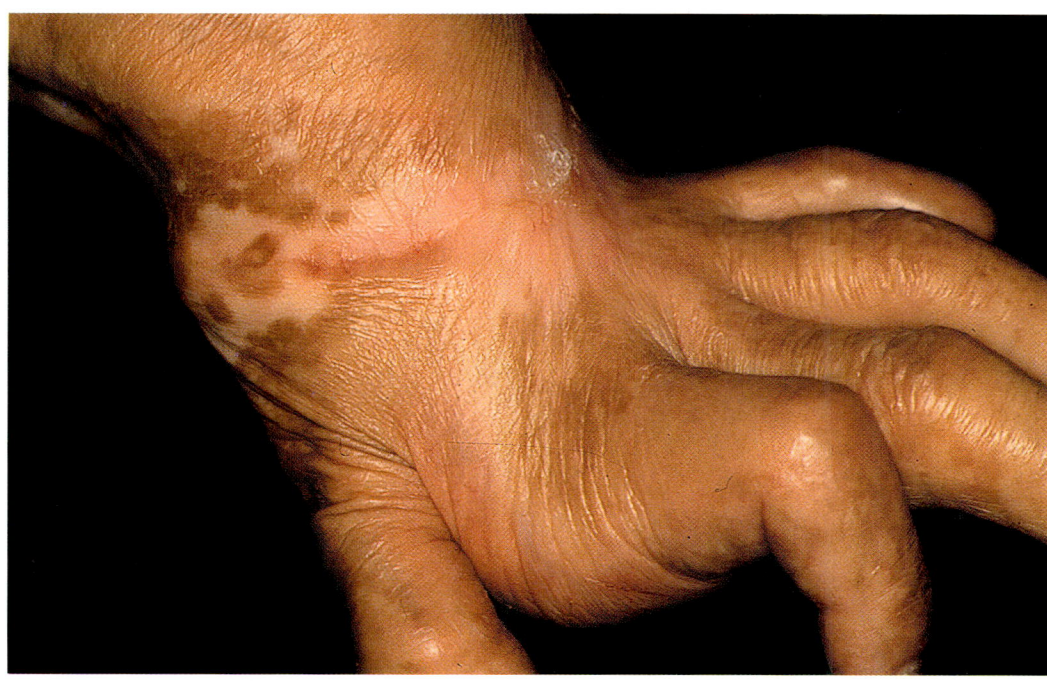

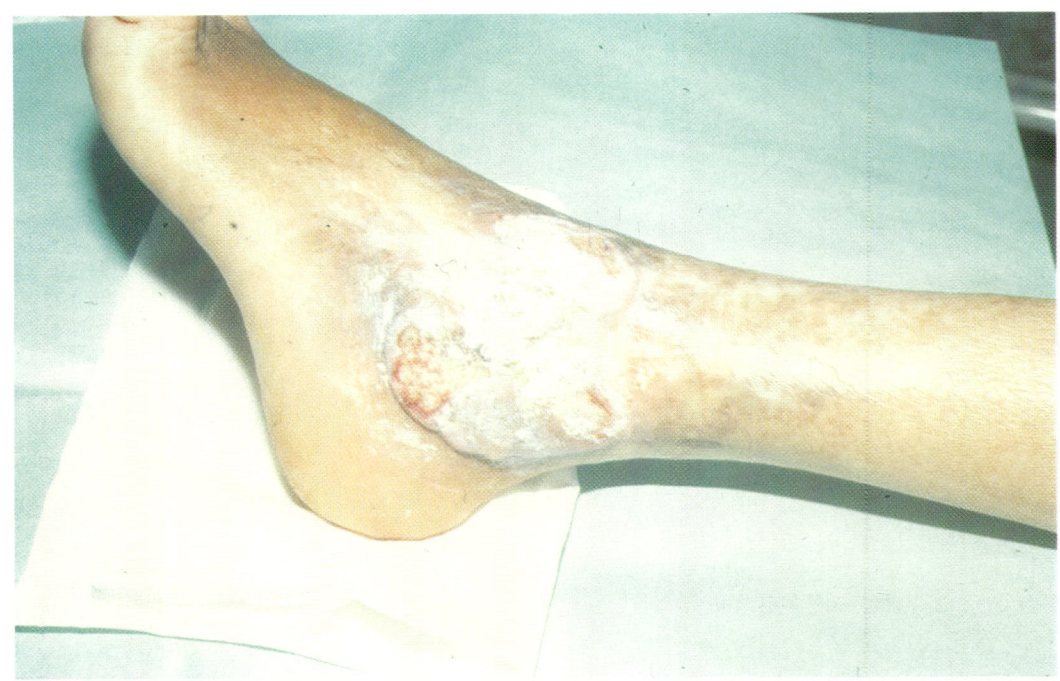

Fig. 11.3.32[2]. Squamous cell carcinoma which had developed on a varicose ulcer. Amputation was proposed (**A**). After cryosurgery, the patient was well for 4 years, had a recurrence in the 5th year, and underwent cryosurgery again (**B**)

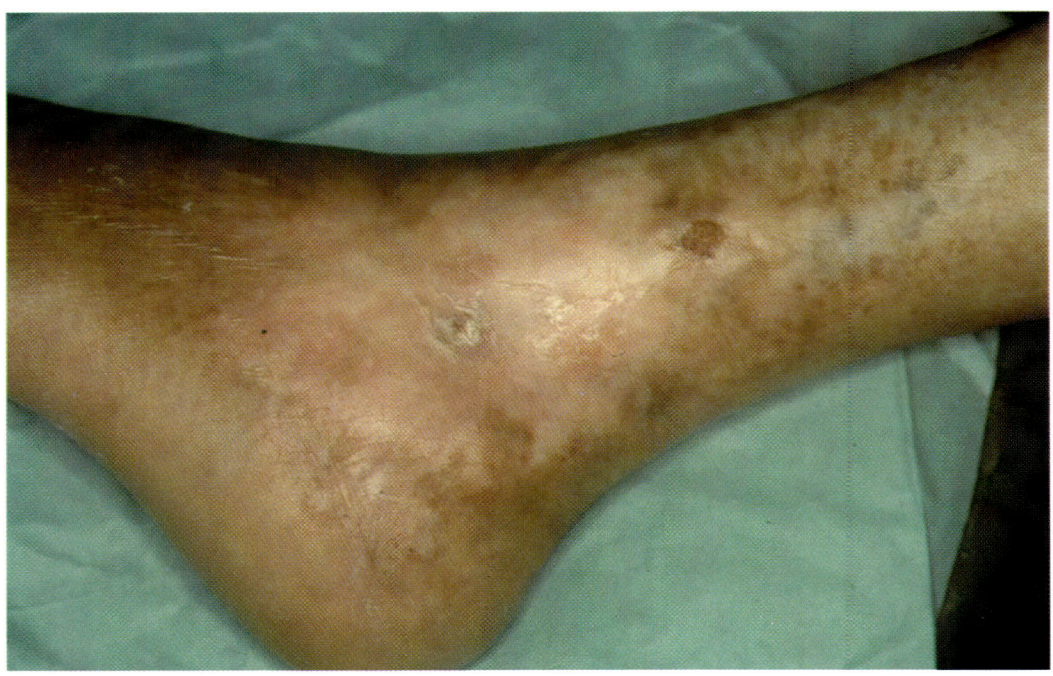

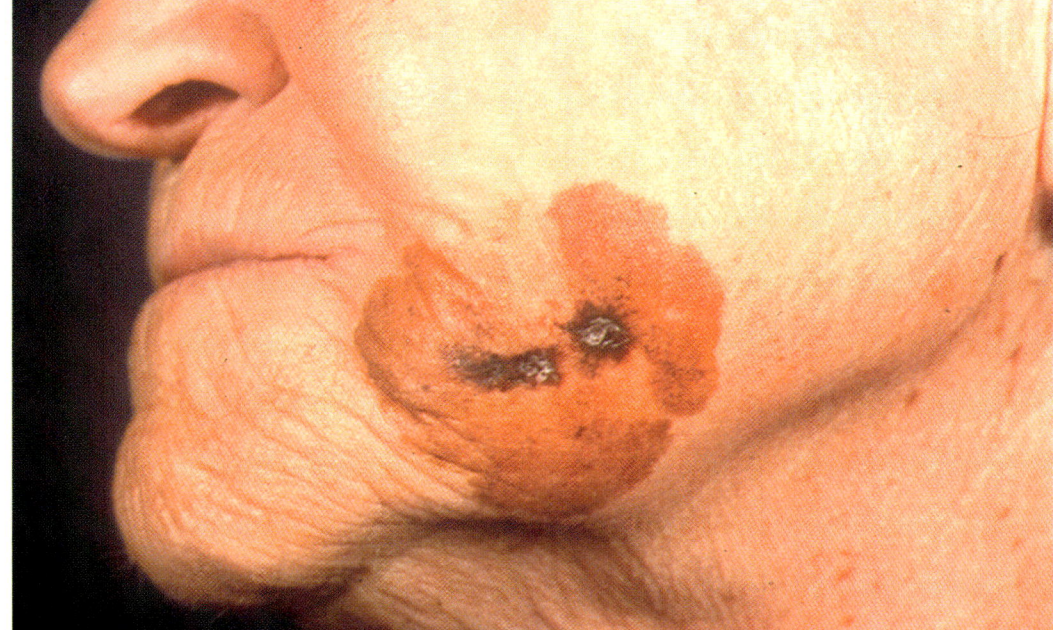

A

Fig. 11.3.33². Melanoma (**A**). After cryosurgery, no recurrence or metastases following a 5-year observation period (**B**)

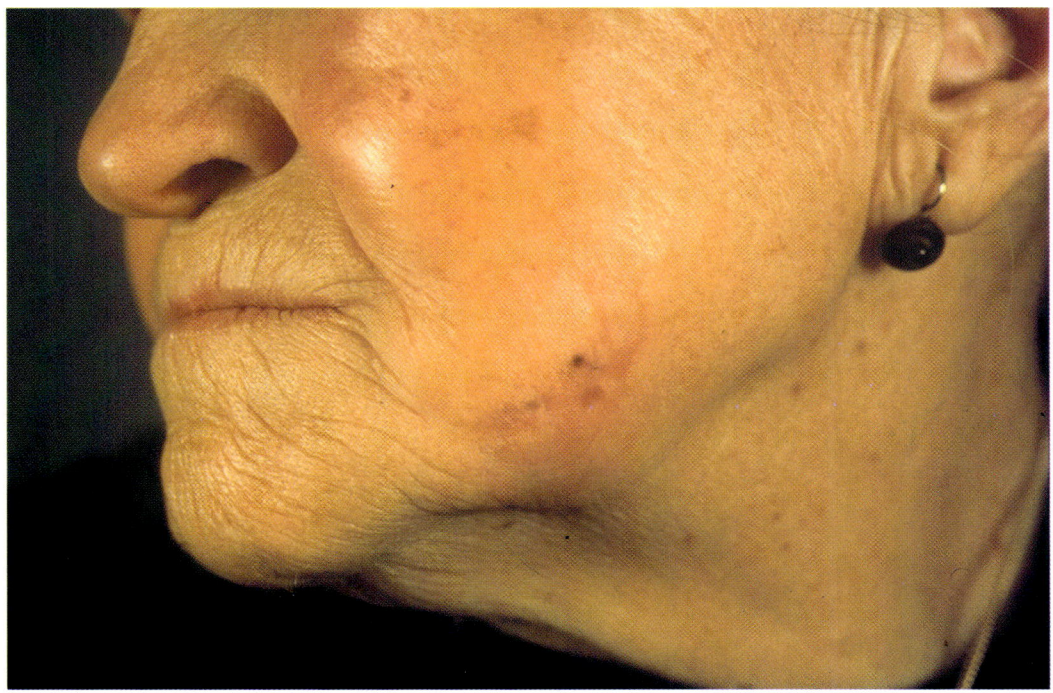

B

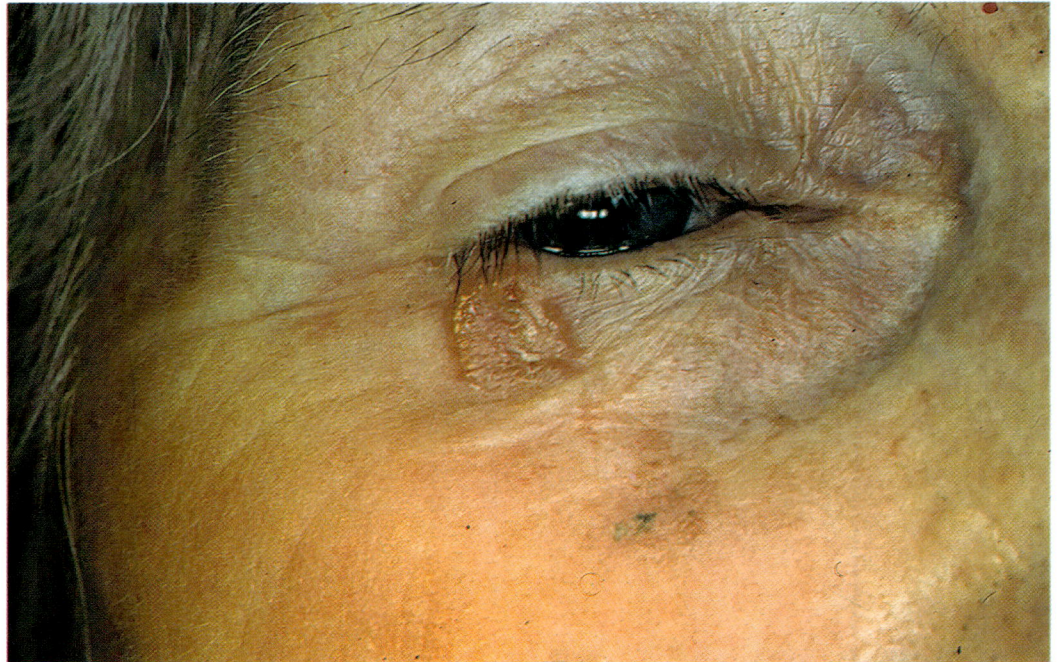

Fig. 11.3.34[3]. Basal cell carcinoma (BCC) of the lower eyelid, measuring 11 × 11 mm. In this case, any conventional plastic surgery technique would have resulted in a visible scar and ultimately in a deformity. The customary cryosurgical technique would inevitably have caused lagophthalmos: 11 mm in diameter plus 3 mm of safety margin would have resulted in an ulceration of at least 17 mm. Cicatrization would have caused an unsightly scar. In order to treat this BCC the author's technique of fractional cryosurgery was used. The first freezing was carried out in the center of the lesion with the intention of reducing the tumor. This procedure was repeated as often as necessary until the diameter of the BCC was less than 10 mm. Subsequently, a standard cryosurgical procedure was performed in two freeze-thaw cycles with an adequate safety margin. In this particular case, one month after the first treatment, the tumor was reduced to 6 × 5 mm and a definitive cryosurgical treatment was performed. One month later a suspicious papule appeared in the center of the treated area, which was again treated cryosurgically

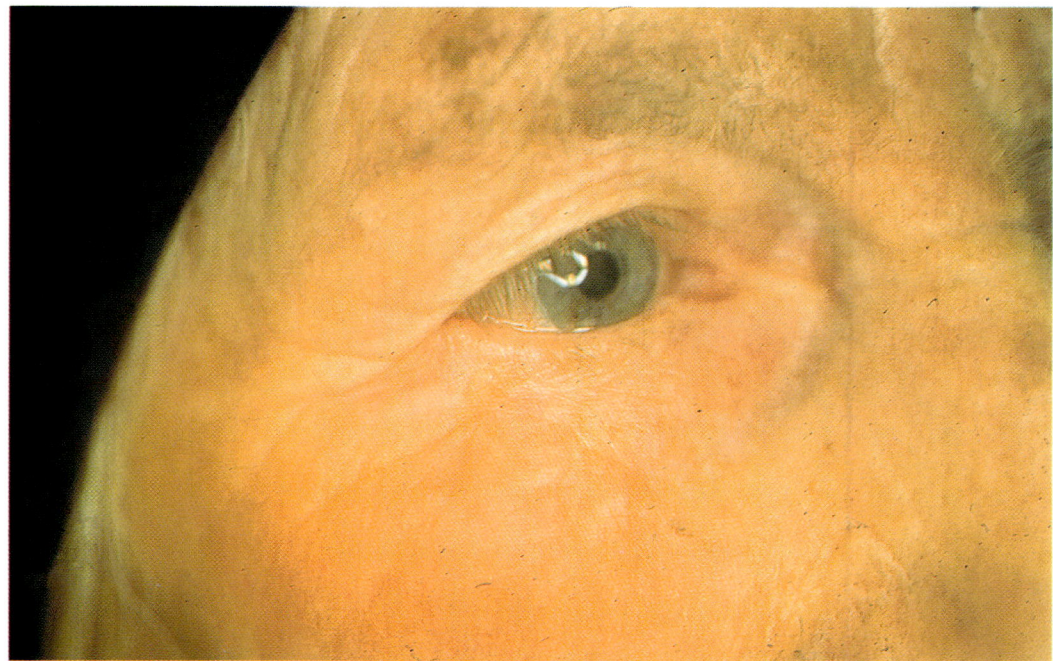

Fig. 11.3.35[3]. Two years after the clinical cure. There is no retraction or visible scar. The patient remained under observation for 5 years without recurrence

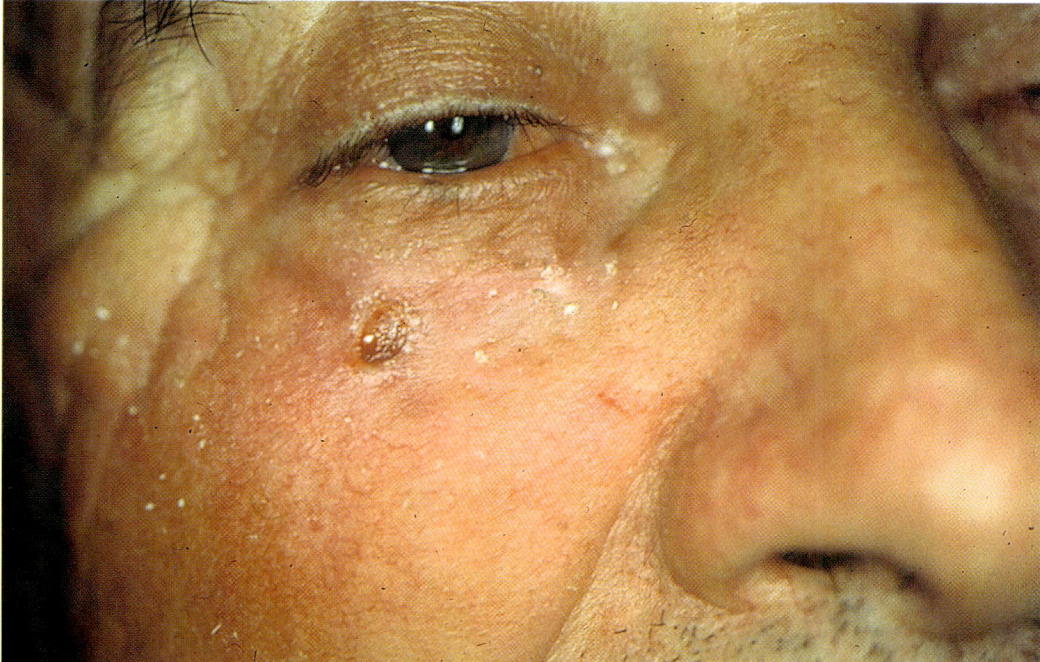

Fig. 11.3.36[3]. Basal cell carcinoma of the lower palpebral region, measuring 25 × 13 mm, that has been present for an indefinite number of years

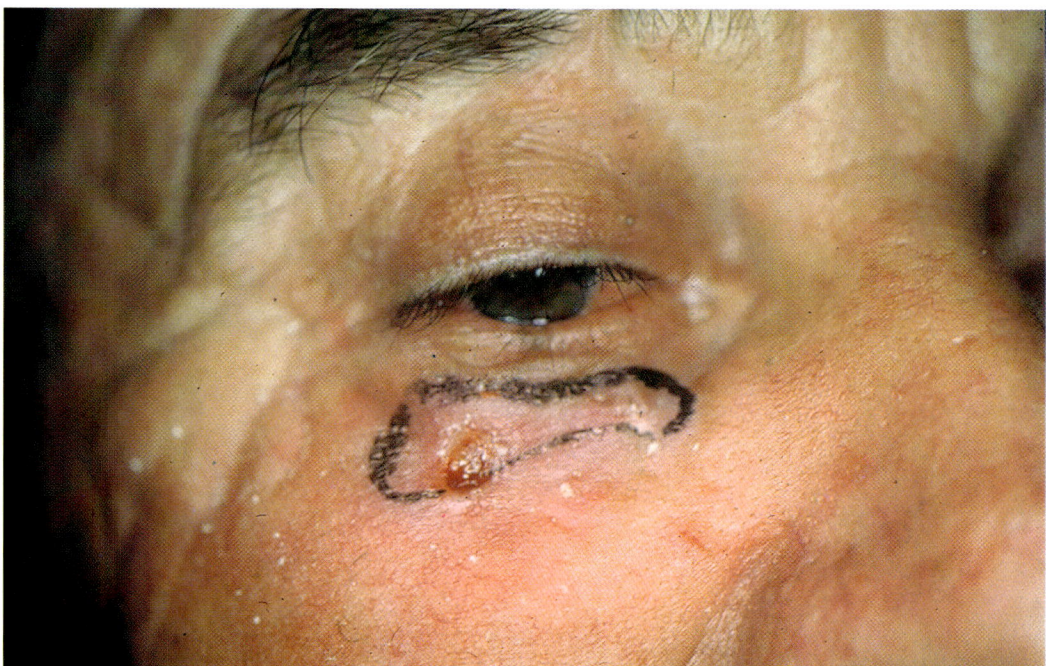

Fig. 11.3.37[3]. The ink contour shows the actual extent of the tumor. The first cryosurgical treatment was carried out on the external limit of the tumor with the Zacarian segmental technique. The BCC was reduced to 21 × 10 mm. Two fractional cryosurgical treatments were subsequently performed

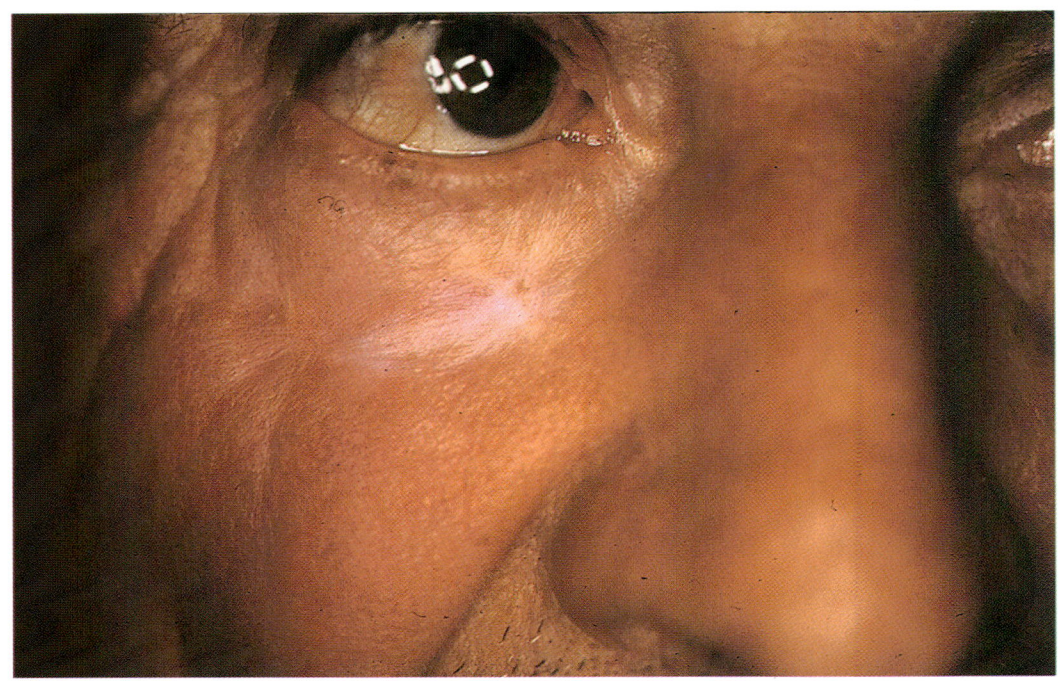

Fig. 11.3.38³. The tumor was clinically cured, leaving a slight scar

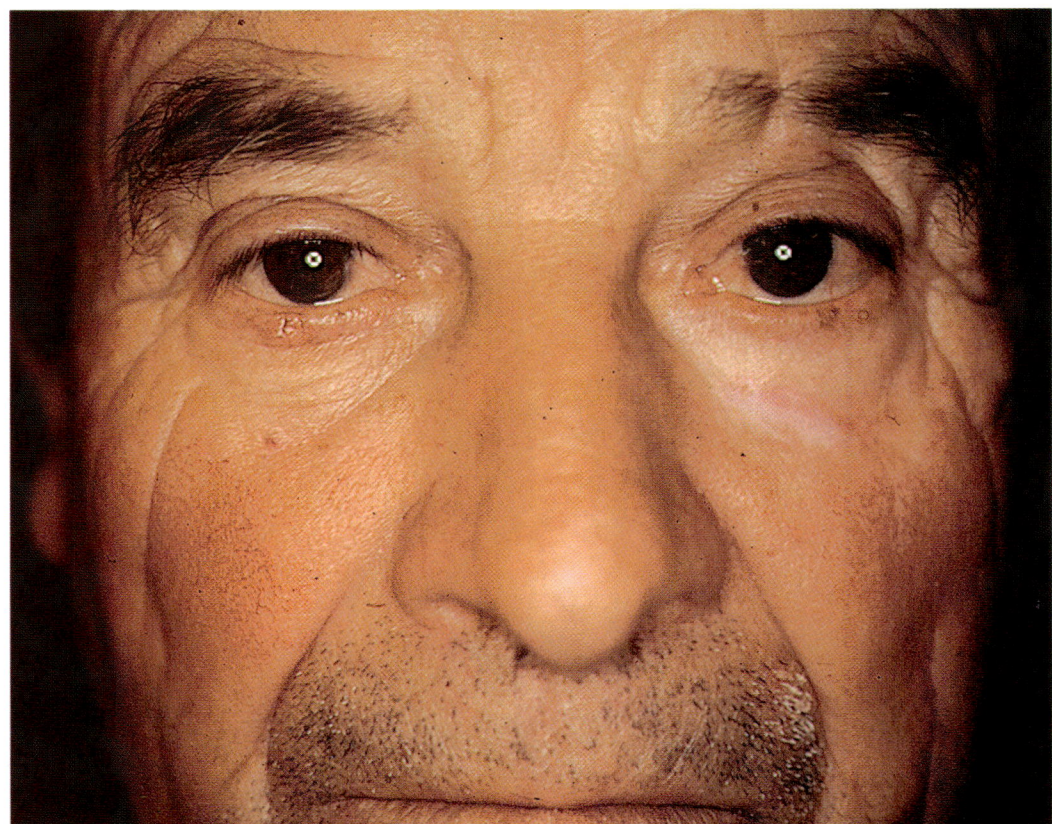

Fig. 11.3.39³. The patient remained under observation for 4 years without recurrence. The symmetry of the eyelids is perfect

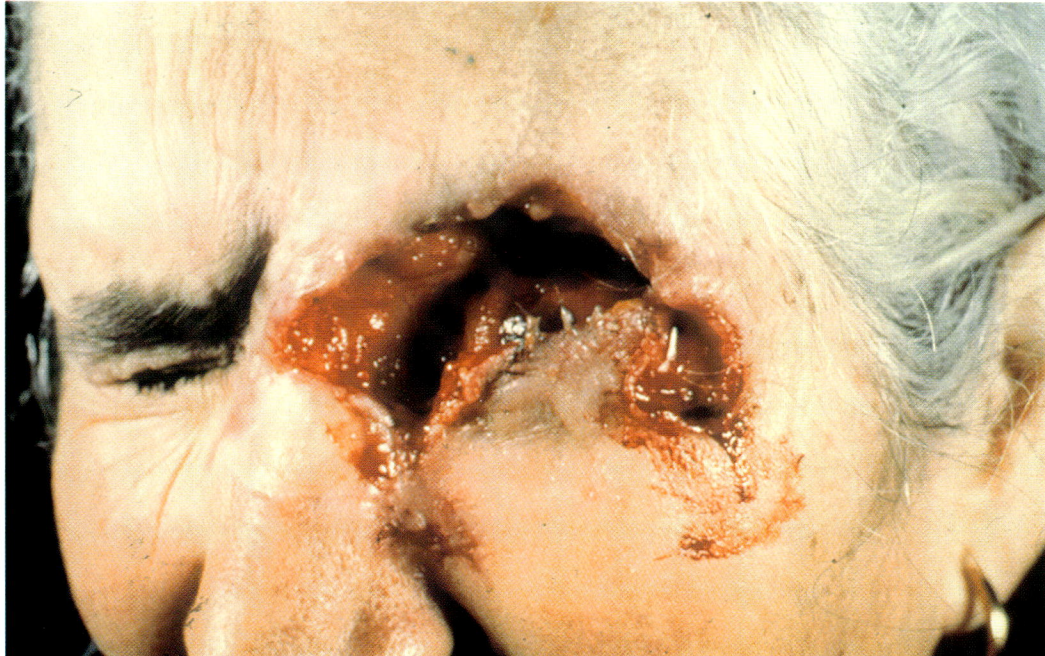

Fig. 11.3.40[3]. When a neglected basal cell carcinoma of the periocular region and, particularly, of the medial canthus, penetrates the orbit, the situation becomes dangerous. It is very difficult to eliminate the tumor, which frequently proves lethal. To deal with this situation, the patient was submitted to general anesthesia; the patient's head was covered with wound dressings, leaving only the orbital region exposed; thermocouples were introduced into the orbits to control the effectiveness of the freezing process until a temperature of −50°C was reached. Freezing was achieved by means of a strong spray of liquid nitrogen

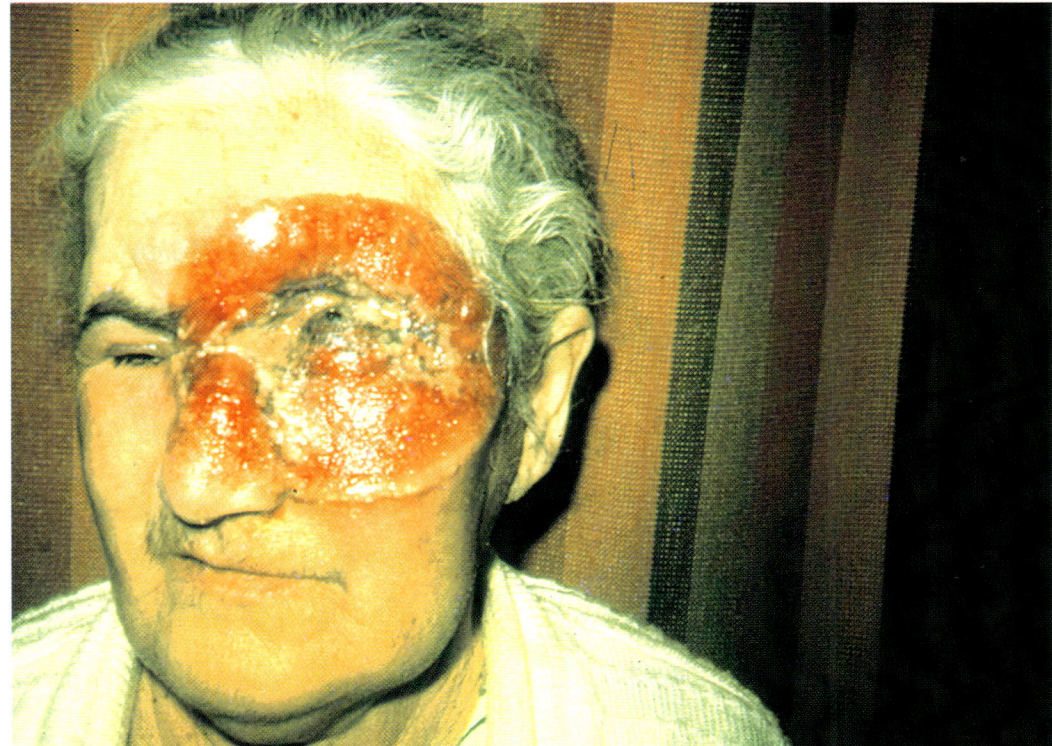

Fig. 11.3.41[3]. The following day, there was a considerable second-degree burn and edema

Chapter 11 Cryosurgical Dermatology

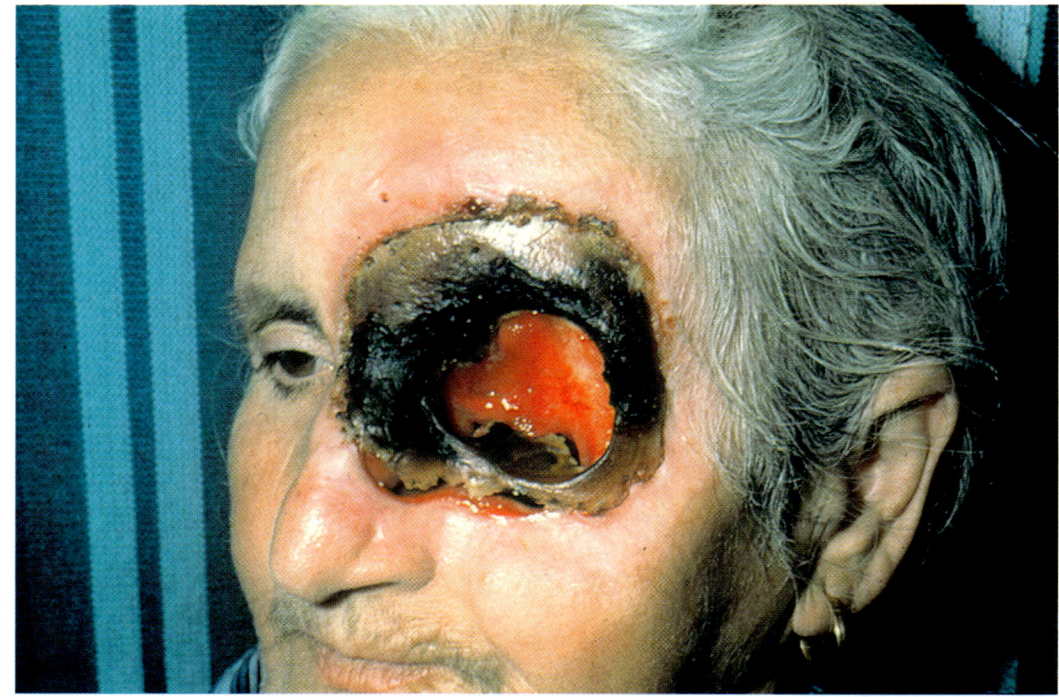

Fig. 11.3.42[3]. Four months later the bone contour of the orbit was necrosed. Later it was sequestered

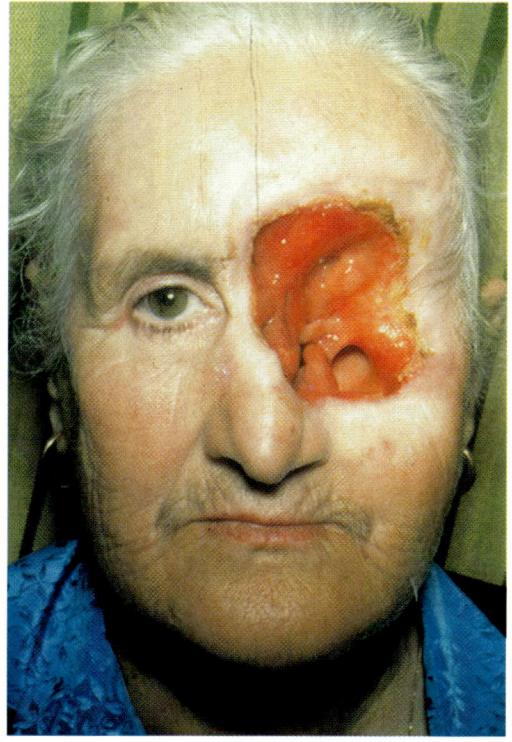

Fig. 11.3.43[3]. Three years after cryosurgery. The patient remained under observation for 12 years without recurrence

Section F Clinical Aspects

Chapter 11
Cryosurgical
Dermatology

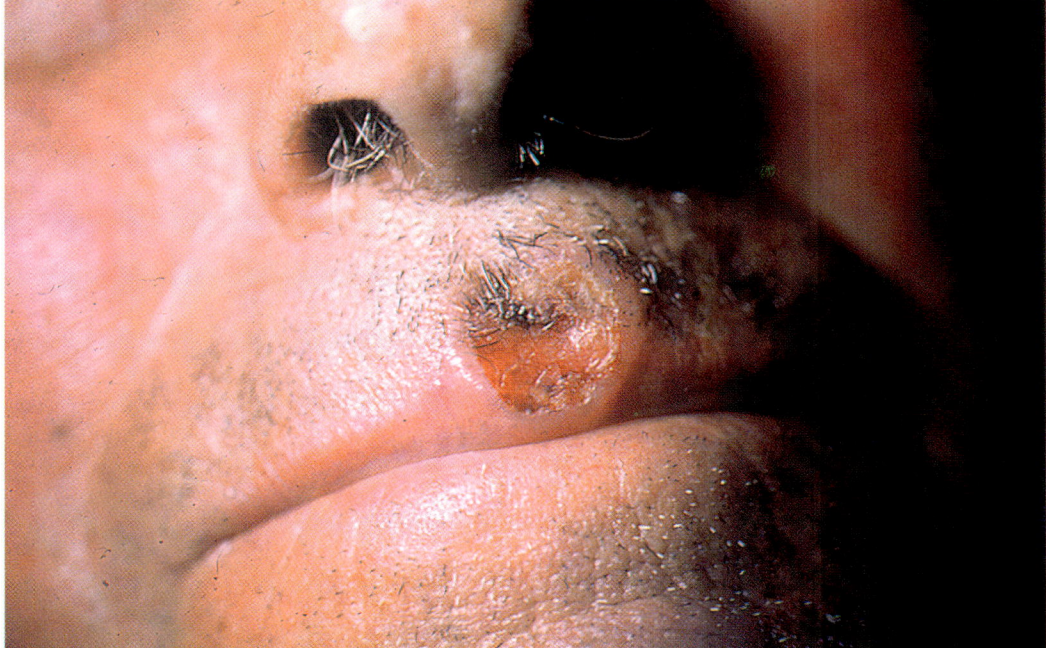

Fig. 11.3.44[3]. The surgical treatment of a large BCC of the upper lip presents substantial cosmetic difficulties. Fractional cryosurgery was particularly successful in this case

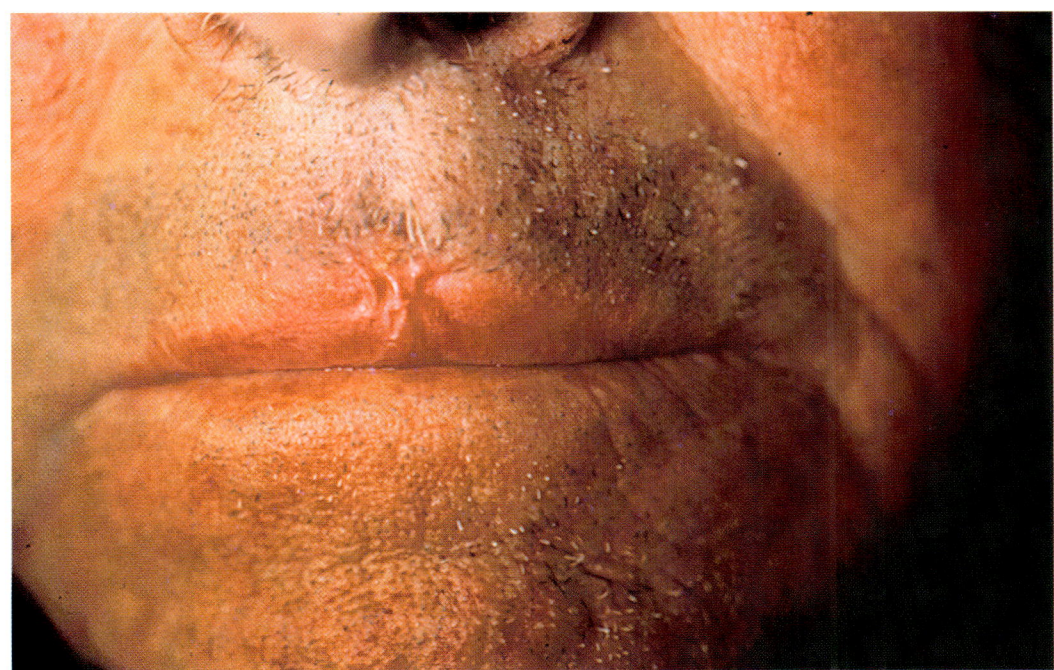

Fig. 11.3.45[3]. Two months later the scar was acceptable

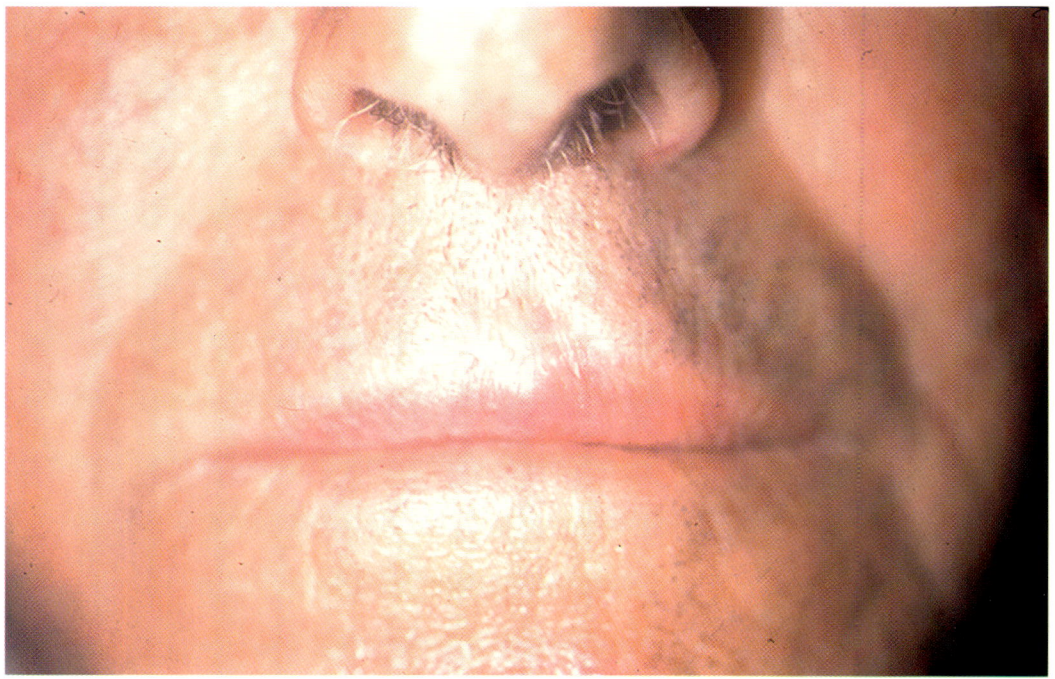

Fig. 11.3.46[3]. Ten months after treatment the scar has completely disappeared. One particular advantage of cryosurgery is that the scars left improve significantly with time

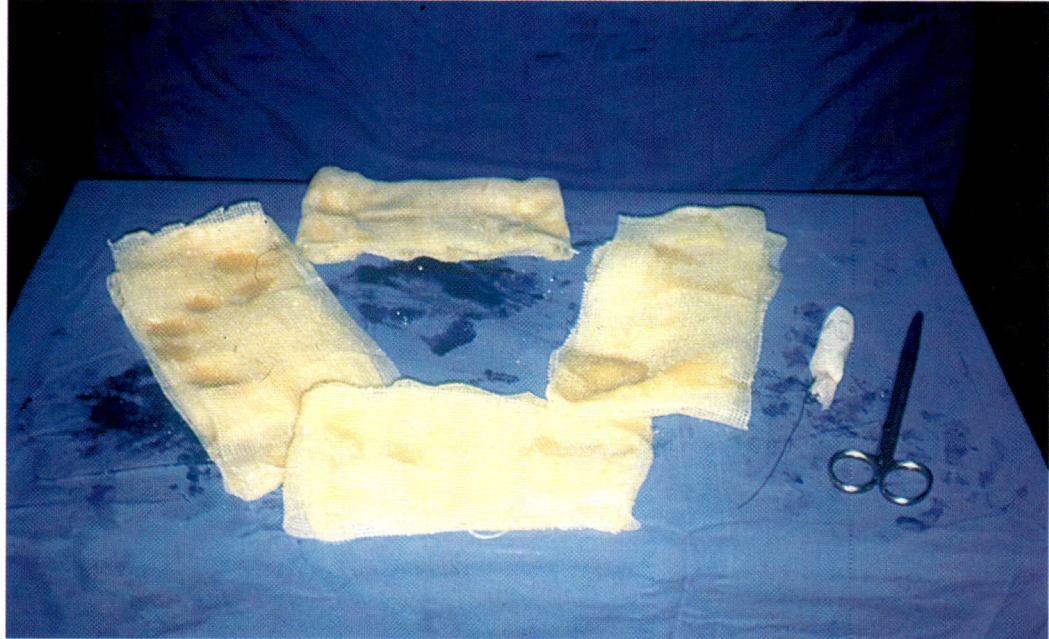

Fig. 11.3.47[3]. In treating advanced external cancers three important technical points must be taken into consideration: the limitation of the target; the monitoring of the progress of the freezing process by means of thermocouples or electric impedance; and the use of a strong spray to remove warmth in the surrounding tissues. In this figure, four flexible plaques of folded paraffinated bandages are shown

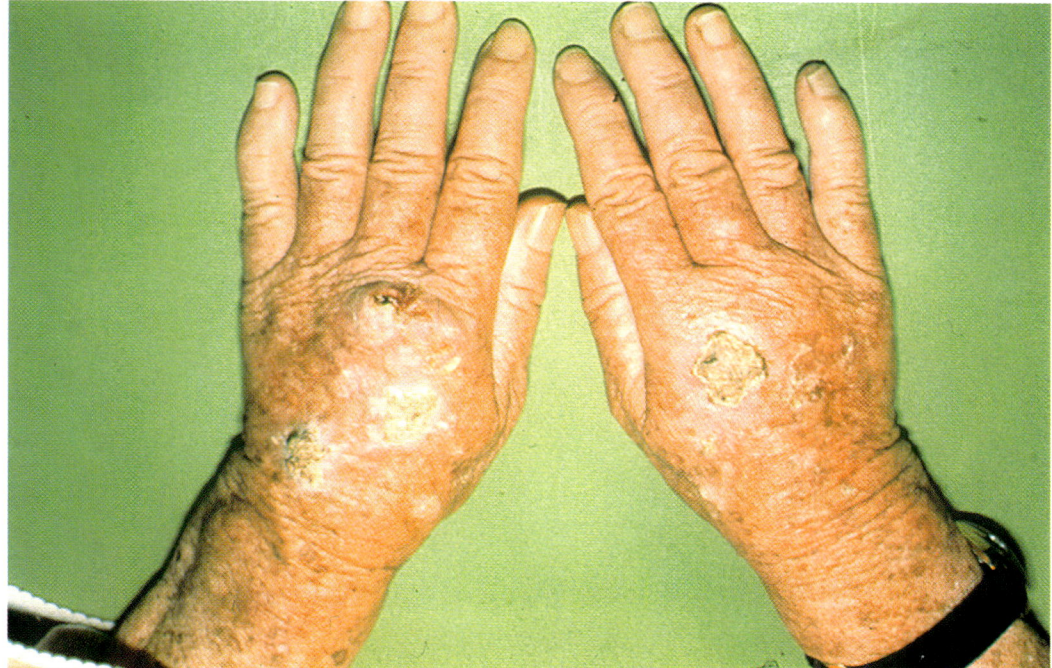

Fig. 11.3.48³. Cryosurgery is medically indicated in the case of inoperable cancer of the extremities. This patient had a large squamous cell carcinoma on the dorsum of the left hand and a smaller one on the other hand. The surgeons of the Department of Surgery proposed the amputation of the right hand. The patient was submitted to general anaesthesia, and many layers of gauze bandages protected the contour of the tumors. These were frozen to −40°C (not lower to avoid damaging the structures of the hand)

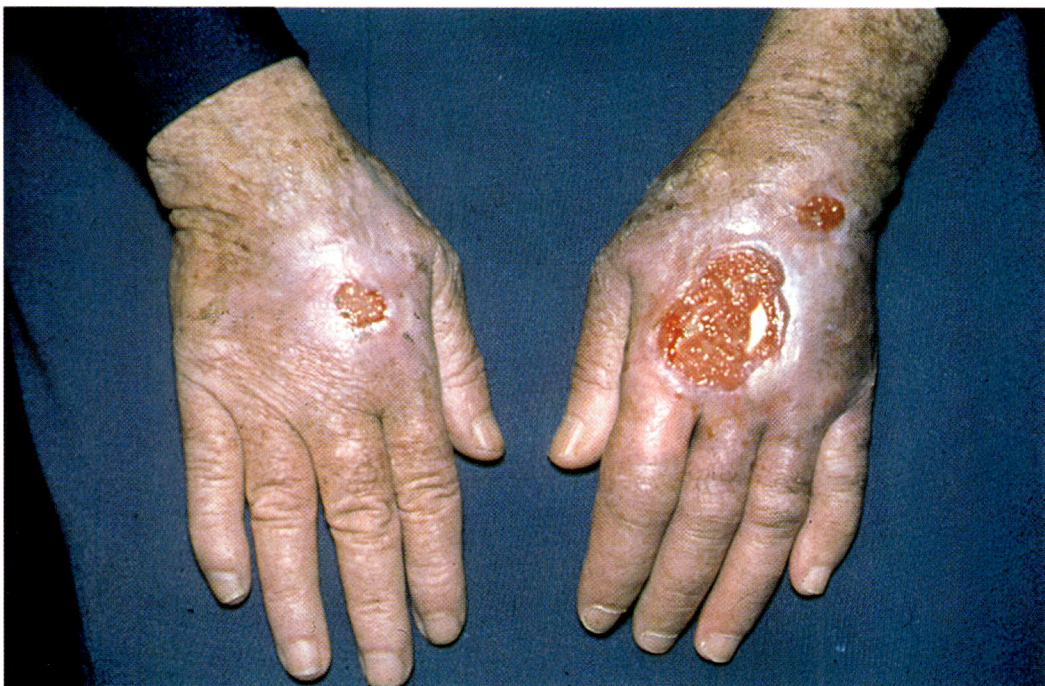

Fig. 11.3.49³. Six weeks later the ulcerations were healing by a second cryosurgical intervention

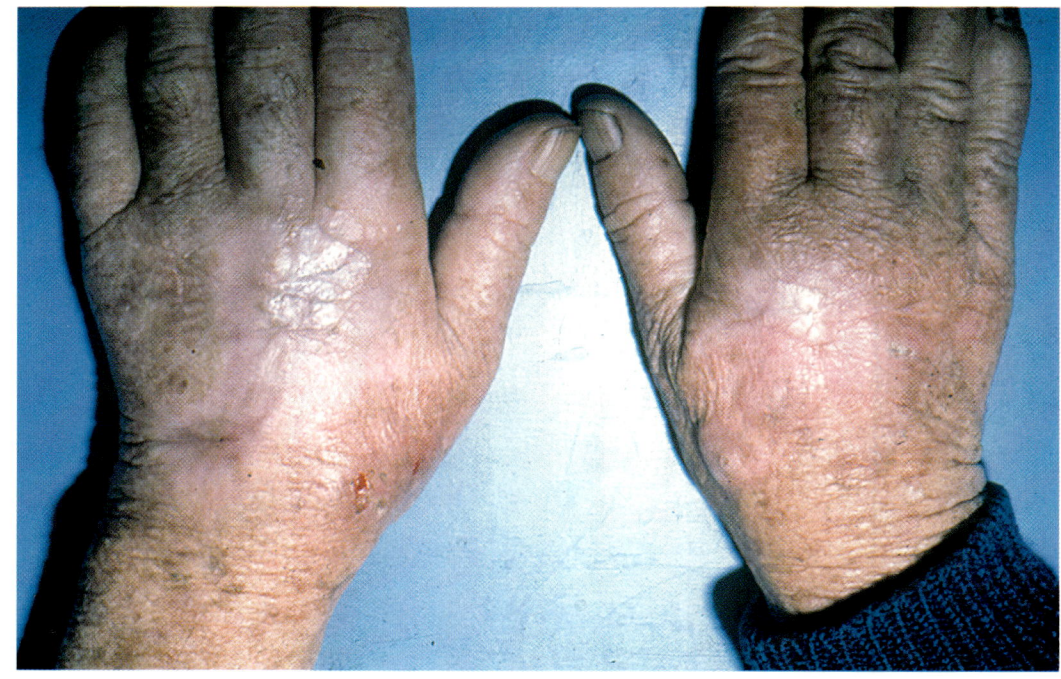

Fig. 11.3.50³. The same patient. Four months after cryosurgery the scars were surprisingly moderate. The functions of the hand had been maintained. The patient remained under observation for 17 months, without recurrence or metastases, and stopped coming to the outpatient department around this time

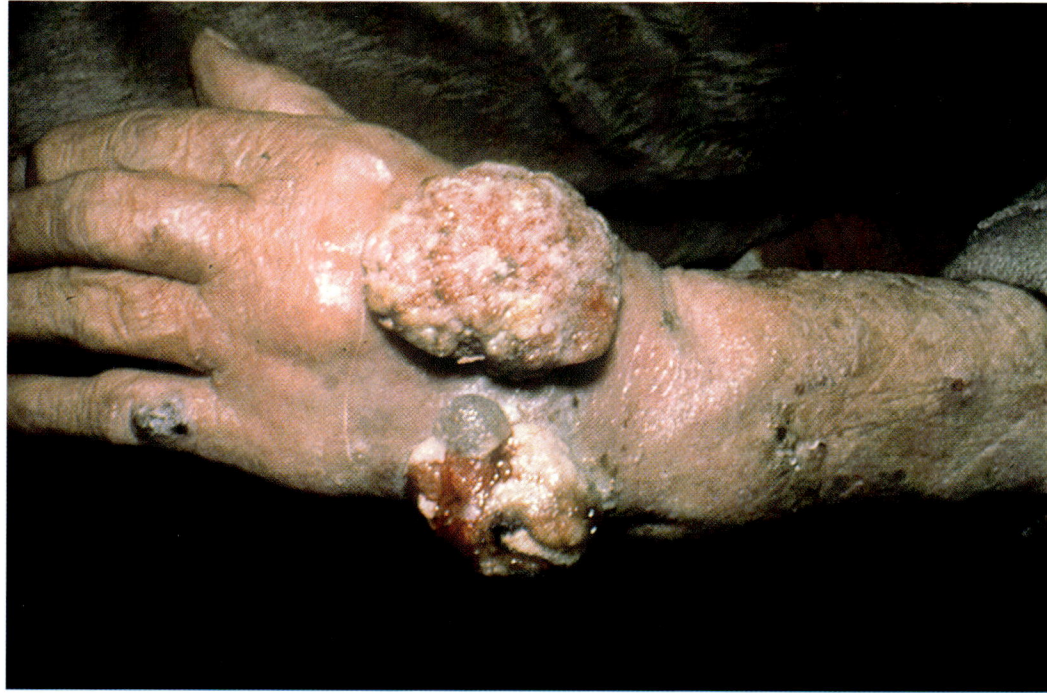

Fig. 11.3.51³. In this case, these huge squamous cell carcinomas seemed incurable

Section F   Clinical Aspects   215

Chapter 11
Cryosurgical
Dermatology

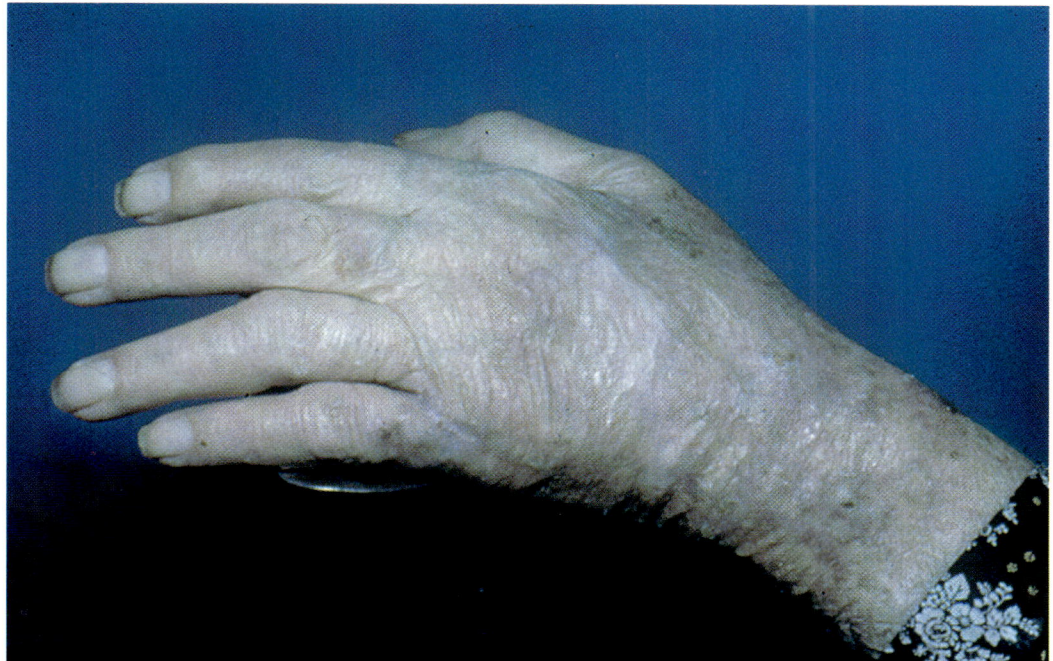

Fig. 11.3.52³. The same patient. This technique achieved a clinical cure. There was no recurrence or metastases. The patient died of unrelated causes 8 months after cryosurgery

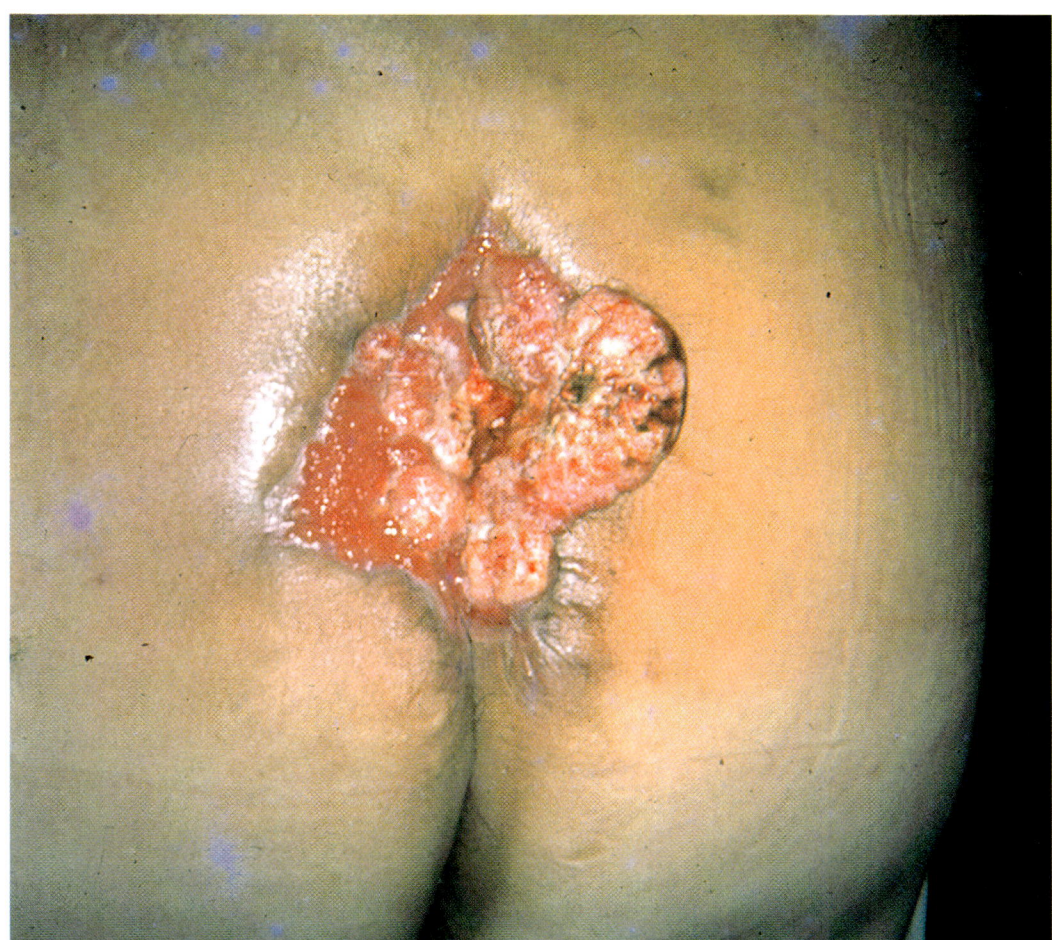

Fig. 11.3.53³. A squamous cell carcinoma developed on a pilonidal sinus and promptly recurred after conventional surgery. The patient underwent cryosurgery with adequate protection of the contour

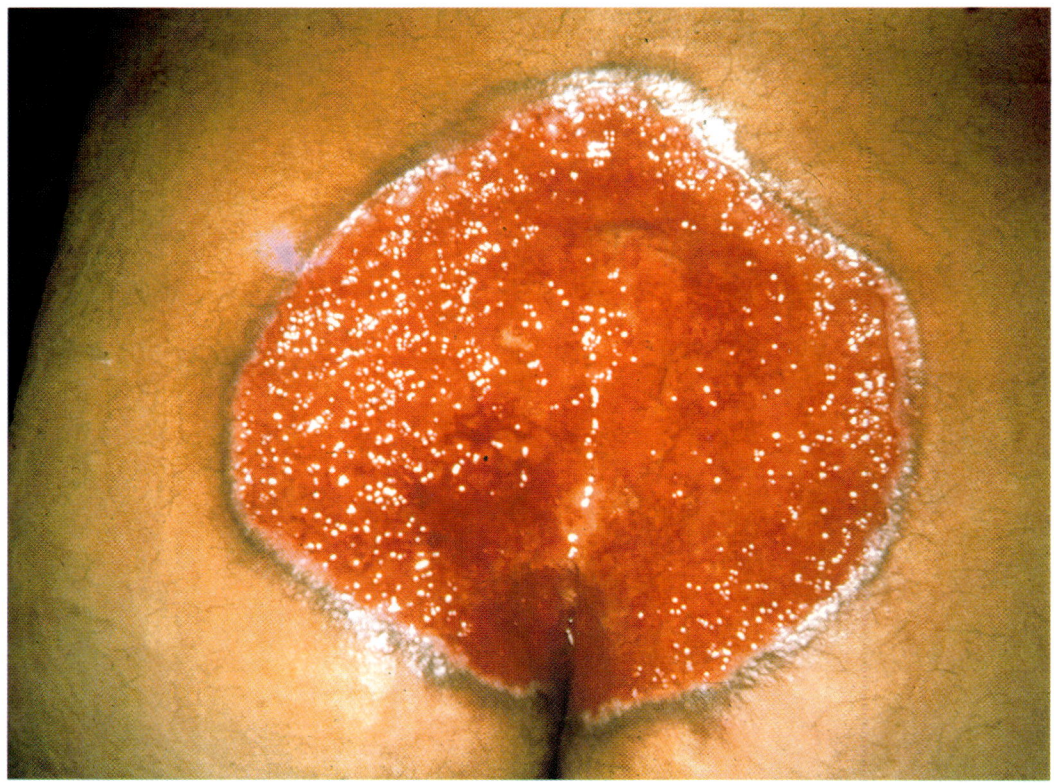

Fig. 11.3.54³. The clean ulceration after removal of the necrotic tissue

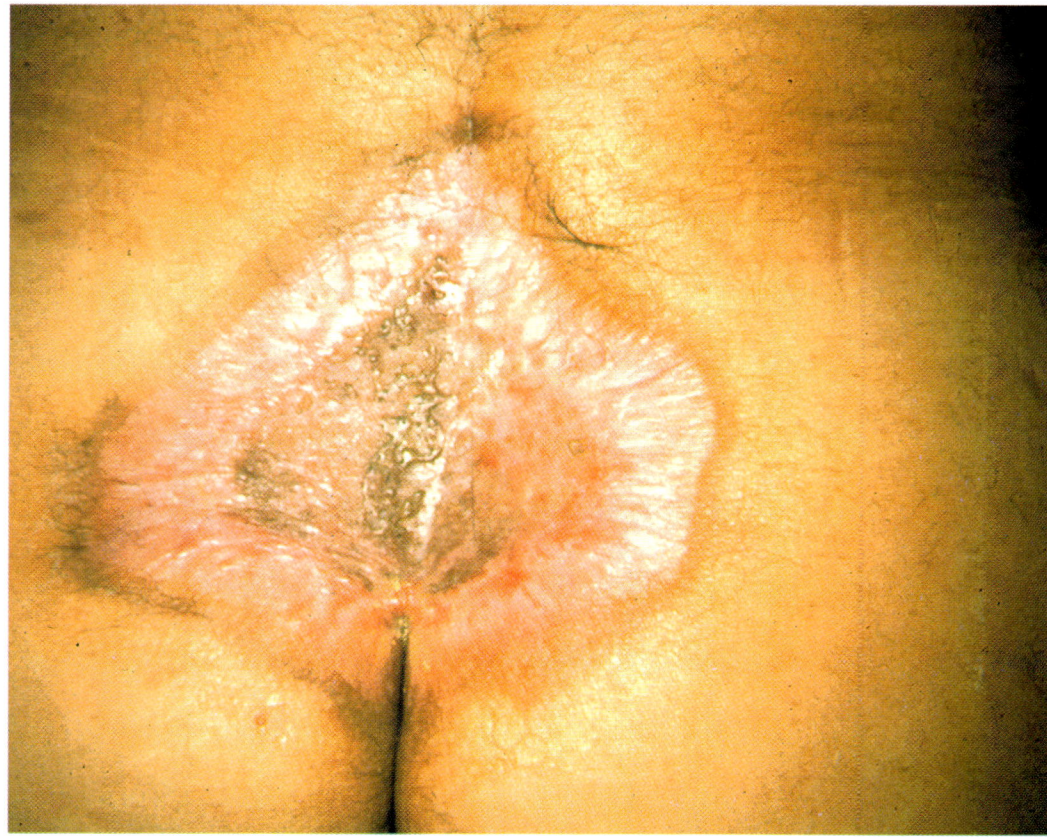

Fig. 11.3.55³. A skin graft was performed to accelerate healing. The patient remained under observation for 14 years without recurrence or metastases

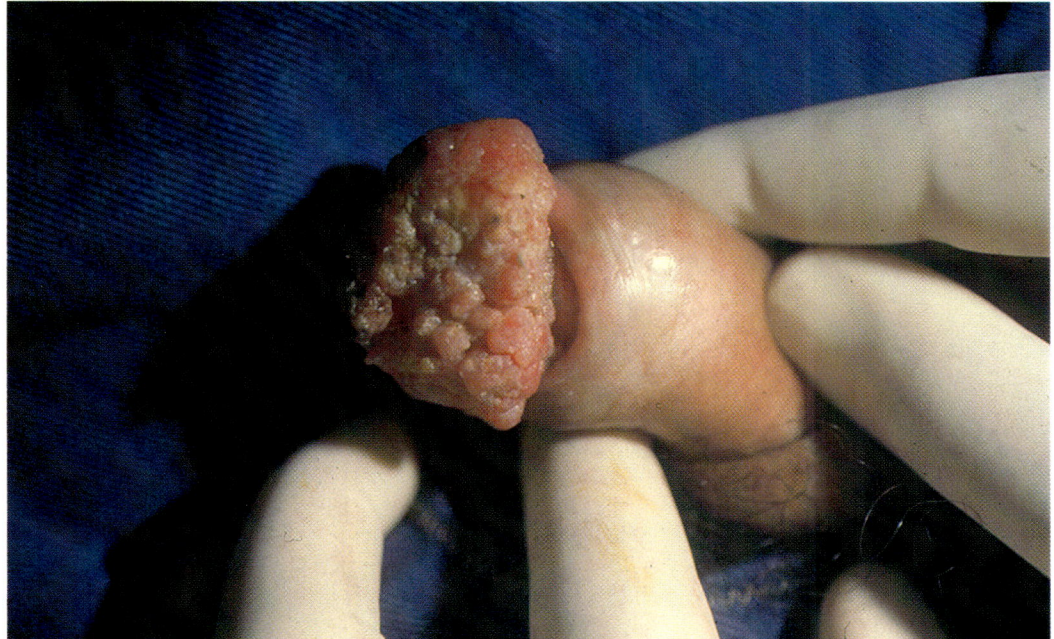

Fig. 11.3.56³. A squamous cell carcinoma of the glans penis. The cryosurgery was performed by probe contact and controlled by two thermocouples. A lymphadenectomy was also performed

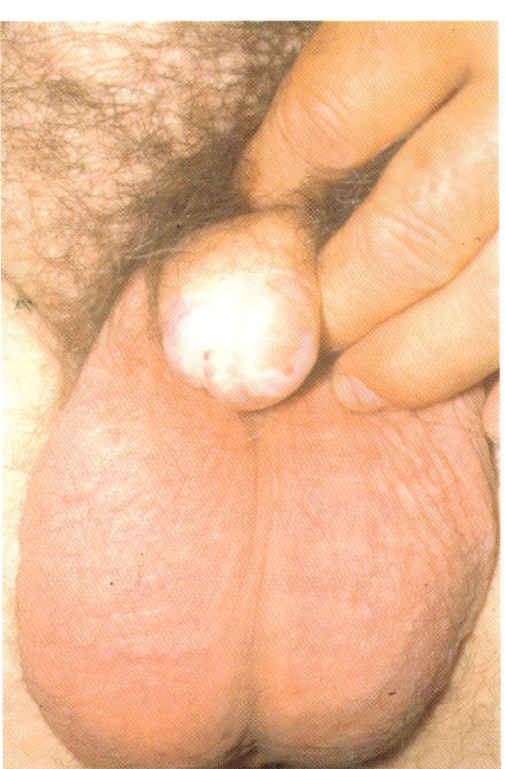

Fig. 11.3.57³. Two years after cryosurgery. Four years later, there is no recurrence or metastases and function is maintained. Cryosurgery is medically indicated in treating advanced cancer of the penis, if it has not invaded the corpora cavernosa

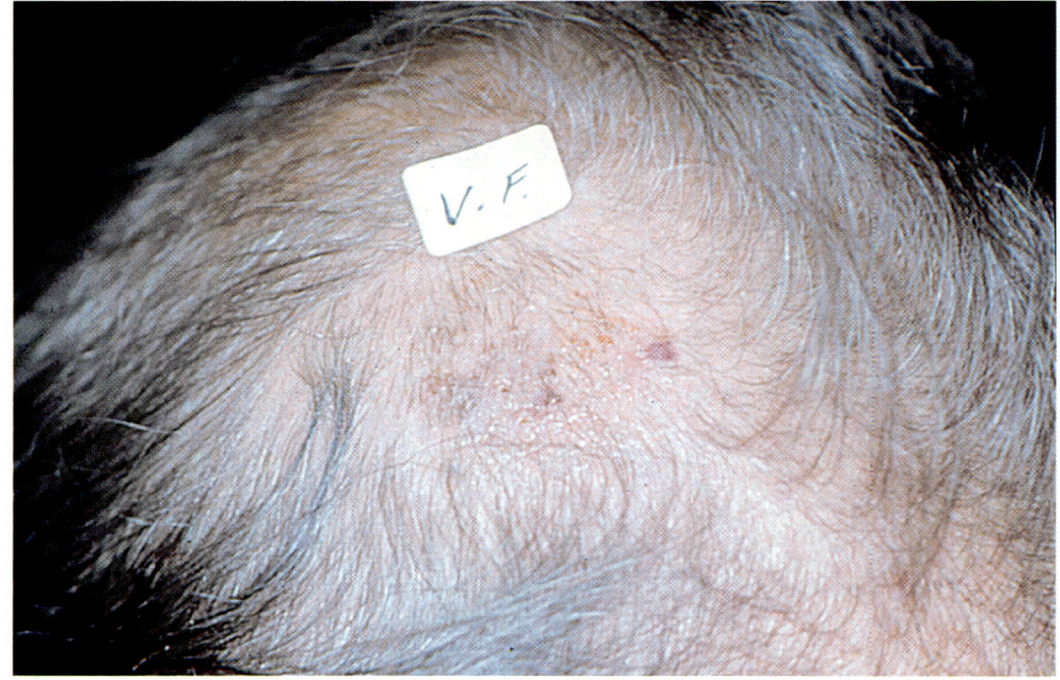

Fig. 11.3.58[4]. Basal cell carcinoma of the scalp (**A**), after 40 days of two cycles each lasting 90 sec. Each of the freezing cycles carried out during a single cryosurgical session (**B**)

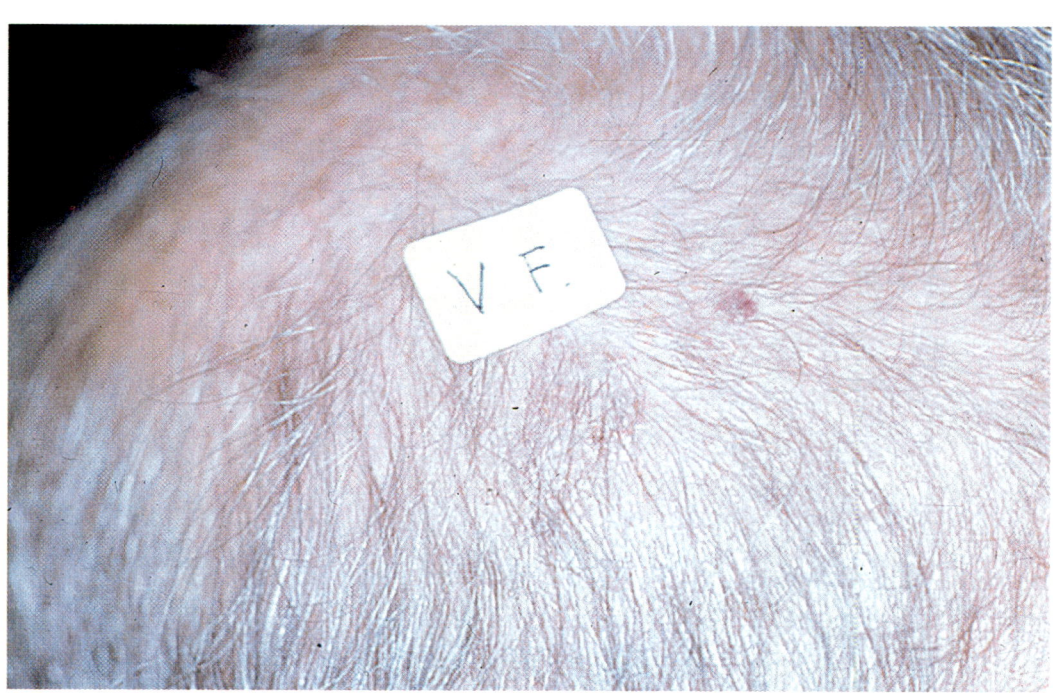

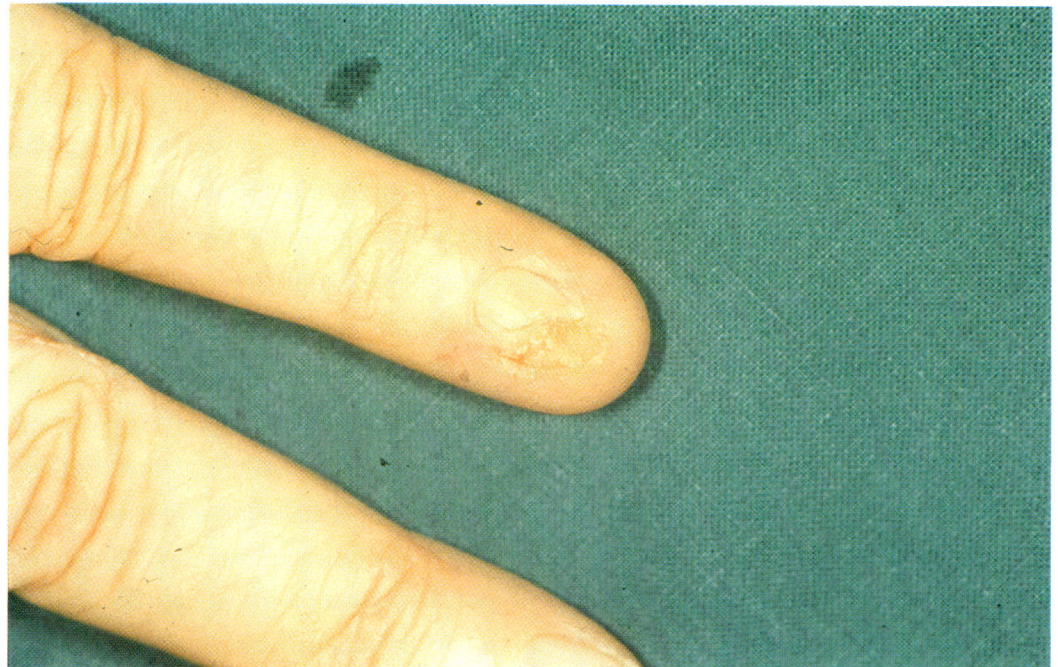

Fig. 11.3.59[5]. A squamous cell carcinoma *in situ* (Bowen's disease) on the subungual area of a finger of the left hand of a female patient born in 1937. In 1995 an incomplete surgical excision had been performed. The surgeon wanted to amputate the distal phalange but the patient was a pianist, and she wanted the finger to remain intact. In 1996 the tumor was treated with curettage-cryosurgery (**A**). After a meticulous curettage the tumor was found to occupy the entire subungual area (**B**). The freezing was carried out with a continuous spray of liquid nitrogen for 25 seconds in a double freeze-thaw cycle. The halo thaw time was more than 60 seconds and the complete thaw time was about 4 minutes (**C**). The finger after 2 weeks (**D**). The result obtained after 6 months, dorsal aspect (**E**). Volar aspect. After 3.5 years the patient had no problems with the finger except absence of the nail (**F**)

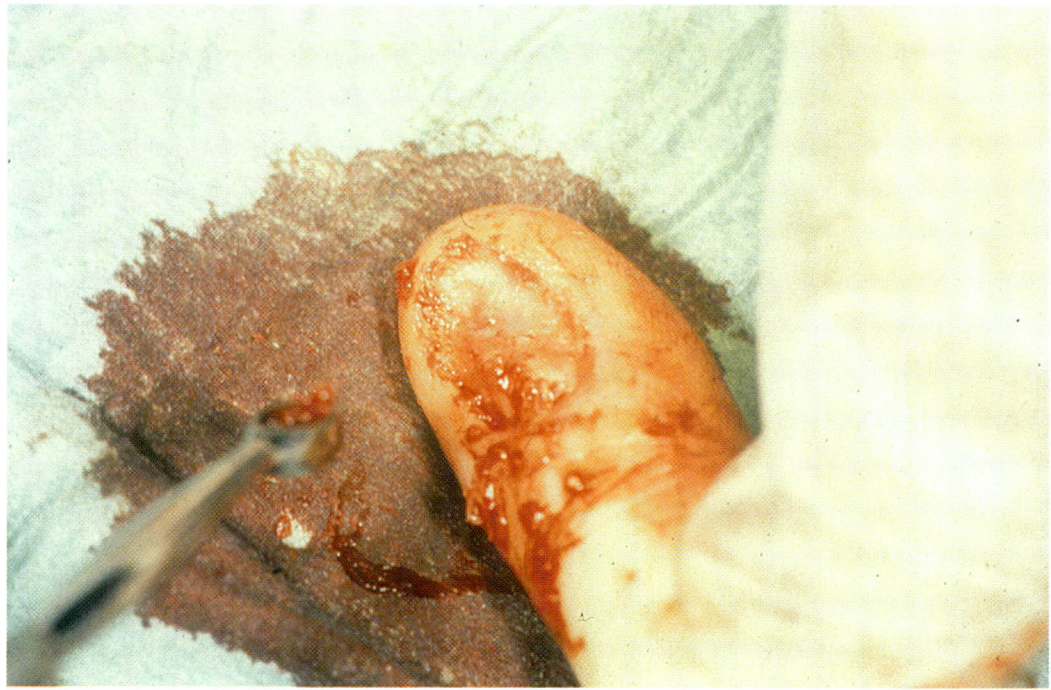

Chapter 11 Cryosurgical Dermatology

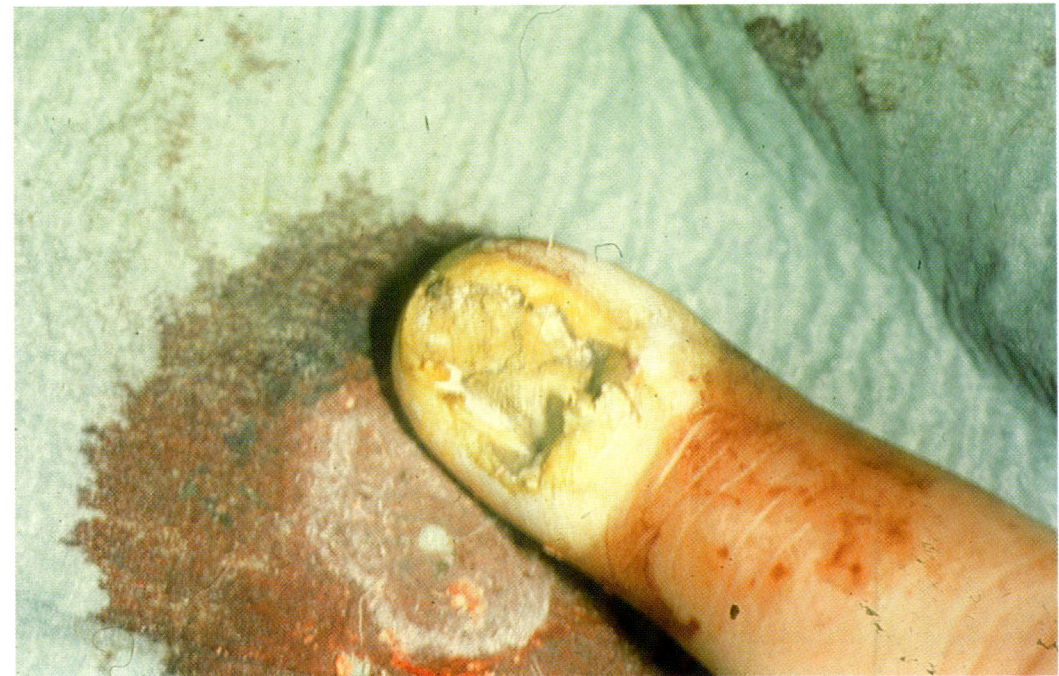

C

Fig. 11.3.59[5]. A squamous cell carcinoma *in situ* (Bowen's disease) on the subungual area of a finger of the left hand of a female patient born in 1937. In 1995 an incomplete surgical excision had been performed. The surgeon wanted to amputate the distal phalange but the patient was a pianist, and she wanted the finger to remain intact. In 1996 the tumor was treated with curettage-cryosurgery (**A**). After a meticulous curettage the tumor was found to occupy the entire subungual area (**B**). The freezing was carried out with a continuous spray of liquid nitrogen for 25 seconds in a double freeze-thaw cycle. The halo thaw time was more than 60 seconds and the complete thaw time was about 4 minutes (**C**). The finger after 2 weeks (**D**). The result obtained after 6 months, dorsal aspect (**E**). Volar aspect. After 3.5 years the patient had no problems with the finger except absence of the nail (**F**)

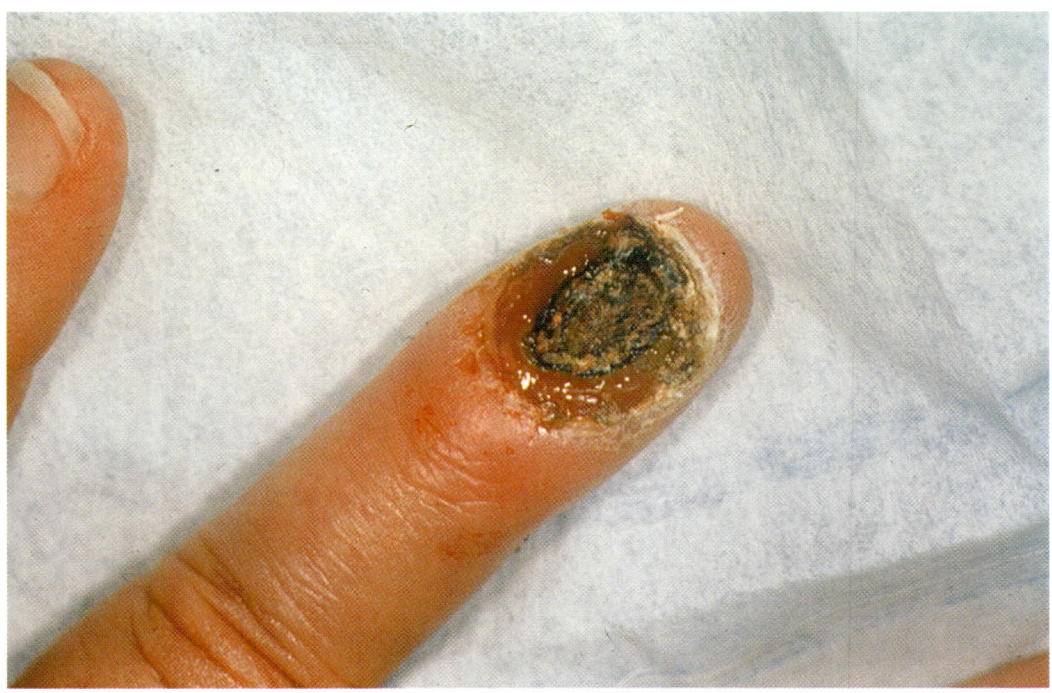

D

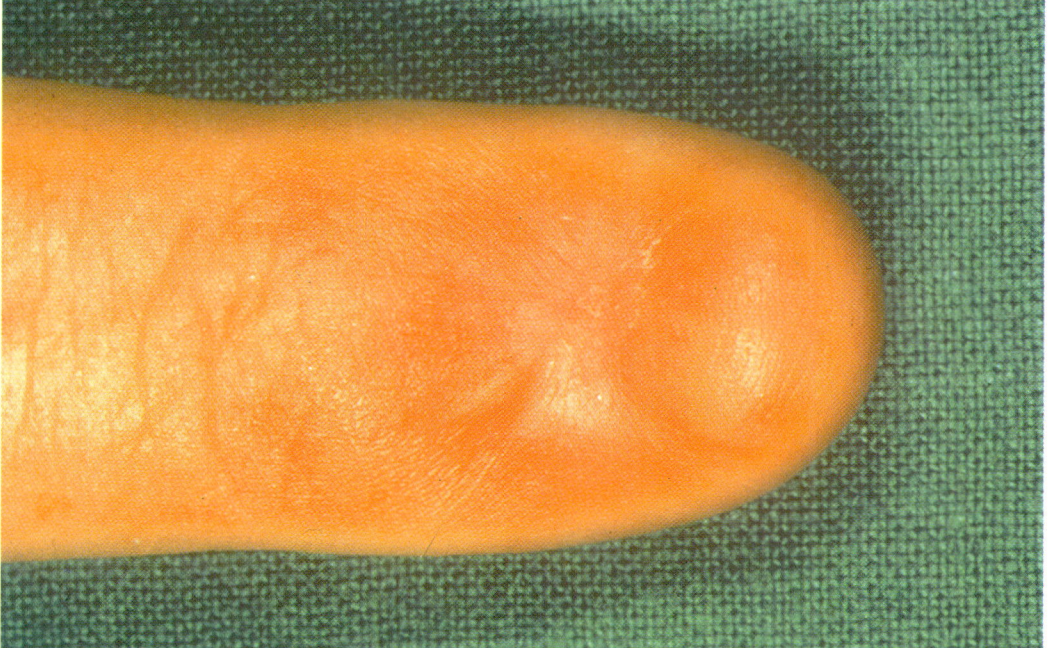

E

Fig. 11.3.59[5]. A squamous cell carcinoma *in situ* (Bowen's disease) on the subungual area of a finger of the left hand of a female patient born in 1937. In 1995 an incomplete surgical excision had been performed. The surgeon wanted to amputate the distal phalange but the patient was a pianist, and she wanted the finger to remain intact. In 1996 the tumor was treated with curettage-cryosurgery (**A**). After a meticulous curettage the tumor was found to occupy the entire subungual area (**B**). The freezing was carried out with a continuous spray of liquid nitrogen for 25 seconds in a double freeze-thaw cycle. The halo thaw time was more than 60 seconds and the complete thaw time was about 4 minutes (**C**). The finger after 2 weeks (**D**). The result obtained after 6 months, dorsal aspect (**E**). Volar aspect. After 3.5 years the patient had no problems with the finger except absence of the nail (**F**)

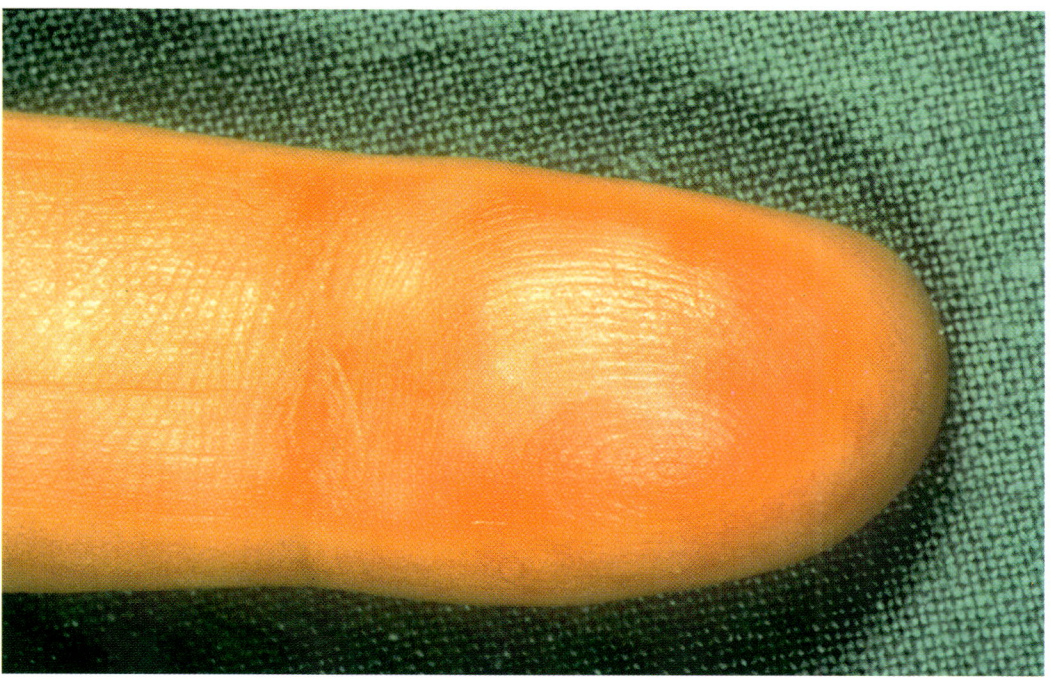

F

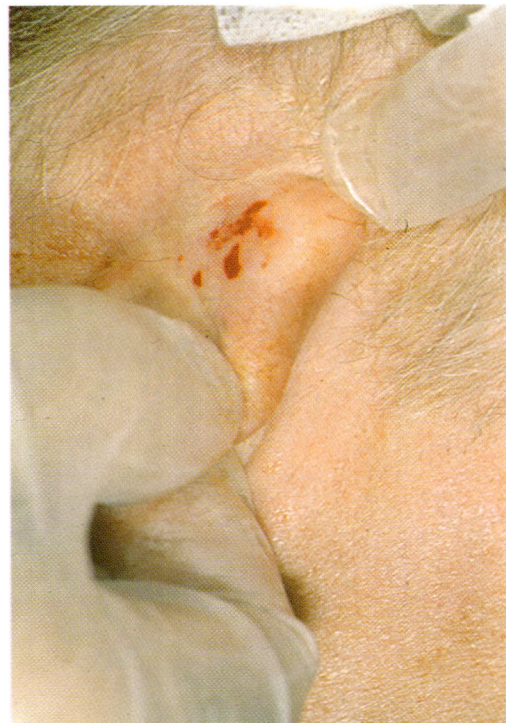

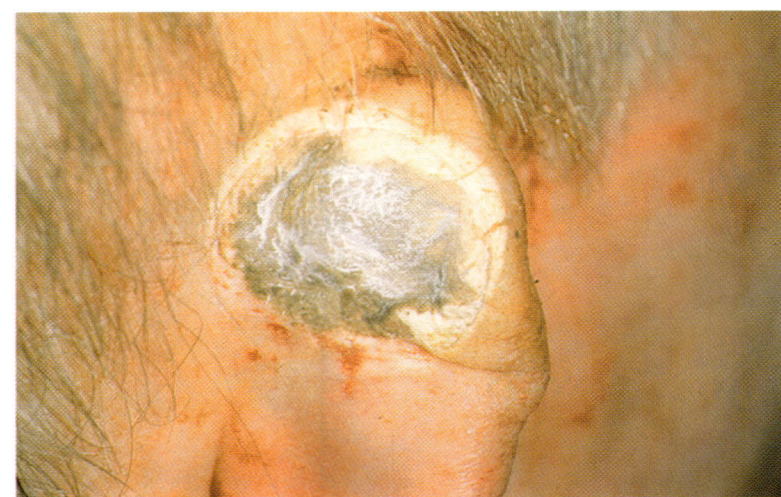

Fig. 11.3.60⁵. In 1996 a clinically ill-defined basal cell carcinoma was found on the dorsal aspect of the right ear of a male patient born in 1920. Histopathological findings from a 3 mm punch biopsy showed an infiltrating non-morphoeiform BCC (**A**). Following a thorough curettage using different sized ring curettes, the freezing was performed. The open cone-spray method in a double freeze-thaw cycle was used. The maximal tumor diameter was 20 mm and a neoprene cone with a diameter of 21 mm fitted well. The freeze halo outside the tumor area was 5–6 mm and the halo thaw time was more than 60 seconds each time. The total thaw time was 3.5–4 minutes (**B**). The result obtained after one year. The condition was unchanged after 3 years (**C**)

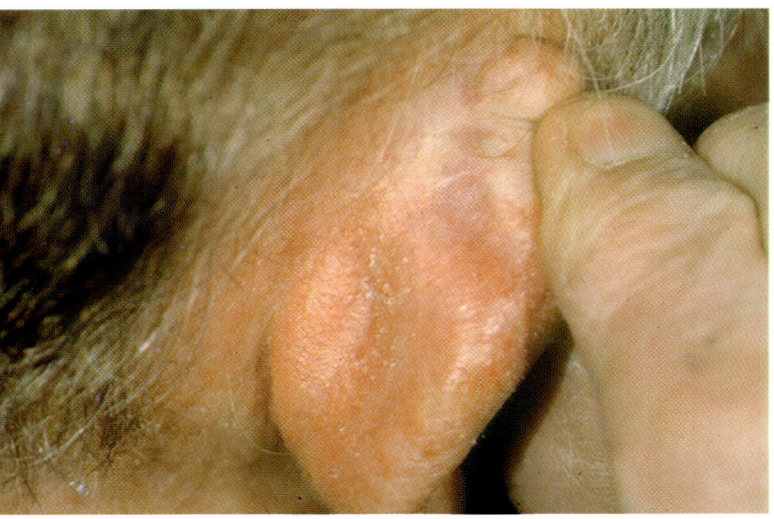

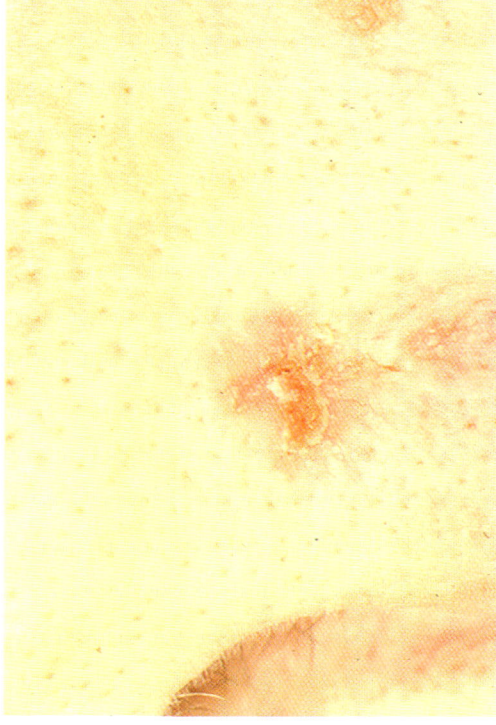

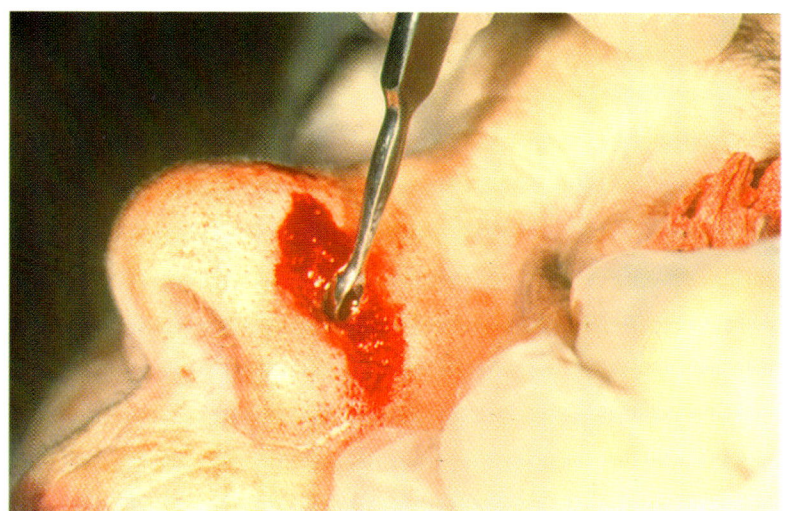

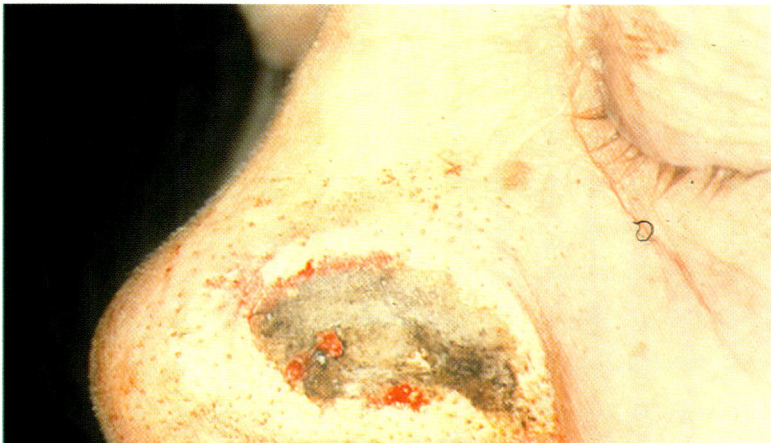

Fig. 11.3.61[5]. An elderly lady born in 1912 with a basal cell carcinoma on her left ala nasi in 1995. Clinically it was considered nodular, the tumor borders were, however, ill-defined (**A**). A meticulous curettage was performed. The tumor was larger than expected with a maximal diameter of 21 mm (**B**). The tumor area frozen with liquid nitrogen. Spray-cone technique in a double freeze-thaw cycle was used (**C**). An oozing wound after 2 weeks (**D**). The result obtained after 4 years (**E**)

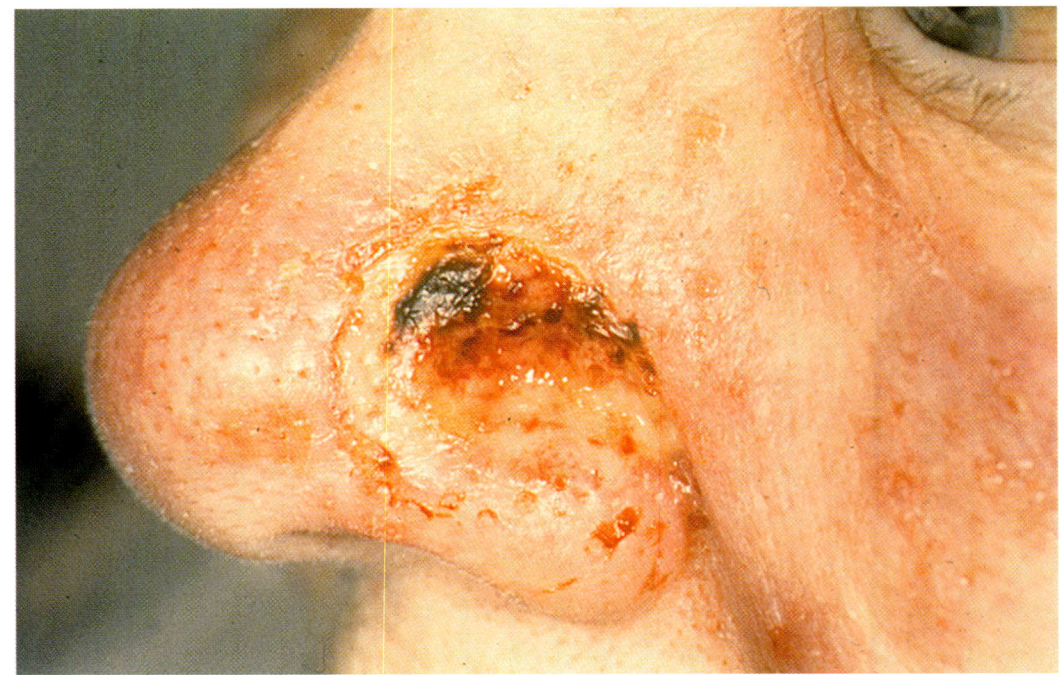

D

Fig. 11.3.61[5]. An elderly lady born in 1912 with a basal cell carcinoma on her left ala nasi in 1995. Clinically it was considered nodular, the tumor borders were, however, ill-defined (**A**). A meticulous curettage was performed. The tumor was larger than expected with a maximal diameter of 21 mm (**B**). The tumor area frozen with liquid nitrogen. Spray-cone technique in a double freeze-thaw cycle was used (**C**). An oozing wound after 2 weeks (**D**). The result obtained after 4 years (**E**)

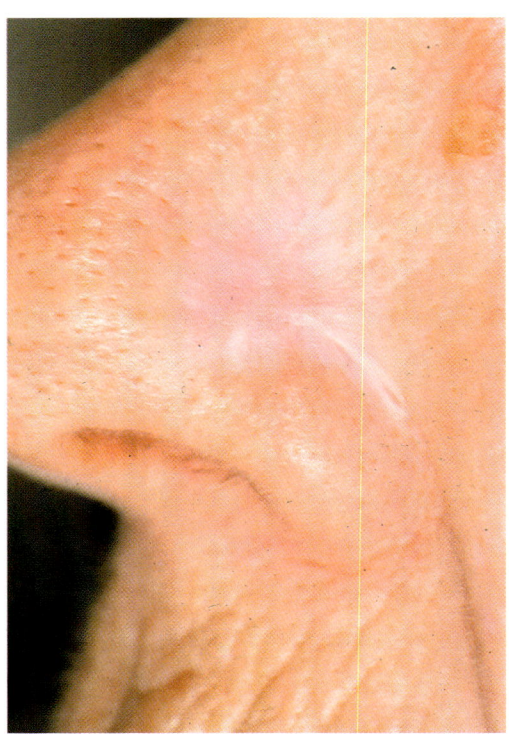

E

Section F   Clinical Aspects   225

Chapter 11
Cryosurgical Dermatology

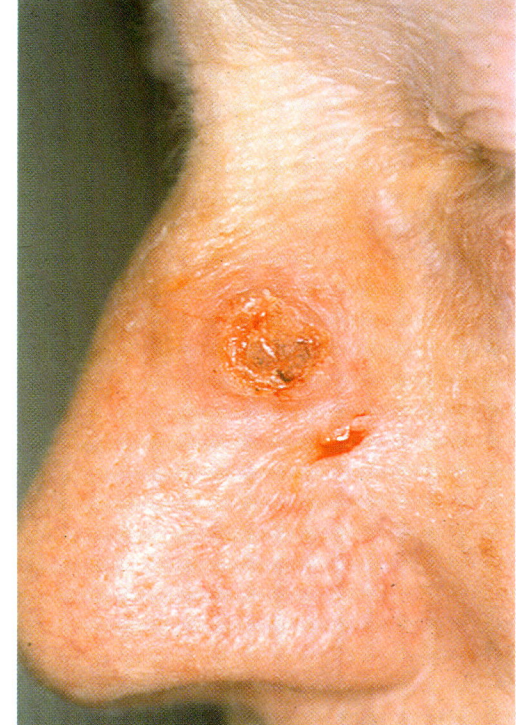

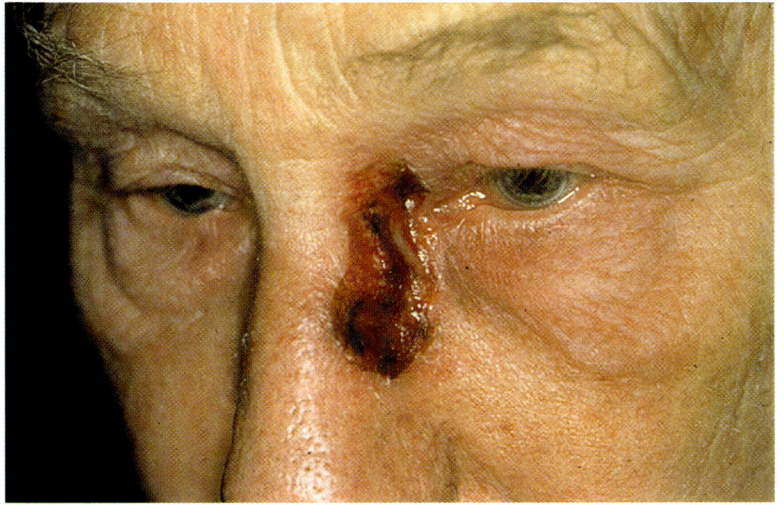

Fig. 11.3.62[5]. A 70-year-old man with a 10 mm well-circumscribed nodular tumor on the bridge of the nose in 1993. The histopathological findings from a 3 mm punch biopsy showed a baso-squamous cancer (**A**). After a meticulous curettage with different sized curettes the extension of the tumor was three times as great as expected. After hemostasis with 50% iron chloride solution, freezing was performed in a double freeze-thaw cycle, using the open-spray technique (**B**). The result obtained after 5 years (**C**)

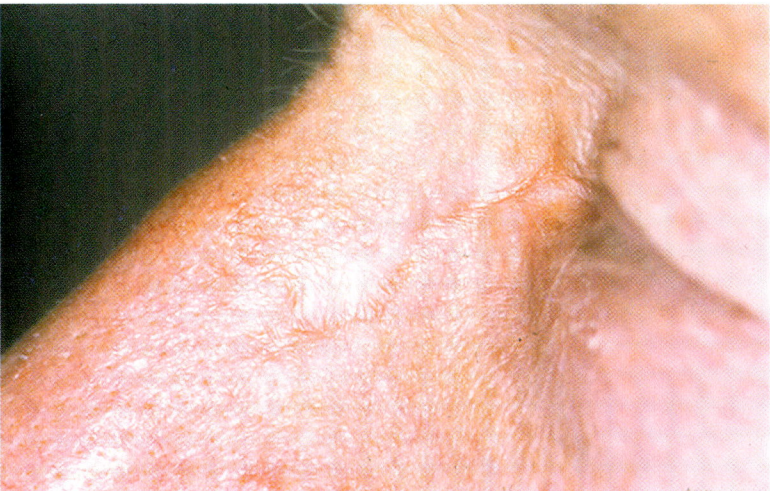

Chapter 11
Cryosurgical
Dermatology

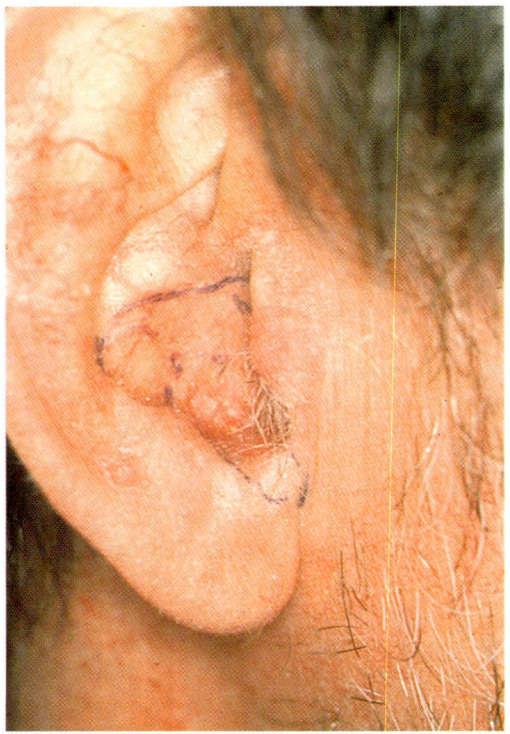

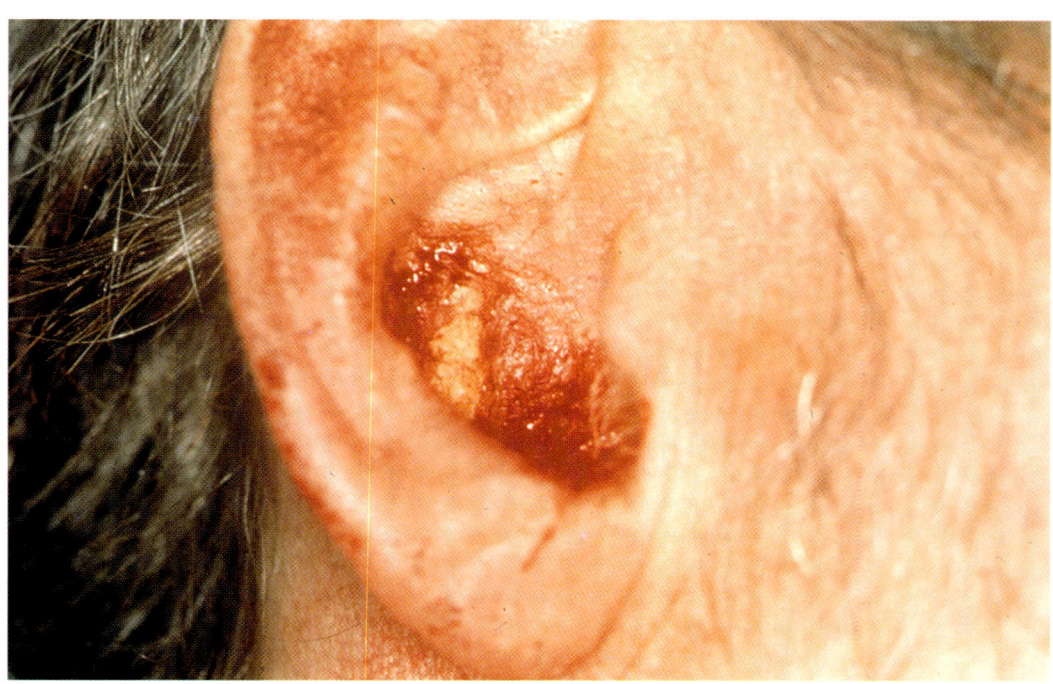

Fig. 11.3.63[5]. A recurrent, clinically ill-defined basal cell carcinoma on the concha of the right ear of a male patient born in 1941. Two incomplete surgical excisions had been performed in 1991 and 1992 (**A**). In 1993 the patient was treated with curettage-cryosurgery. After a thorough curettage the maximal diameter was 30 mm. The tumor grew in some places as far as the cartilage, which, however, was not affected. The freezing was performed with the open spray technique in a double freeze-thaw cycle with a freeze zone of at least 5 mm outside the tumor area. This meant freezing through the cartilage in order to destroy any remaining tumor. The auditory canal was protected by means of soft cotton (**B**). After 2 weeks the patient had an oozing wound but no pain (**C**). The result obtained after 5 years. No local recurrence (**D**)

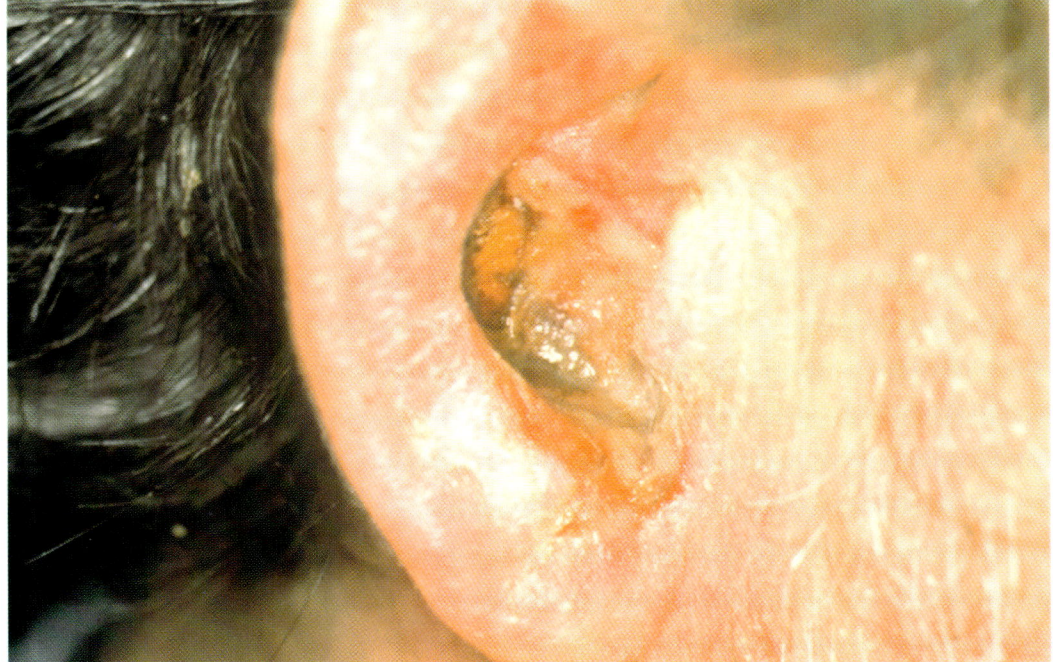

Fig. 11.3.63[5]. A recurrent, clinically ill-defined basal cell carcinoma on the concha of the right ear of a male patient born in 1941. Two incomplete surgical excisions had been performed in 1991 and 1992 (**A**). In 1993 the patient was treated with curettage-cryosurgery. After a thorough curettage the maximal diameter was 30 mm. The tumor grew in some places as far as the cartilage, which, however, was not affected. The freezing was performed with the open spray technique in a double freeze-thaw cycle with a freeze zone of at least 5 mm outside the tumor area. This meant freezing through the cartilage in order to destroy any remaining tumor. The auditory canal was protected by means of soft cotton (**B**). After 2 weeks the patient had an oozing wound but no pain (**C**). The result obtained after 5 years. No local recurrence (**D**)

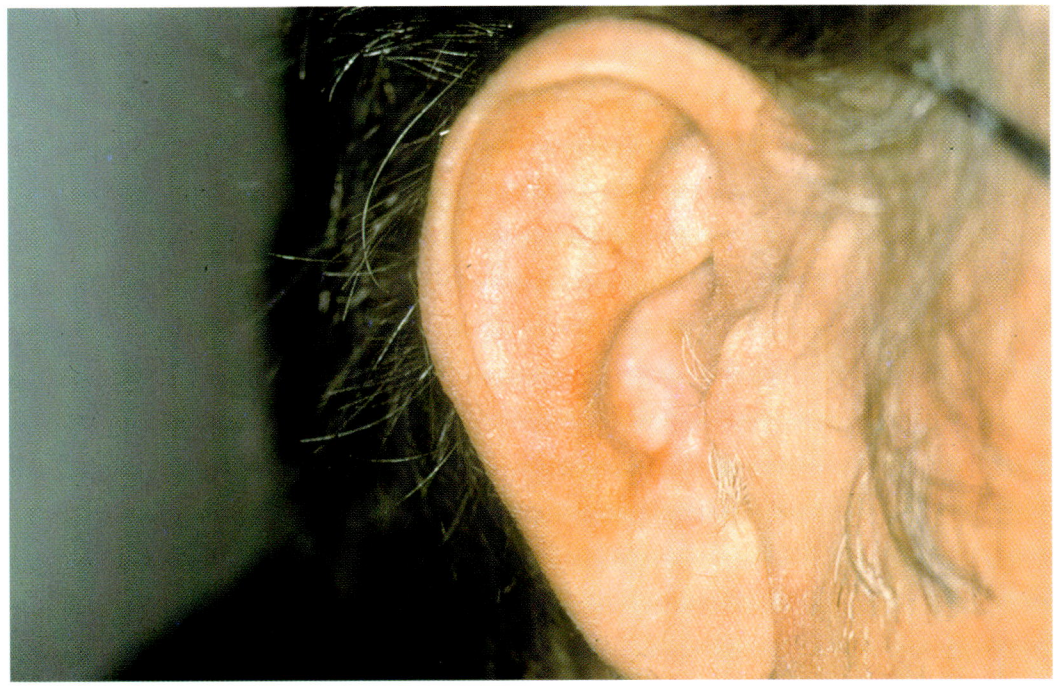

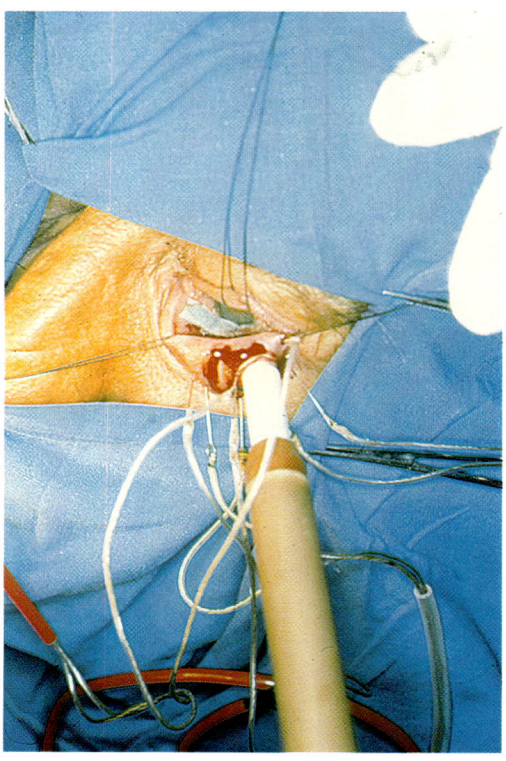

Fig. 11.3.64[6]. Treatment of tumor under eye: Step 1

Fig. 11.3.65[6]. Treatment of tumor under eye: Step 2

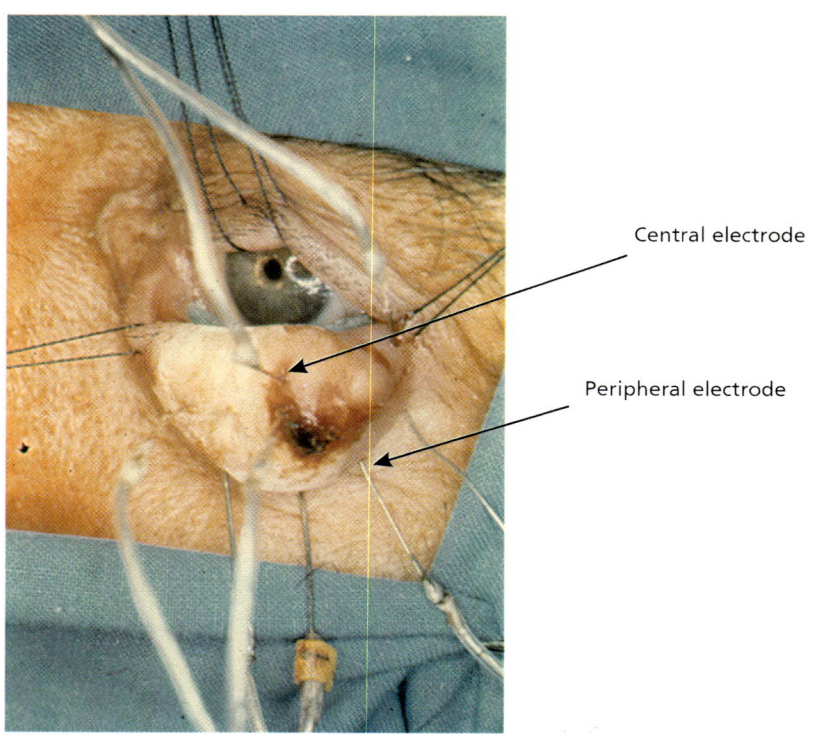

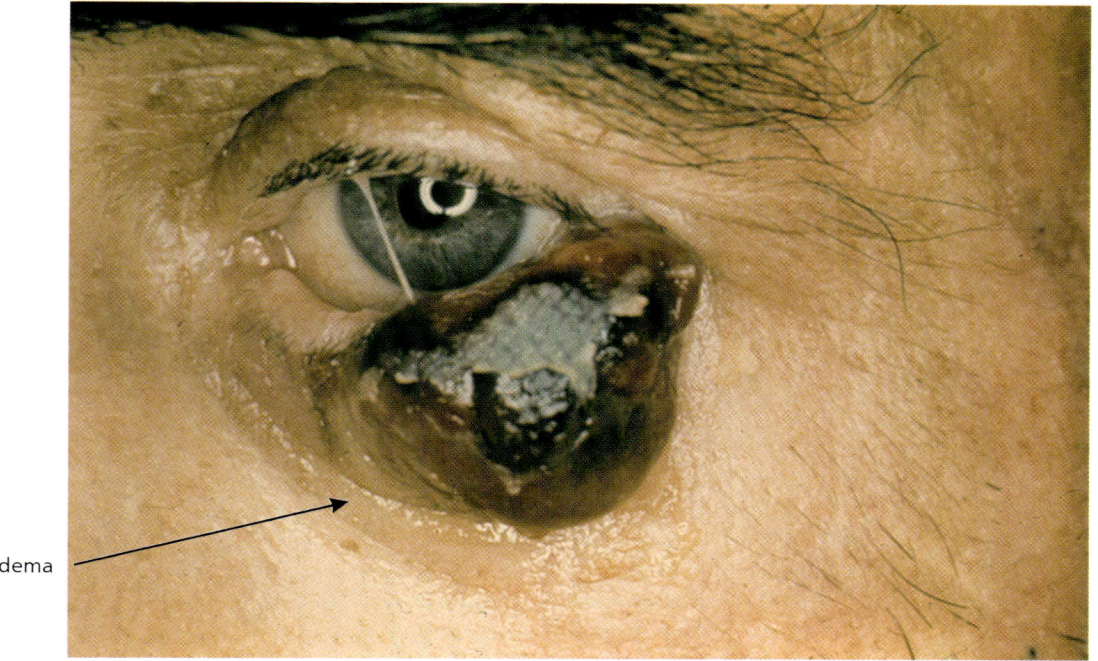

Fig. 11.3.66⁶. Treatment of tumor under eye: Step 3

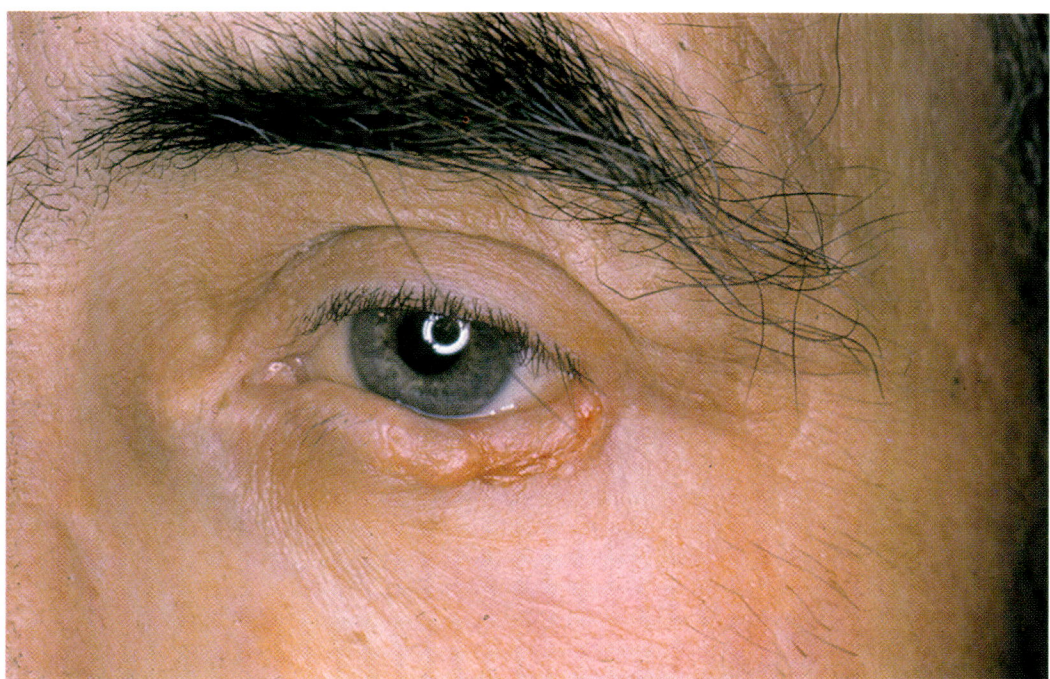

Fig. 11.3.67⁶. Treatment of tumor under eye: Step 4

Chapter 11
Cryosurgical
Dermatology

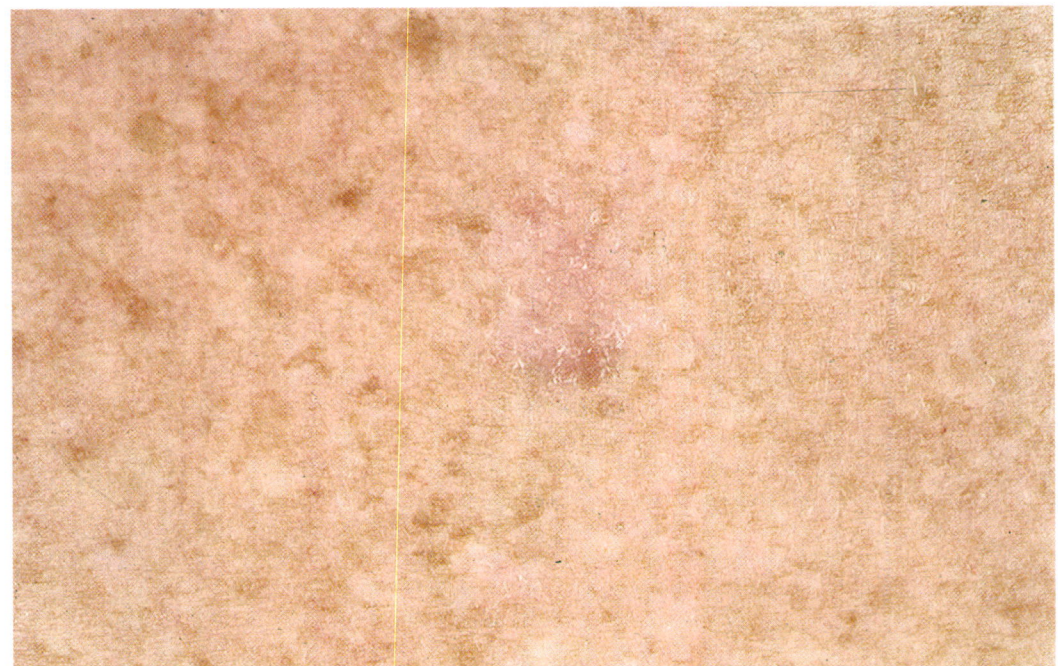

A

Fig. 11.3.68[7]. This set of photographs (**A–D**) shows single freeze-thaw cycle using the fixed spot freeze technique for the treatment of superficial basal cell carcinoma (BCC) on the back of a patient (**A**) with the marked tumor area and a surrounding 5 mm margin of normal-appearing skin (**B**). The cryogun is held 1 cm from the patient and the centre of the lesion is sprayed continuously until the ice ball extends to the edge of treatment field (**C**). Spraying is stopped while the ice-ball is palpated between the thumb and the index finger (**D**). When the lesion is frozen, timing begins. The centre of the BCC is intermittently carefully sprayed for 30 sec, keeping the ice ball the same size

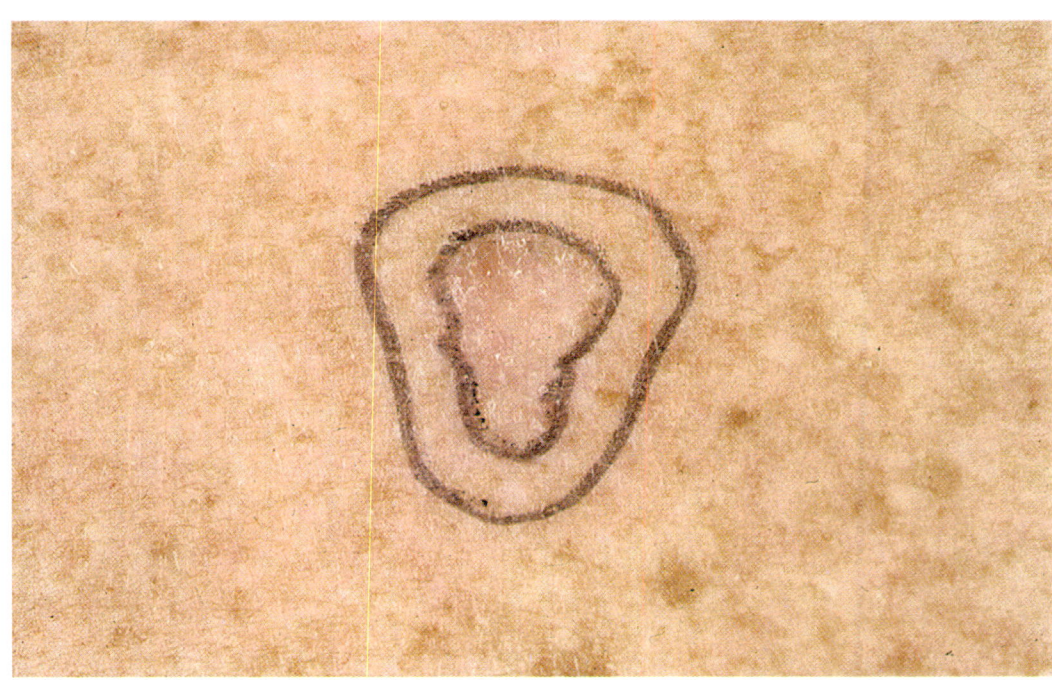

B

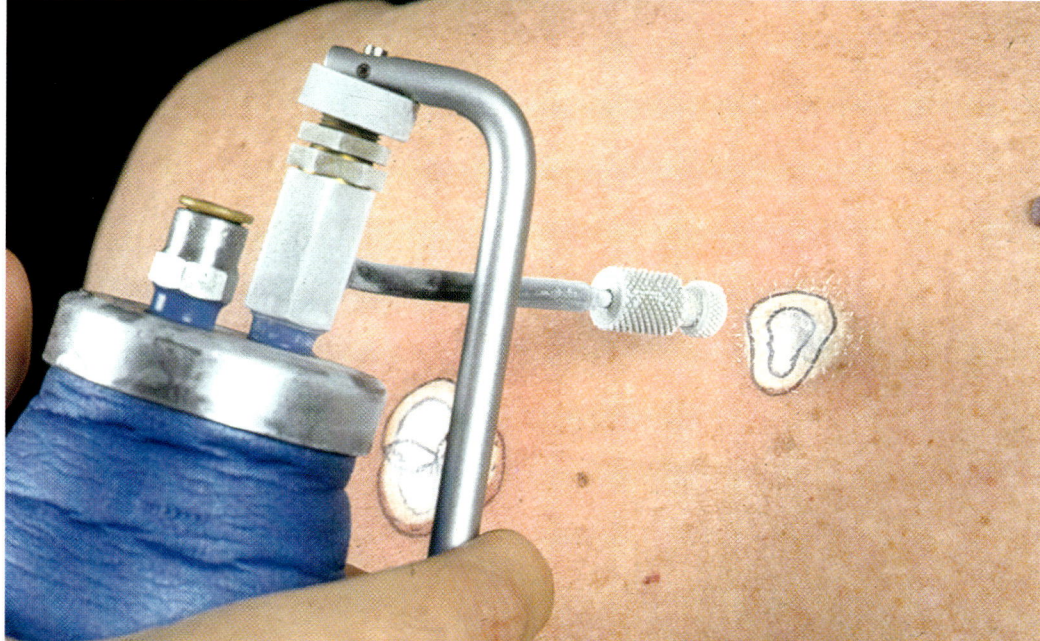

C

Fig. 11.3.68[7]. This set of photographs (**A–D**) shows single freeze-thaw cycle using the fixed spot freeze technique for the treatment of superficial basal cell carcinoma (BCC) on the back of a patient (**A**) with the marked tumor area and a surrounding 5 mm margin of normal-appearing skin (**B**). The cryogun is held 1 cm from the patient and the centre of the lesion is sprayed continuously until the ice ball extends to the edge of treatment field (**C**). Spraying is stopped while the ice-ball is palpated between the thumb and the index finger (**D**). When the lesion is frozen, timing begins. The centre of the BCC is intermittently carefully sprayed for 30 sec, keeping the ice ball the same size

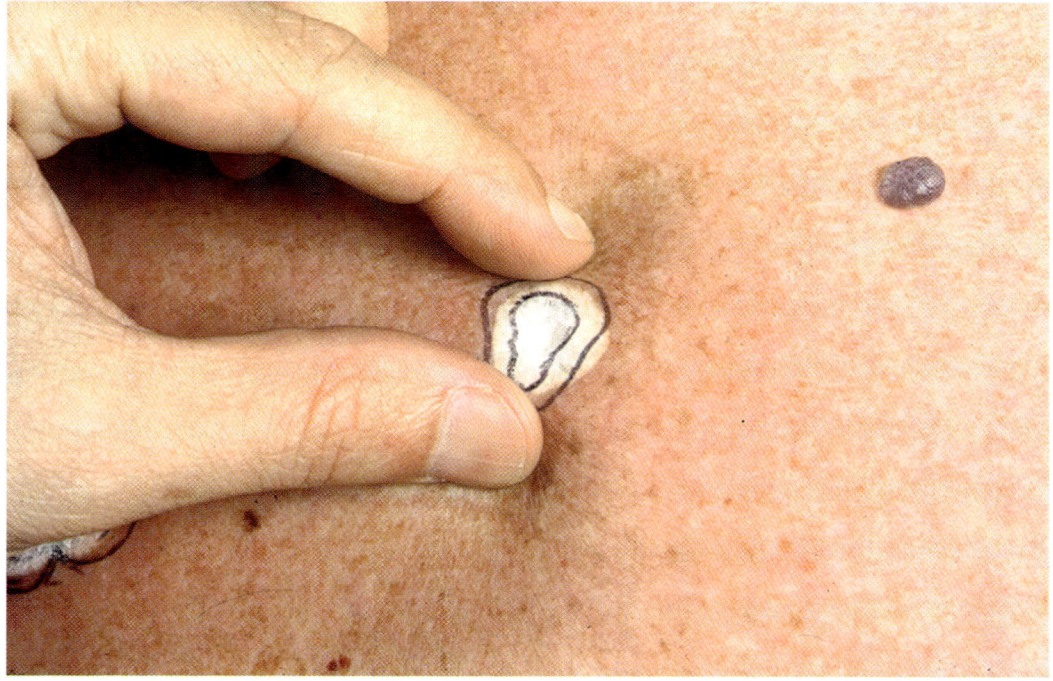

D

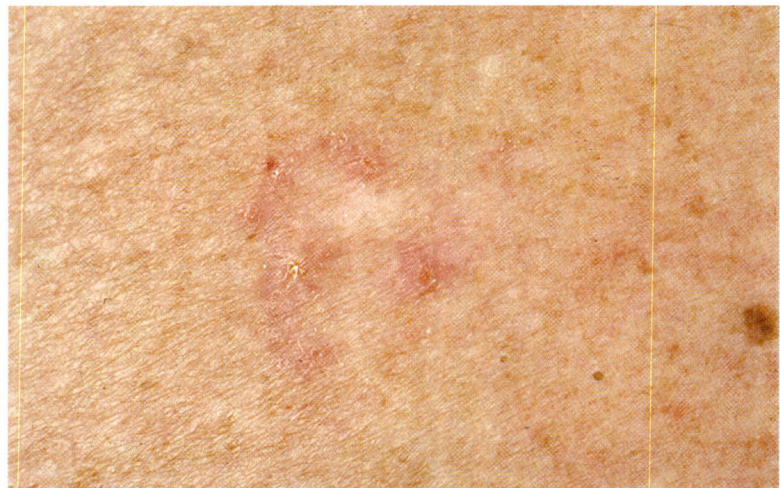

A

B

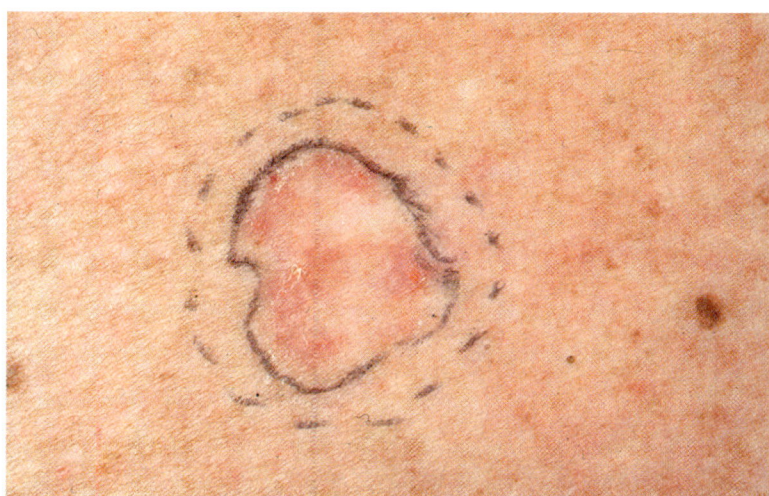

Fig. 11.3.69[7]. The second set of photographs (**A–F**) shows the use of the same overlocking field technique for a larger BCC. The second BCC on the back of the same patient (**A**) is too large to be treated in a single field and a 5 mm surrounding margin of normal skin is drawn on the patient (**B**). Overlapping 2 cm fields are marked out (**C**). The first field is treated as for small lesion 1 (**D**). The lesion is palpated before beginning to time the 30 sec (**E**). The other two fields are then treated in sequence (**F**)

C

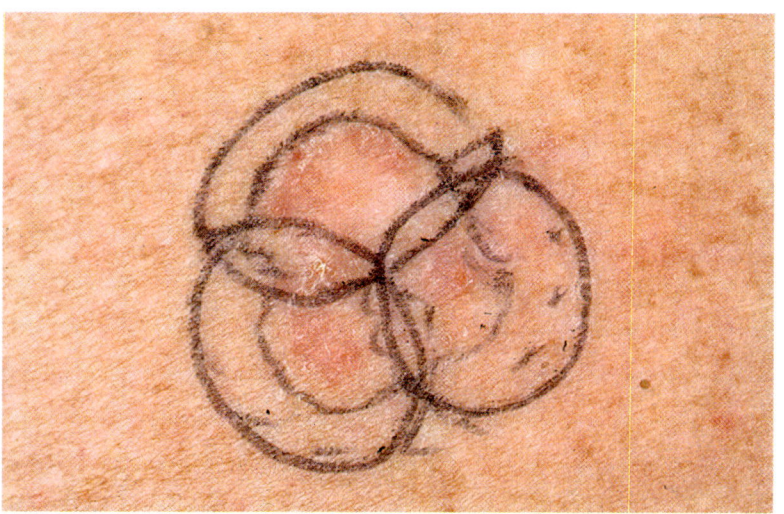

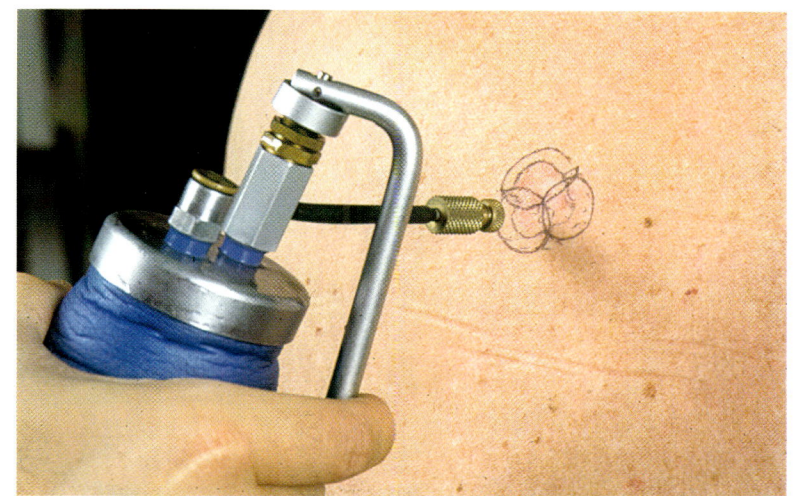

D

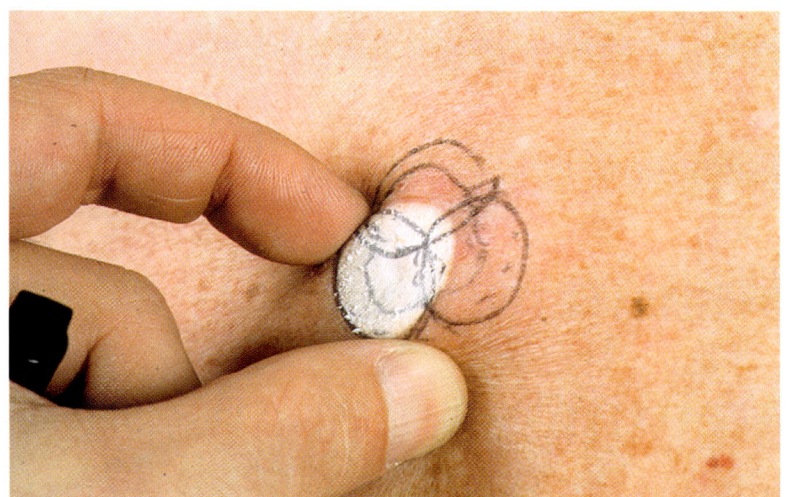

E

Fig. 11.3.69[7]. The second set of photographs (**A–F**) shows the use of the same overlocking field technique for a larger BCC. The second BCC on the back of the same patient (**A**) is too large to be treated in a single field and a 5 mm surrounding margin of normal skin is drawn on the patient (**B**). Overlapping 2 cm fields are marked out (**C**). The first field is treated as for small lesion 1 (**D**). The lesion is palpated before beginning to time the 30 sec (**E**). The other two fields are then treated in sequence (**F**)

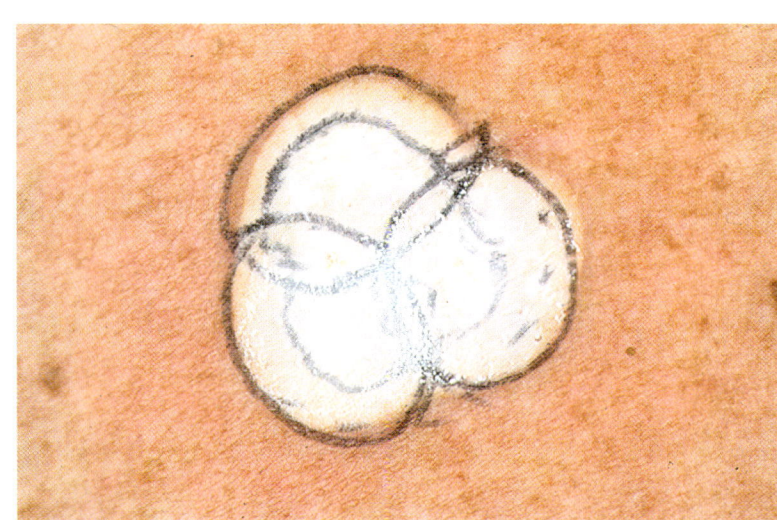

F

Abdominal Cryosurgery: Hepatic Cryosurgery

Nikolai N. Korpan[1] with contributions by
Boris I. Alperovich[2],
Gerhard Hochwarter[1],
Franz Sellner[1] and Ved R. Tandan[3]

12.0 Introduction

Hepatic cryosurgery is at present successfully used in medical practice both as an independent treatment and as a component of other treatments in the field of oncology. Tumors are destroyed by shock-freezing. New scientific research on freezing techniques in the fields of biology and medicine, as well as numerous theoretical and experimental studies *in vitro* and *in vivo*, indicate which mechanisms are activated when low temperatures are applied to the tissue. They also describe the impairment and destruction of cells which occur under cryoinfluence.

In recent years, cryosurgery has become a promising new way of treating primary and metastatic carcinomas of the liver. Liver cryosurgery treats unresectable liver cancer by *in situ* ablation of liver tumors through freezing with liquid nitrogen. Approximately 25% or less of patients with isolated liver metastases have tumors that are resectable by conventional surgical techniques, and only 20% to 35% survive for five or more years. Patients with primary hepatocellular carcinoma also face low resectability rates.

The important advantage of treating non-resectable liver tumors cryosurgically, compared with other methods (laser ablation, tumor heat treatment), is that all the tumor cells are mechanically fixed during the process of their being destroyed, so that no dissemination of tumor cells can take place during the operation. However, only with state-of-the-art equipment can the method be successfully applied.

It is generally held that cryoablation should be performed in cases involving liver tumors that are deemed unresectable: i.e., central tumor localization straddling the line of demarcation between right and left lobes, multiple tumors in both lobes (bilobar involvement), vessel infiltration and very large tumor size. Although conventional resection is still the treatment of first choice, cryosurgery offers significant hope to patients with unresectable disease.

Several studies have demonstrated the advantages of using intraoperative liver ultrasonography to guide the cryoprobe safely into the tumor region, thus facilitating central placement of the probe, and monitoring of the freeze-thaw process.

12.1 Hepatic Cryosurgery for Small Liver Metastases

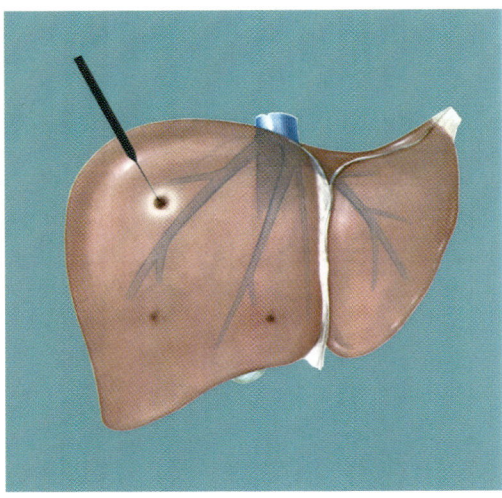

Fig. 12.1.1[1]. A single needle, measuring at least 2 mm to maximally 22 mm, is implanted directly in the tumor mass using the Seldinger approach with the help of ultrasound monitoring (see. Fig. 8.1.2.3a–f)

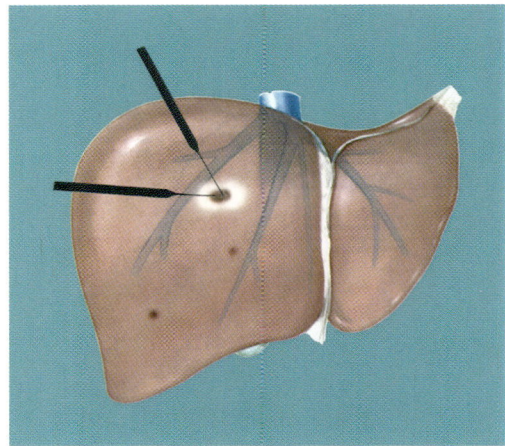

A

B

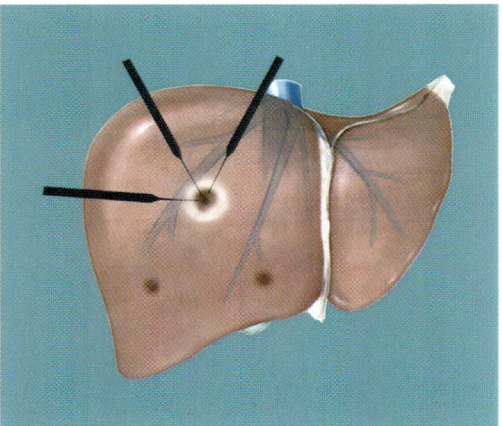

Fig. 12.1.2[1] A–B. Two (**A**) or three (**B**) needles can be implanted in a small liver metastasis

12.2 Hepatic Cryosurgery for Large Liver Metastatic Tumors (Cancer)

Chapter 12
Abdominal Cryosurgery: Hepatic Cryosurgery

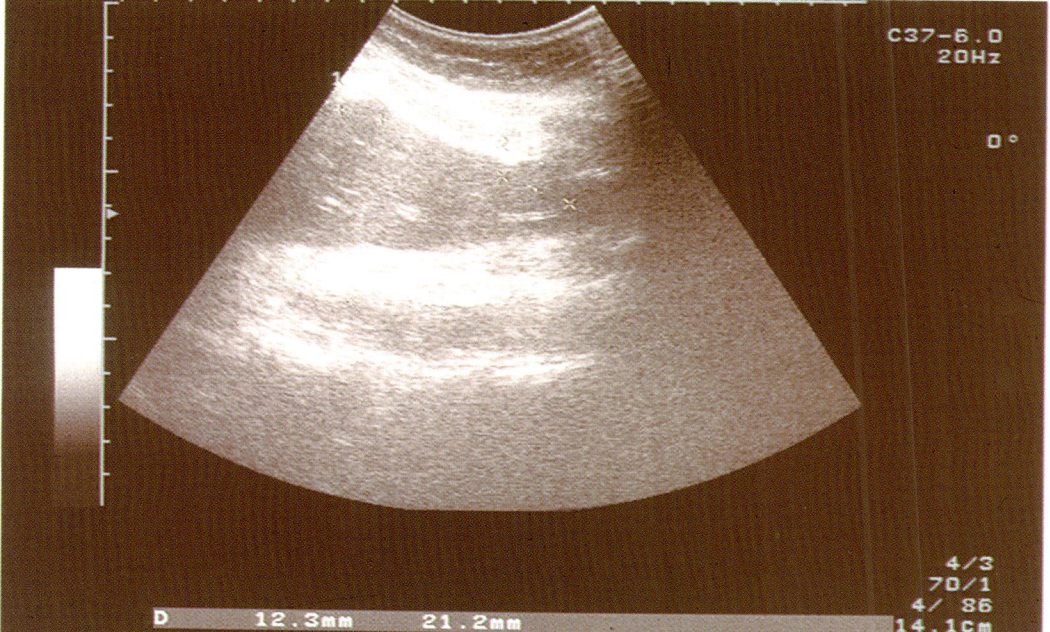

A

Fig. 12.2.1[1] A–D. Metastatic colon carcinoma. Multiple liver metastases are seen in this sagittal view of the right lobe (segment IV, IV/V, V/VIII) in preoperative ultrasound of the liver. A total of three liver metastases, measuring between 20 mm and 44 mm, can be made out

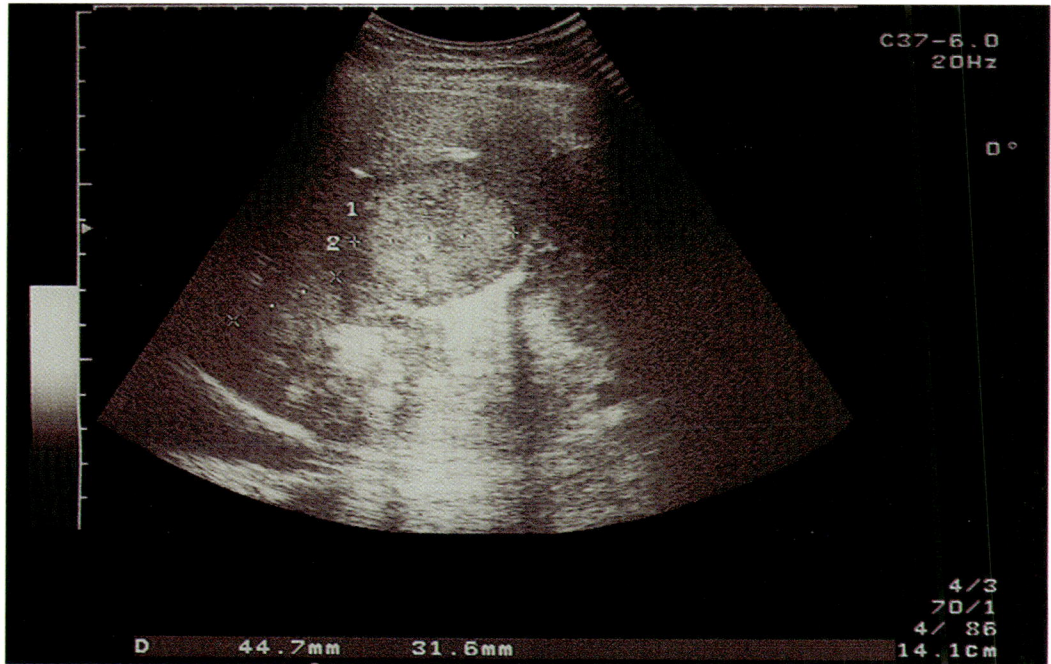

B

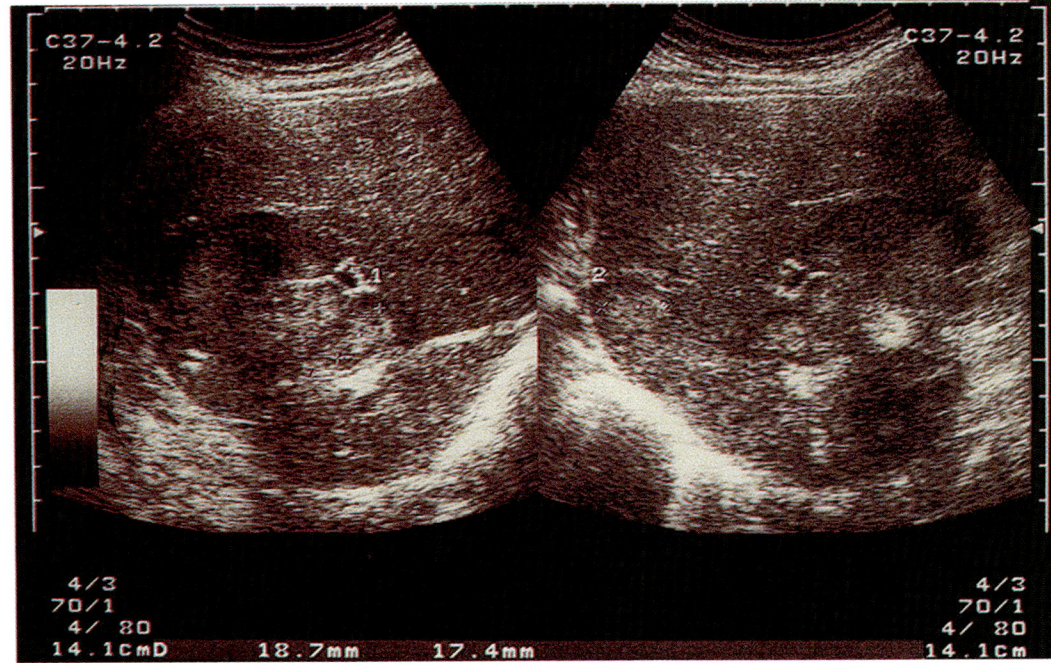

C

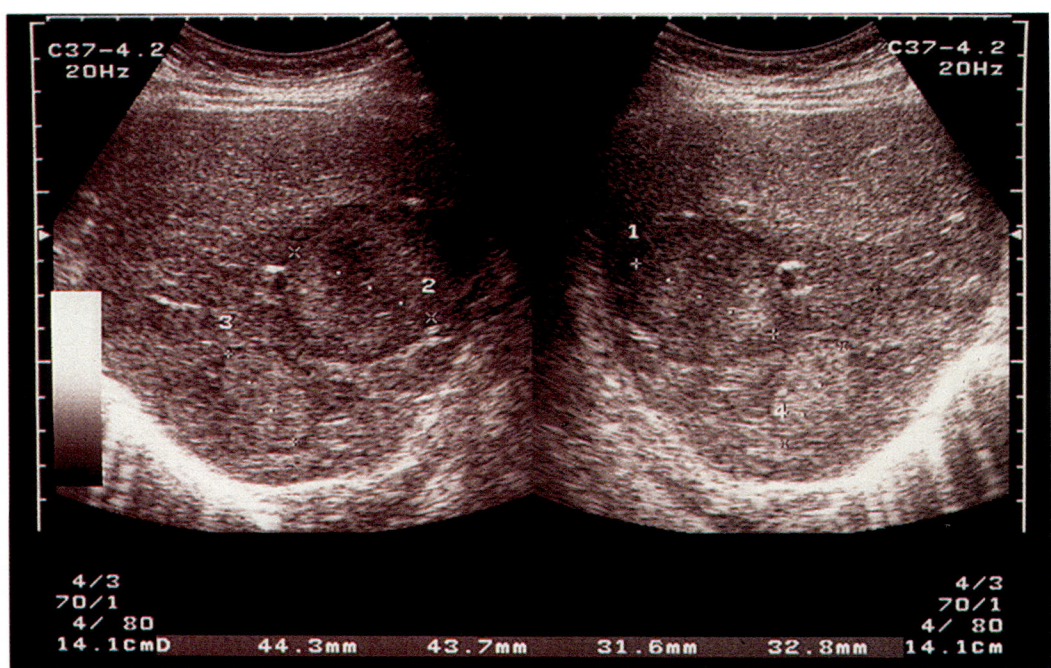

D

Fig. 12.2.1[1] A–D. Metastatic colon carcinoma. Multiple liver metastases are seen in this sagittal view of the right lobe (segment IV, IV/V, V/VIII) in preoperative ultrasound of the liver. A total of three liver metastases, measuring between 20 mm and 44 mm, can be made out

Section F Clinical Aspects 239

Chapter 12
Abdominal
Cryosurgery:
Hepatic
Cryosurgery

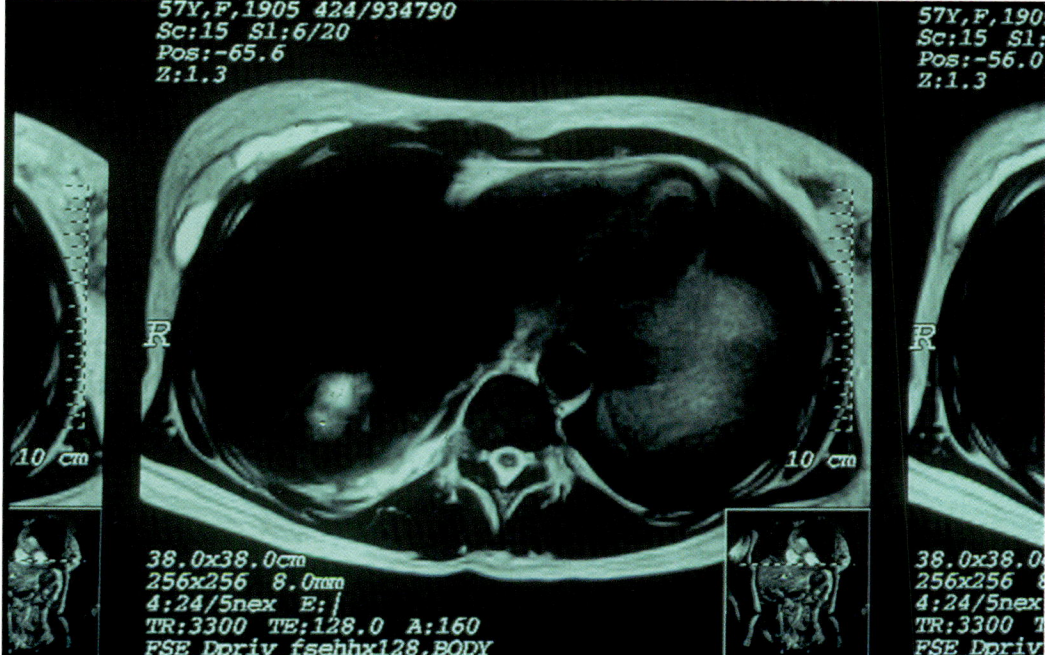

A

Fig. 12.2.2[1] A–D. Typical preoperative findings in magnetic resonance imaging (MRI) which shows multiple liver metastases 2–4-cm in diameter in the right lobe

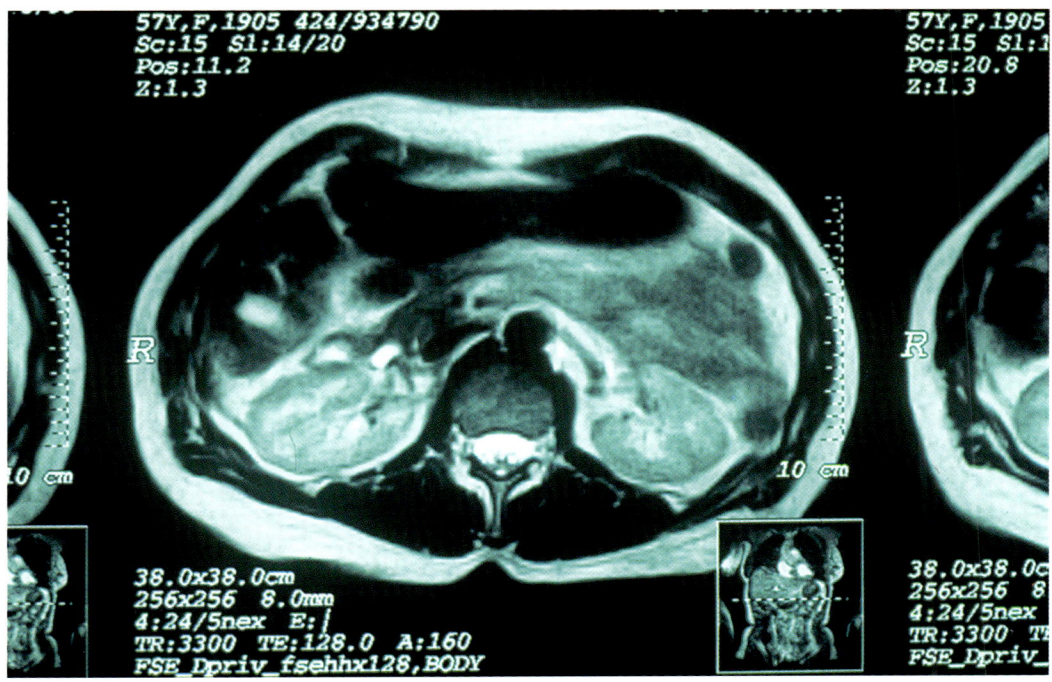

B

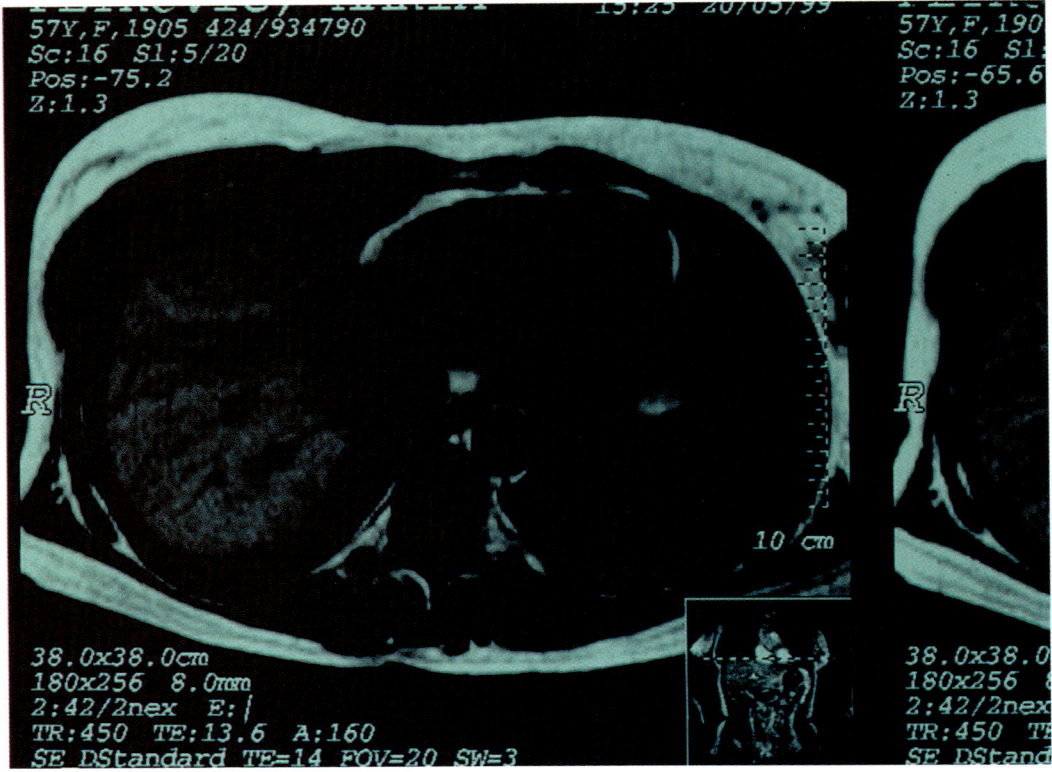

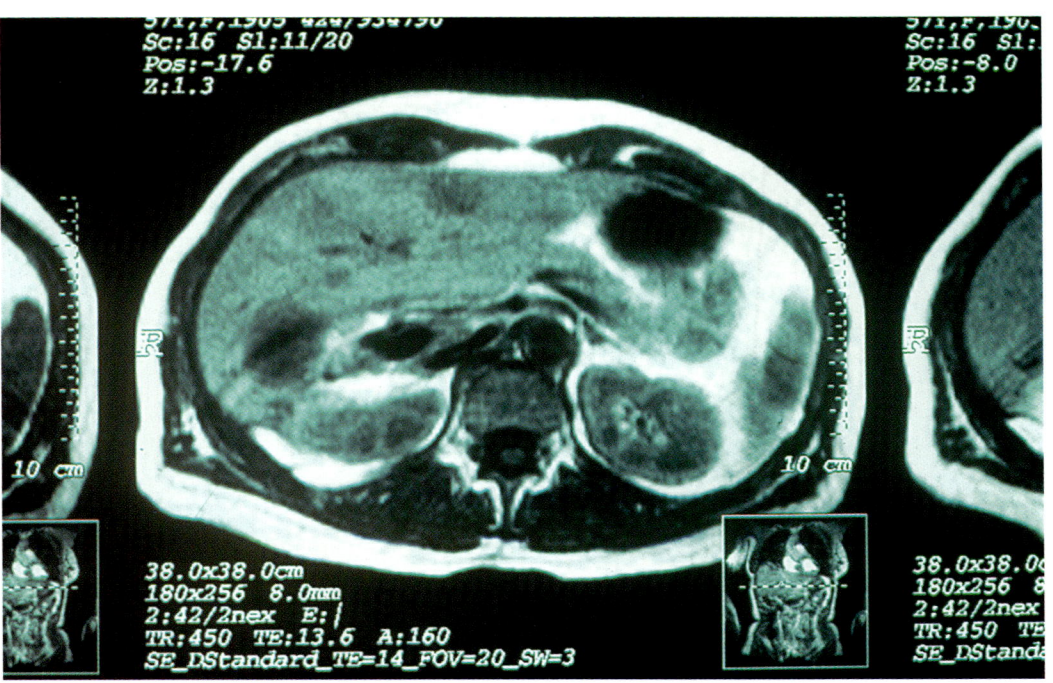

Fig. 12.2.2[1] A–D. Typical preoperative image findings in magnetic resonance imaging (MRI) which shows multiple liver metastases 2–4-cm in diameter in the right lobe

Section F Clinical Aspects 241

Chapter 12
Abdominal
Cryosurgery:
Hepatic
Cryosurgery

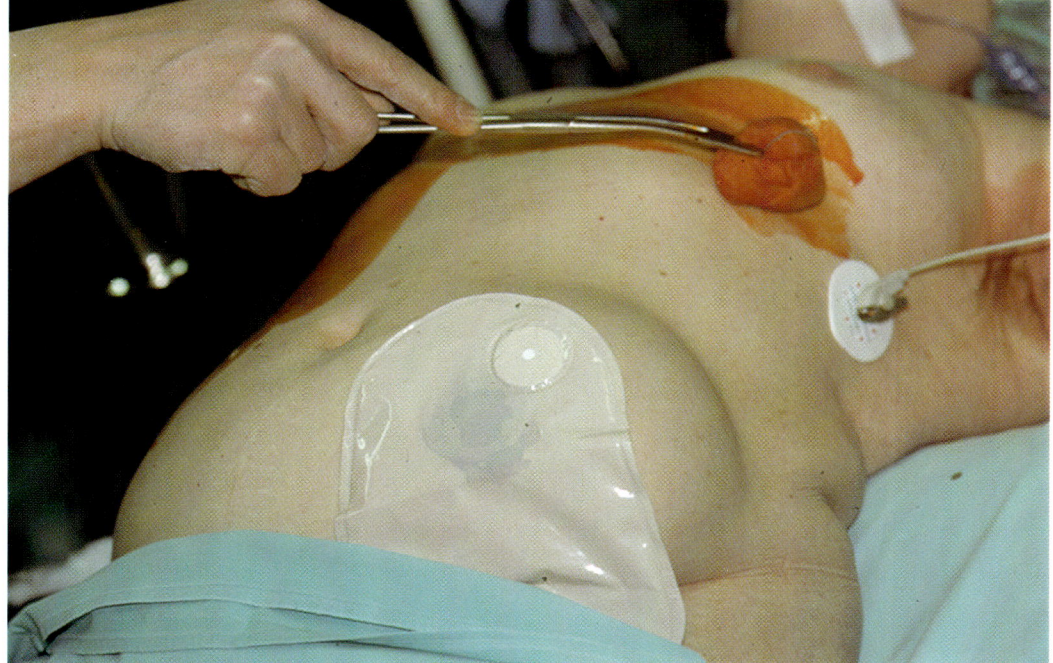

Fig. 12.2.3[1]. Position of the patient for open hepatic cryosurgery (OHC). The patient is placed in a supine position on an operating table over the kidney rest

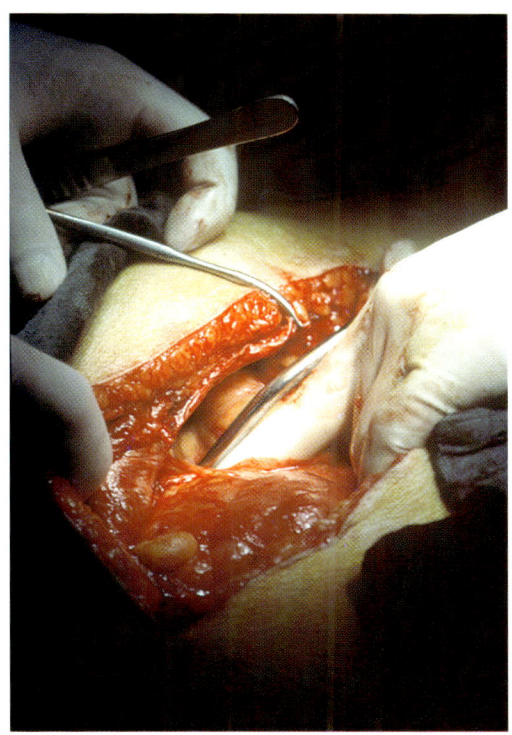

Fig. 12.2.4[1]. The initial incision is in the right subcostal area, which permits detailed exploration of the abdomen. If no extrahepatic disease is identified, the incision is extended to the left, just beyond the rectus abdominis muscle, and to the right, just to the lateral peritoneal flank. This maneuver makes it possible to move and completely examine the liver

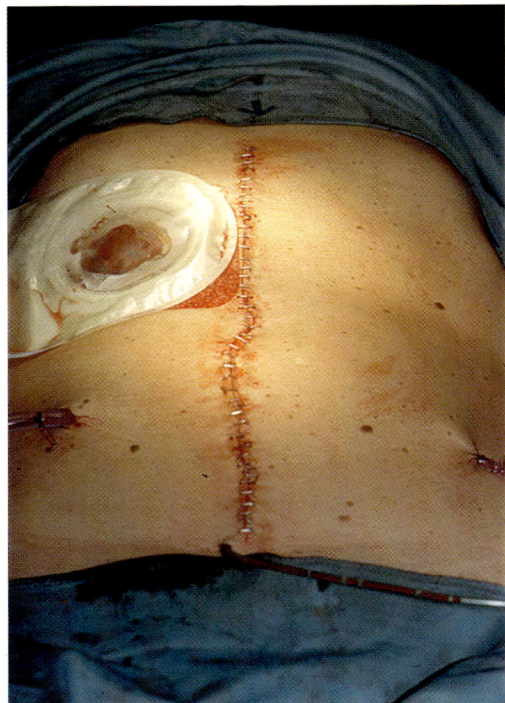

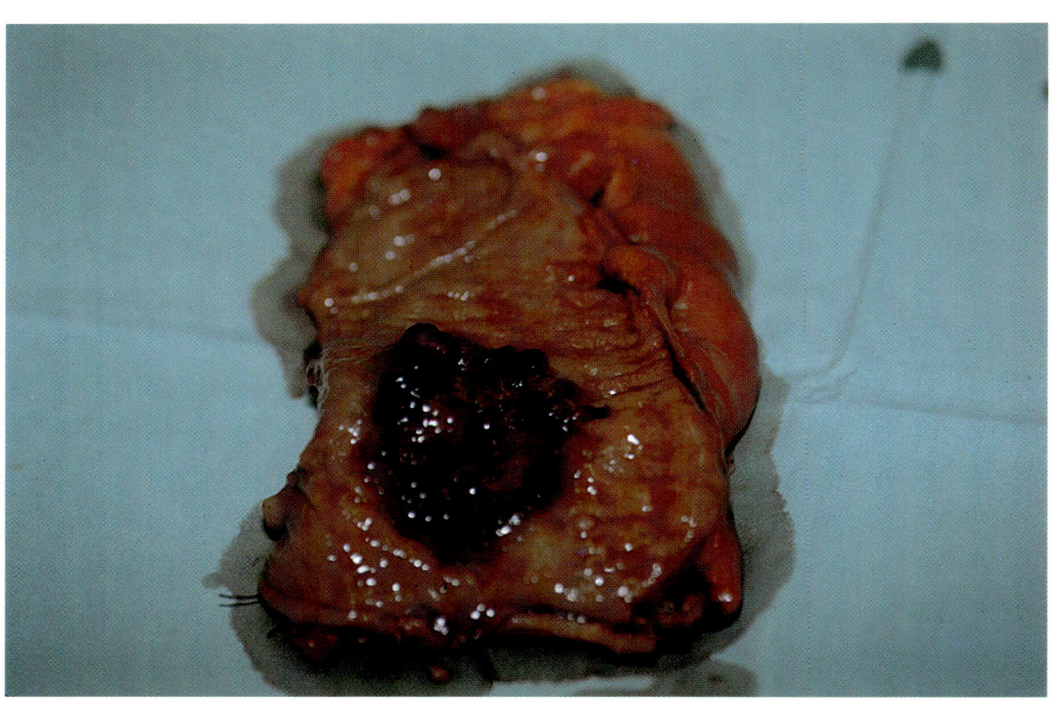

Fig. 12.2.5[1] A, B. In some cases the initial incision is the abdominal laparotomy (**A**) for ease of access to the rectum, sigmoid, and the left colon. In patients with colorectal liver metastases from primary colorectal cancer (**B**), conventional colorectal resection is performed and followed by liver cryosurgery

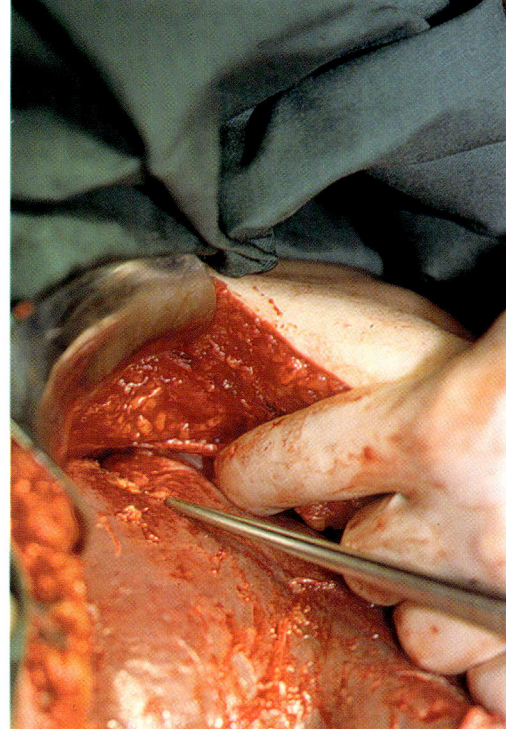

Fig. 12.2.6[1] A–H. View of livers of different cancer patients with multiple large metastases before cryosurgical procedure. The large metastases can be seen in liver segments II (**A**), II/IV (**B**), IV (**C**), IV/V (**D**), V (**E**), VI (**F**), and VII (**G, H**) intraoperatively

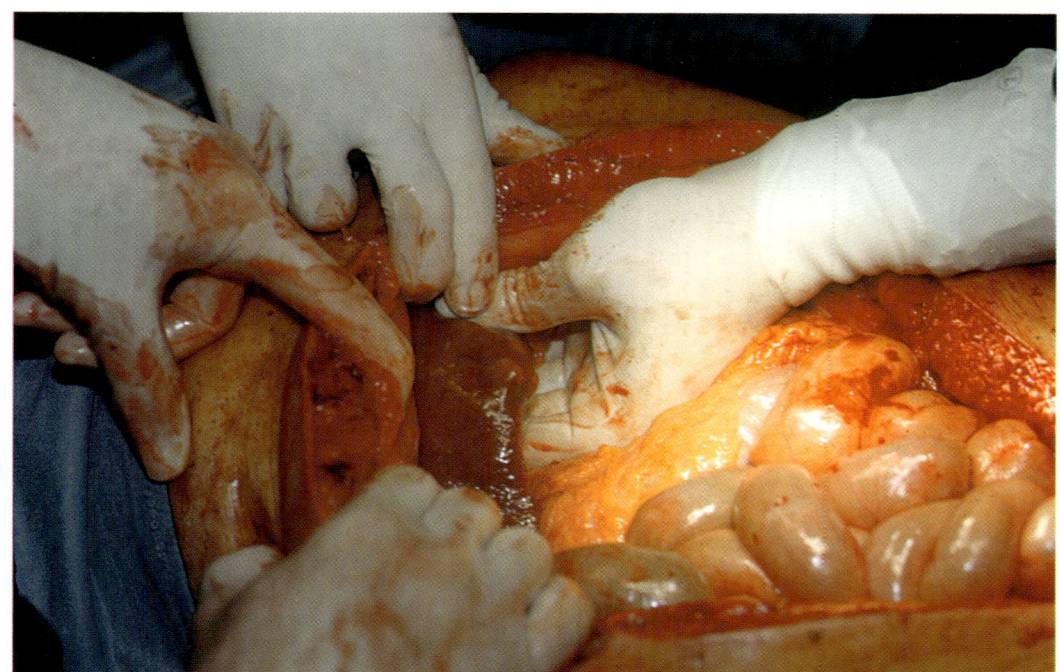

C

Fig. 12.2.6[1] A–H. View of livers of different cancer patients with multiple large metastases before cryosurgical procedure. The large metastases can be seen in liver segments II (**A**), II/IV (**B**), IV (**C**), IV/V (**D**), V (**E**), VI (**F**), and VII (**G**, **H**) intraoperatively

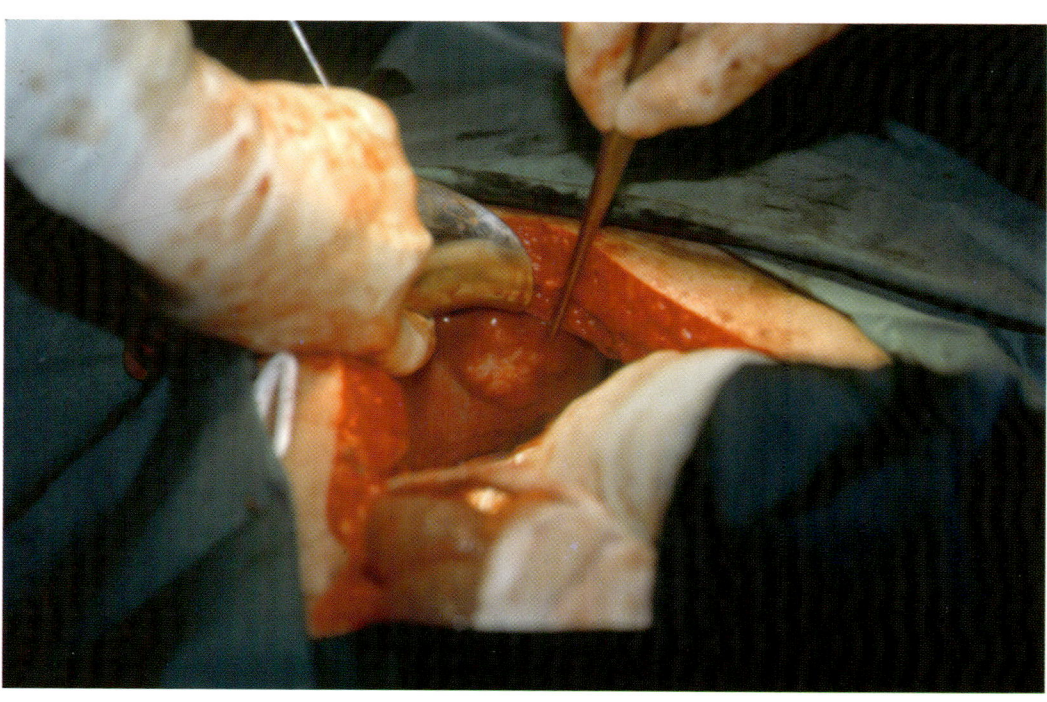

D

Section F　　Clinical Aspects

Chapter 12
Abdominal
Cryosurgery:
Hepatic
Cryosurgery

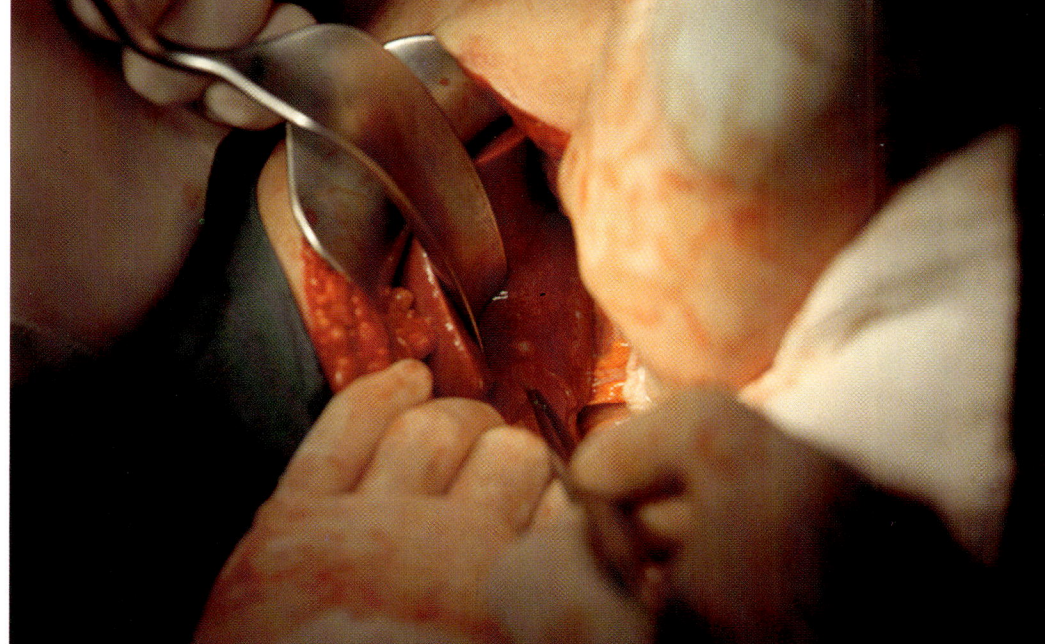

E

Fig. 12.2.6[1] **A–H.** View of livers of different cancer patients with multiple large metastases before cryosurgical procedure. The large metastases can be seen in liver segments II (**A**), II/IV (**B**), IV (**C**), IV/V (**D**), V (**E**), VI (**F**), and VII (**G, H**) intraoperatively

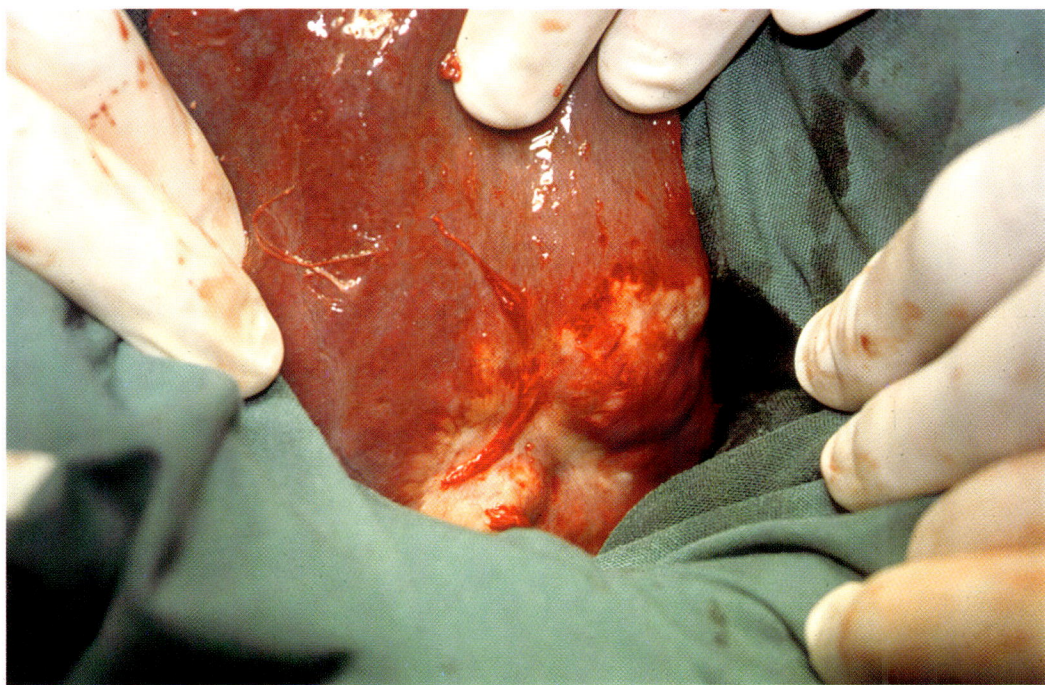

F

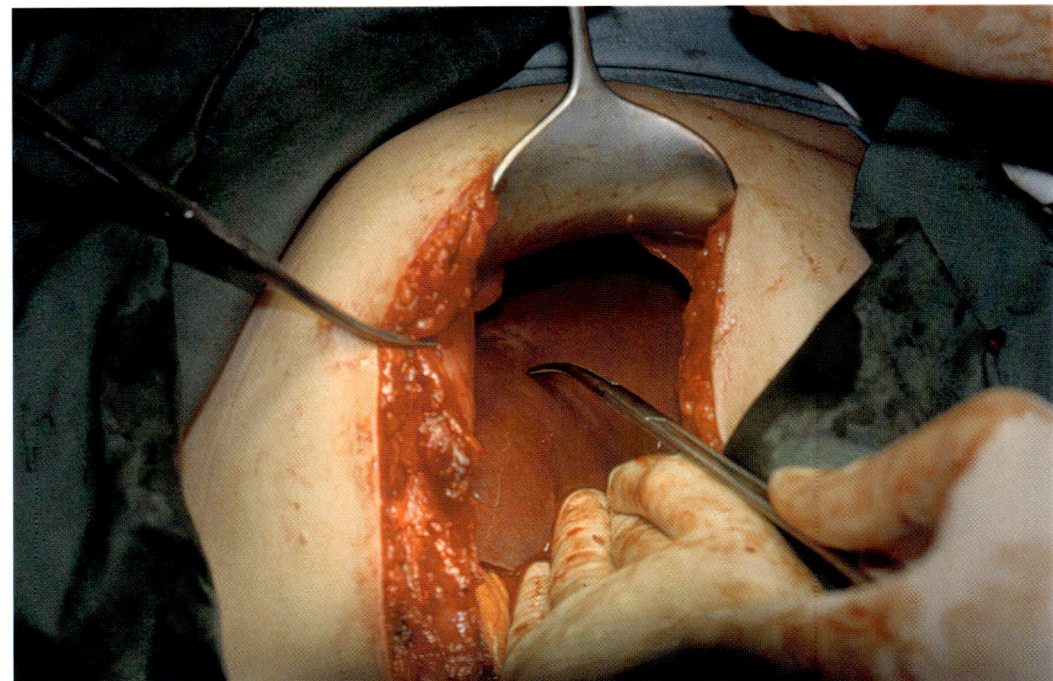

G

Fig. 12.2.6[1] A–H. View of livers of different cancer patients with multiple large metastases before cryosurgical procedure. The large metastases can be seen in liver segments II (**A**), II/IV (**B**), IV (**C**), IV/V (**D**), V (**E**), VI (**F**), and VII (**G, H**) intraoperatively

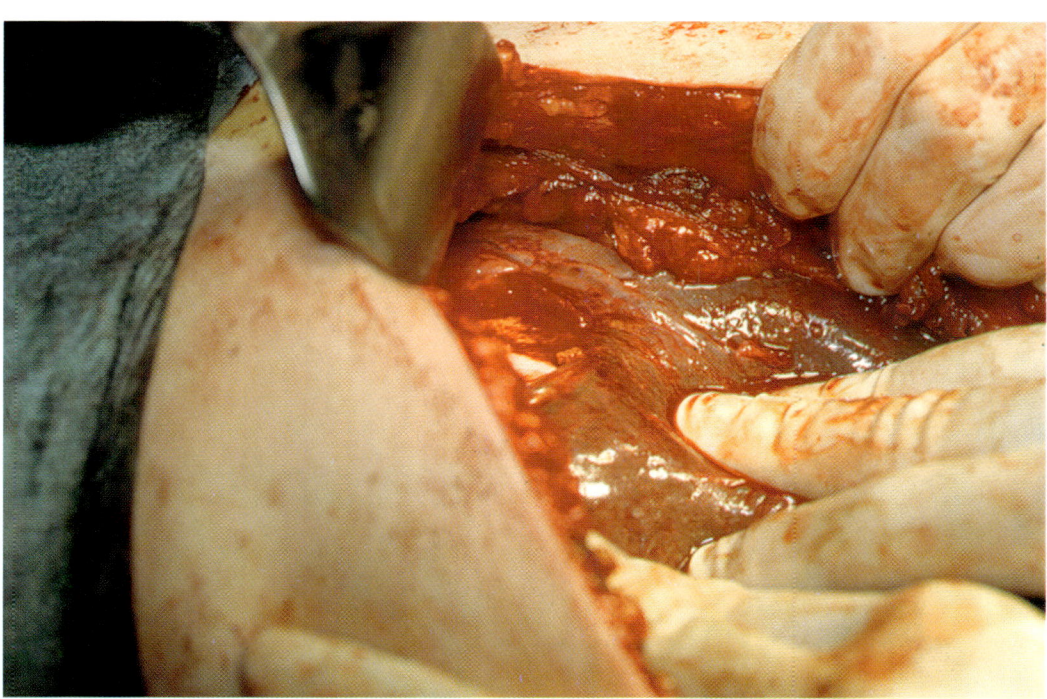

H

Section F　　　　　　　　　　　　　Clinical Aspects　　　　　　　　　　　　　247

Chapter 12
Abdominal
Cryosurgery:
Hepatic
Cryosurgery

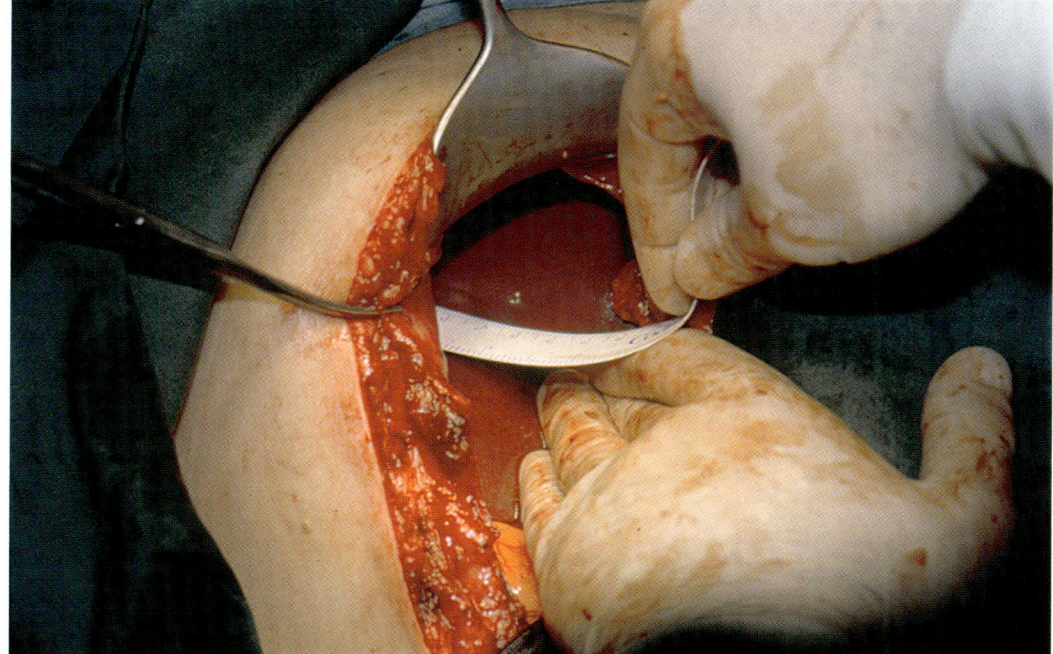

Fig. 12.2.7[1]. After surgical inspection of the abdomen, each liver metastasis is measured and a biopsy is made

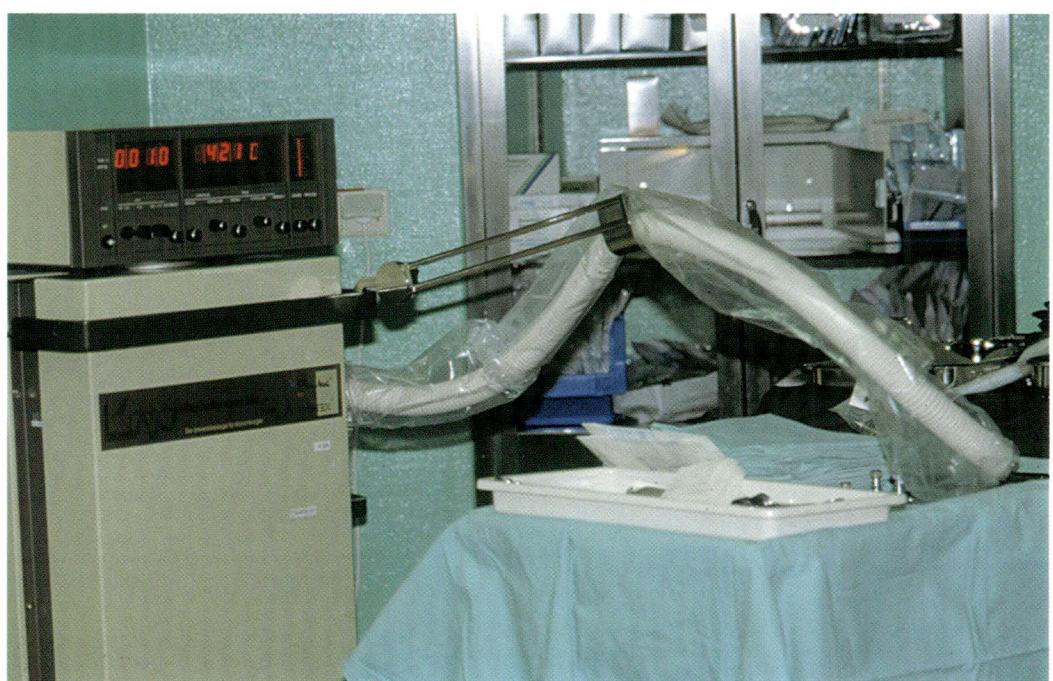

Fig. 12.2.8[1]. Liver cryosurgical equipment. The cryosurgical device is prepared before the abdomen is explored

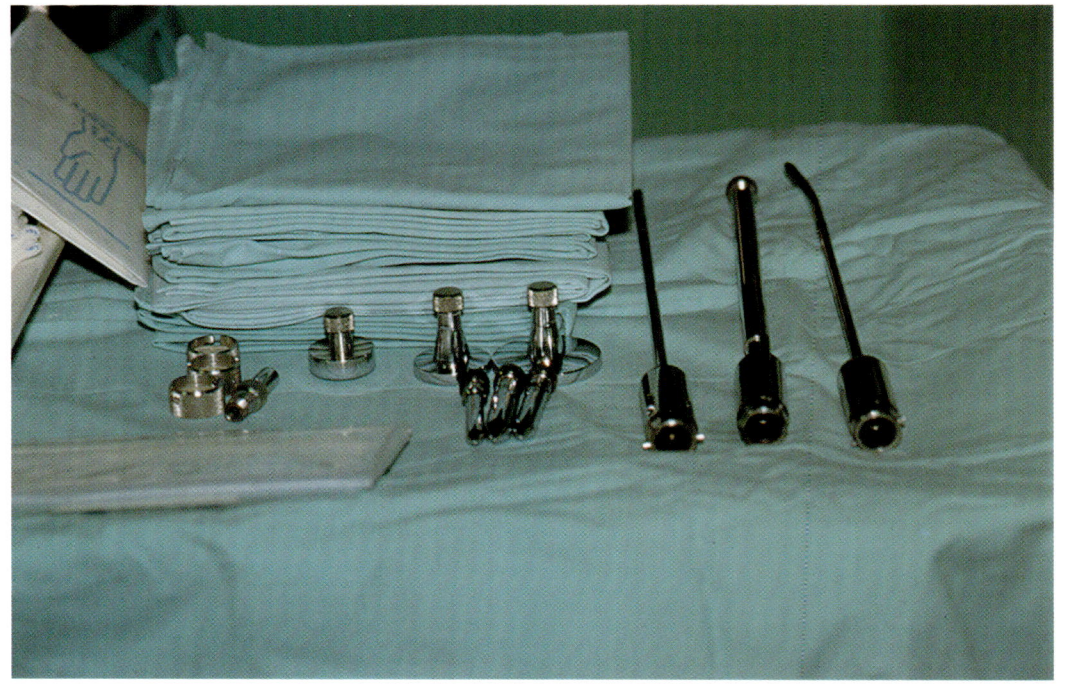

Fig. 12.2.9[1] A, B. Liver cryosurgical equipment. A set of cryosurgical instruments with cryoprobes and needles (**A**) is prepared together with a set of surgical instruments for conventional abdominal surgery (**B**)

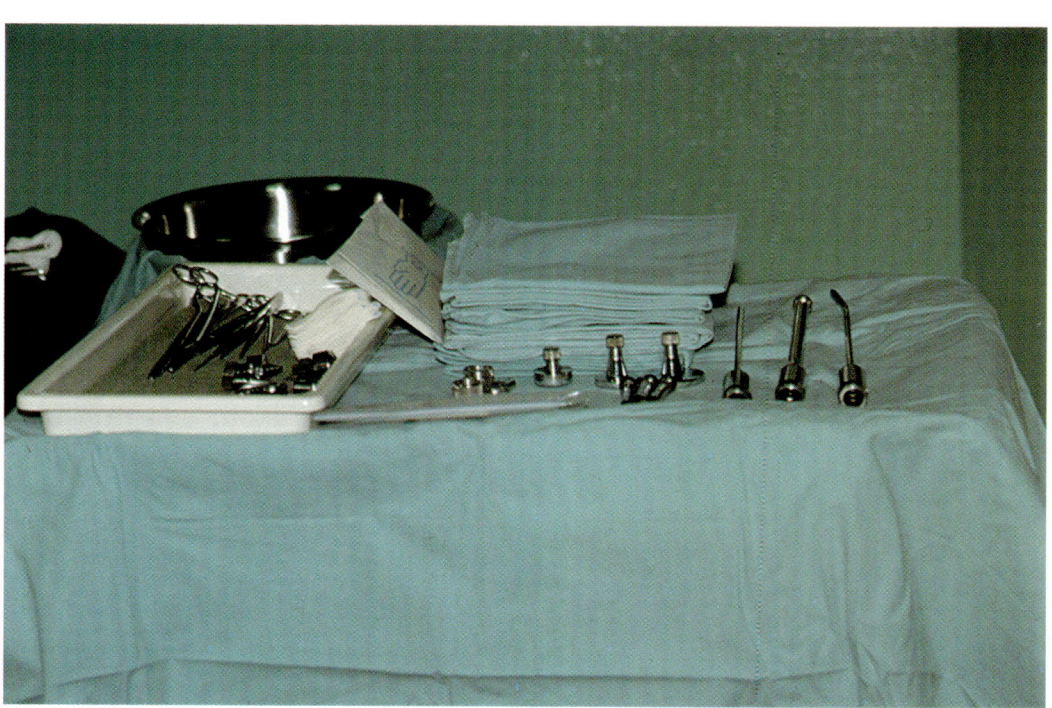

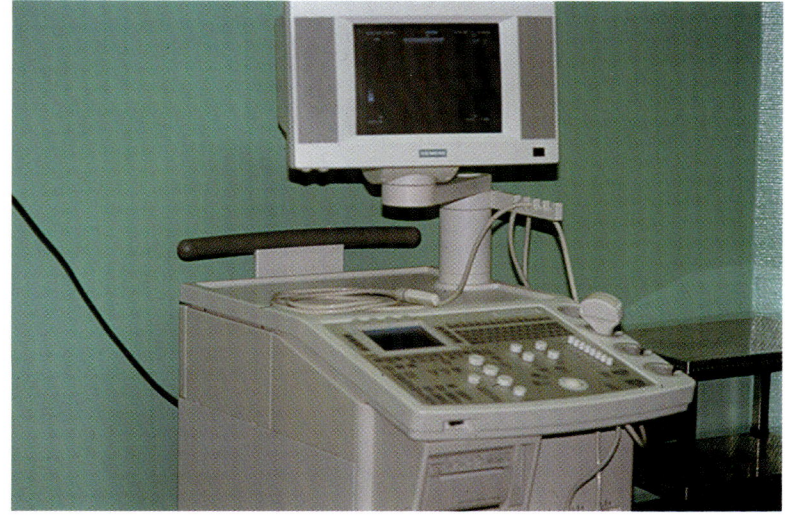
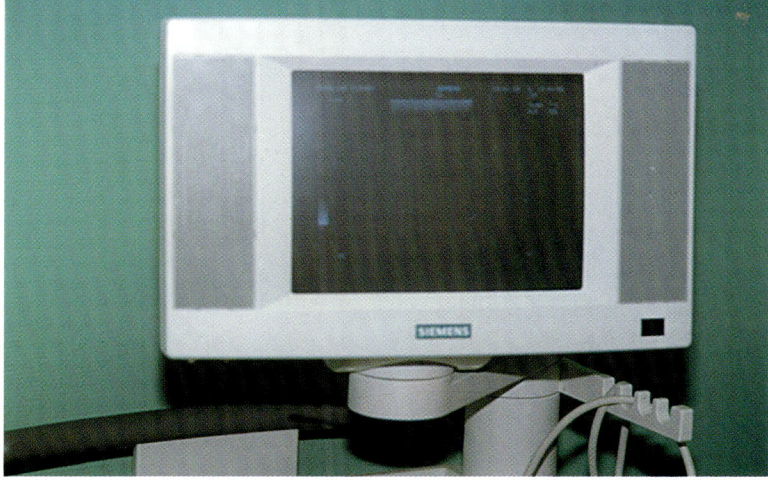

Fig. 12.2.10[1] A, B. Intraoperative ultrasound of the liver. Intraoperative ultrasound is essential for detecting metastatic tumors or primary neoplasms in order to carry out liver cryosurgery and to observe and control ice ball formation in the liver during the freeze-thaw cycle on the liver (cryosurgery monitoring). View of the device for intraoperative ultrasound (**A**) with display (**B**)

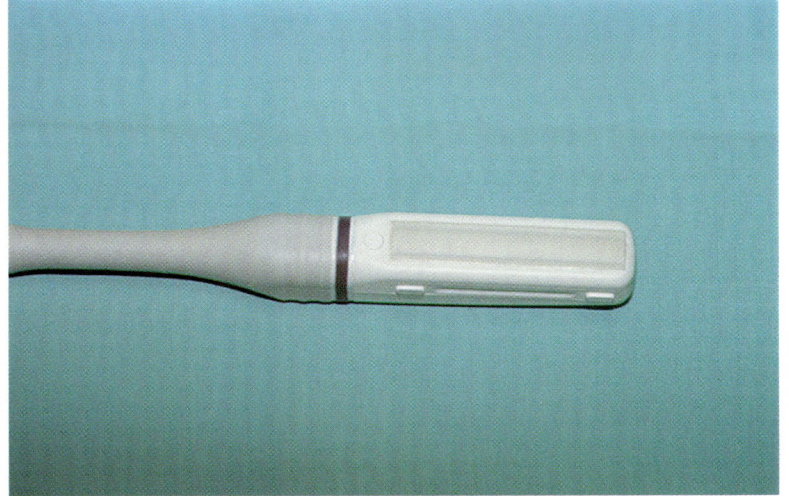
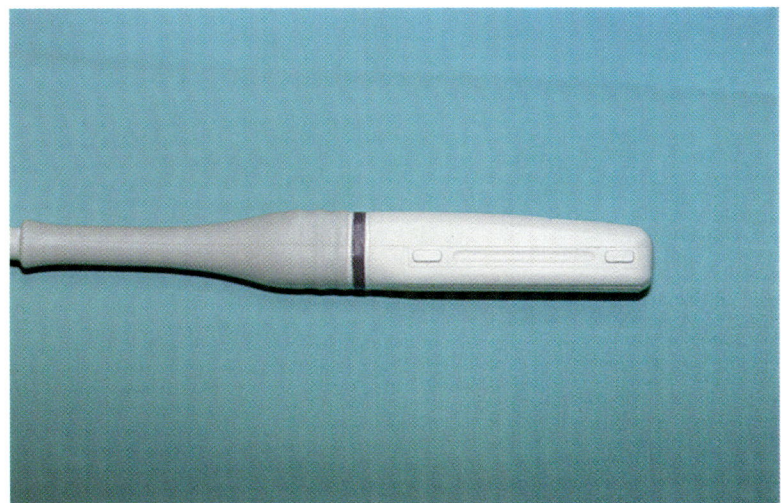

Fig. 12.2.11[1] A, B. The standard intraoperative transducers for liver cryosurgery monitoring

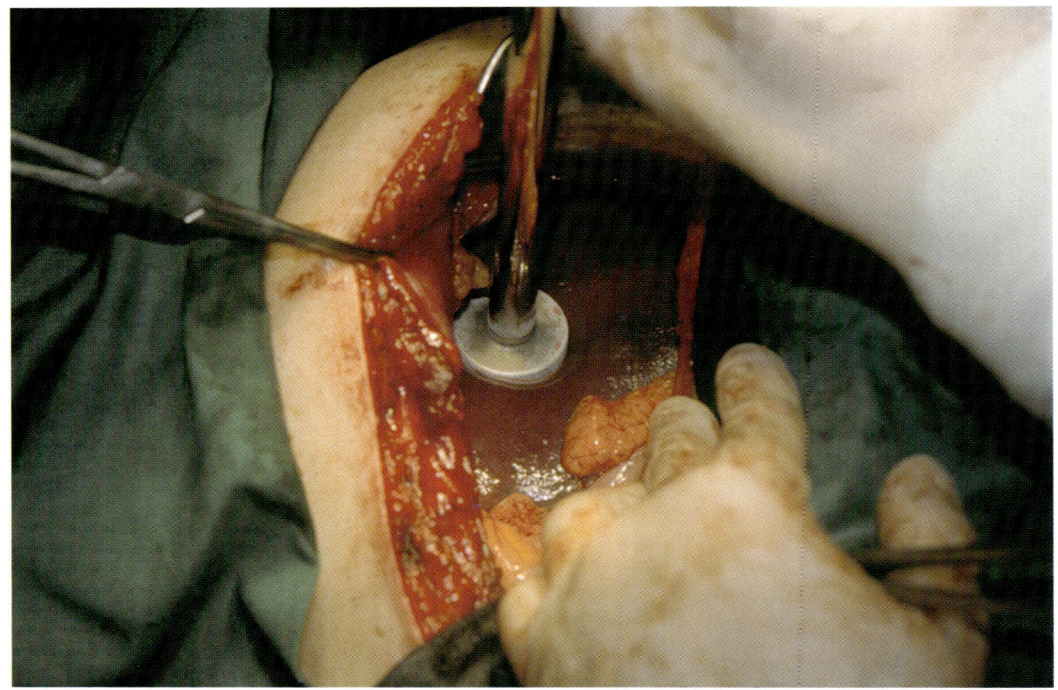

A

Fig. 12.2.12[1] A, B. Open liver cryosurgical technique. Cryoprobes of varying diameters, for example, of 20 mm (**A**) and 55 mm (**B**), are placed on the liver tumor mass at a temperature of −180°C for 9 min

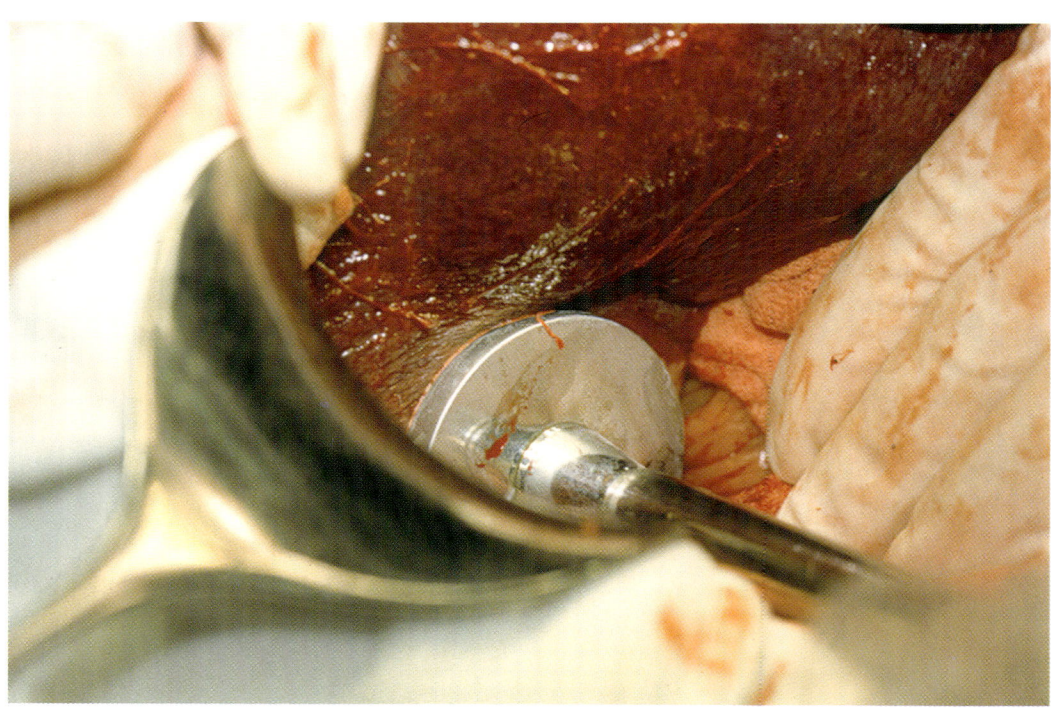

B

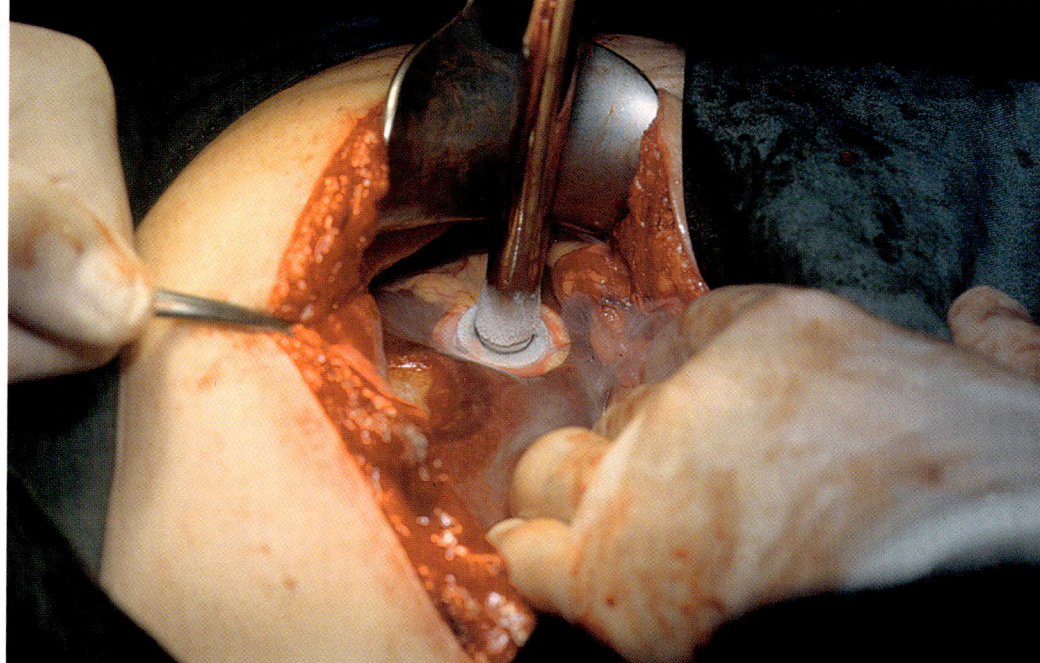

Fig. 12.2.13[1] A–D. Liver cryosurgery. A single freeze-thaw cycle to induce aseptic liver tumor cryonecrosis in segment IV (**A**), V (**B**), IV/V (**C**), and VI (**D**) in a patient with multiple liver metastases

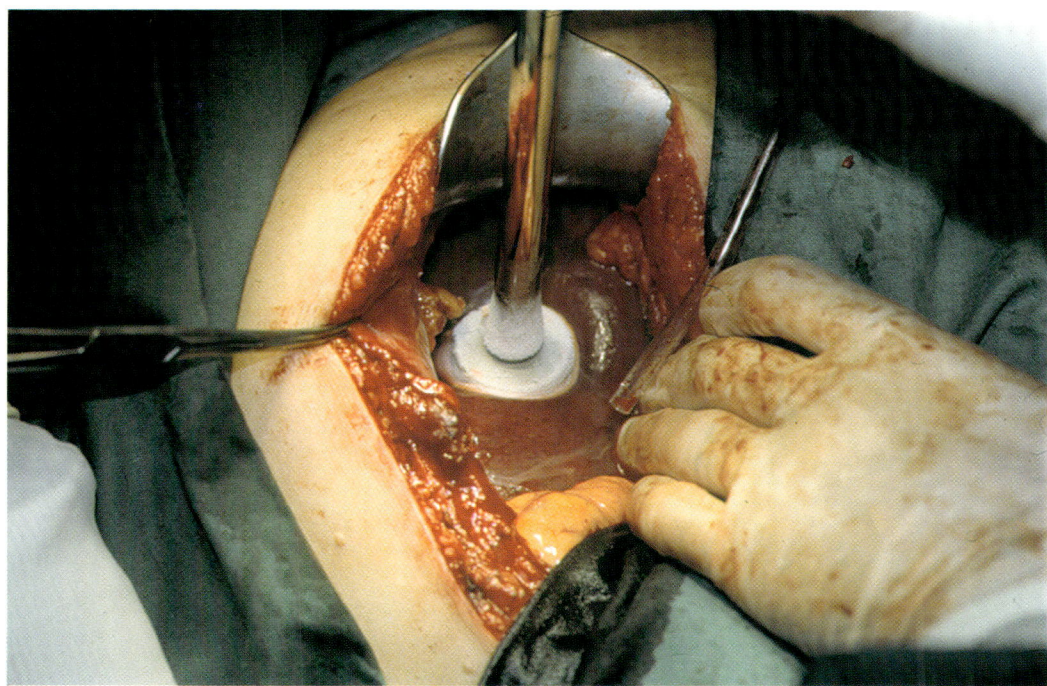

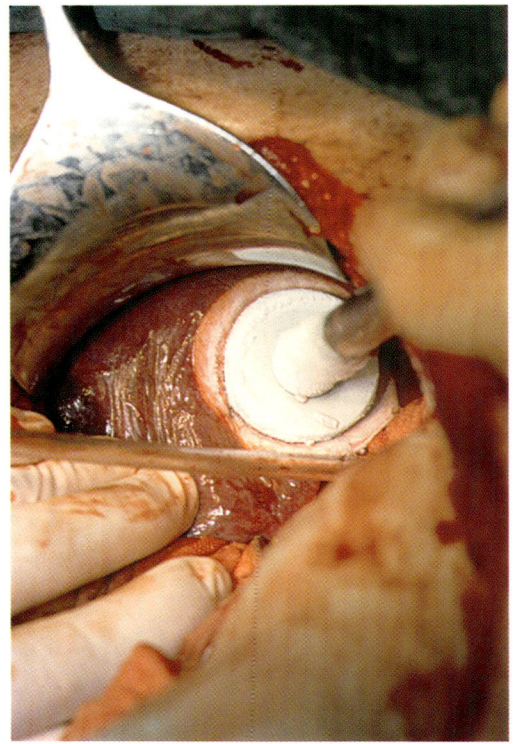

C

Fig. 12.2.13[1] A–D. Liver cryosurgery. A single freeze-thaw cycle to induce aseptic liver tumor cryonecrosis in segment IV (A), V (B), IV/V (C), and VI (D) in a patient with multiple liver metastases

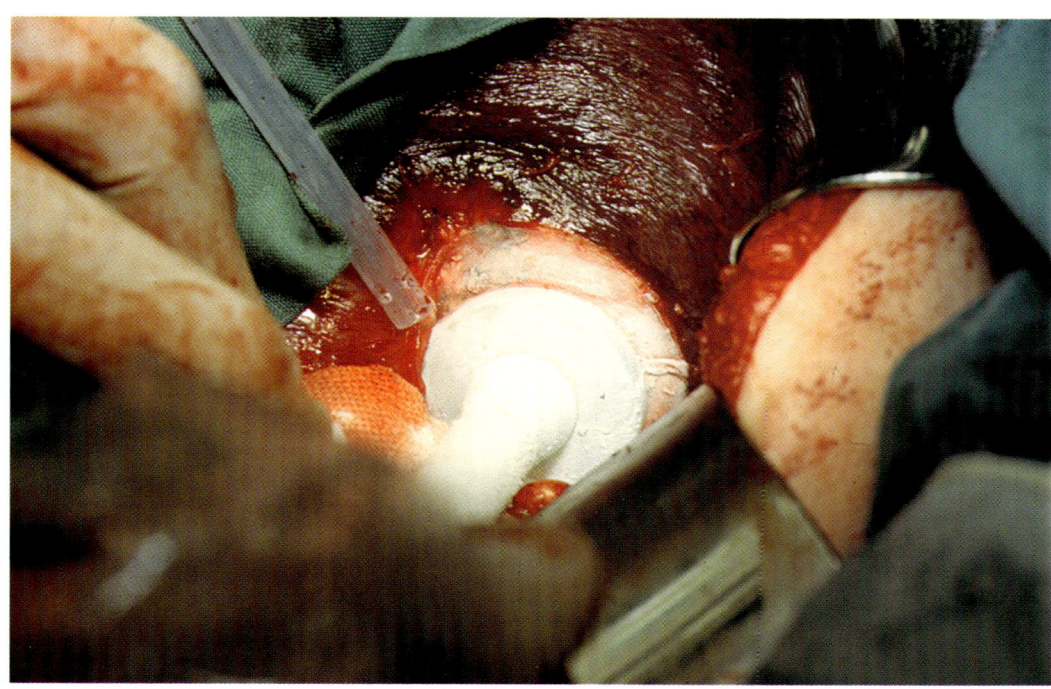

D

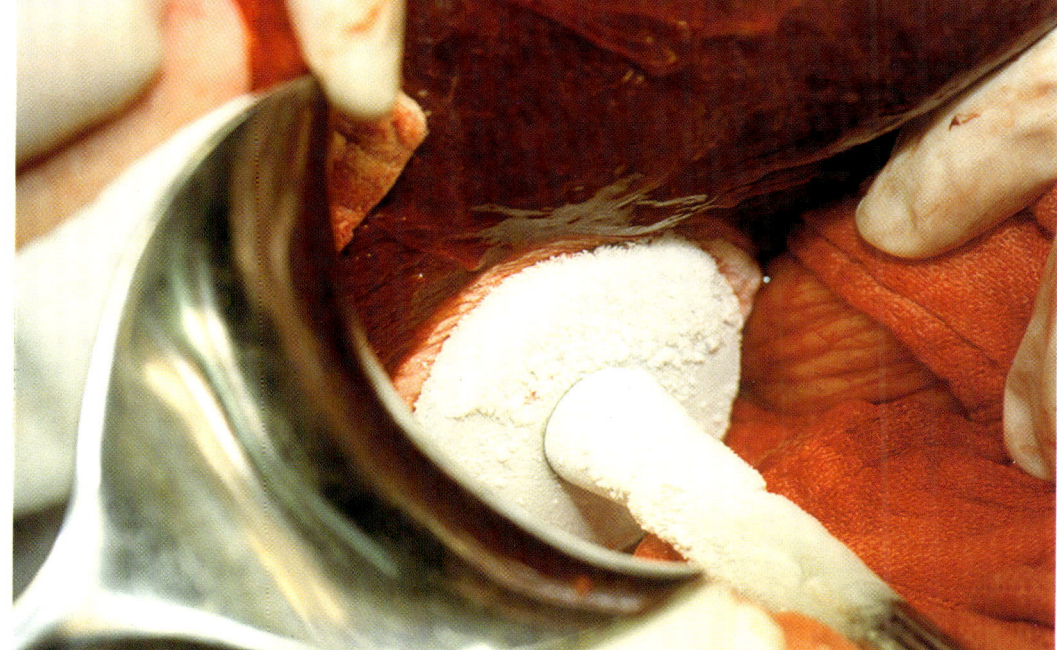

Fig. 12.2.14¹ A, B. The technique of liver cryosurgery, showing a disc probe and the cryosurgical rim of the cryozone, which forms the demarcation line between cryonecrosis and the healthy liver parenchyma (**A**). During a single freeze-thaw cycle at a freeze temperature of −180°C lasting 9 min, a 12 mm margin forms between the cryozone and the normal-appearing liver parenchyma

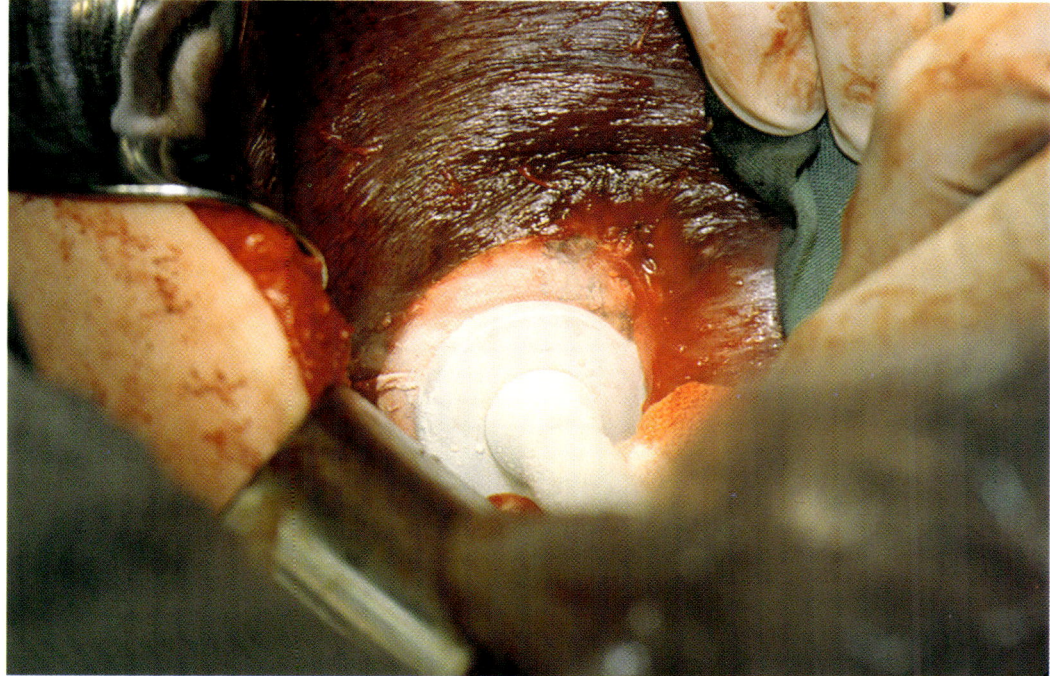

Chapter 12
Abdominal
Cryosurgery:
Hepatic
Cryosurgery

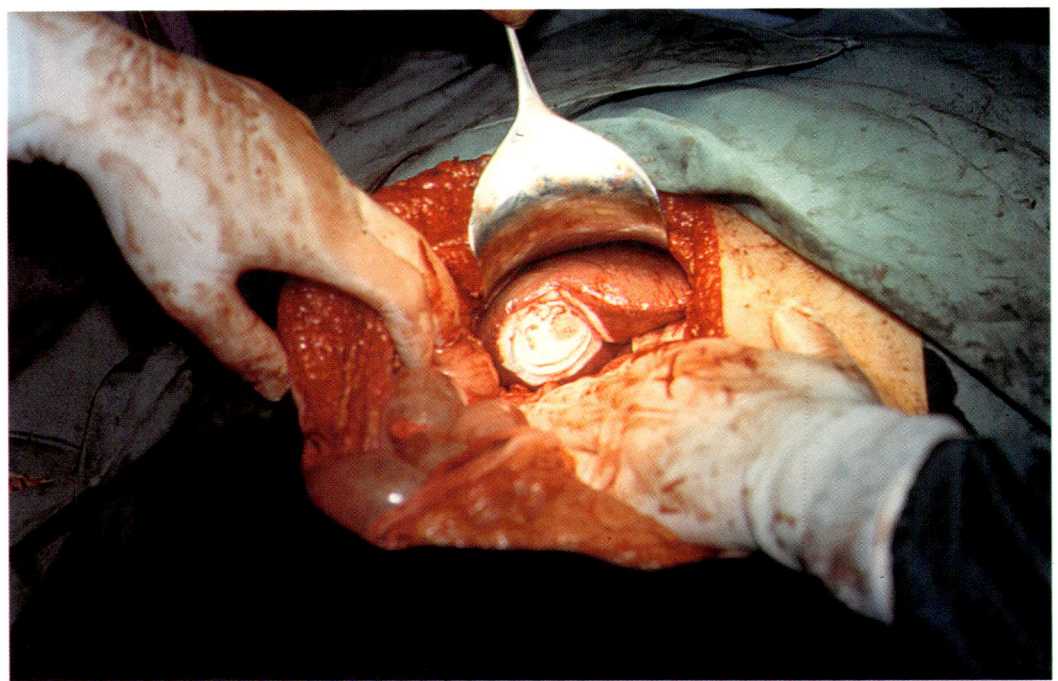

Fig. 12.2.15[1] A, B. Liver cryosurgery. The post-cryosurgical zone formed and its demarcation are clearly visible. With a 20 mm cryoprobe (**A**), a 9 mm margin, and with a 55 mm cryoprobe (**B**) a 12 mm margin are created between the cryozone and the healthy liver parenchyma

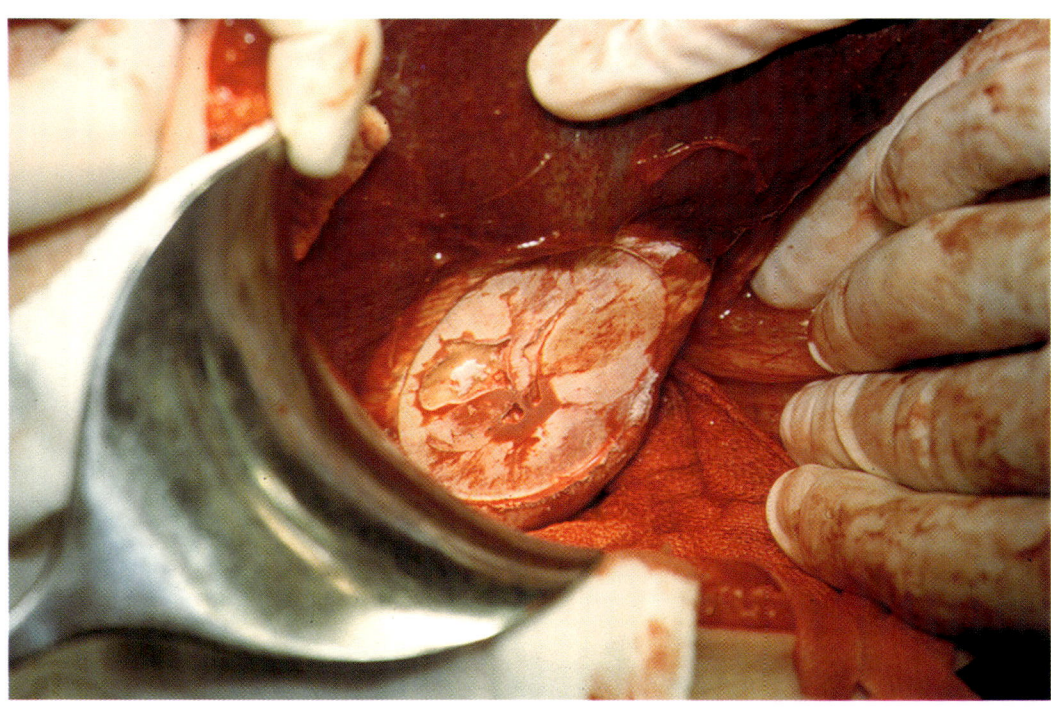

Chapter 12
Abdominal
Cryosurgery:
Hepatic
Cryosurgery

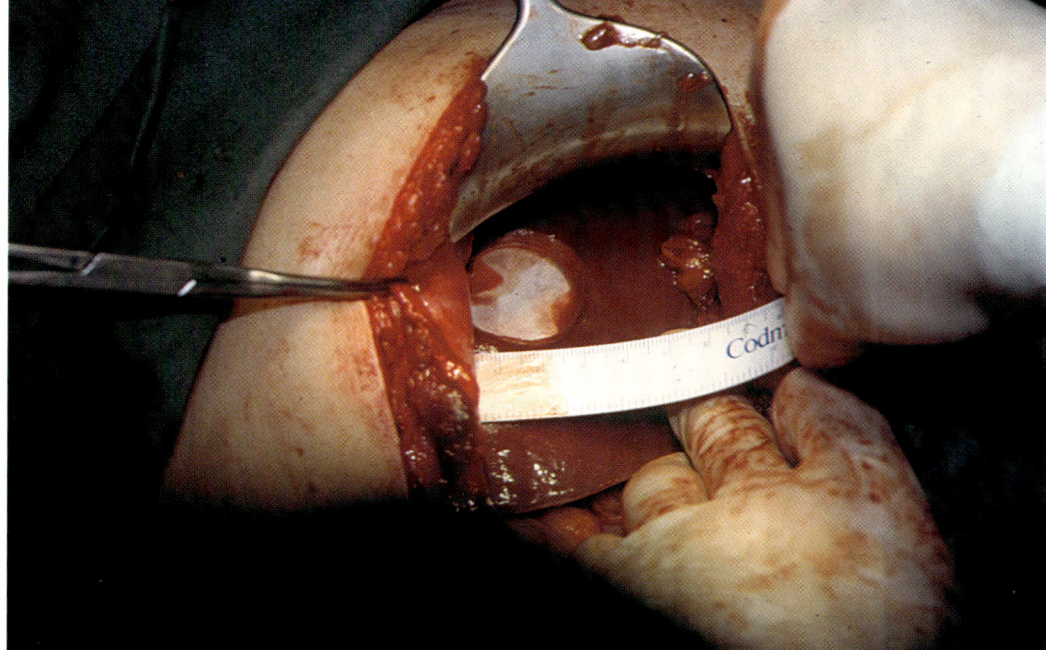

A

Fig. 12.2.16[1] A, B. Liver cryosurgery. Post-cryosurgical view of a cryozone with the ice crater in the middle, and of the ice margin with the line of demarcation, immediately after a single cryosurgical session. After a single freeze-thaw cycle at a temperature of −180°C applied for 9 min, the cryozone measures 38 mm in diameter when the disc probe has a diameter of 20 mm (**A**). When the disc probe has a diameter of 55 mm the cryozone measures 67 mm in diameter (**B**)

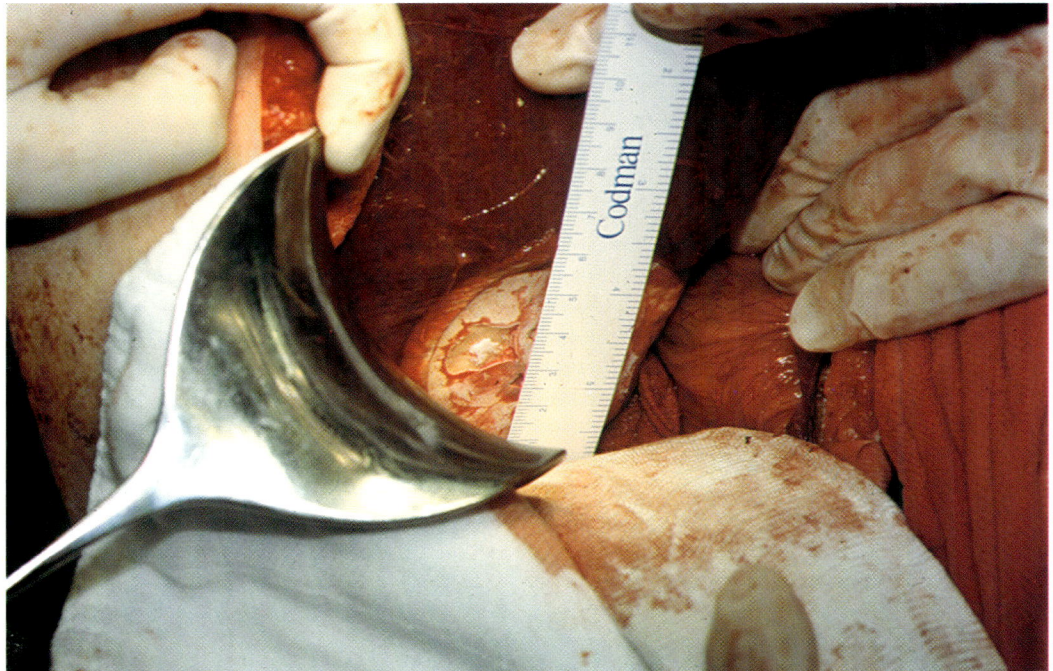

B

Chapter 12
Abdominal
Cryosurgery:
Hepatic
Cryosurgery

A

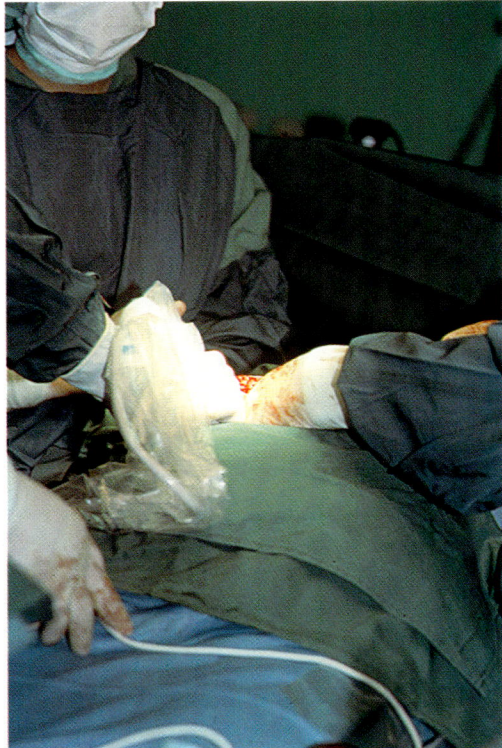

B

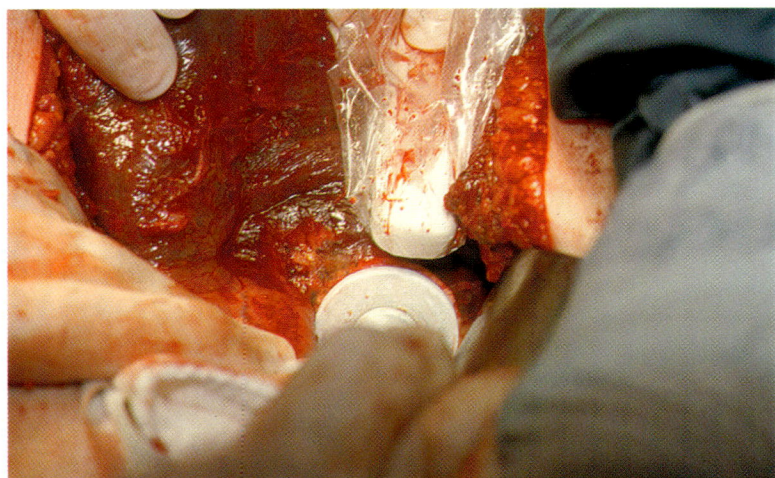

Fig. 12.2.17[1] A–C. Intraoperative ultrasound monitoring of hepatic cryosurgery: before (**A**), during (**B**), and after (**C**) liver cryosurgery

C

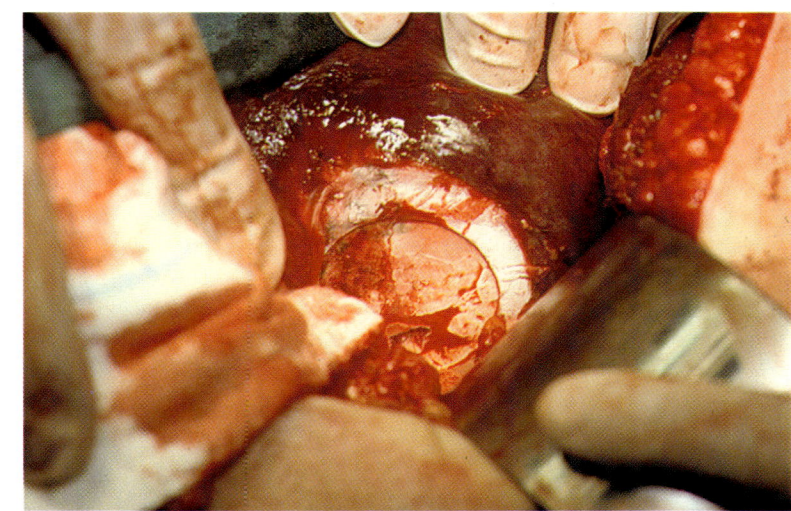

Section F   Clinical Aspects   **257**

Chapter 12
Abdominal
Cryosurgery:
Hepatic
Cryosurgery

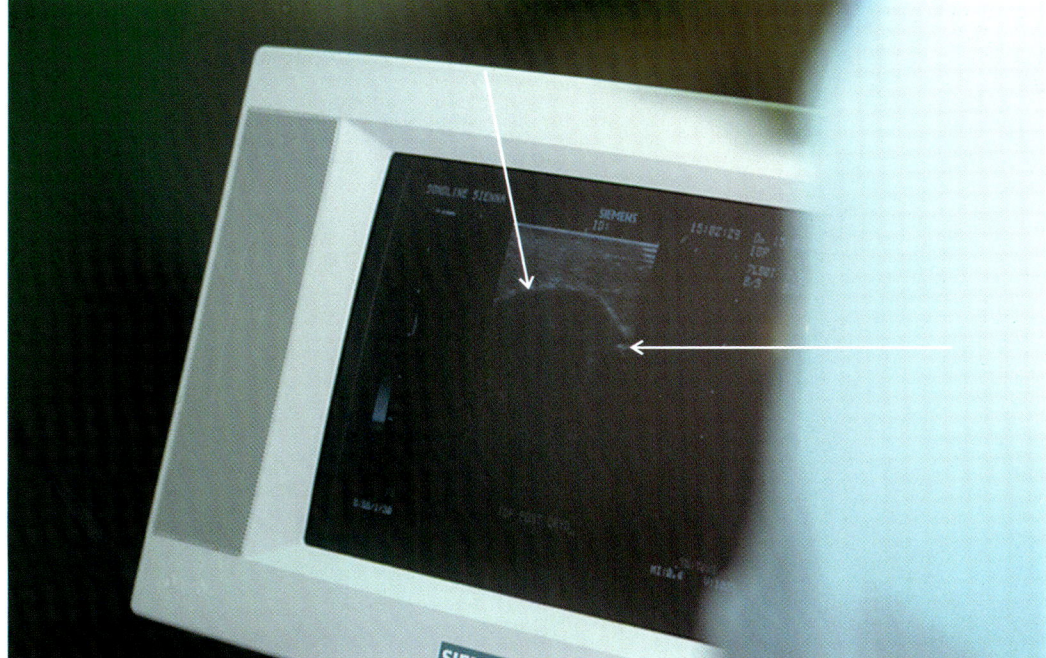

A

Fig. 12.2.18[1] **A, B.** Intraoperative ultrasound monitoring of hepatic cryosurgery. The ice balls are characterized by bright, echogenic interfaces of ice formation, which correlates with complete tissue destruction. At a temperature of $-180\,°C$ at the end of a 9 min single freeze-thaw cycle the ice ball measures 38 mm in diameter when a disc probe with a diameter of 20 mm is used (**A**), and with a disc probe 55 mm in diameter the ice ball measures 67 mm in diameter (**B**)

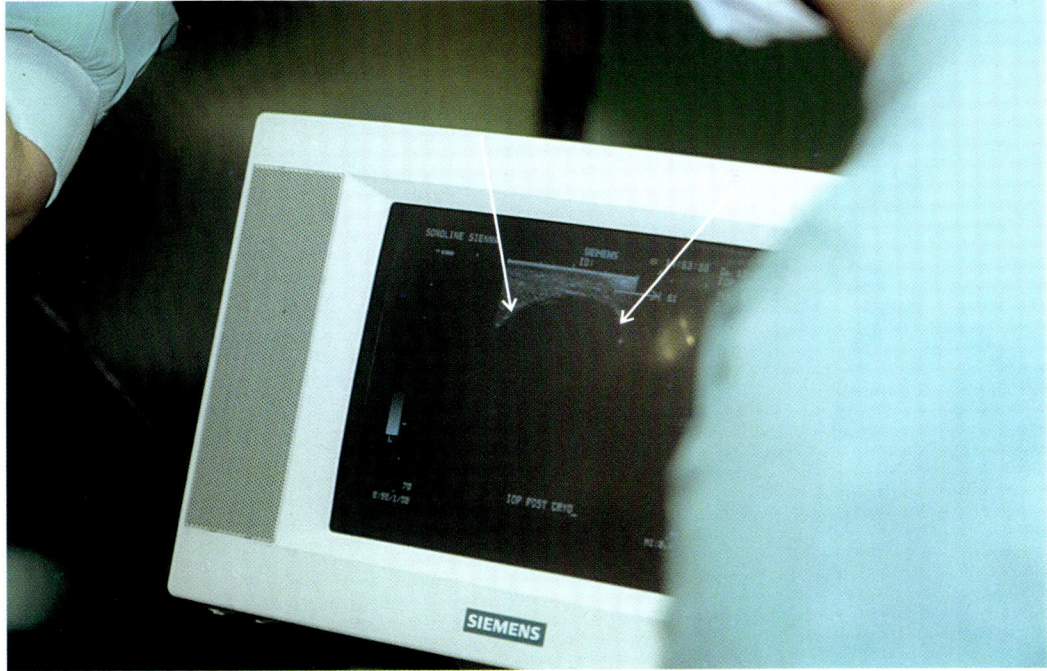

B

Chapter 12
Abdominal Cryosurgery: Hepatic Cryosurgery

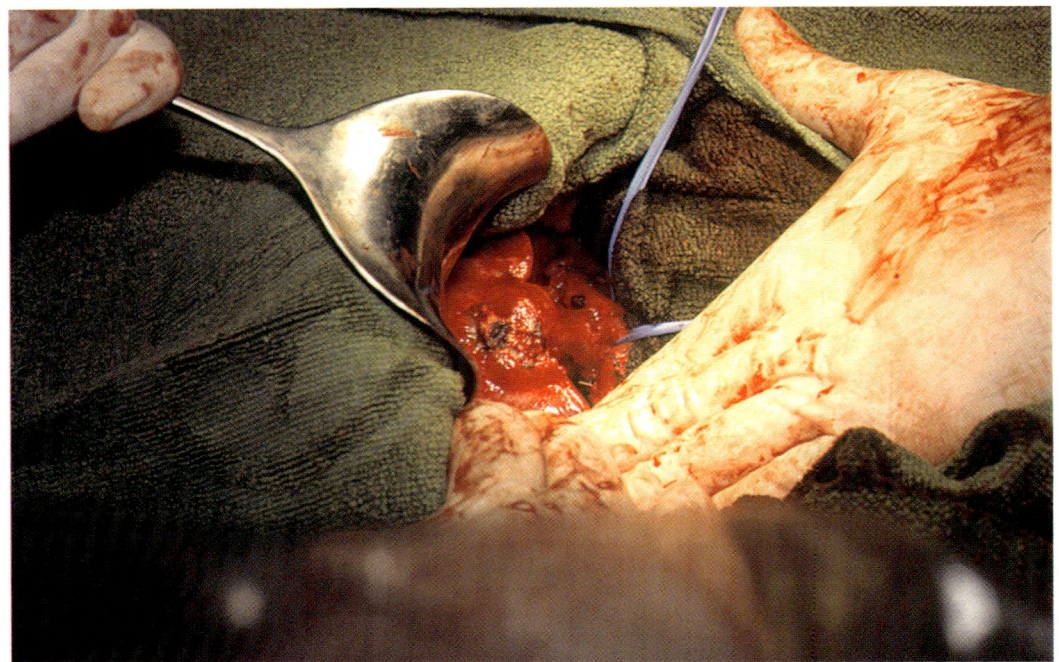

A

Fig. 12.2.19[1] A, B. Arterial Port-A-Cath system (Arterial Titanium System) placement. After liver cryosurgery and elective cholecystectomy elimination to avert the problem of chemical cholecystitis in the postoperative period, an arterial catheter (arterial systems only) can be placed in an artery using the standard surgical technique to deliver regional intrahepatic chemotherapy to a tumor or metastases in the liver. One of the most common arteries for catheter placement is the gastroduodenal artery for perfusion of the liver. After the hepatic artery (a. hepatica communis) has been prepared, the gastroduodenal artery and all the other branches are carefully identified and ligated to prevent extrahepatic distribution of drugs (**A**). The catheter is inserted surgically into the gastroduodenal artery for hepatic artery infusion. A close-up view of the catheter position is shown intraoperatively (**B**)

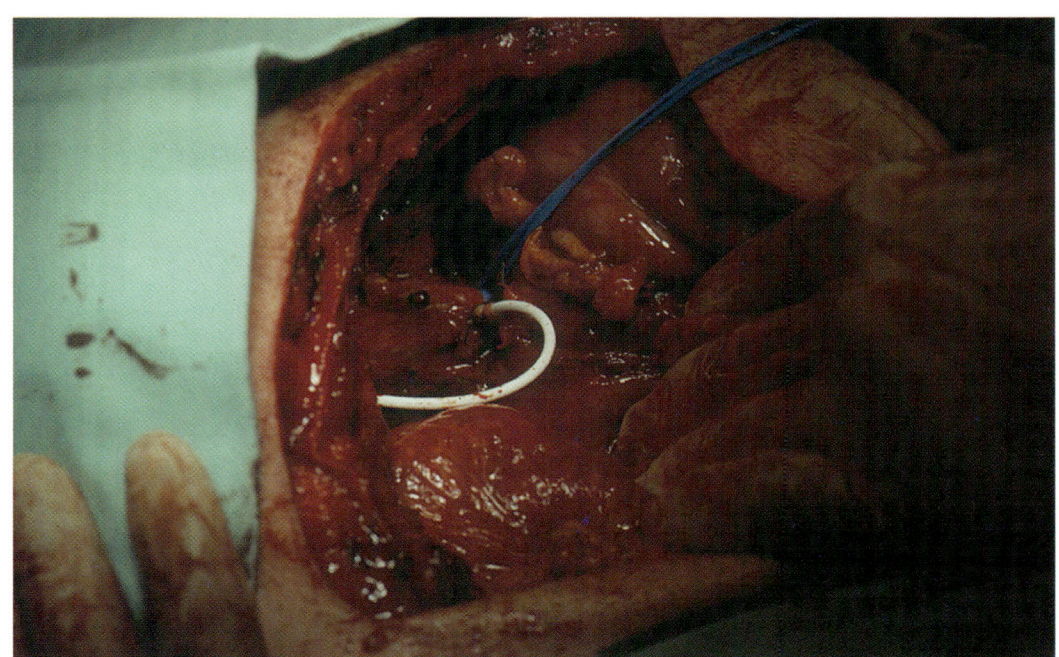

B

Section F Clinical Aspects 259

Chapter 12
Abdominal
Cryosurgery:
Hepatic
Cryosurgery

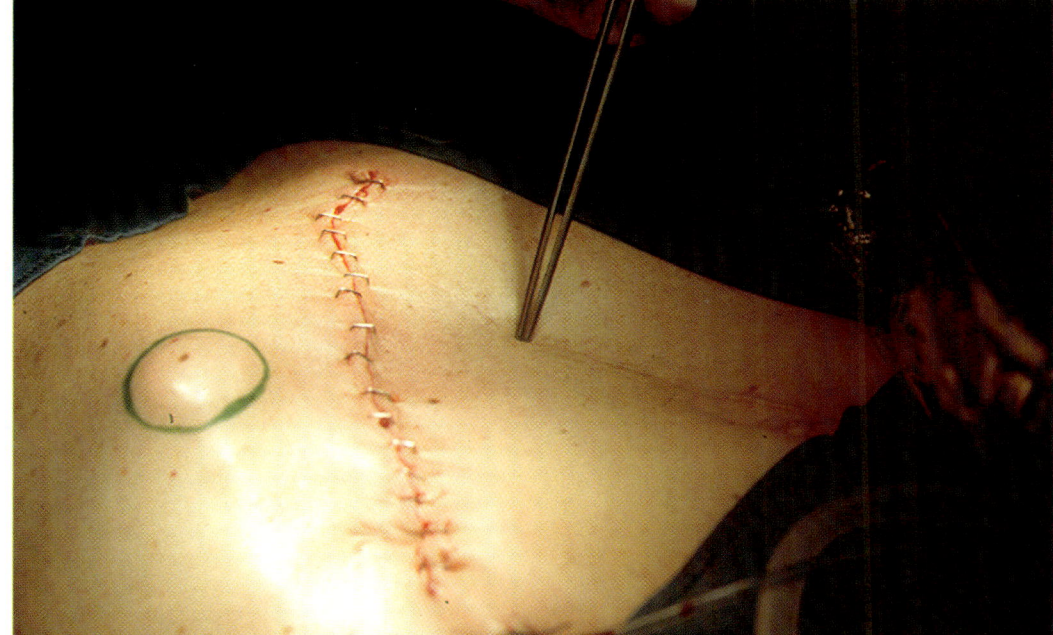

A

Fig. 12.2.20[1] **A, B.** Arterial Port-A-Cath system (Arterial Titanium System) placement. Postoperative view immediately after the operation. The port is positioned in the right lower quadrant of the abdomen. A horizontal port position is marked on the skin (**A**). Confirmation by X-ray that the distal tip of the catheter is positioned at the desired site (**B**)

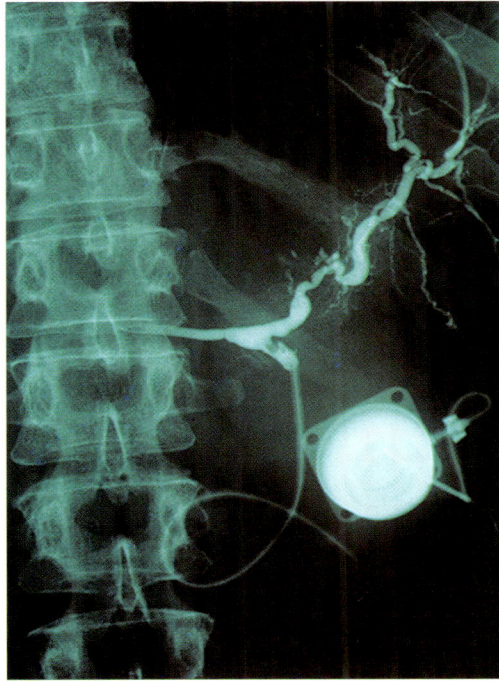

B

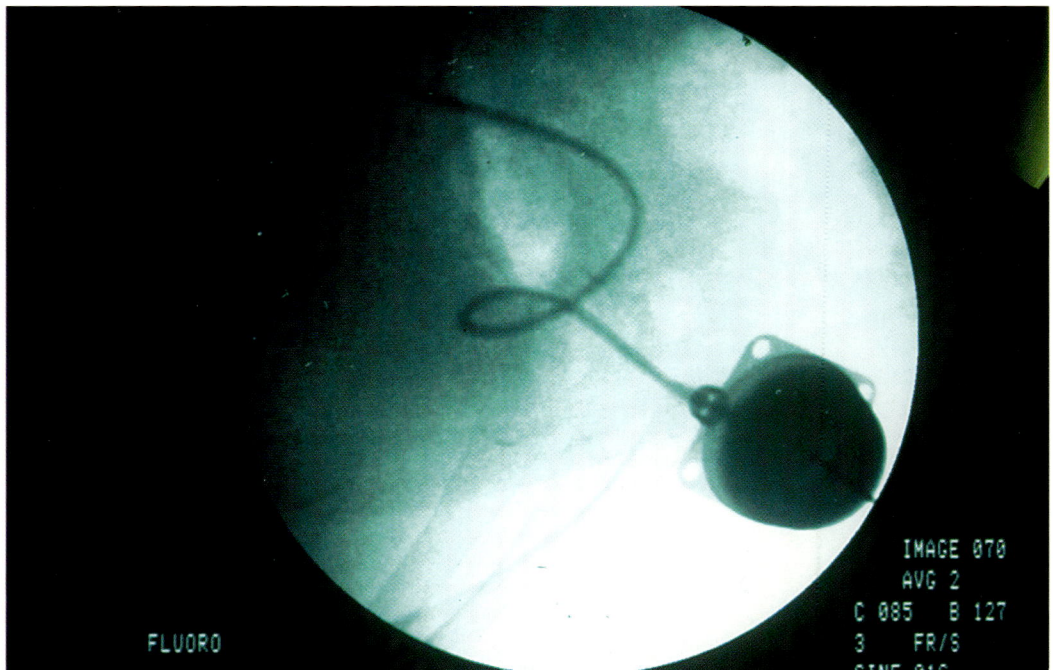

Fig. 12.2.21[1] A, B. Arterial Port-A-Cath system (Arterial Titanium System) placement. Control by X-ray 1 (**A**) and 2 (**B**) years after catheter placement in the gastroduodenal artery for perfusion of the liver. An X-ray is recommended to determine whether there are problems with the system, for example, catheter embolization or drug extravazation

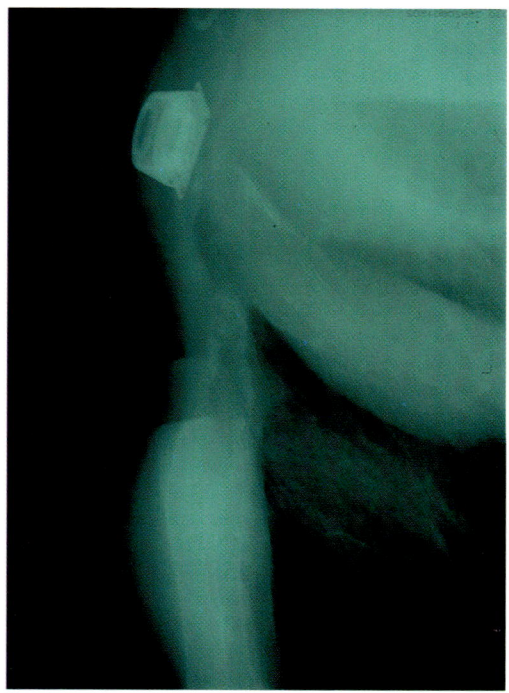

Section F Clinical Aspects

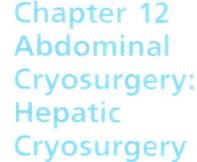
Chapter 12
Abdominal
Cryosurgery:
Hepatic
Cryosurgery

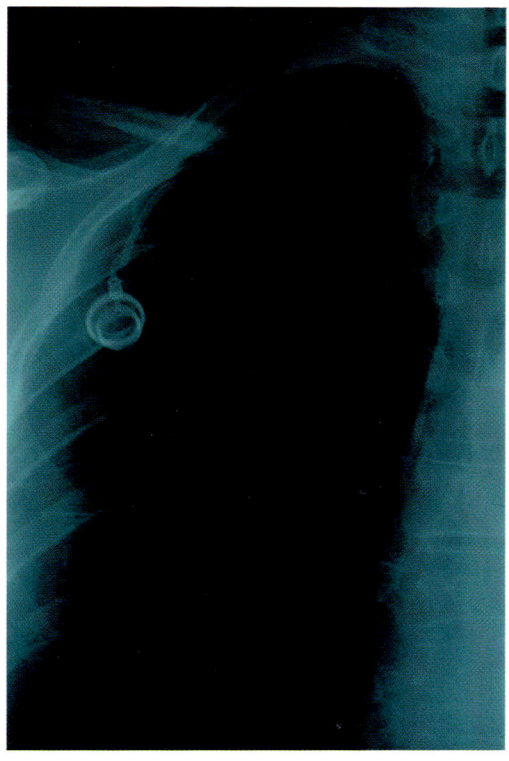
A

Fig. 12.2.22[1] A, B. Venous Port-A-Cath system (Vascular Access Systems) placement. Port-A-Cath venous implantable access system is designed to permit repeated access to the vascular system for the parenteral delivery of medications (systemic chemotherapy) in the treatment of hepatic metastases. The port is implanted subcutaneously against the chest wall just superficial to the pectoralis fascia and pectoralis major muscle, in an infraclavicular position, in standard technique. A postoperative X-ray control of subcutaneous placement of a venous Port-A-Cath system in patients with multiple liver metastases after hepatic cryosurgery: subcutaneous insertion of the catheter via the subclavian vein (**A**) and position of the catheter tip at the lower end of the superior vena cava just above the right atrium (**B**)

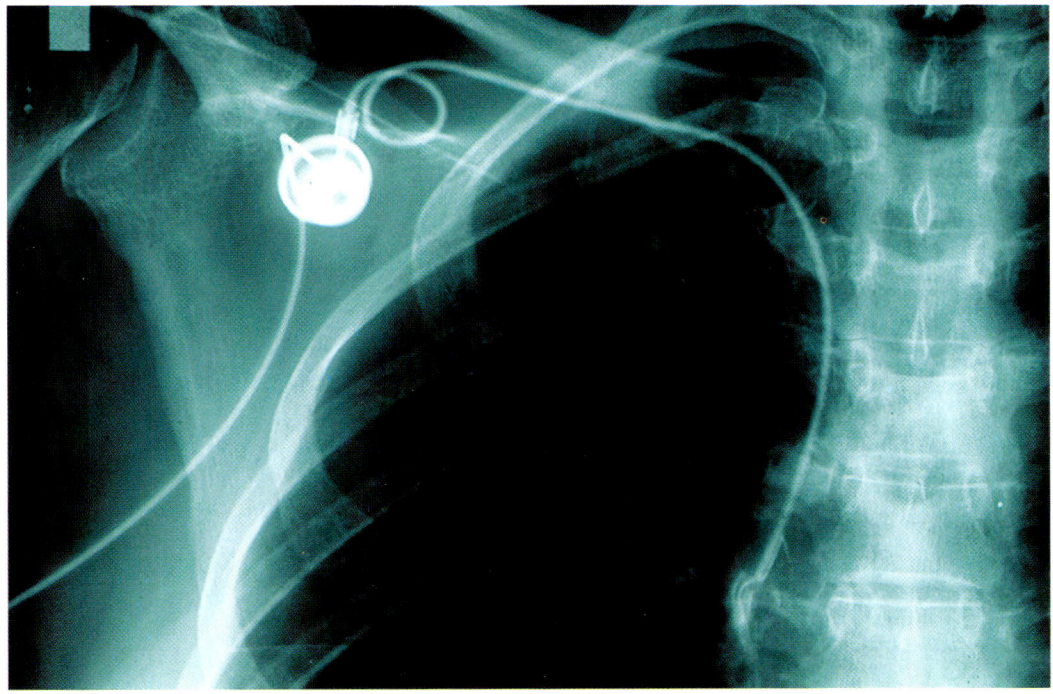
B

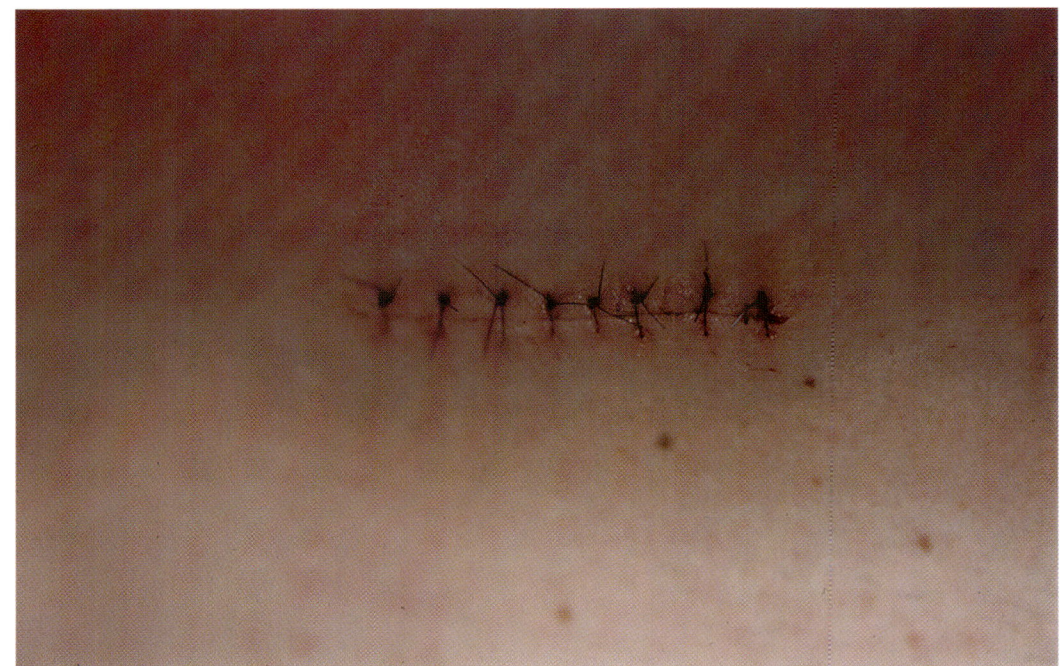

Fig. 12.2.23[1] A, B. Arterial Port-A-Cath system placement. If the arterial or venous Port-A-Cath system is no longer used or needs to be revised intraoperatively, a port can be removed or changed using standard technique. Postoperative view: wound healing on the first (**A**) and seventh (**B**) days

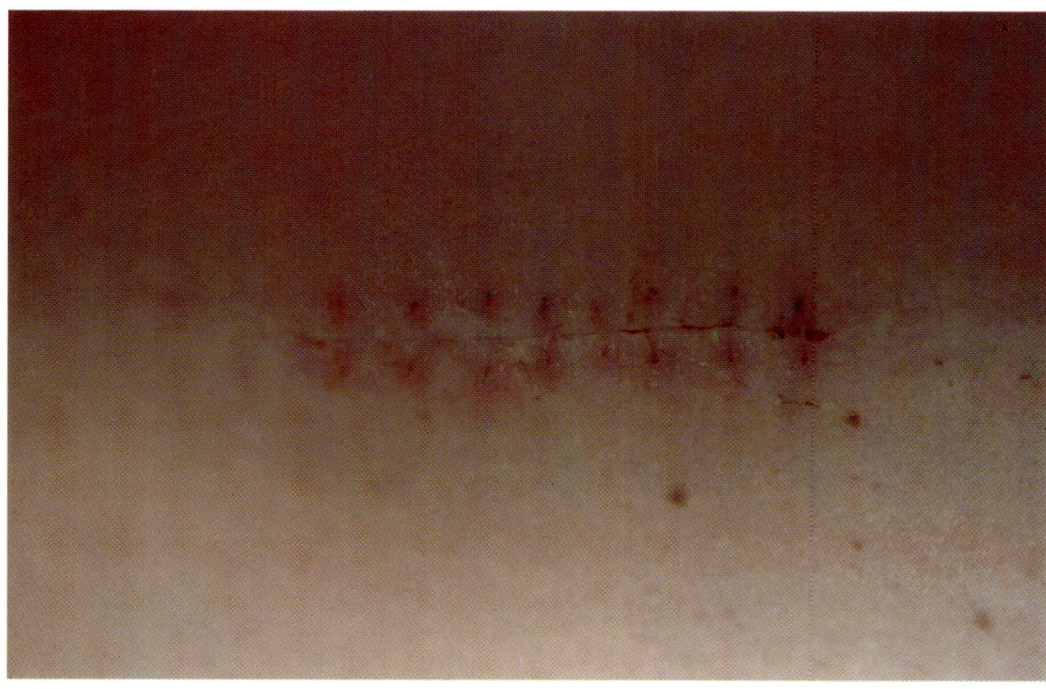

Section F Clinical Aspects **263**

**Chapter 12
Abdominal
Cryosurgery:
Hepatic
Cryosurgery**

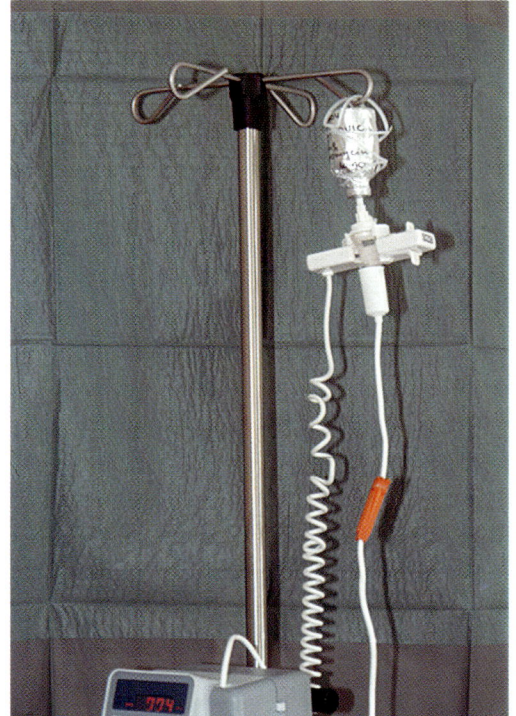

A

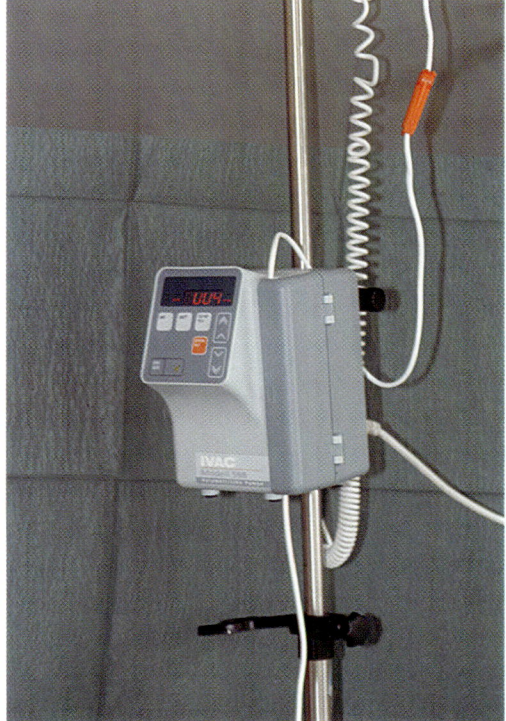

B

Fig. 12.2.24[1] **A, B, C.** Arterial Port-A-Cath system. Repeated regional hepatic artery chemotherapy: the liver with multiple large metastases is perfused by way of a catheter positioned in the gastroduodenal artery two weeks after hepatic cryosurgery. View of the delivery system for chemotherapy (**A**), a volumetric pump (**B**), and the Port-A-Cath Needle (Gripper) positioned into the port (**C**)

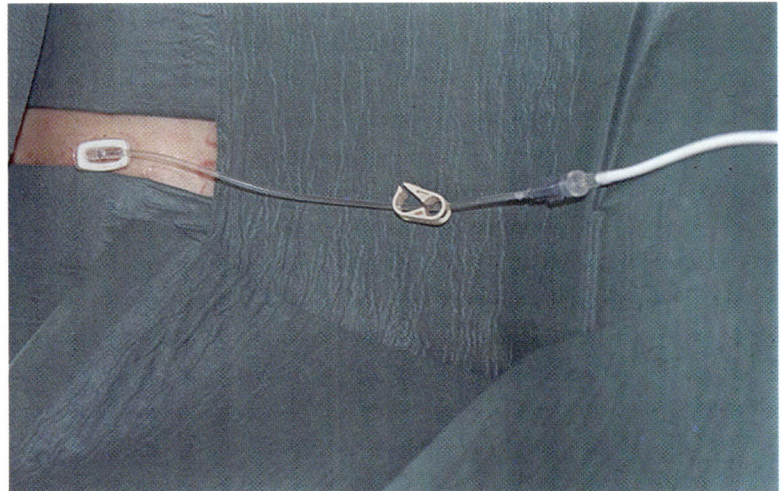

C

Chapter 12
Abdominal Cryosurgery: Hepatic Cryosurgery

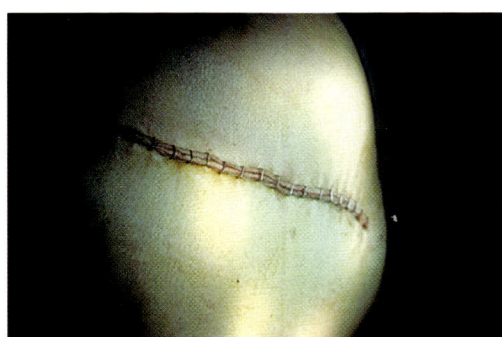

A

Fig. 12.2.25[1] A, B. After hepatic cryosurgery the abdomen is usually closed without drain (**A**) or seldom with a drain (**B**)

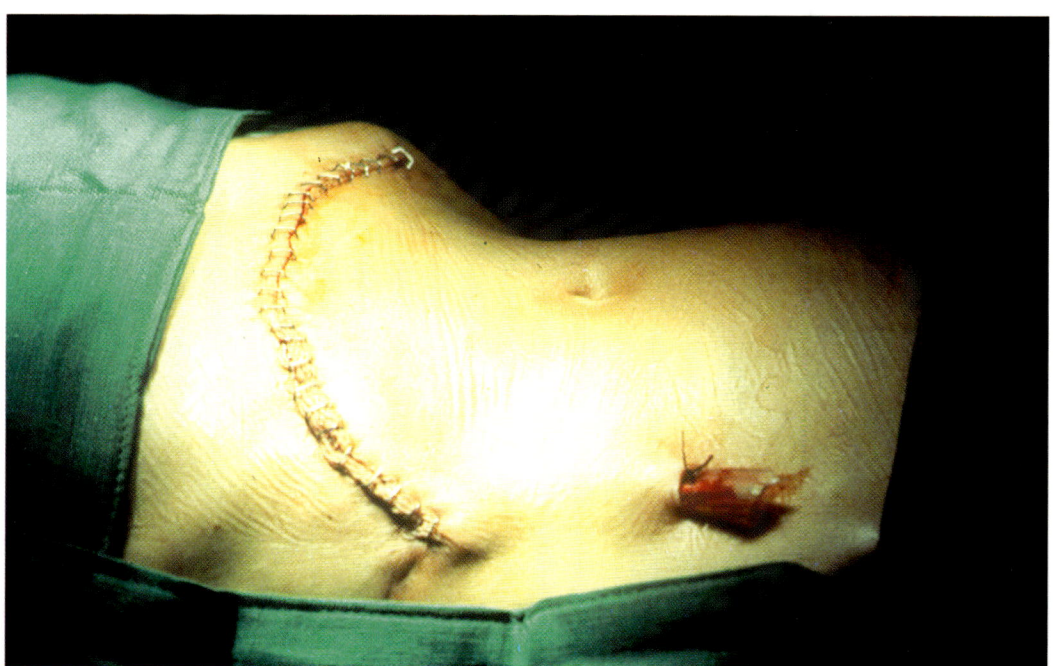

B

Section F Clinical Aspects 265

Chapter 12
Abdominal
Cryosurgery:
Hepatic
Cryosurgery

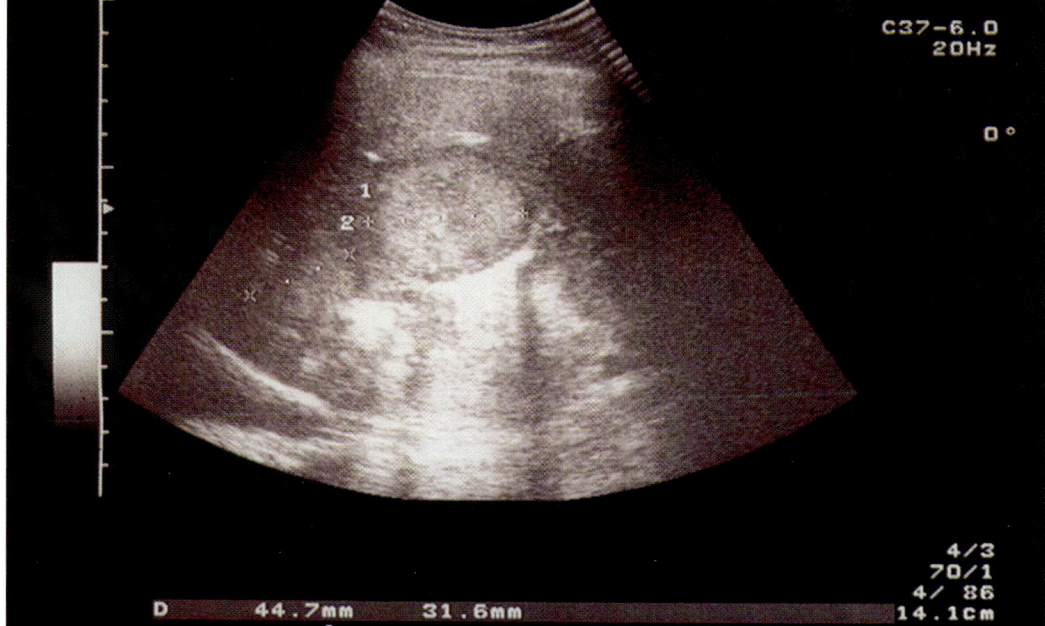

A

Fig. 12.2.26[1] A, B. Typical postoperative post-cryosurgical appearance of the liver one week after hepatic cryosurgery. A The sagittal view from the linear array probe (abdomen ultrasound) shows the area of hypoechoic liver tissue (segment IV/V), measuring 44 mm, and defines the borders of the treated liver metastasis with a thin rim of hypoechoic tissue. B A spiral CT scan shows a well-defined post-cryosurgical tumor area in the liver (arrow), and demonstrates an avascular cryolesion in the same patient

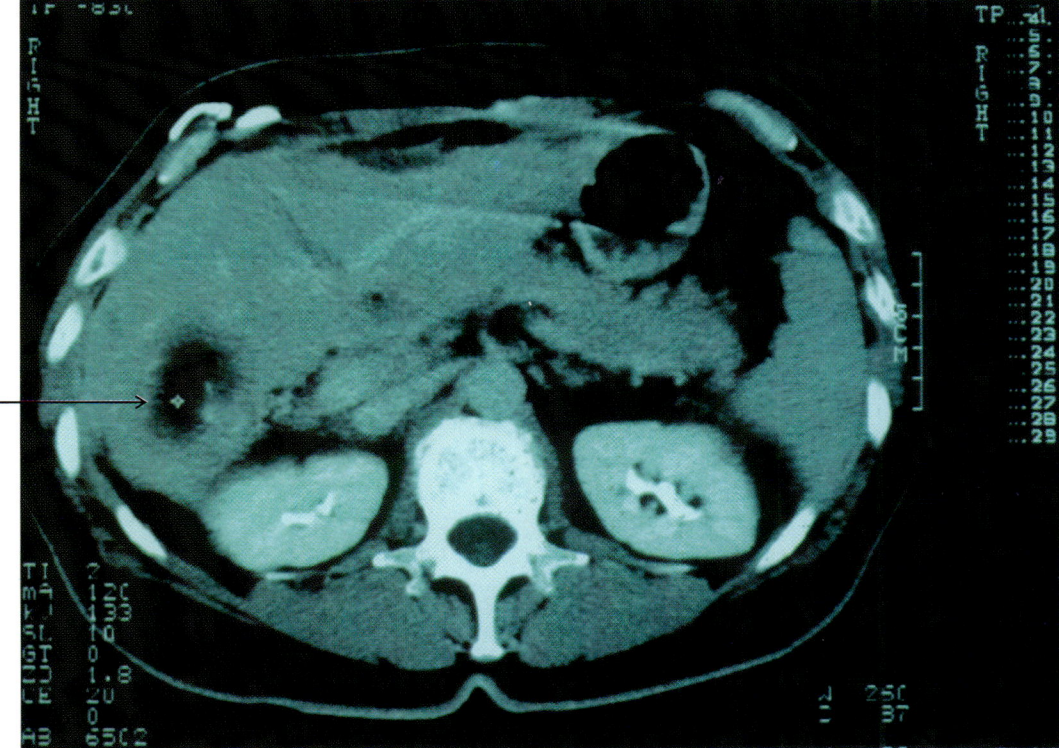

B

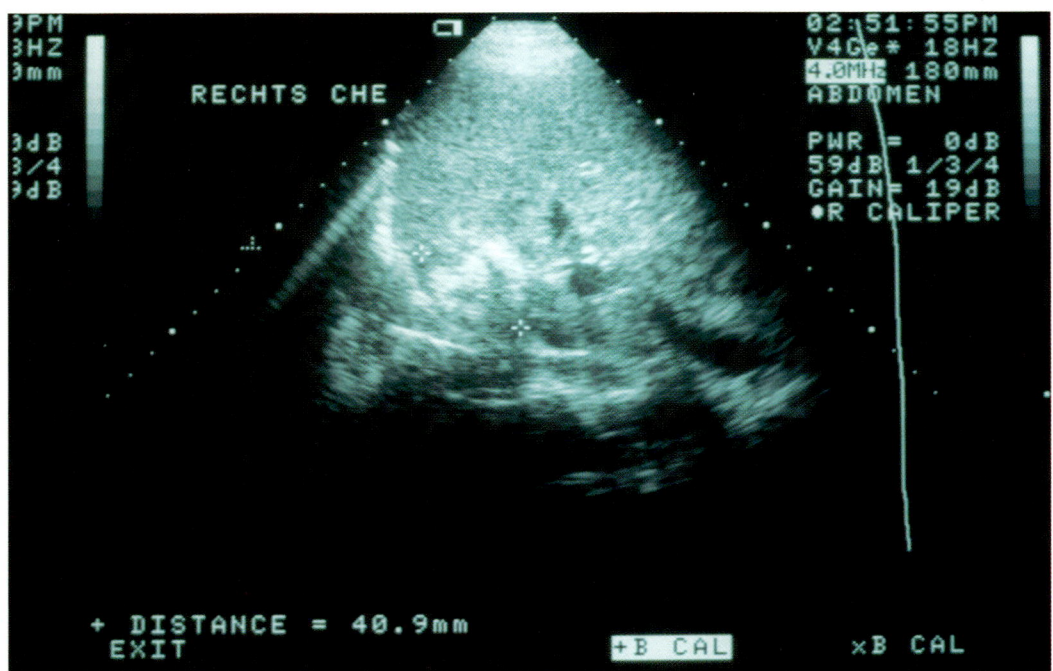

Fig. 12.2.27[1] A, B. The same patient. Typical postoperative post-cryosurgical findings three months after hepatic cryosurgery. There are residual subcapsular fluid collection and a low density post-cryosurgical zone. Ultrasound (A) and enhanced spiral computed tomography (B) three months after surgery show a decrease in the amount of subcapsular fluid and the post-cryosurgical area measuring 40.9 mm

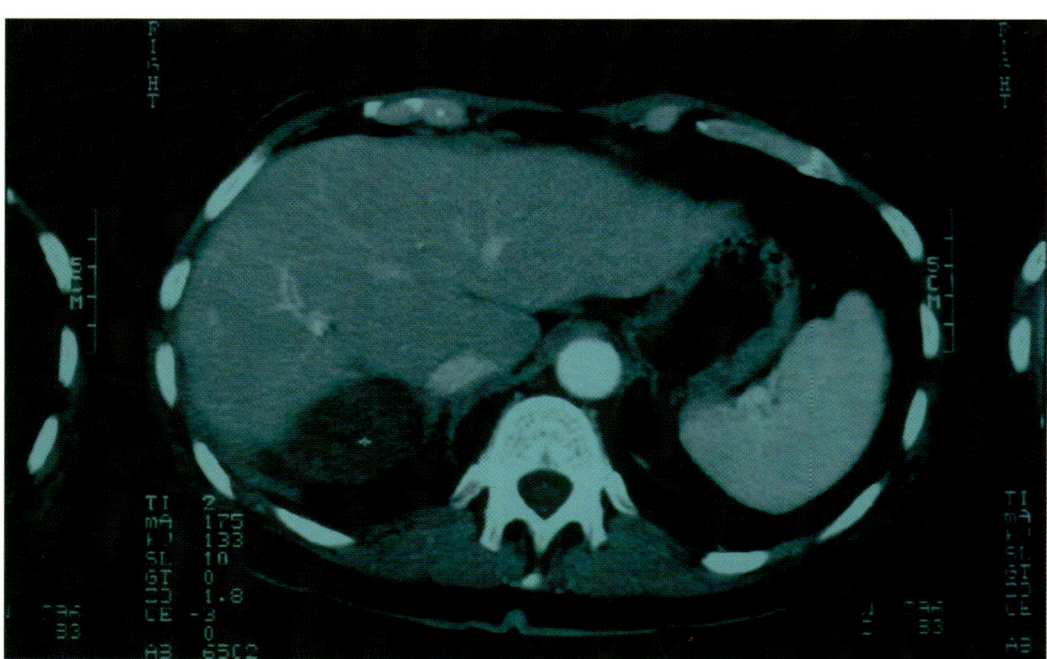

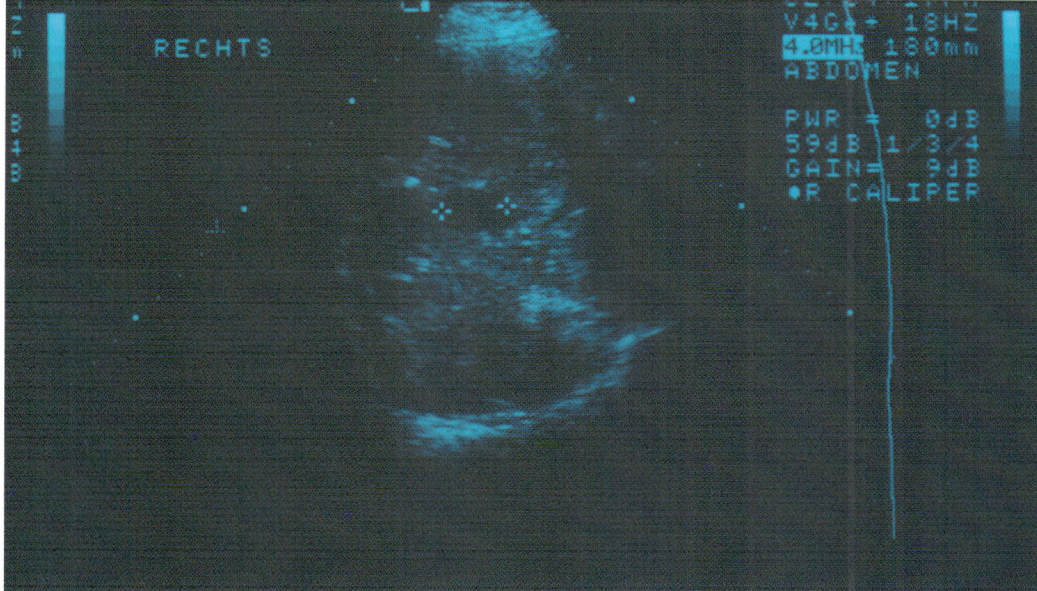

Fig. 12.2.28[1] A, B. Typical postoperative post-cryosurgical view six months after hepatic cryosurgery in the same patient. Ultrasound (A) and abdominal MRI (B) six months after surgery show resorption of the cryolesion and no evidence of a residual tumor. The shrunk post-cryosurgical area with the subcapsular fluid has decreased in size to 21.0 mm

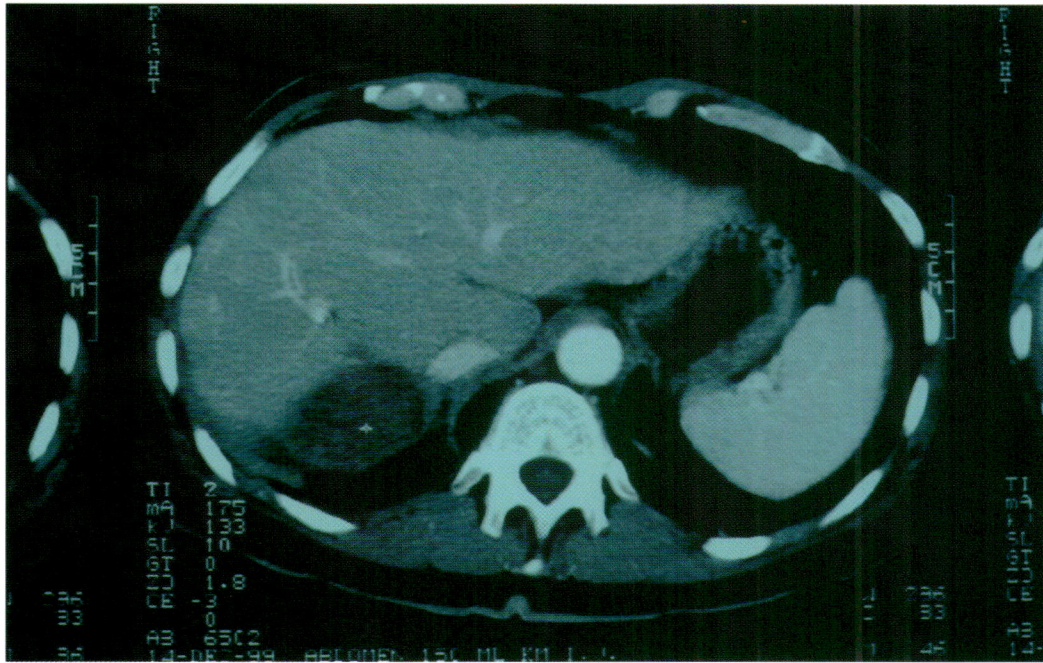

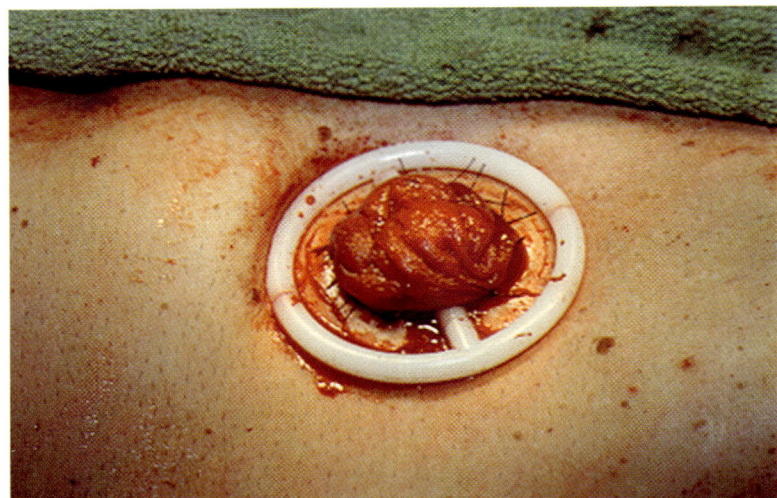

A

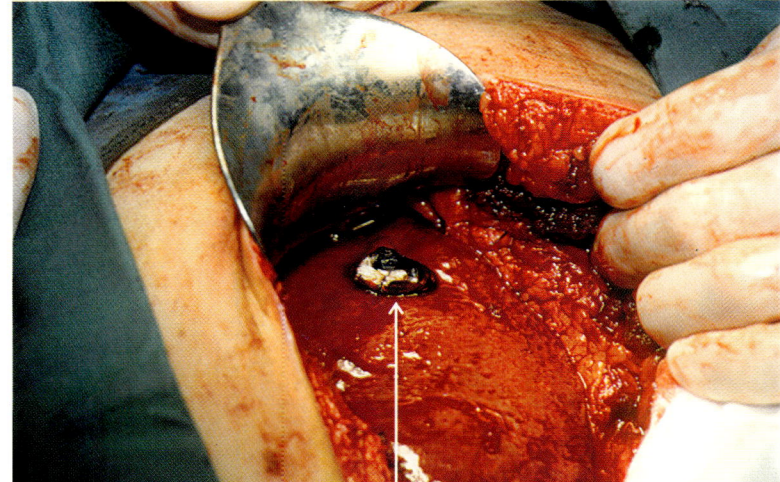

B

Fig. 12.2.29[1] **A–C.** In some patients with multiple liver metastases after hepatic cryosurgery and colon resection, a temporary colostomy (**A**) is created, which is closed 2–3 months later. During the second operation, when the colostomy is closed, the areas of the cryoextirpated liver metastases are inspected and a biopsy taken intraoperatively. After removing the hemostatic plate (**B**), which is usually placed over the cryozone after each cryosurgical operation on the liver in order to prevent hemorrhageing, the post-cryoextirpated liver area, which is free of cancer cells, is visible (**C**)

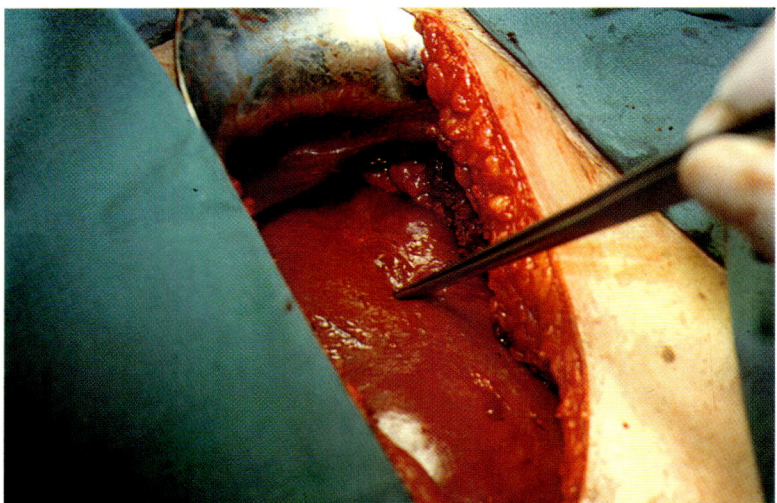

C

12.3 Cryosurgical Avascular Tumor Phenomenon (CAT-Phenomenon)

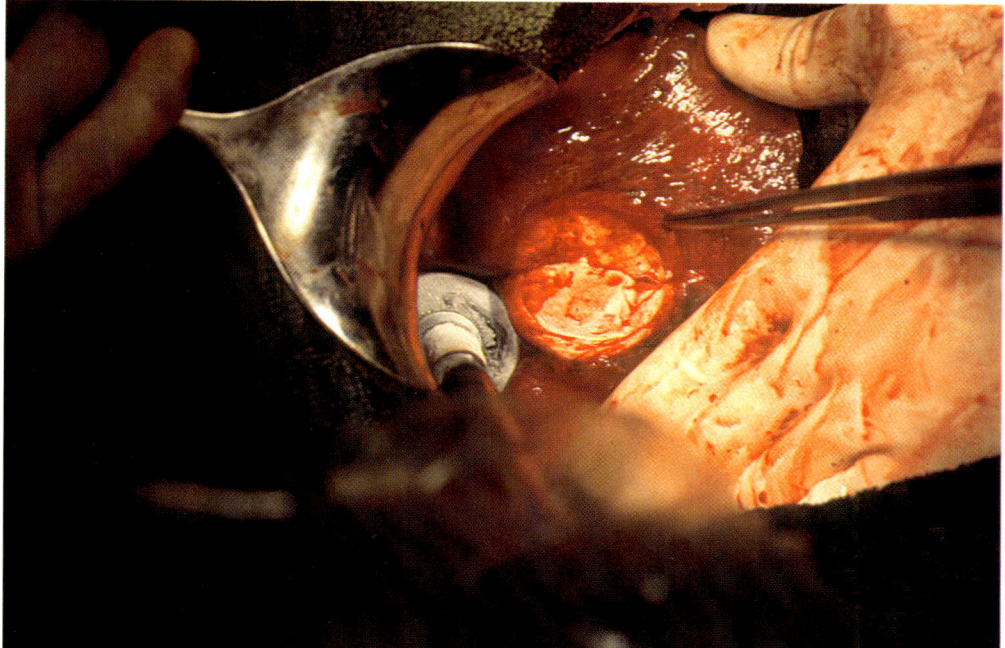

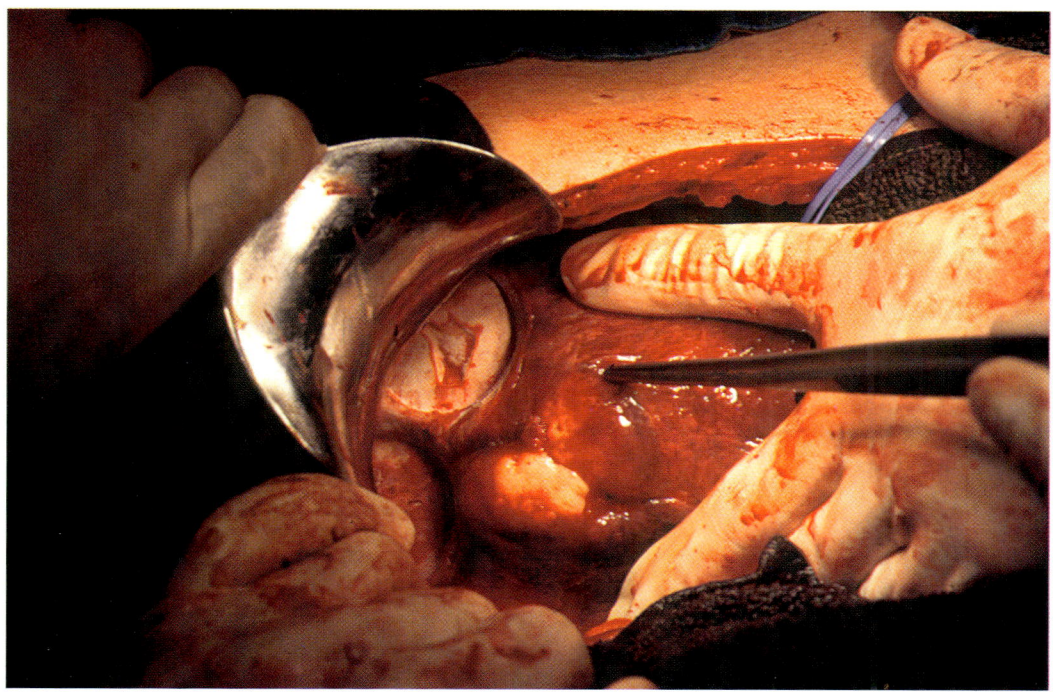

Fig. 12.3.1[1] **A, B.** CAT-Phenomenon. Multiple liver metastases. Liver cryosurgery for the second large liver metastasis with the post-cryosurgical zone of the first liver metastasis (**A**). Post-cryosurgical view of both cryozones with the ice crater in the middle, and of the ice margin with the line of demarcation, immediately after a single cryosurgical session (**B**)

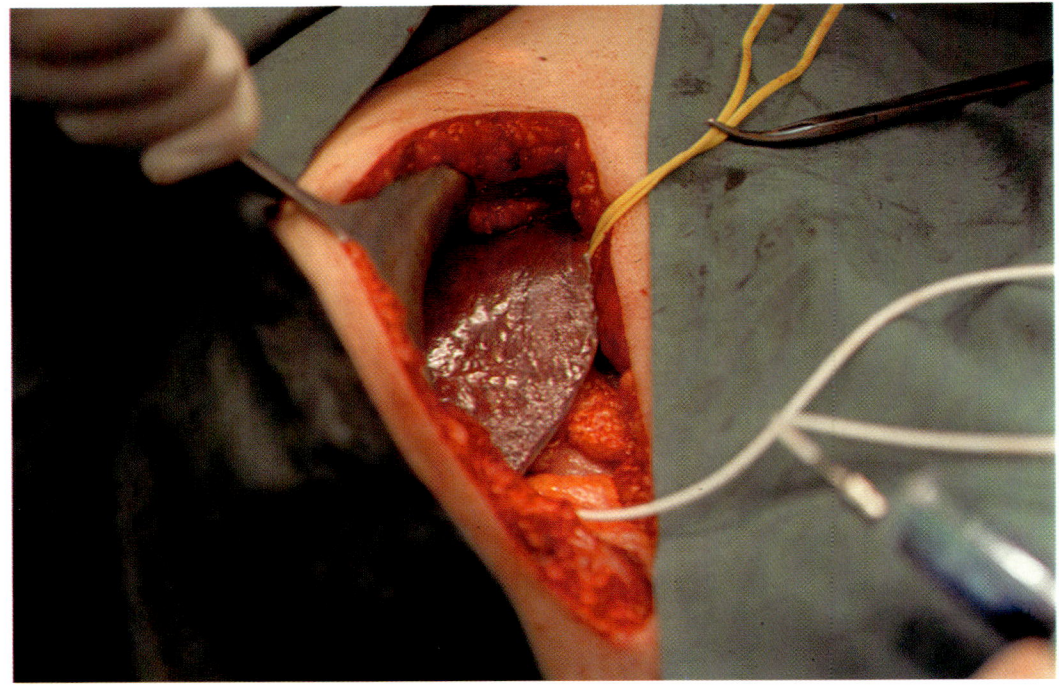

Fig. 12.3.2[1]. CAT-Phenomenon. The liver with multiple large metastases is perfused with methylene blue via a catheter positioned in the gastroduodenal artery immediately after a hepatic cryosurgical session

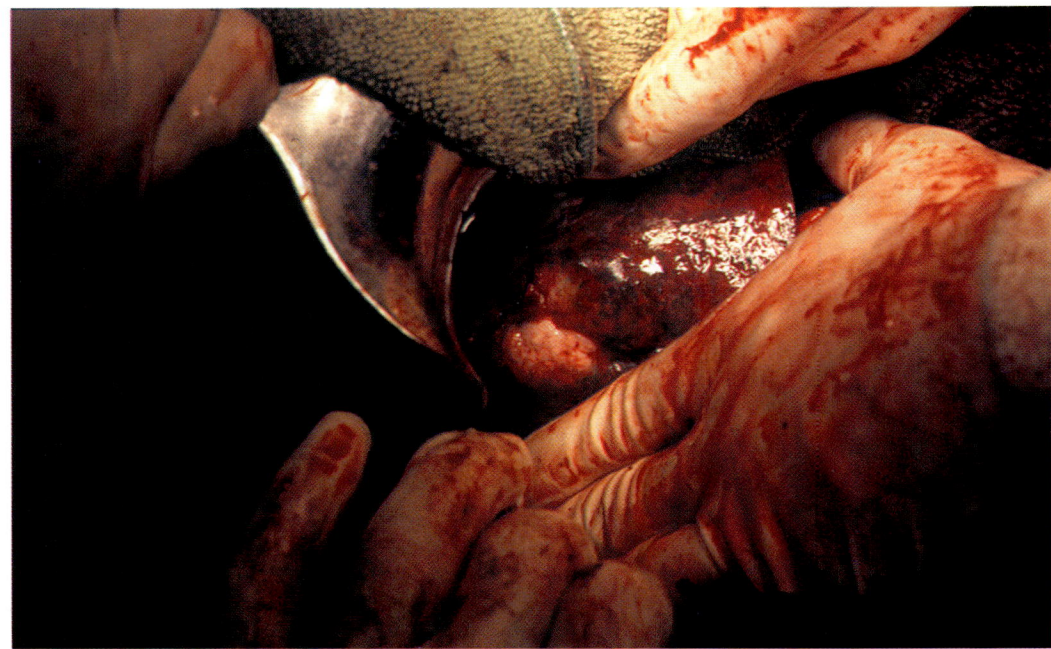

Fig. 12.3.3[1]. CAT-Phenomenon. View of multiple liver metastases after liver cryosurgery and liver perfusion with methylene blue

Chapter 12
Abdominal Cryosurgery: Hepatic Cryosurgery

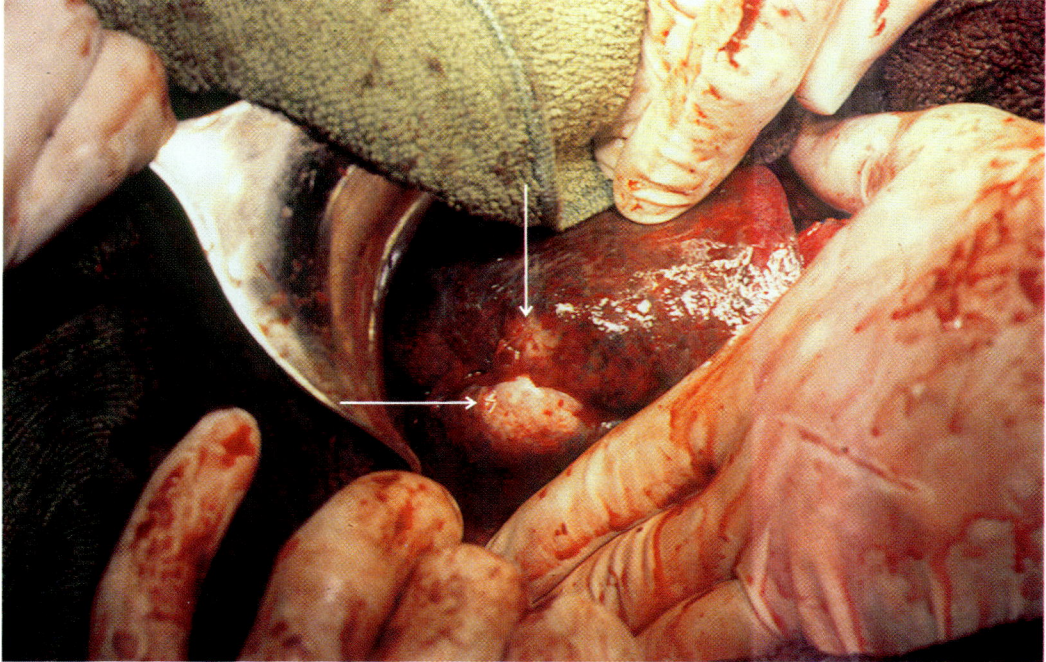

Fig. 12.3.4[1]. CAT-Phenomenon. When the cryosurgical freeze-thaw cycle is finished and the cryozones with the ice crater in the middle, and the ice margin with the line of demarcation are thawed, the liver parenchyma has taken on the color of the dye, but the two cryoextirpated liver metastases have not, both cryoextirpated liver metastases are not dyed (arrow)

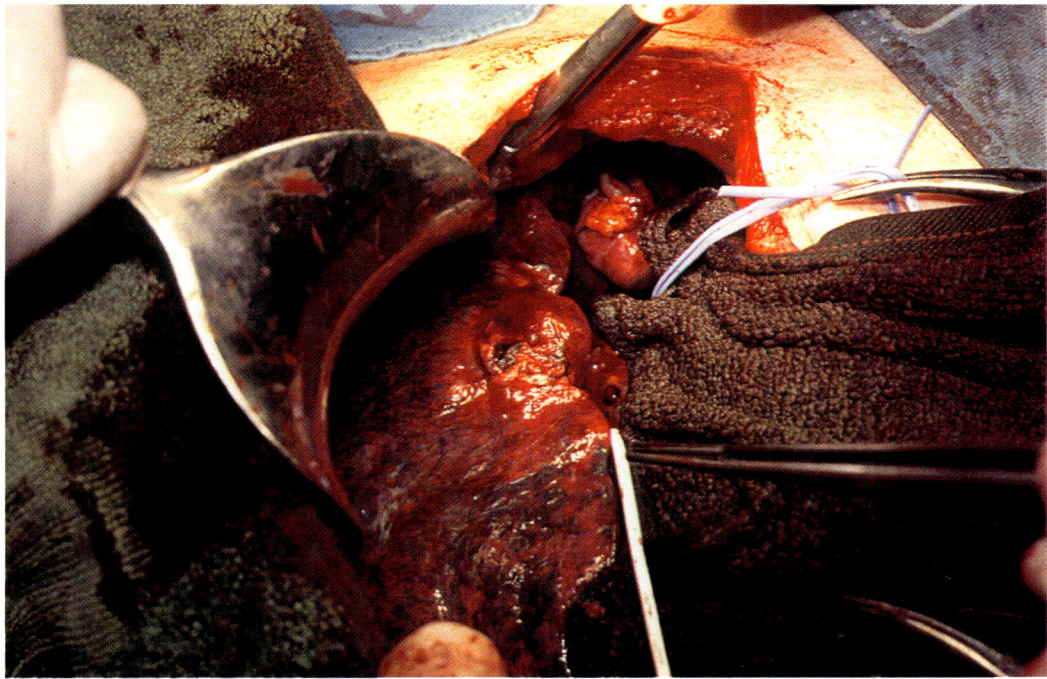

Fig. 12.3.5[1]. CAT-Phenomenon. Only the healthy hepatic parenchyma is sensitive to color, but large liver metastasis with the post-cryosurgical zone is not sensitive to color. The absence of dye indicates a post-surgical avascular tumor area. Post-cryosurgical view of both, immediately after a single cryosurgical session

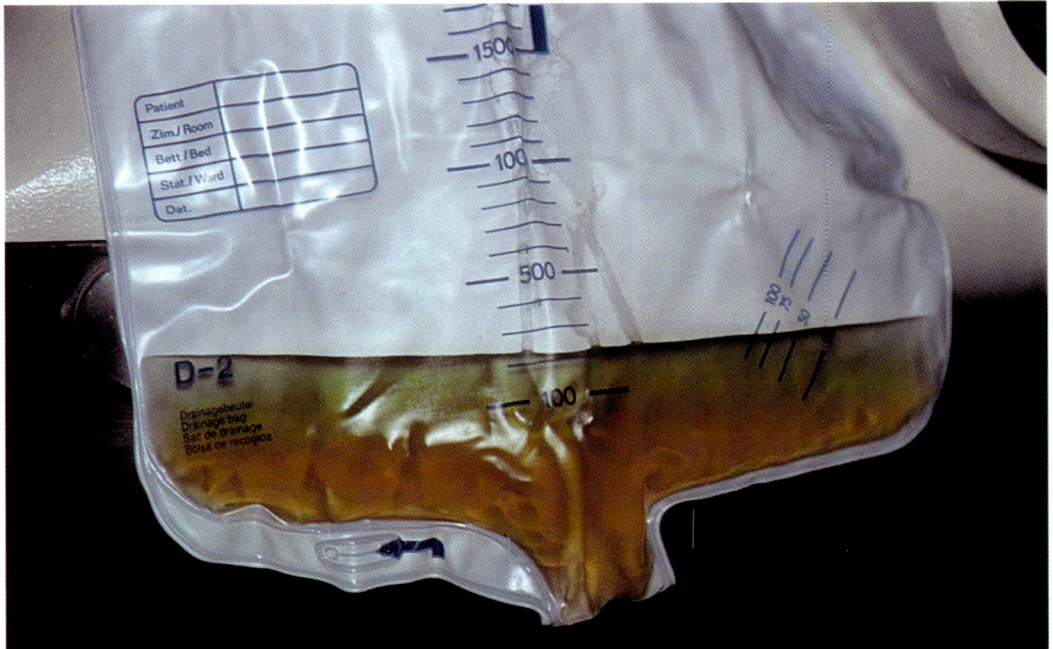

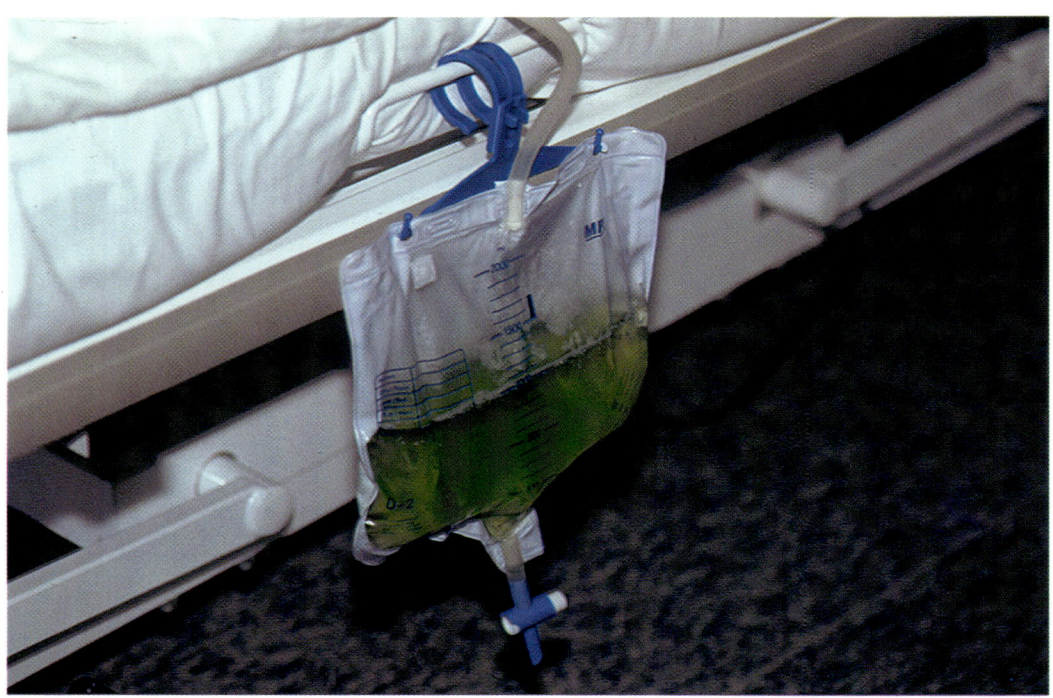

Fig. 12.3.6[1] **A, B.** CAT-Phenomenon. Green colored urine excretion after hepatic perfusion with methylene blue: at first (**A**) and on second postoperative day (**B**). The urine is usually a normal color on the third postoperative day after perfusion of the liver with a coloured fluid (e.g., methylene blue) by way of a catheter positioned in the gastroduodenal artery

Section F Clinical Aspects

12.4 Laparoscopic Liver Cryosurgery

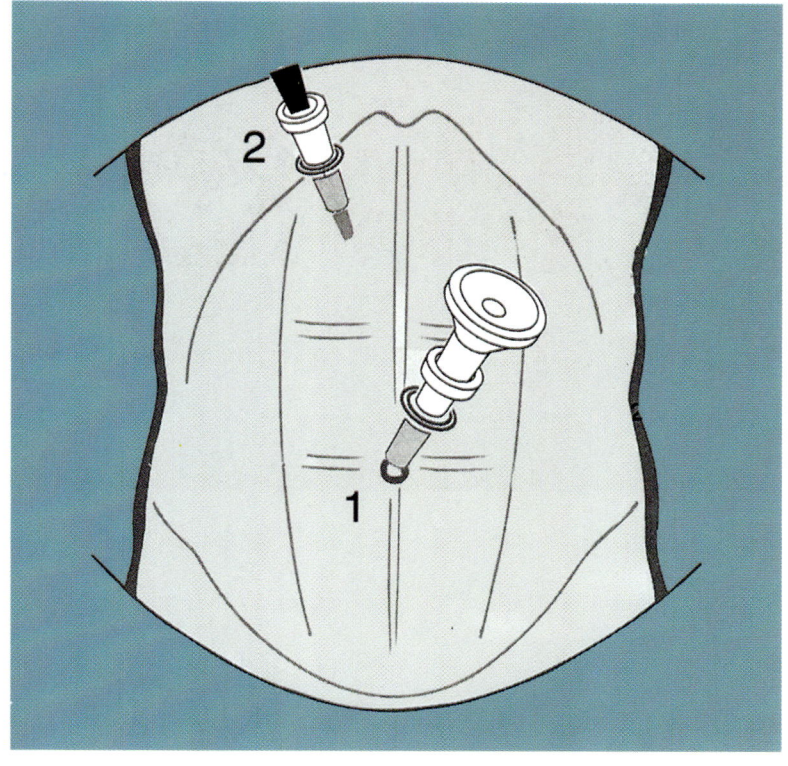

A

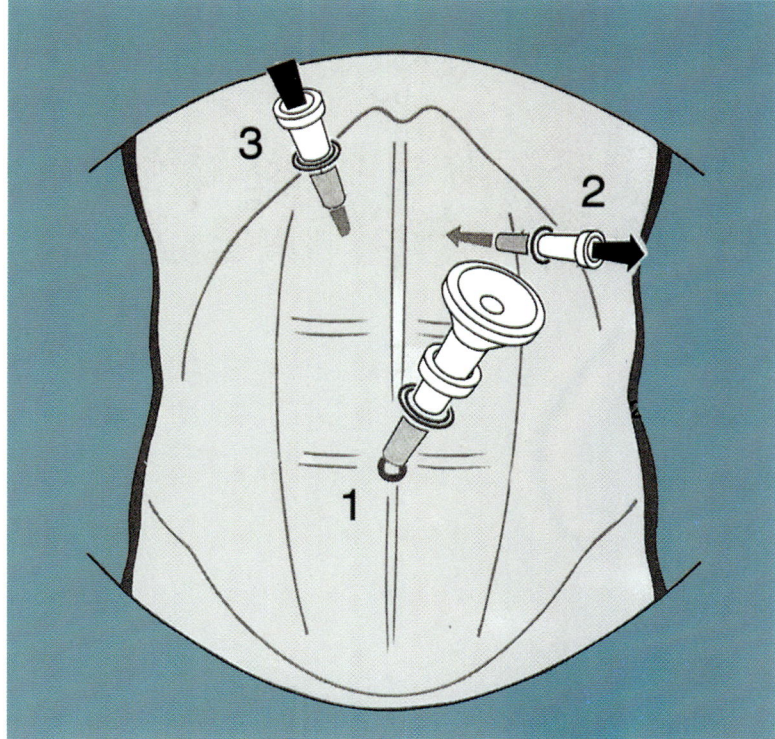

B

Fig. 12.4.1[1] **A, B.** Puncture points for the trocar cannulas for laparoscopic liver cryosurgery. **A**: 11 mm trocar cannulas for an optic trocar (1) and cryosurgical instruments (2). **B**: 11 mm rigid trocar cannulas for an optic trocar (1) and cryosurgical instruments (3); 8 mm flexible trocar cannula (2)

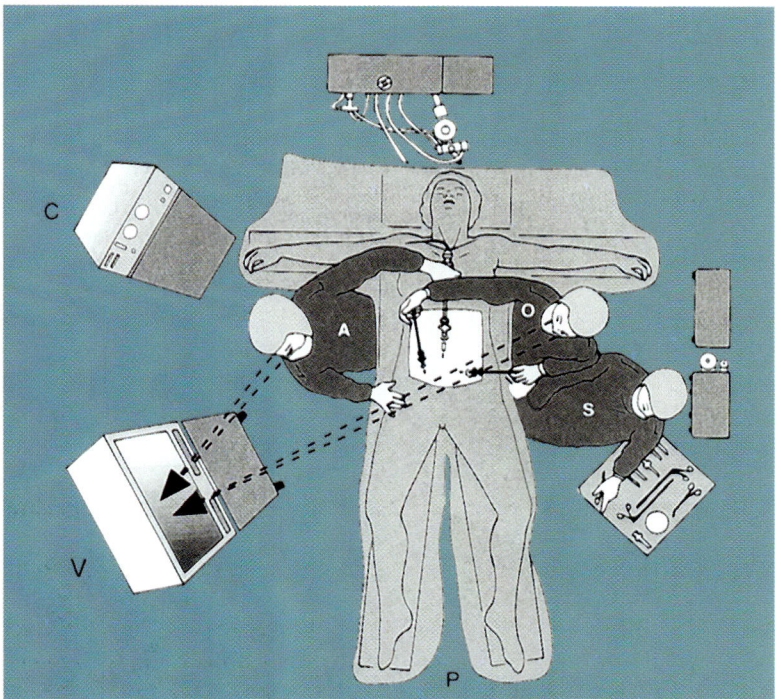

Fig. 12.4.2[1]. Operating design for laparoscopic liver cryosurgery. The operating surgeon (**O**) and operating nurse (**S**) stand at the patient's (**P**) left side, oriented to the patient's head. The assisting surgeon (**A**) stands at the right side of patient. The video equipment (**V**) which is used for endoscopic surgery is also used for laparoscopic liver cryosurgery. The cryosurgical device (**C**) is placed opposite the operating surgeon on the patient's right side

Chapter 12
Abdominal Cryosurgery: Hepatic Cryosurgery

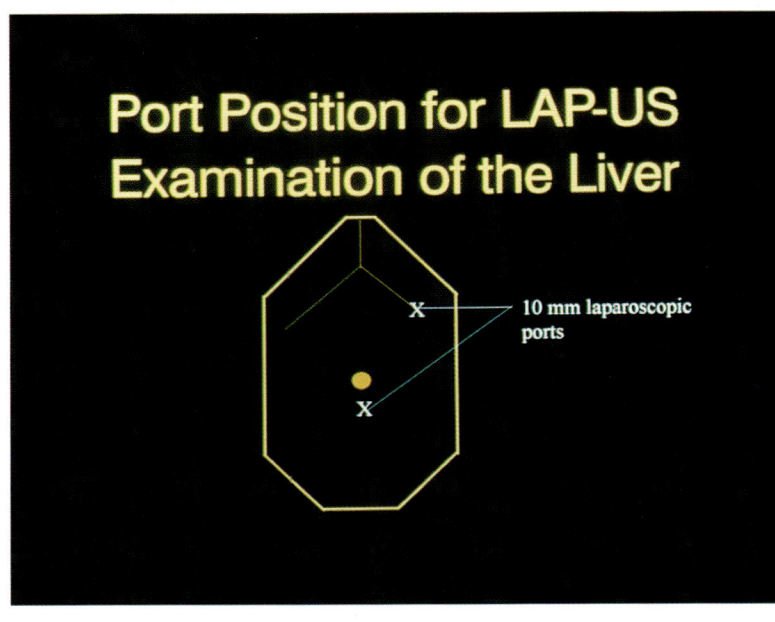

Fig. 12.4.3[3]. A schematic showing of the port position which can be used for laparoscopic ultrasound examination of the liver. Laparoscopic cryosurgery port position would clearly depend on the location of the lesion in the liver

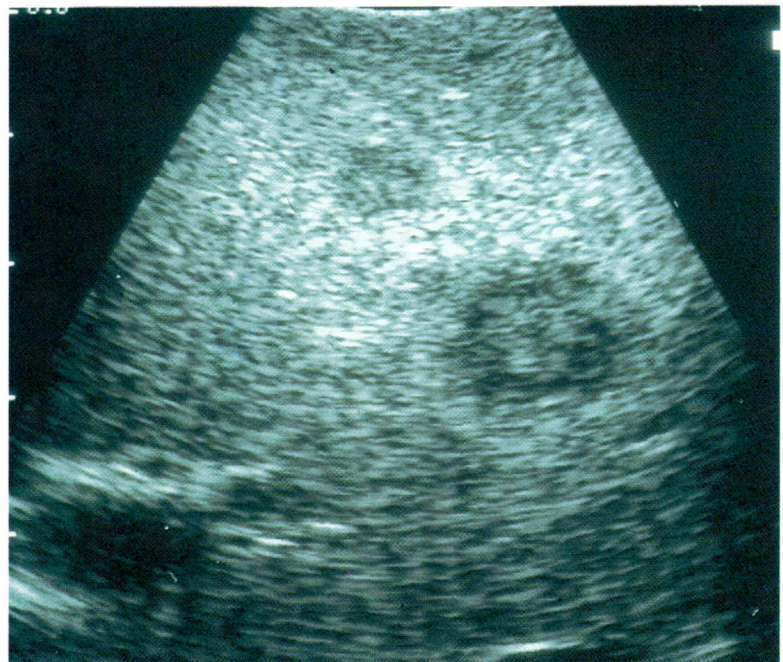

Fig. 12.4.4[3]. An image taken with laparoscopic intraoperative ultrasound identifying 2 small hepatic metastases originating from colorectal cancer

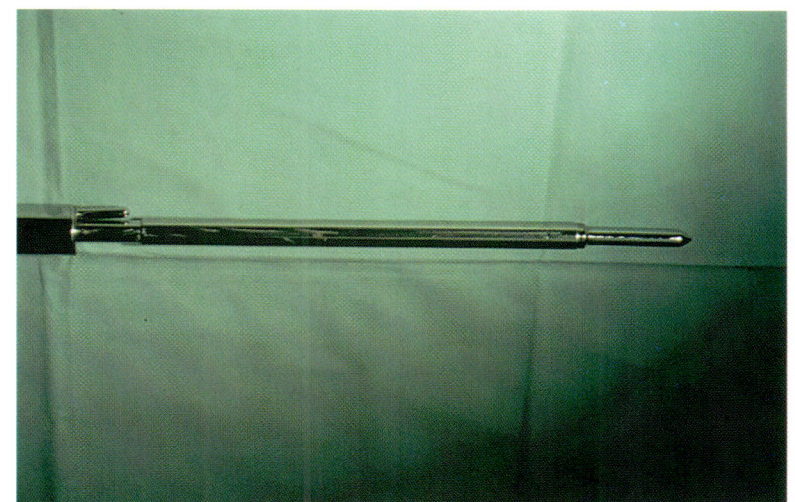

A

B

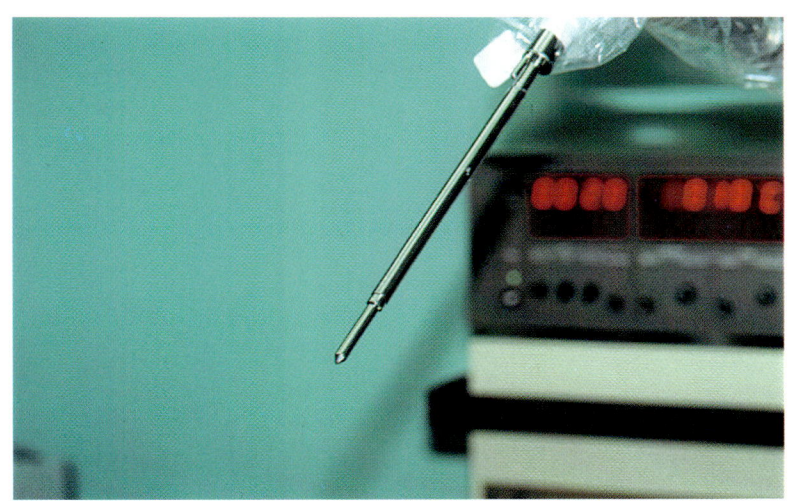

Fig. 12.4.5[1] **A, B.** A laparoscopic cryosurgical needle (**A**) connected to a universal cryosurgical device (**B**) for laparoscopic liver cryosurgery (LLC)

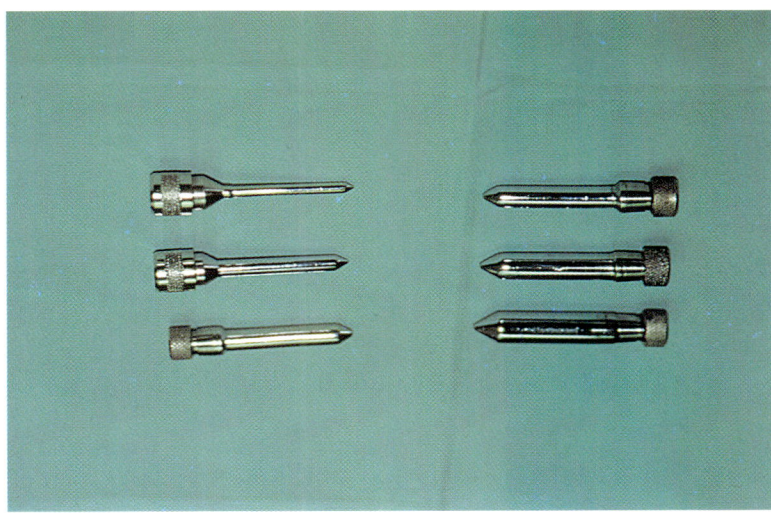

Fig. 12.4.6[1]. A set of basic universal cryosurgical needles with diameters of between 4 mm and 12 mm for LLC

Chapter 12
Abdominal Cryosurgery: Hepatic Cryosurgery

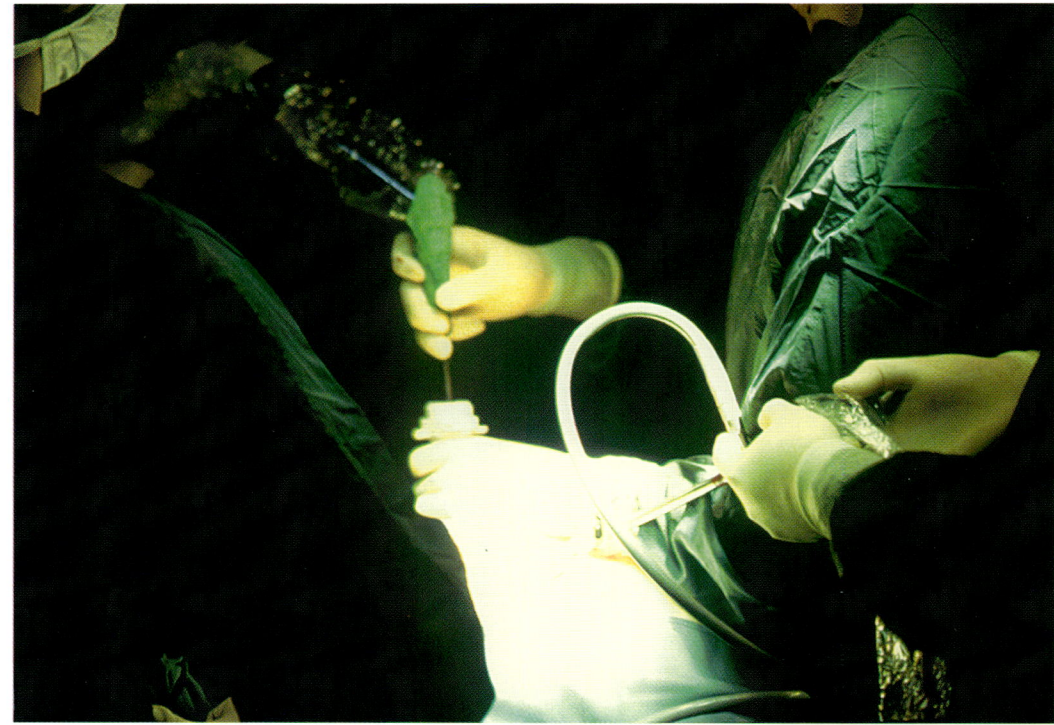

Fig. 12.4.7[1]. In the operating theatre. Standard position of the operating surgeon with operating team used an optic trocar with cryosurgical needle for LLC in patient with liver metastases

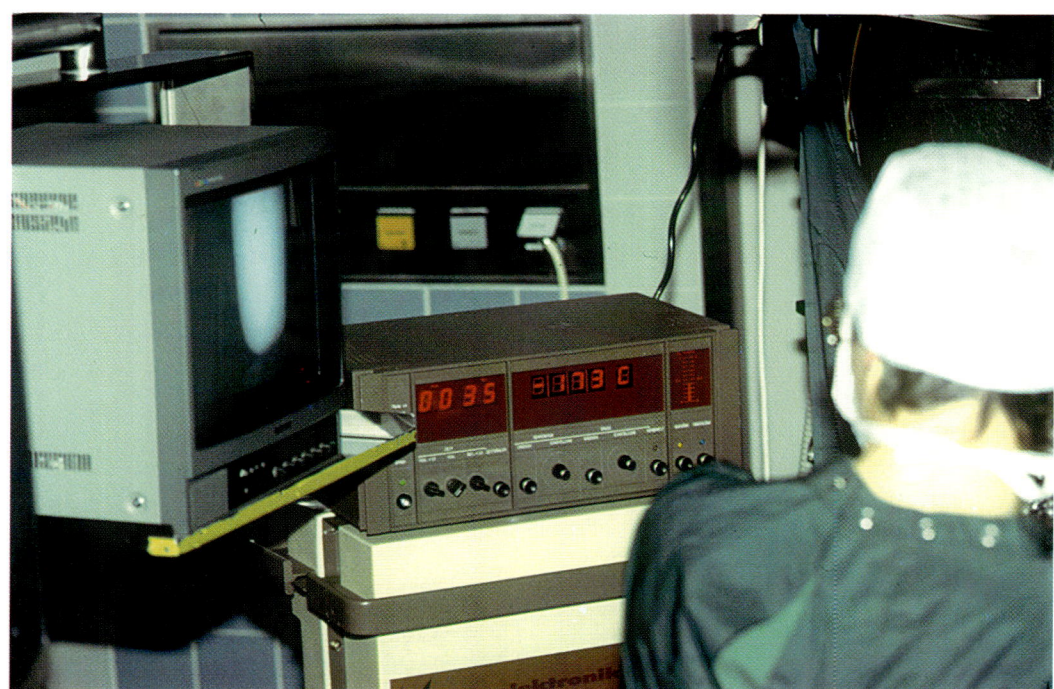

Fig. 12.4.8[1]. Video monitor (left) and display of the universal cryosurgical device (right) during the LLC

Clinical Aspects

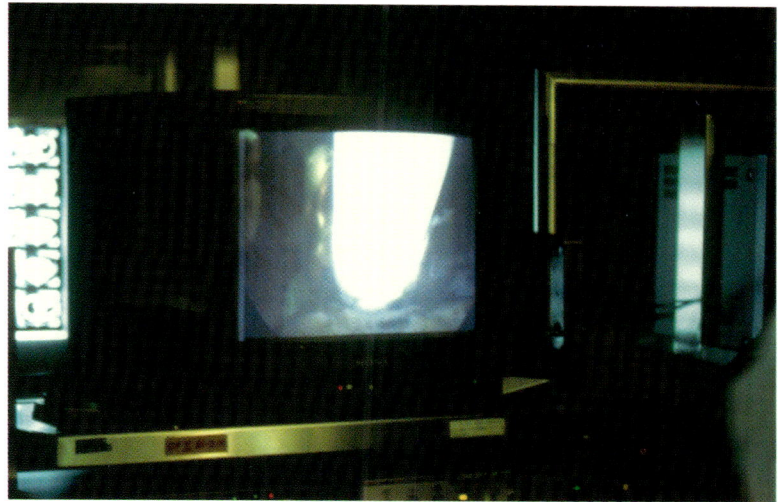

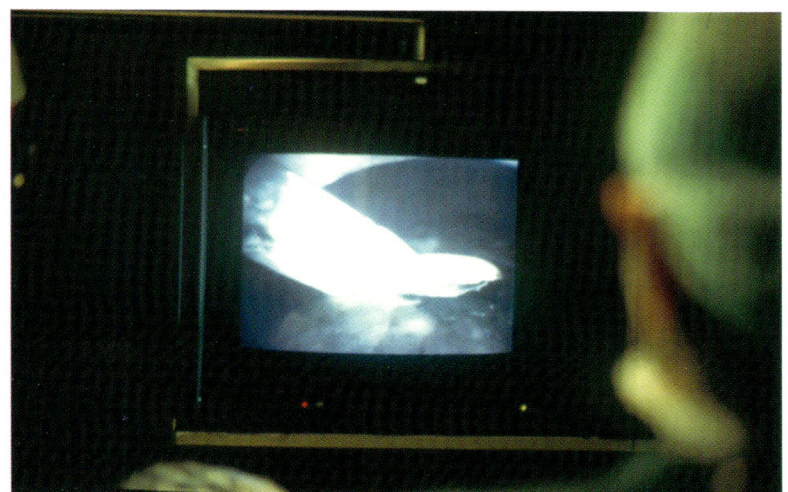

Fig. 12.4.9[1] A, B. Video image of the single freeze cycle during laparoscopic liver cryosurgery using the universal cryosurgical unit "Mobile Cryosurgical System" at a temperature of −180°C (**A**). Cryozone formation in the area of the liver metastasis (**B**)

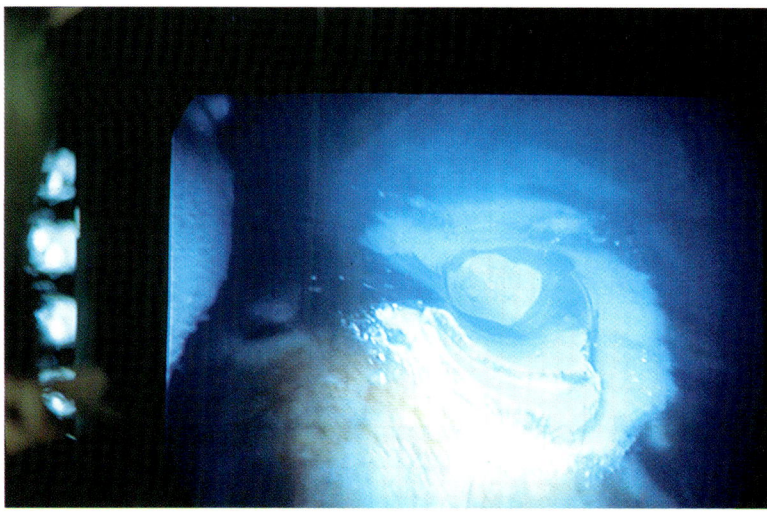

Fig. 12.4.10[1]. 'Dense clouds' in the abdominal cavity after thawing during laparoscopic liver cryosurgery with the cryozone in the middle of the video monitor

Chapter 12 Abdominal Cryosurgery: Hepatic Cryosurgery

12.5 Cryosurgery for Liver Echinococcal Cystic Disease of the Liver

The aim of surgery in patients with echinococcal cystic disease of the liver is to remove the parasitic cyst with its contents from the liver and to prevent the recurrence of the disease. In patients who have a liver cyst in a marginal location, liver resection is possible. In patients with multiple cysts an echinococcectomy can be performed by means of a cystectomy with removal of the fibrous capsule. These operations, especially the echinococcectomy, are rather traumatic. But echinococcotomy by way of cystectomy with treatment of the walls of the fibrous capsule is often preferred for this disease. The cystectomy can only be radically performed if the walls of the fibrous capsule are 'sterilized', which means that they must be free of echinococcosis, which in most cases is difficult to eliminate, because the walls of the fibrous capsule consist of elements of echinococcosis, e.g., scolex.

The new surgical technique for treating liver echinococcal cystic disease is hepatic cryosurgery. It is necessary to use cryosurgical equipment with sub-zero temperatures ranging from $-160°C$ to $-180°C$ to overcome parasitic liver disease, because of the high blood circulation in the liver, and treatment can only have the desired radical effect if very low sub-zero temperatures are applied.

Cryosurgical operations on patients with echinococcal cystic disease of the liver can be performed in two ways. First, by liver cryoresection using a cryoscalpel to prevent liver bleeding and avoid recurrence of the disease. Secondly, by cryoechinococcotomy.

We have successfully performed 22 cryosurgical operations on patients with echinococcal cystic disease of the liver and no deaths occurred. This operation appears to be a very safe and effective operative technique for treating echinococcal cystic disease of the liver.

Section F   Clinical Aspects   279

Chapter 12
Abdominal
Cryosurgery:
Hepatic
Cryosurgery

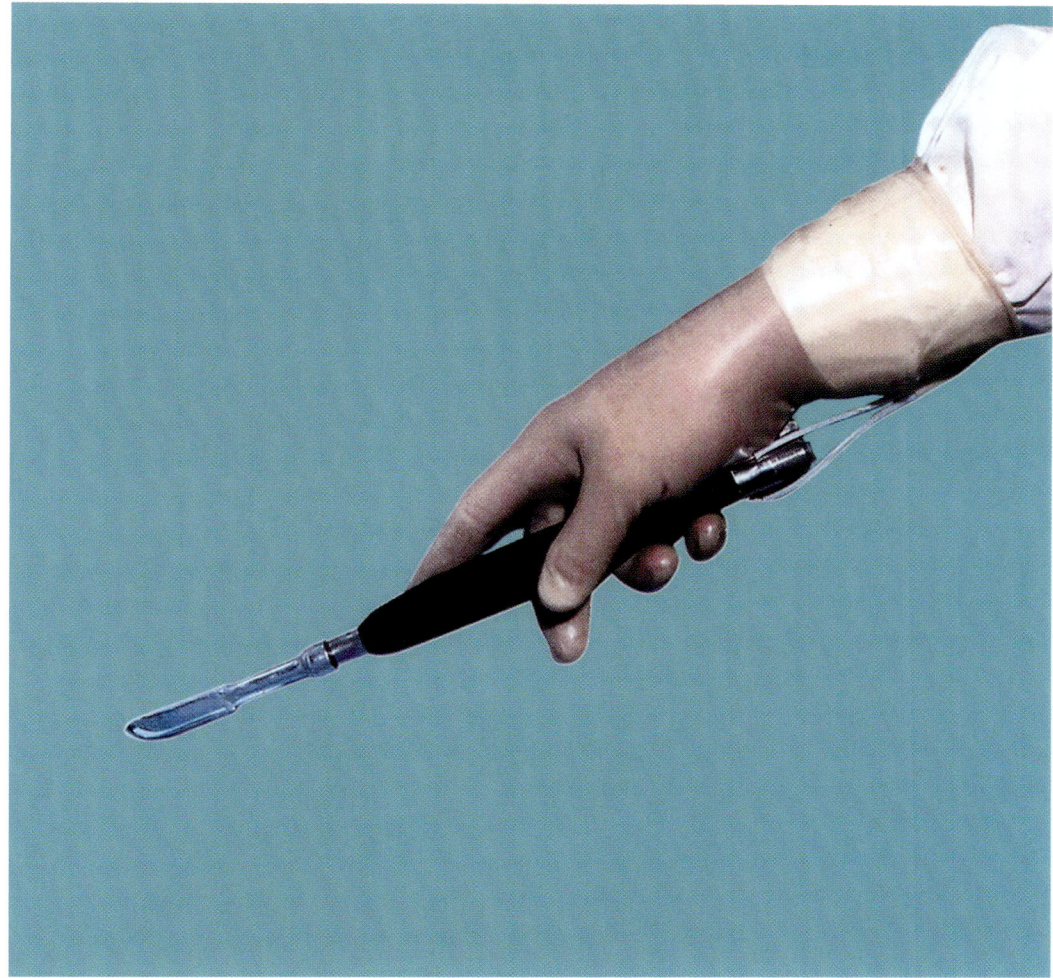

A

Fig. 12.5.1[2] A, B. Cryoscalpel: general view (A) and schematic view (B)

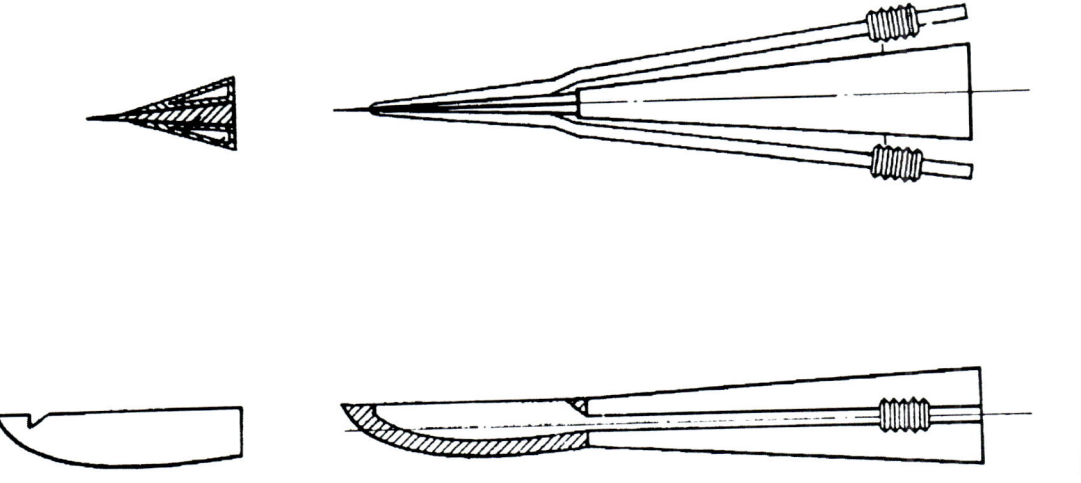

B

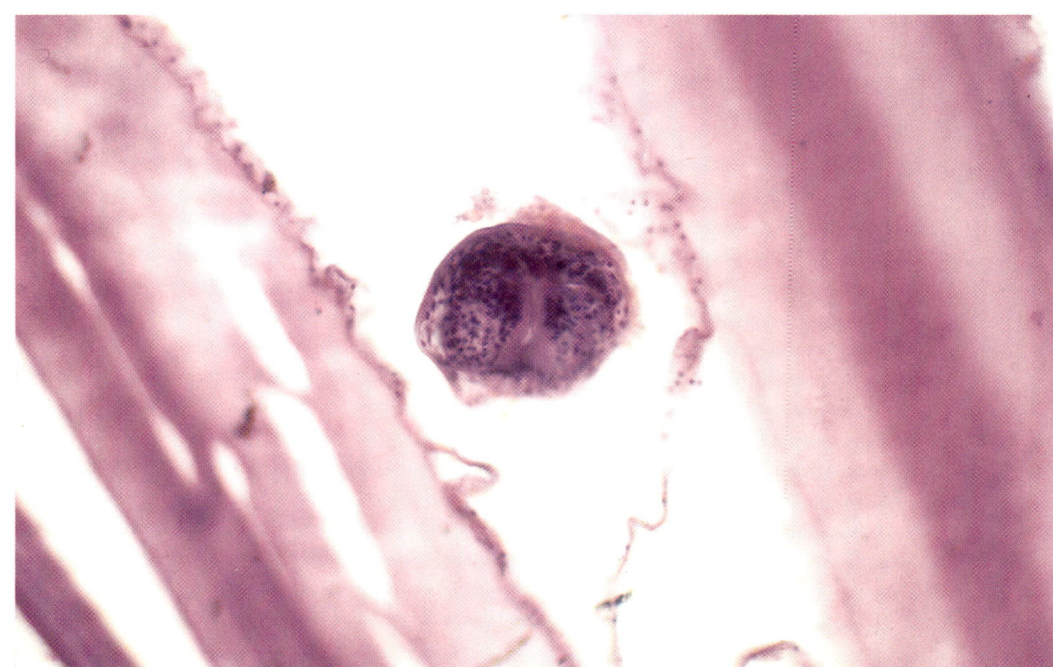

Fig. 12.5.2². Echinococcal cystic disease of the liver. In the wall of the fibrous capsule there are elements of echinococcosis: scolex. Haematoxylin and eosin stain, magnification ×200 (**A**) and ×600 (**B**)

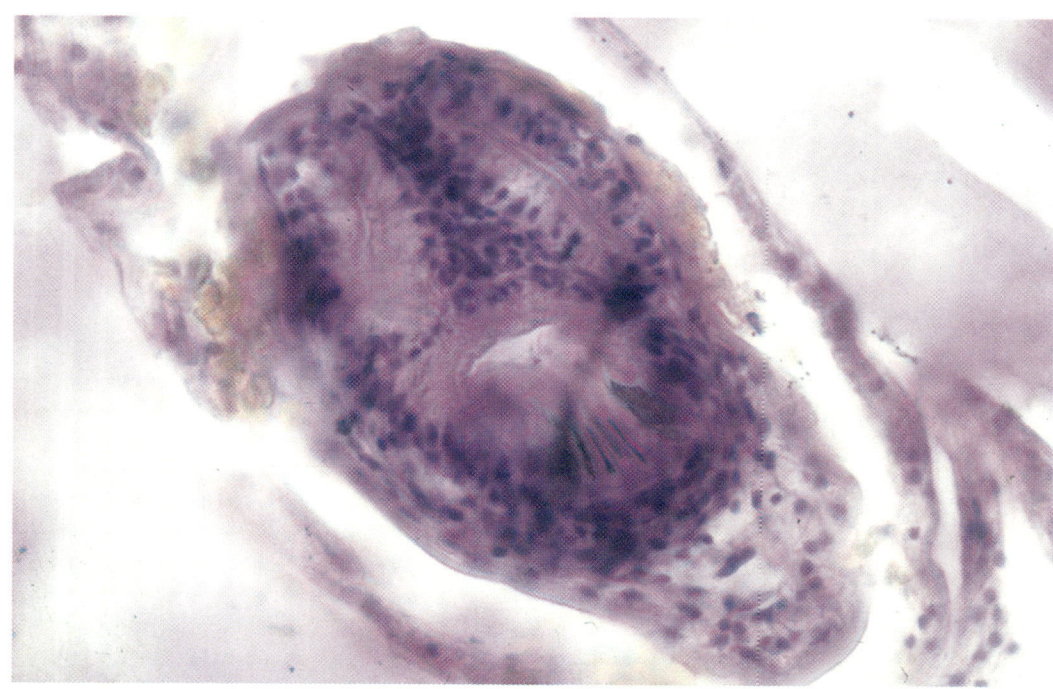

Section F Clinical Aspects 281

Chapter 12
Abdominal
Cryosurgery:
Hepatic
Cryosurgery

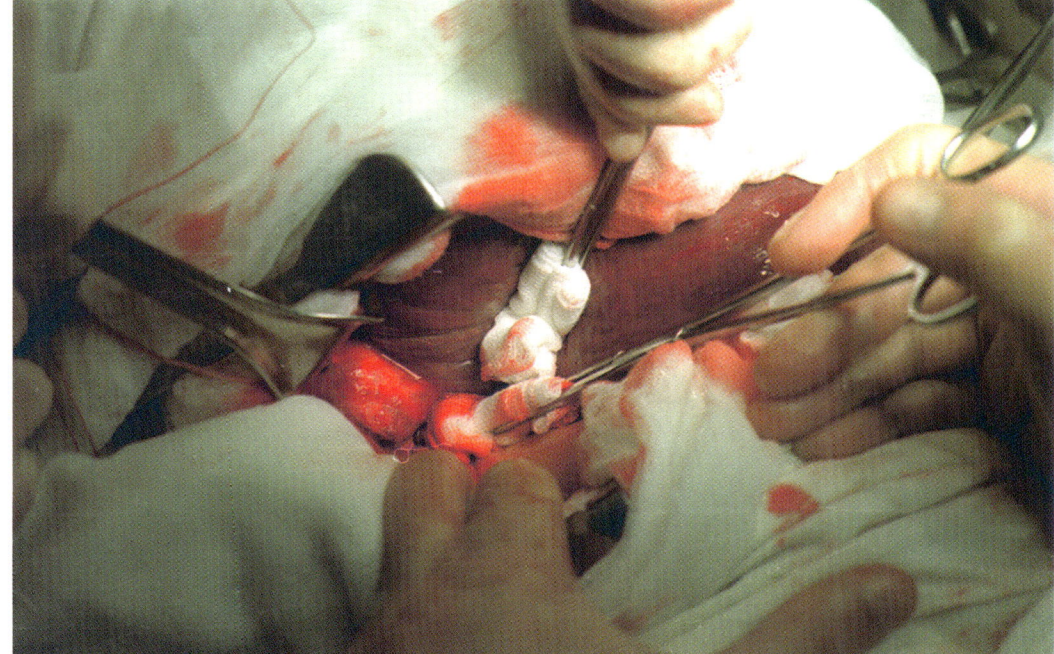

A

Fig. 12.5.3². Echinococcal cystic disease of the liver. Intraoperative appearance of echinococcosis (**A**) and during its puncture (**B**)

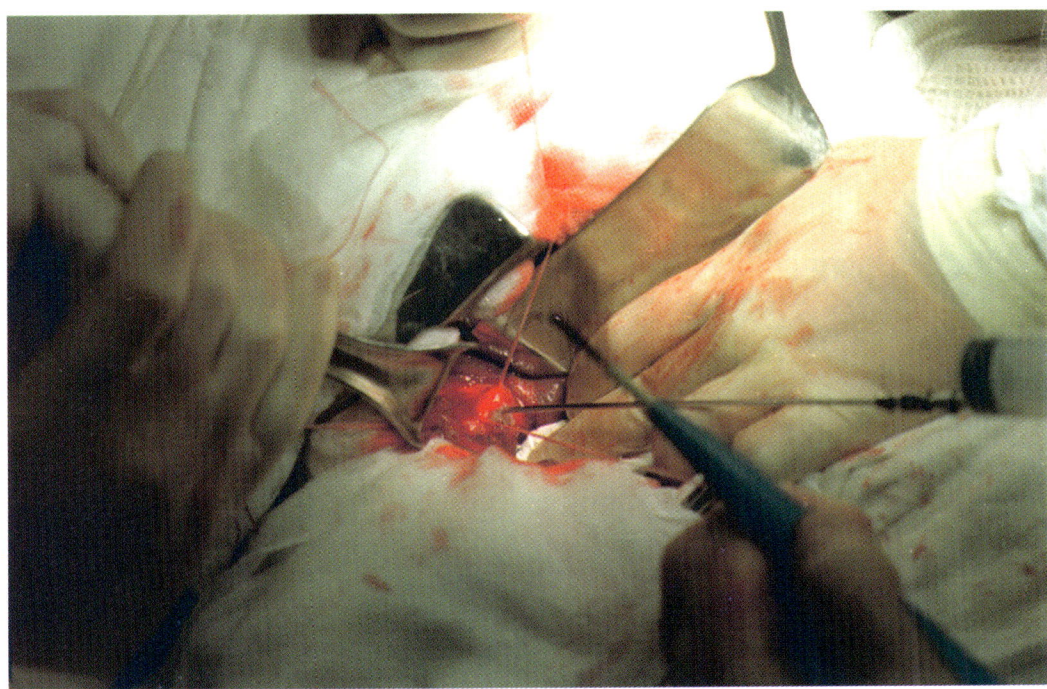

B

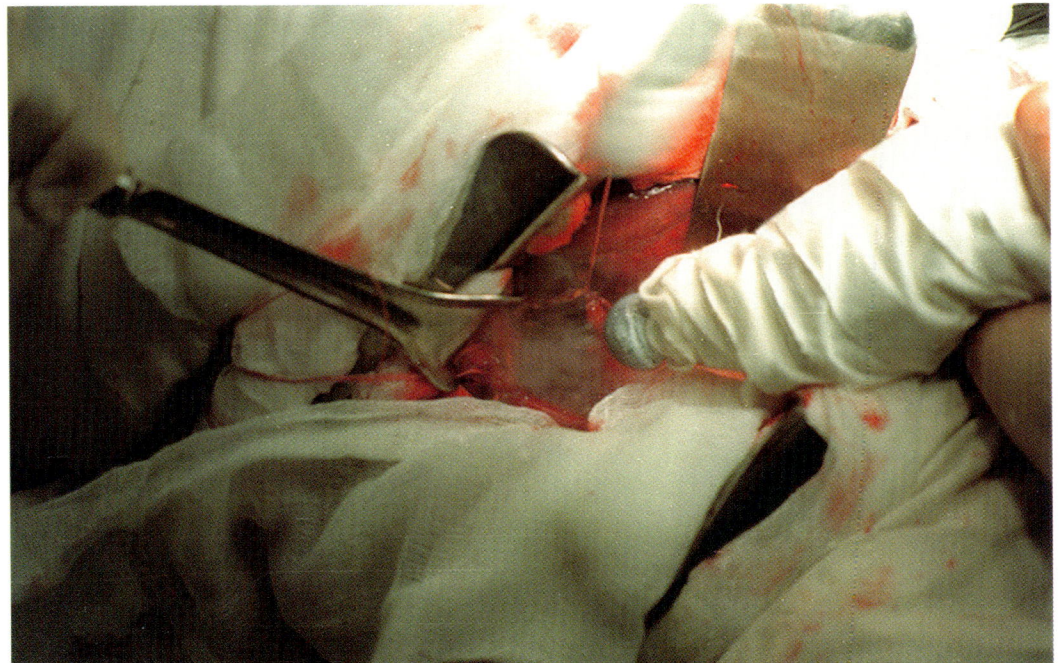

Fig. 12.5.4². Echinococcal cystic disease of the liver: intraoperative view. Cryosurgical session on the echinococcal fibrous capsule (**A, B**)

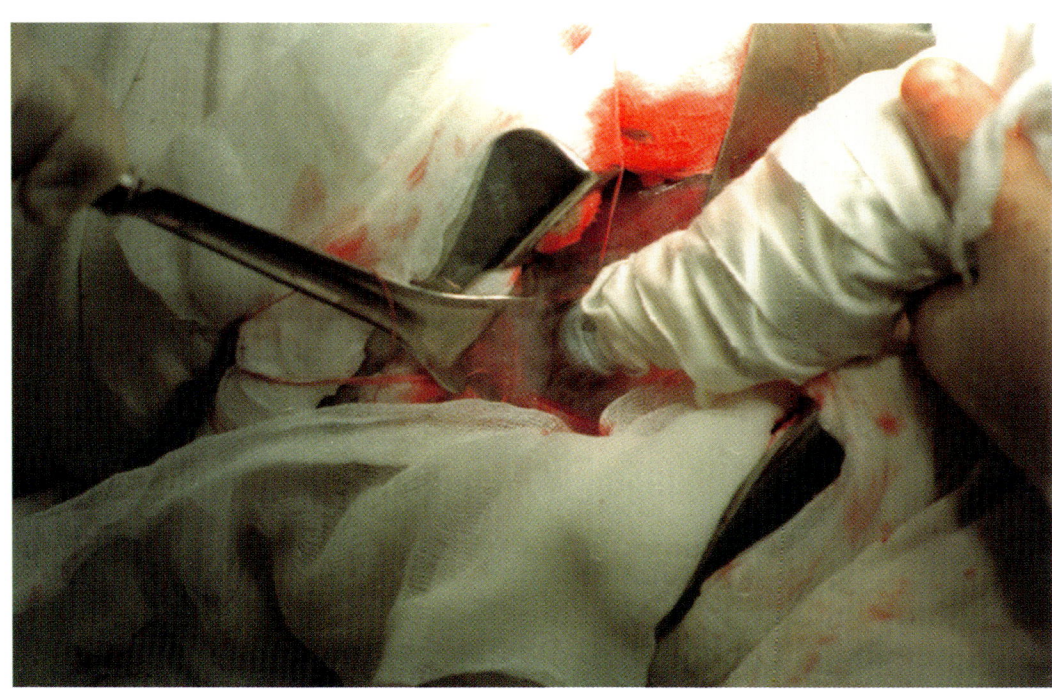

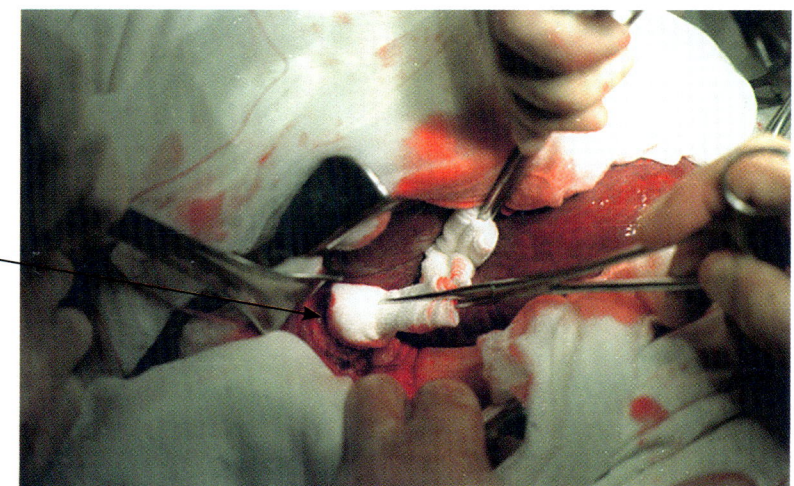

Fig. 12.5.5[2]. Echinococcal cystic disease of the liver: immediately after the cryosurgical session. (Arrow points to cryotreated cyst)

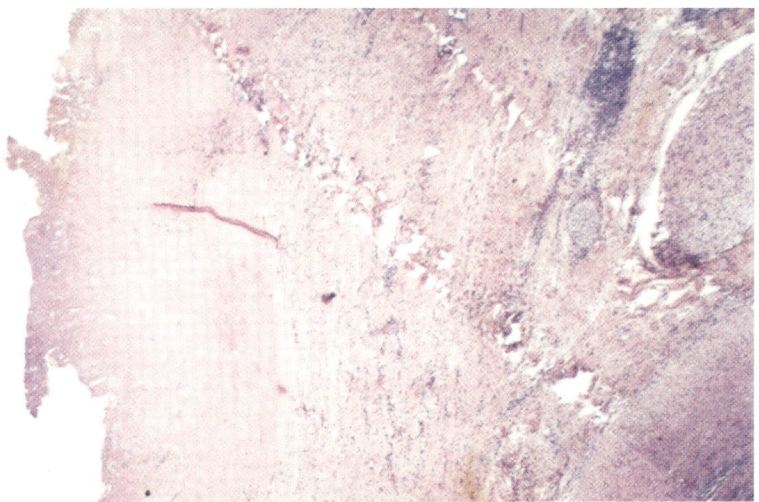

A

B

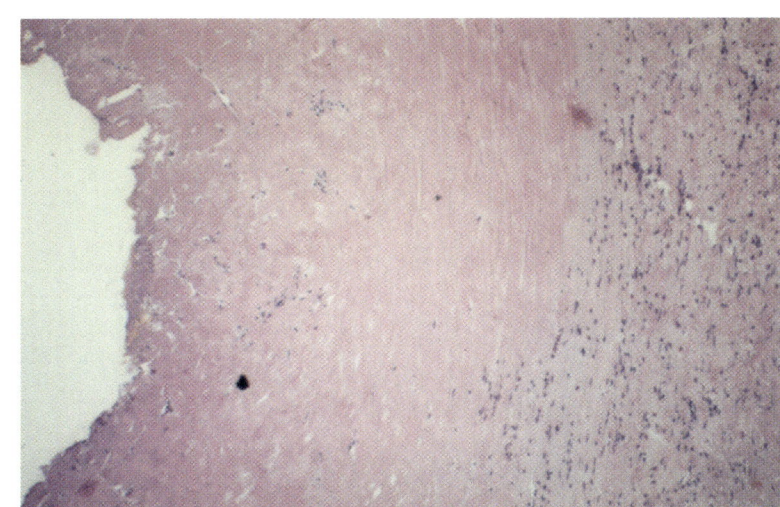

Fig. 12.5.6[2]. Echinococcal cystic disease of the liver. Necrosis of fibrous capsule. Intraoperative biopsy immediately after the cryosurgical session. Haematoxylin and eosin stain, magnification ×40 (**A**) and ×100 (**B**) under the microscope

12.6 Cryosurgery of Liver Alveococcosis

Cryosurgery is especially valuable treating liver alveococcosis, as this disease is similar to a malignant liver tumor in its growth. Local recurrence and germination into the surrounding tissue are often observed. Liver alveococcosis frequently leads to metastases.

Experimental and clinical investigations have proved that the alveococcal tissue can be destroyed by sub-zero temperatures lower than $-80°C$.

For the treatment of liver alveococcosis, the following variety of cryosurgical operations can be performed:

1. Cryosurgical liver resection as a radical operation. The liver cryoresection is performed with a cryoscalpel. It is also possible, after a conventional liver resection, to carry out a cryosurgical session on the resected liver. This cryosurgical measure can prevent recurrence of the disease.
2. Palliative liver resection followed by a cryosurgical session on the remaining parts of the parasitic tissue, especially in germination areas, near the inferior vena cava or structures of the porta hepatis.
3. Cryosurgery carried out on the walls of the parasitic alveococcal cavern after its evacuation.

A total of 22 radical liver resections using the cryosurgical technique, and 35 palliative liver resections followed by cryosurgical sessions on the remaining parts of the parasitic tissue were performed without any of the patient deaths. The long-term results of these cryosurgical operations are good.

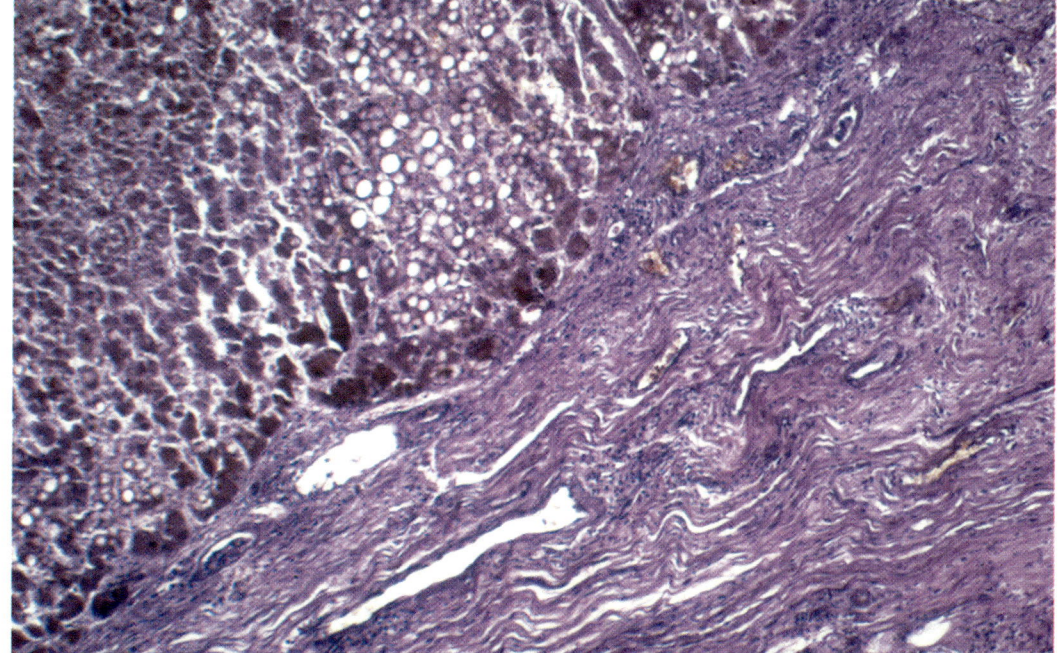

Fig. 12.6.1². Liver alveococcosis. Pre-treatment intraoperative biopsy. Haematoxylin and eosin stain, magnification ×200 (**A**) and ×600 (**B**) under the microscope

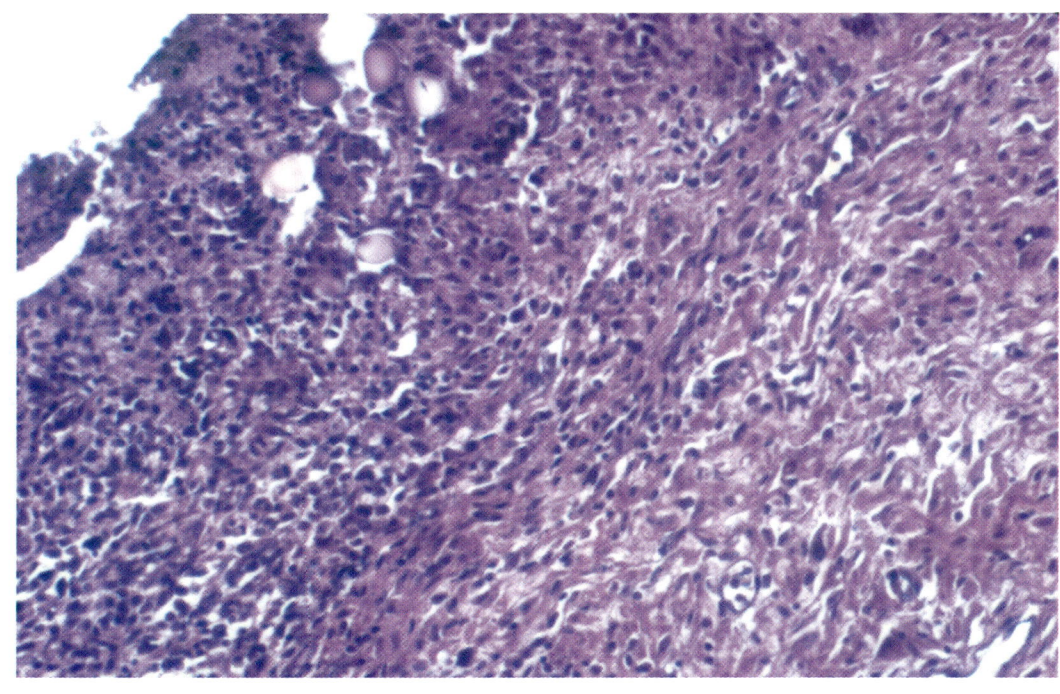

Chapter 12
Abdominal Cryosurgery: Hepatic Cryosurgery

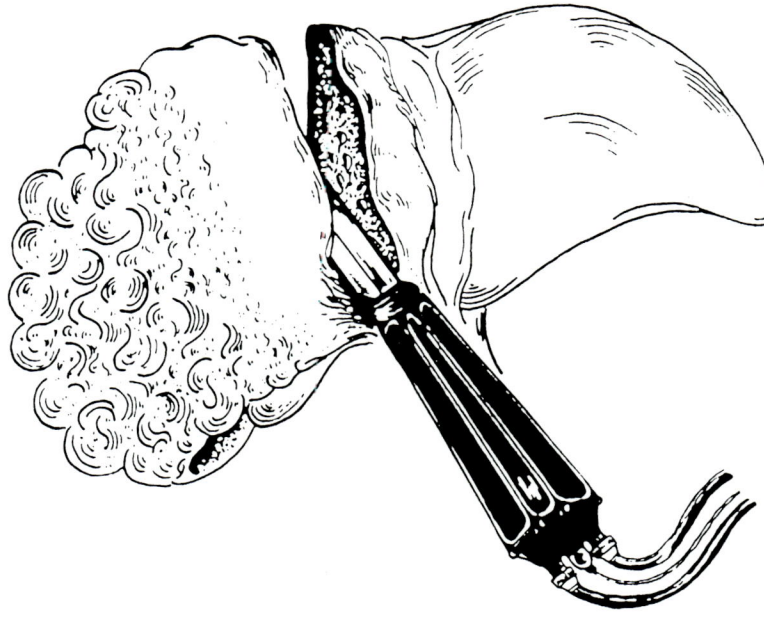

Fig. 12.6.2². Liver alveococcosis. Schematic radical liver cryosurgical resection

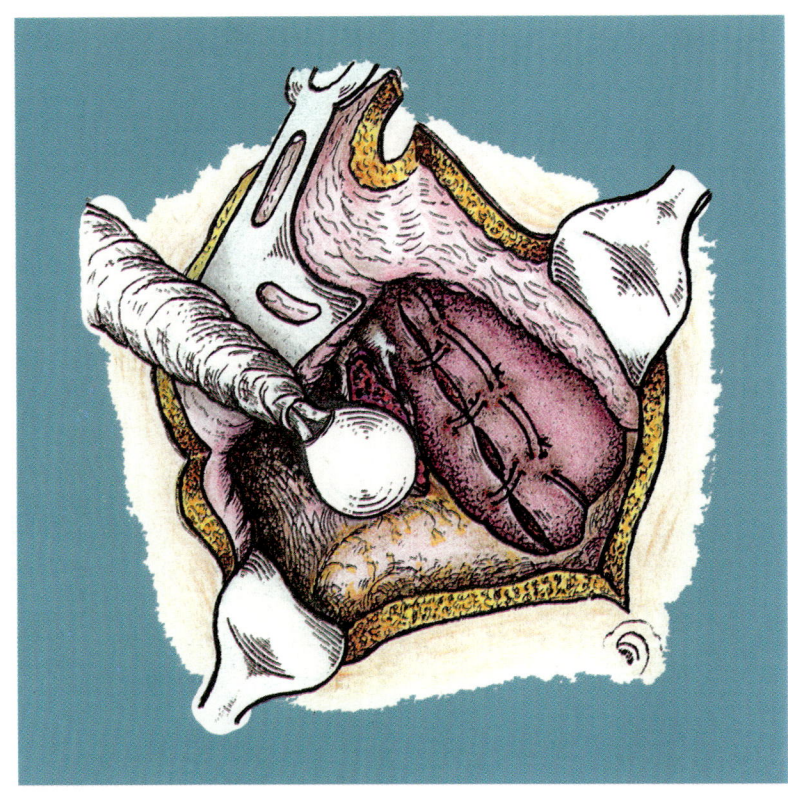

Fig. 12.6.3². Liver alveococcosis. Palliative liver resection with cryosurgical session on the remaining parts of the parasitic tissue in the 'dangerous' liver areas (scheme)

Section F Clinical Aspects

**Chapter 12
Abdominal
Cryosurgery:
Hepatic
Cryosurgery**

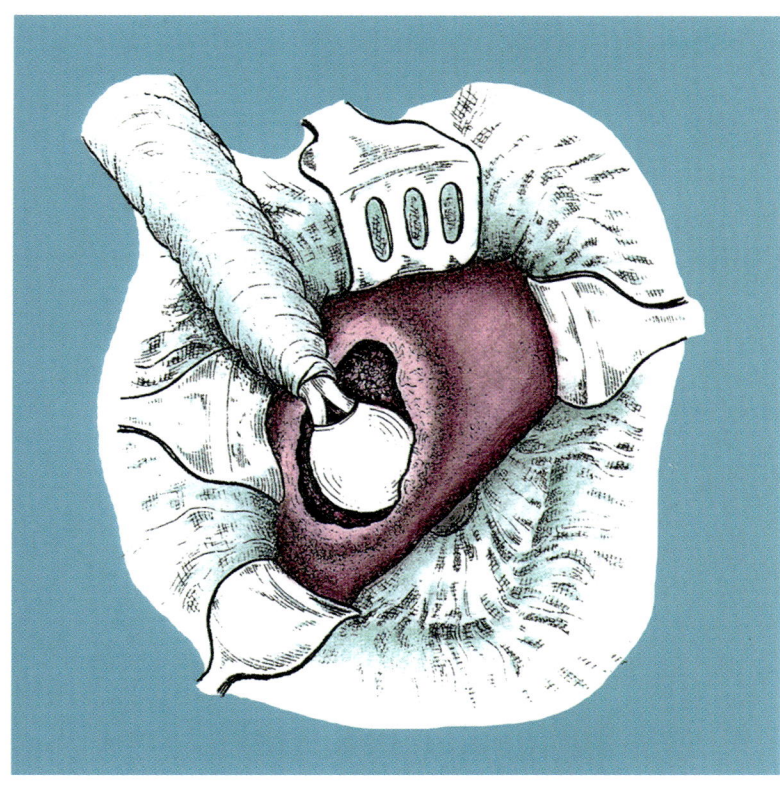

Fig. 12.6.4[2]. Liver alveococcosis. Cryosurgery applied to the walls of the parasitic alveococcal cavern (scheme)

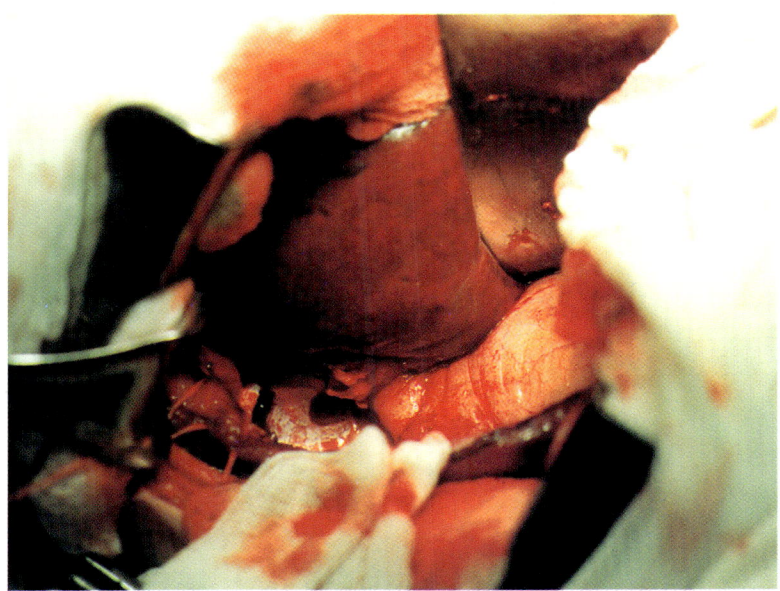

Fig. 12.6.5[2]. Liver alveococcosis. View of the liver after a cryosurgical session

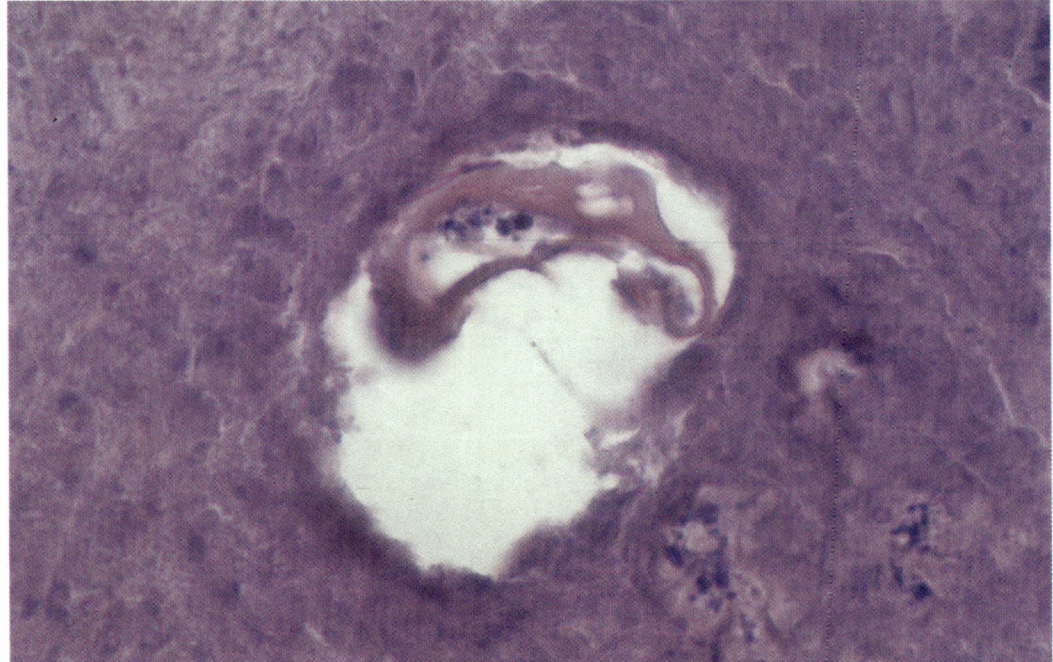

Fig. 12.6.6². Liver alveococcosis. 21 days after a cryosurgical session, all the parasitic tissue had disappeared. Extremely granulated tissue. Haematoxylin and eosin stain, magnification ×100 (**A**) and ×200 (**B**) under the microscope

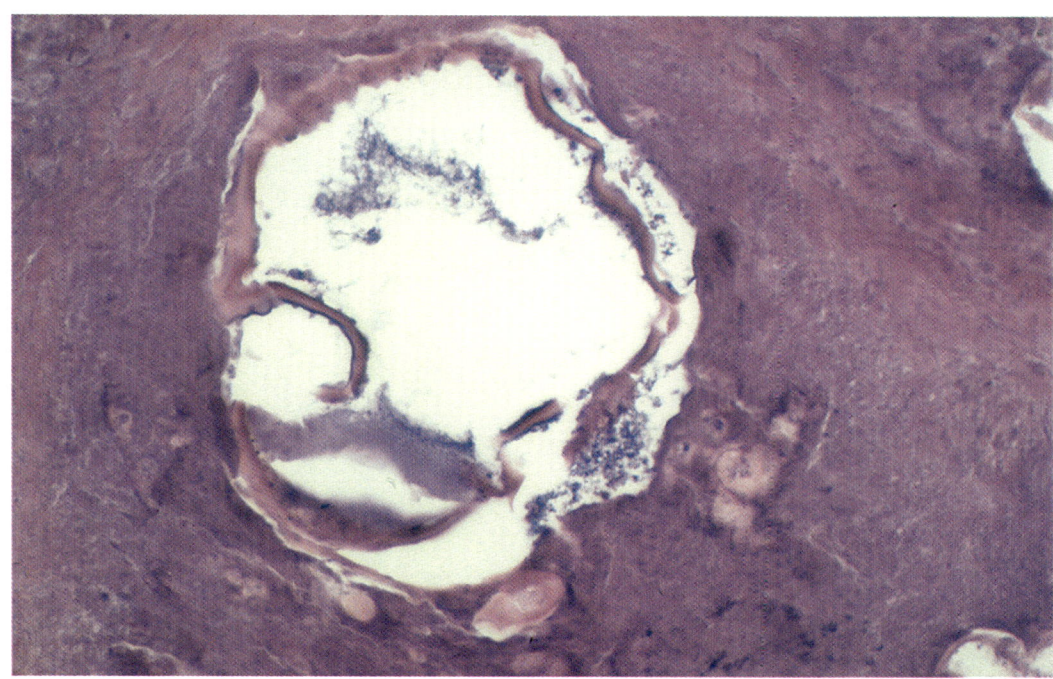

Abdominal Cryosurgery: Pancreas Cryosurgery

Nikolai N. Korpan[1] with contributions by Gerhard Hochwarter[1], Tatjana B. Komkova[2], Franz Sellner[1]

13.0 Introduction

Years of experience with cryosurgery for the removal of benign and malignant tumors have shown that it is possible successfully to convert a tumor into a solid necrotic mass, thus facilitating its removal. This makes avascular resection of the tumor possible, without removing it, and with little or no blood loss during this procedure.

Carcinoma of the pancreas is on the increase worldwide as well as in Austria, where the linear trend shows an increase to 15.1 per 100 000 compared to the WHO average of 7.9 per 100 000. Compared with other malignant tumors 42% of all cases have reached the disseminating stage when they are first diagnosed.

Early diagnosis is difficult because pancreas tumours are clinically inconspicuous and develop relatively slowly until the tumour reaches a considerable size. The success of both curative and palliative therapy is not satisfactory. As alarming symptoms do not appear until late, the prognosis is bad. The five-year survival rate after surgical resection of a pancreas carcinoma is less than 5% in many medical institutions. After detailed reports on pancreas carcinoma had been published by the WHO and the Japanese Pancreatic Society, surgeons were for the first time able to make postoperative prognoses of pancreas carcinoma at various stages. It soon became obvious that only a very small percentage of the patients who had extensive resections profited from surviving their operations. What most patients actually need is minimally invasive palliative therapy, which guarantees a good quality of life and only brief stays in hospital for the short time that remains of their lives.

New scientific findings in the fields of biological research and experimental surgery, as well as modern technological developments, have opened up an important and at the same time fascinating outlook on the treatment strategy for advanced stages of liver and pancreas tumors. For patients with pancreas carcinoma, which is incurable by conventional pancreas resection, cryosurgery is motivating and promising.

Clinical application of the cryosurgical technique in patients with diseases of the pancreas, especially with chronic pancreatitis, was preceded by experimental research carried out on the pancreases of dogs. Morphological changes in the removed post-cryosurgical pancreas tissue were studied. Cryolysis was carried out by means of a cryoprobe of original design at a temperature of −180°C. Numerous vessels and nerve-endings could still be seen microscopically after cryosurgery on the pancreas. The investigation of tissue specimens under different conditions after the operation showed that glandular tissue is subject to aseptic necrosis with the subsequent formation of connective tissue of a cicatrix in the zone of cryodestruction. In neural conductors and intramural nerve endings degenerative and destructive changes take place, that are the morphological basis for cryolysis. In the small calibre blood vessels stasis and clotting with subsequent

Chapter 13
Abdominal Cryosurgery: Pancreas Cryosurgery

canalization of vessels develop. The pancreatic secretory passages are not subjected to morphological changes.

The purpose of the operation in patients with chronic pancreatitis is to interrupt the pain and prevent the development of destructive pancreatitis in the long-term postoperative period. Anatomic-physiological features of the constitution of the nerve fibers and intramural nerve endings have determined the location of a 'key point' for cryoprobe application in the transition zone of the pancreas head where it joins the body. The body of the pancreas is also subjected to cryodestruction at two or three freely selected points.

The essence of operations on patients with pancreatic cysts consists of ablation of the pathological center and preventive measures against the recurrence of the disease. One group of operations consists of excision of a cyst wall while sparing healthy tissue, and ablation of the contents of the cyst with subsequent cryolysis of the pancreas bed.

In the field of pancreatic cryosurgery new cryosurgical instruments must be developed to enable different cryosurgical operations to be performed on patients with different inflammatory and malignant diseases of the pancreas.

13.1 Chronic Pancreatitis

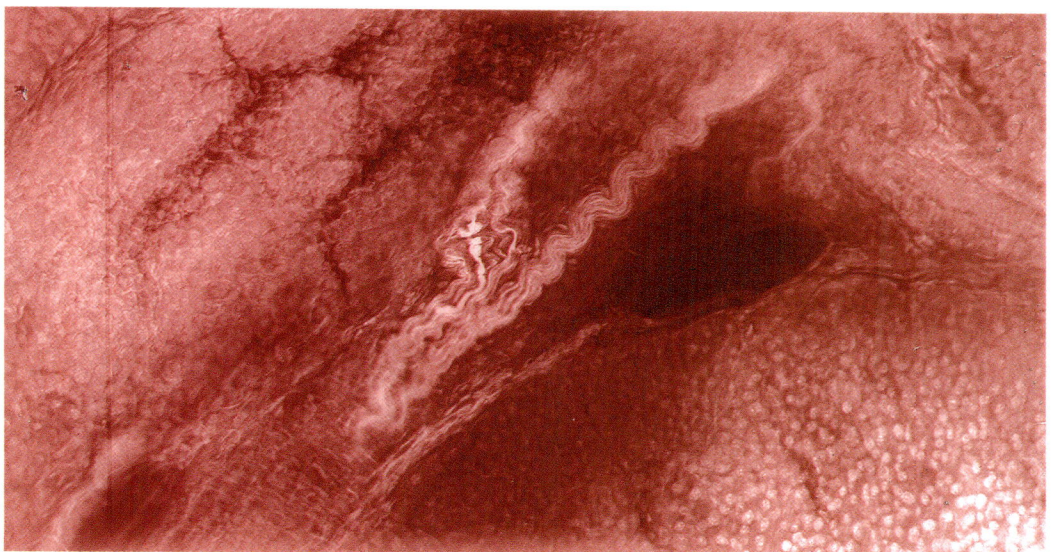

Fig. 13.1.1[2]. The development of fibrous cicatrices in the zone of aseptic necrosis. 20th day after experimental cryosurgical application on pancreas in dog with chronic pancreatitis. Temperature −180°C, exposure time 10–30 sec. Haematoxylin and eosin stain, magnification ×400

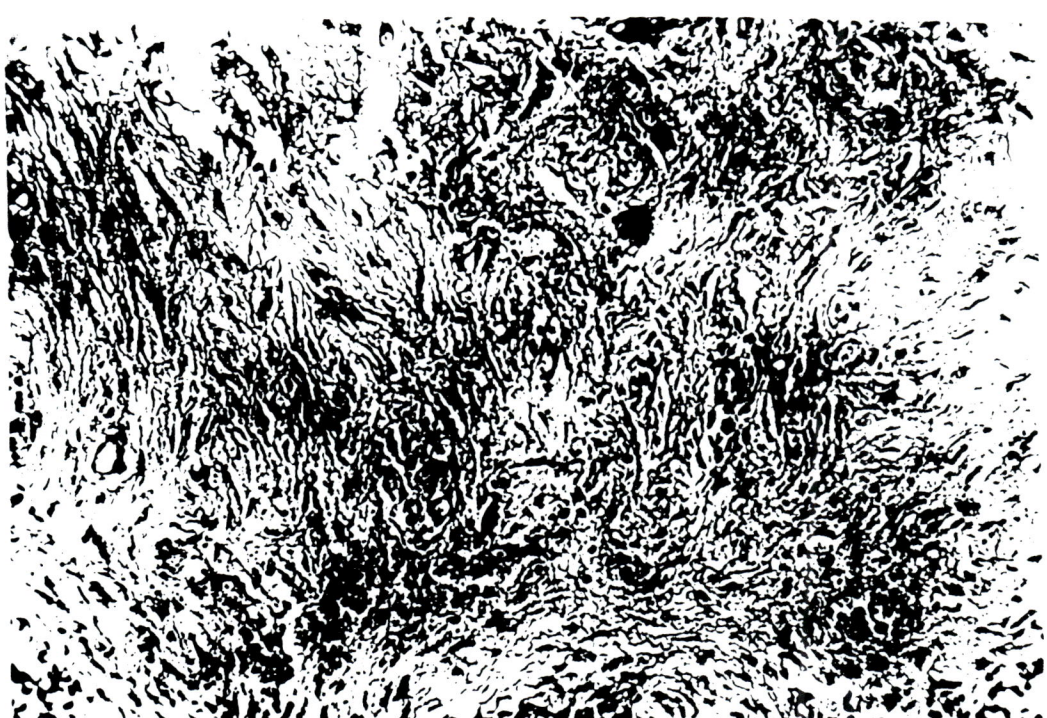

Fig. 13.1.2[2]. Degenerative and destructive changes in neural conductors of pancreas. The 20th day after the experiment. Magnification ×600

**Chapter 13
Abdominal
Cryosurgery:
Pancreas
Cryosurgery**

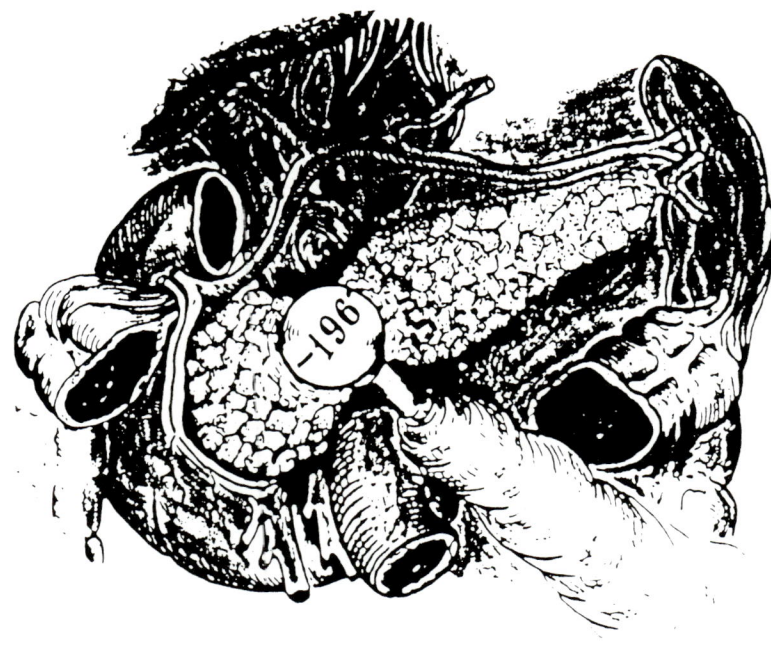

Fig. 13.1.3². 'Key point' for cryosurgery in patients with chronic pancreatitic pain. Schematic view

Fig. 13.1.4². 'Key point' for pseudotumorous pancreatitis and pancreas tumor. Schematic view

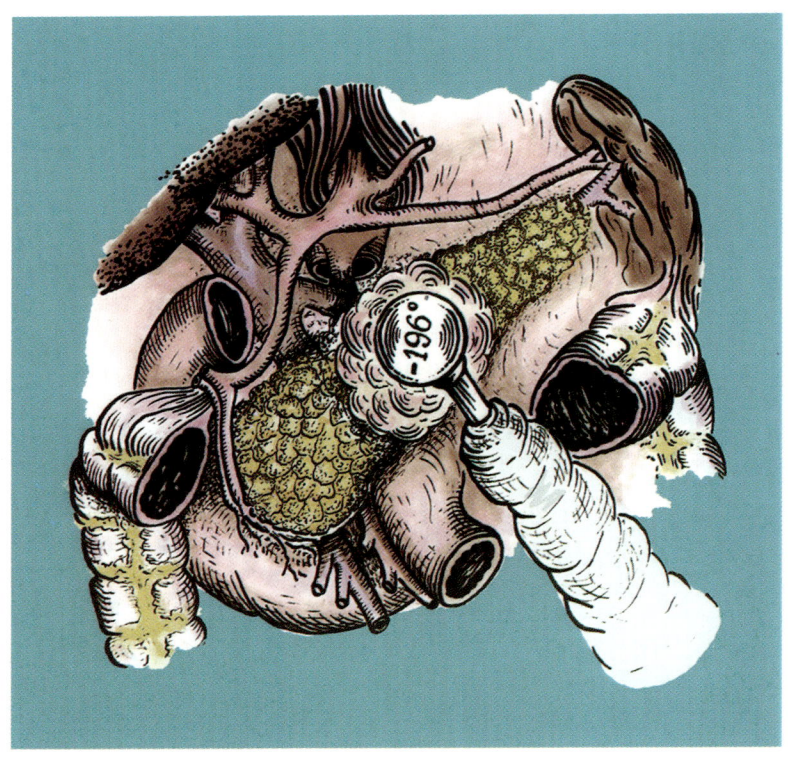

Section F   Clinical Aspects   **293**

**Chapter 13
Abdominal
Cryosurgery:
Pancreas
Cryosurgery**

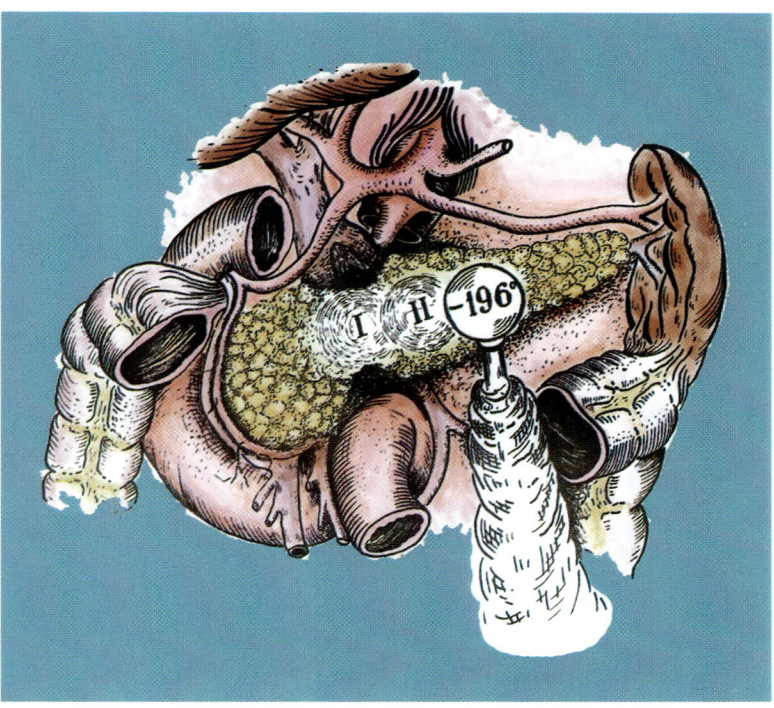

Fig. 13.1.5². Additional points for cryosurgical application in patients with chronic pain due to pseudotumorous pancreatitis. Schematic view

Fig. 13.1.6². Excision of the cyst bed. Schematic view

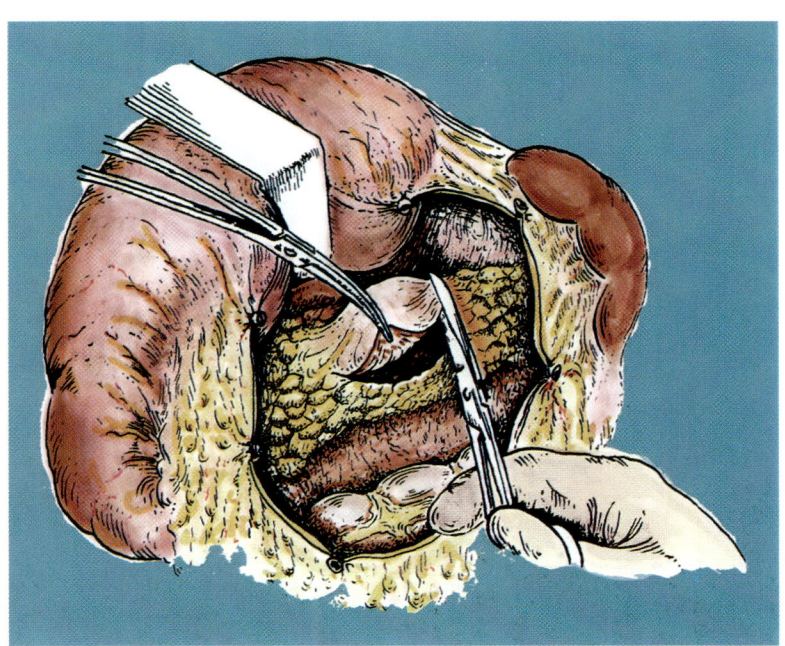

Chapter 13
Abdominal Cryosurgery: Pancreas Cryosurgery

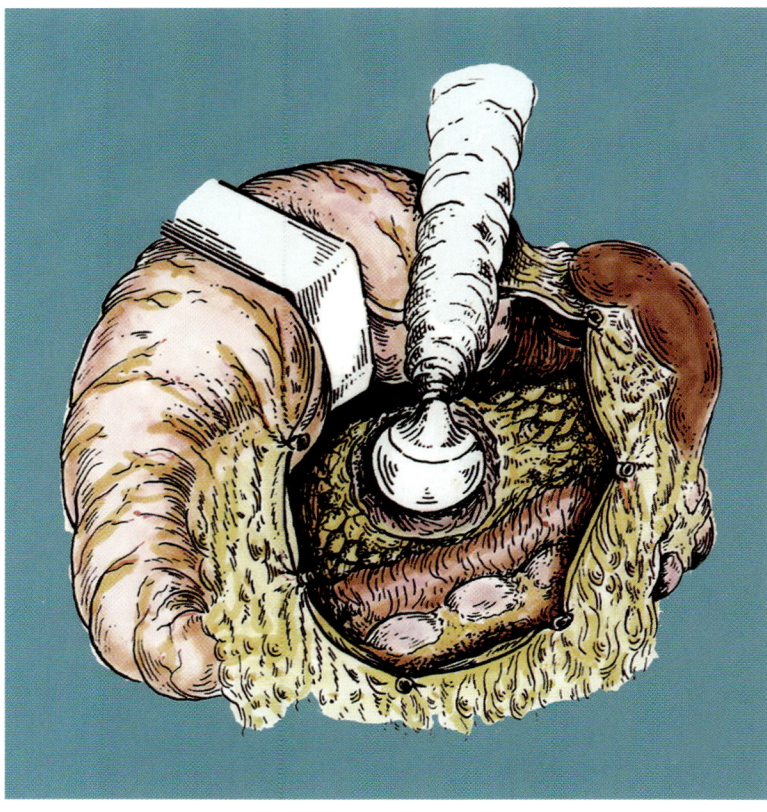

Fig. 13.1.7². Cryodestruction of the cyst bed. Schematic view

Fig. 13.1.8². Tamponade of the epiploon. Schematic view

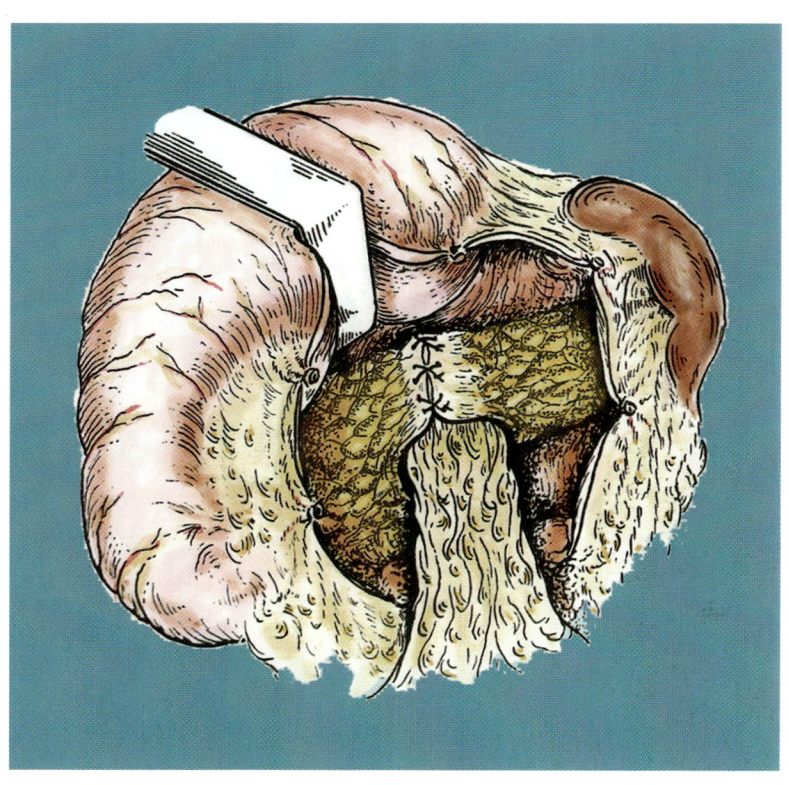

Section F   Clinical Aspects   295

Chapter 13
Abdominal
Cryosurgery:
Pancreas
Cryosurgery

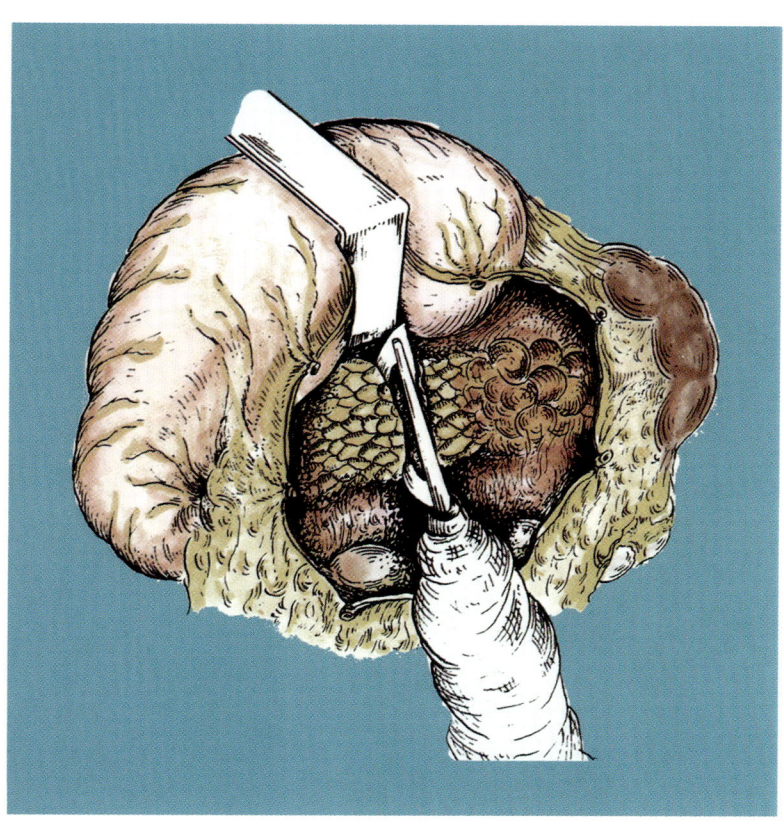

Fig. 13.1.9[2]. Cryoresection of the pancreas. Schematic view

Fig. 13.1.10[2]. Cryodestruction of the remaining part of the pancreas. Schematic view

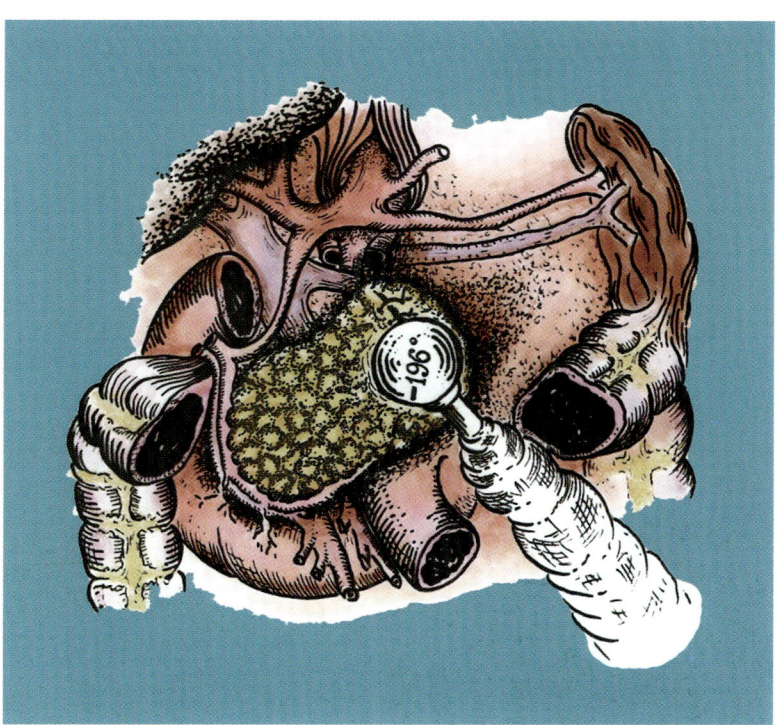

13.2 Advanced Pancreatic Cancer

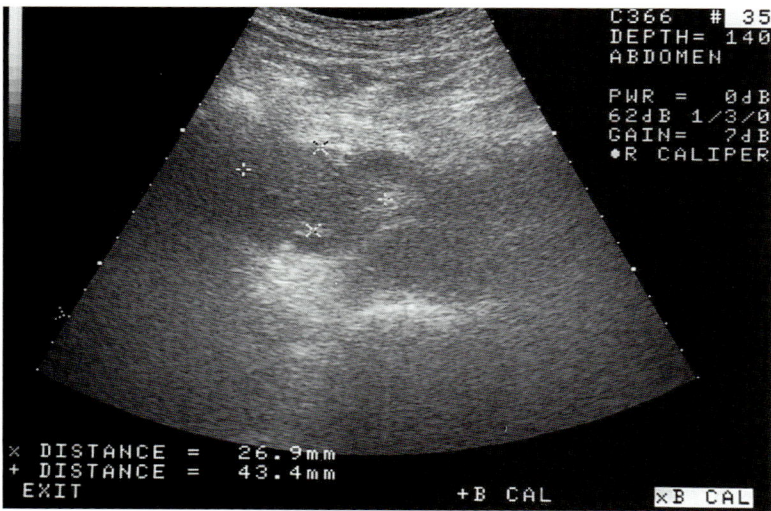

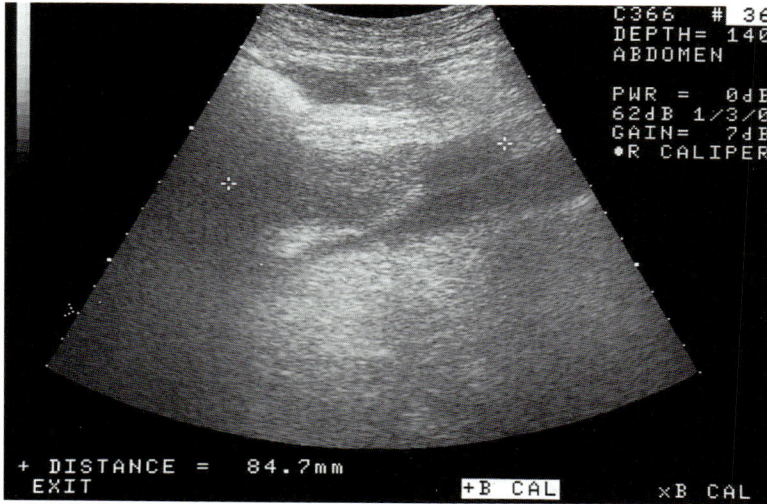

Fig. 13.2.1[1]. Patient with a large pancreas head tumor which is not resectable. Only a palliative hepato-jejunostomy and a gastro-enterostomy was carried out. Prior to the operation a space of approximately 4.3 × 2.7 cm was observed in the area of the pancreas head during a sonography of the upper abdomen (**A**), which extended to the right on the caudal side slightly ventral of the v.cava inferior and measured roughly 9 cm in the cranio-caudal diameter (**B**). The v.cava is somewhat compromised as a result

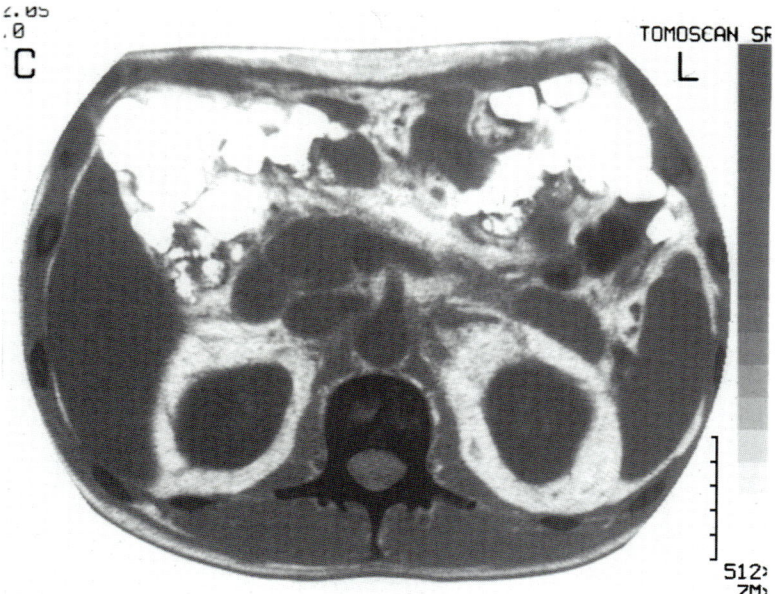

Fig. 13.2.2[1]. Computed tomography (CT) is the mainstay of diagnostic confirmation and evaluation of the extent of cancer of the pancreas. A pancreas tumor is easily demarcated. As shown on the ultrasound, the tumour is located primarily in the head or in the processus ulcinatus area of the pancreas. Obvious mass on CT scan, shown to have normal pancreatic duct

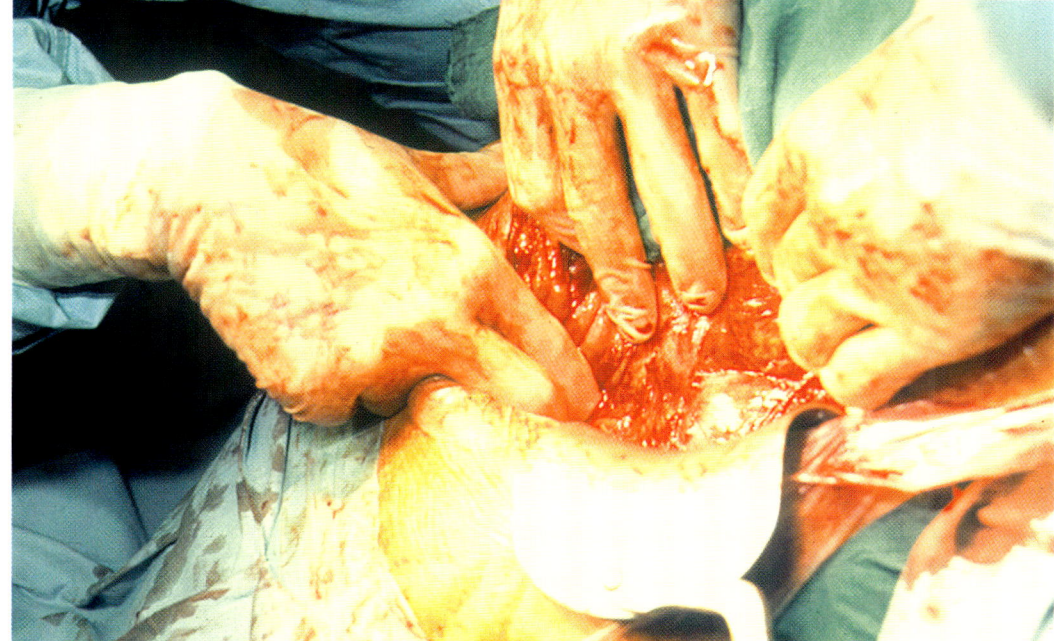

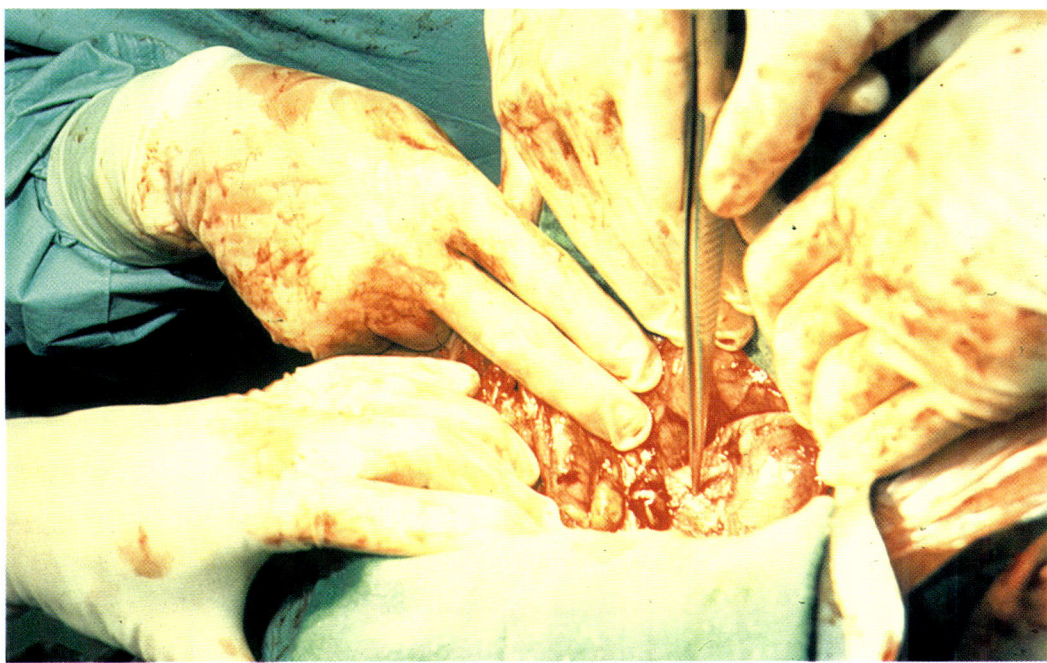

Fig. 13.2.3[1]. A bilateral subcostal incision is used. The abdomen is explored, and metastatic disease of the liver or peritoneal surfaces is ruled out. An extensive Kocher maneuver is performed which permits assessment of the local extent of the tumor in the pancreas head. Intraoperative view (**A–D**)

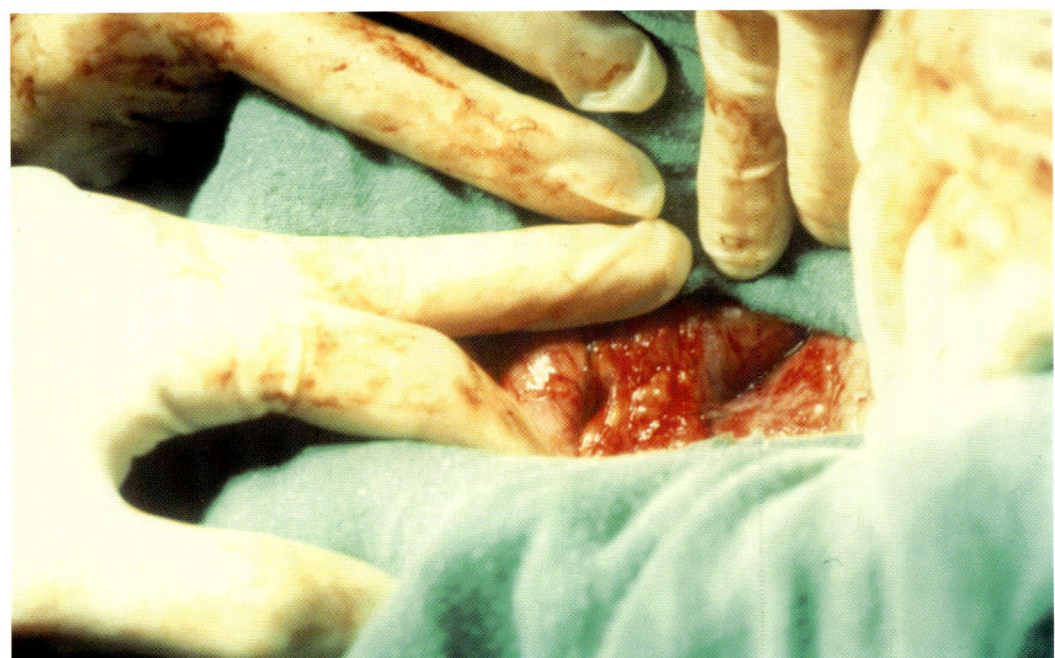

C

Fig. 13.2.3[1]. A bilateral subcostal incision is used. The abdomen is explored, and metastatic disease of the liver or peritoneal surfaces is ruled out. An extensive Kocher maneuver is performed which permits assessment of the local extent of the tumor in the pancreas head. Intraoperative view (**A–D**)

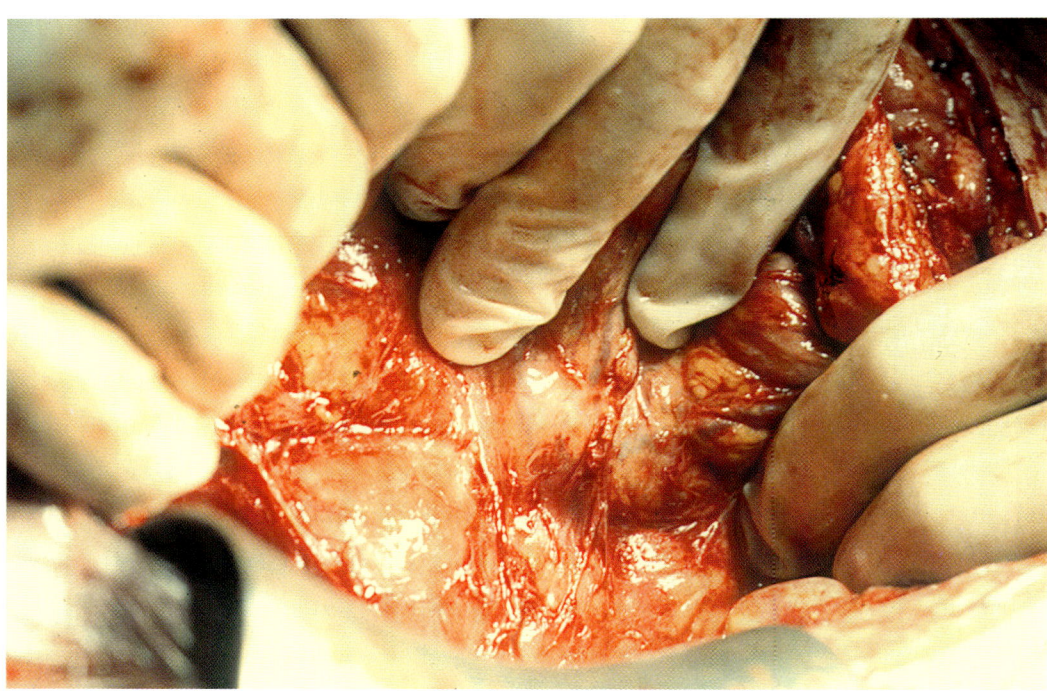

D

Chapter 13 Abdominal Cryosurgery: Pancreas Cryosurgery

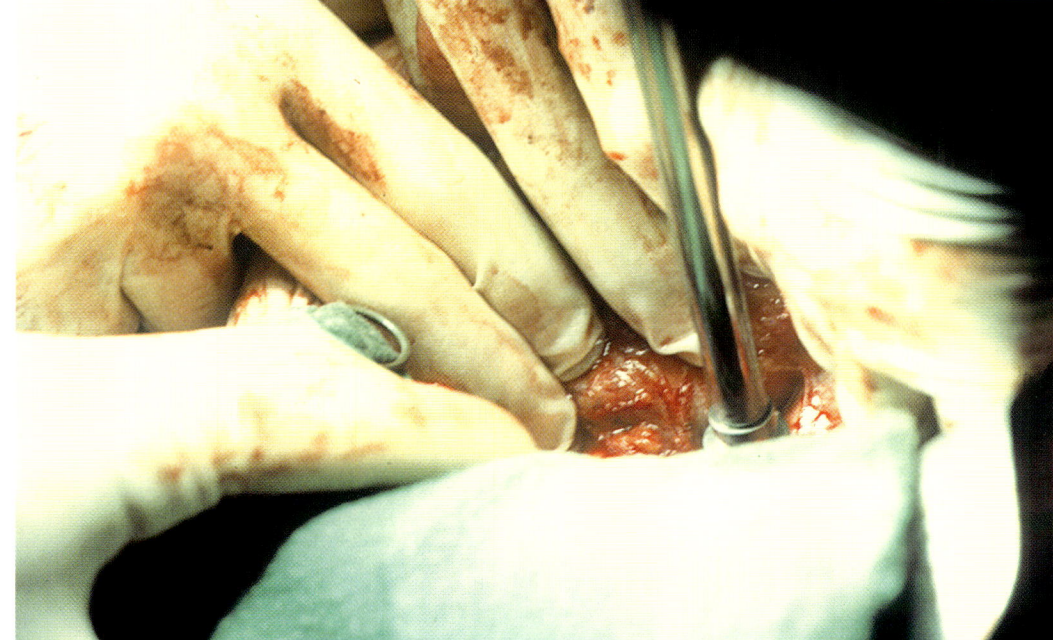

Fig. 13.2.4[1] A, B. Pancreas cryosurgery. A cryoprobe 30 mm in diameter is placed on the tumor mass of the pancreas head at a temperature of −180°C for 10 sec. A single freeze-thaw cycle is used to induce aseptic pancreas tumor cryonecrosis in a patient with advanced, unresectable pancreas head carcinoma

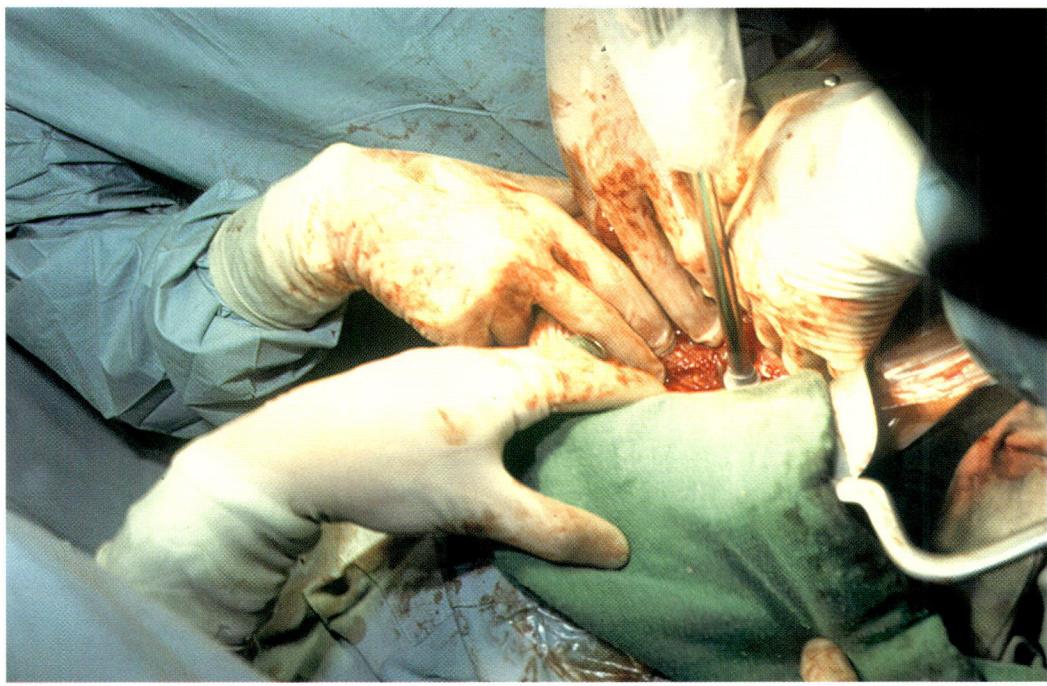

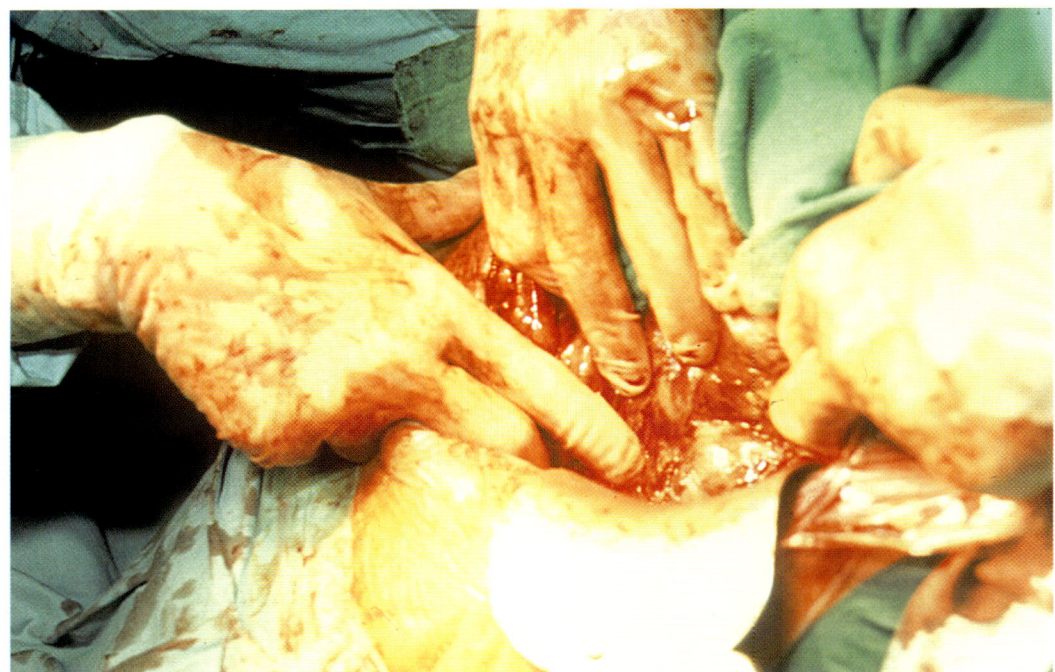

Fig. 13.2.5[1] A, B. Pancreas cryosurgery. Post-cryosurgical view of a cryozone with the ice crater in the middle, and the ice margin with the line of demarcation, immediately after the single cryosurgical session

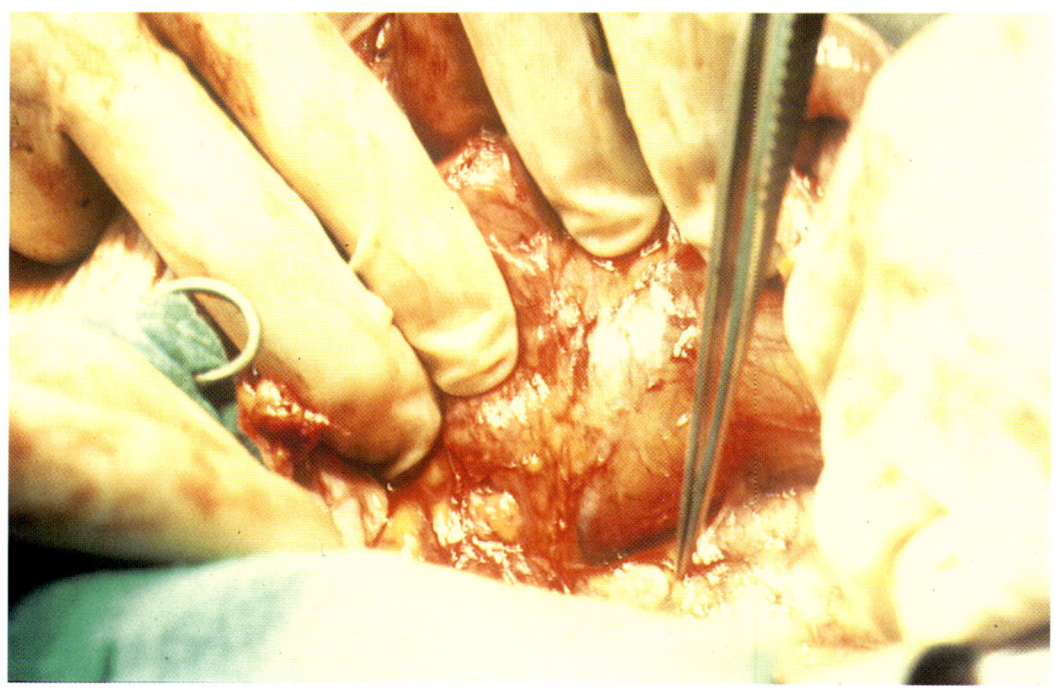

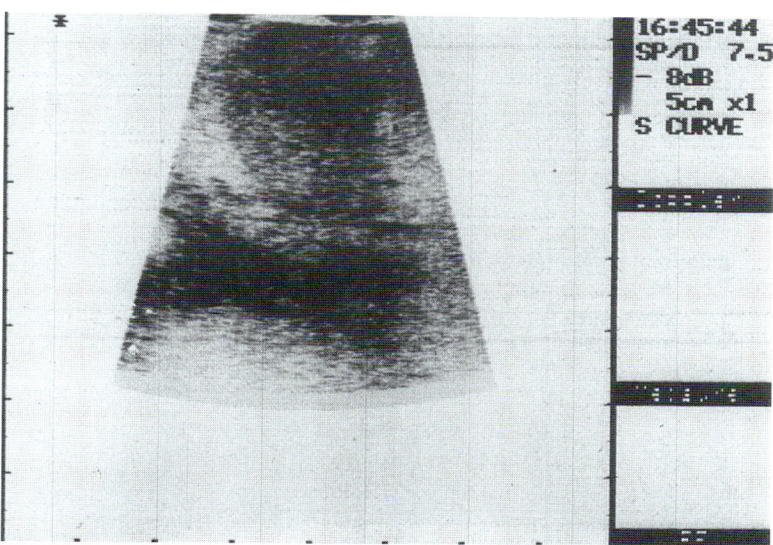

Fig. 13.2.6[1]. Pancreas cryosurgery. Intraoperative ultrasound monitoring of pancreas cryosurgery helps to observe and to control ice ball formation during the freeze-thaw cycle on the pancreas. The ice ball is characterized by bright, echogenic interfaces of ice formation, which correlates with complete tissue destruction

Chapter 13 Abdominal Cryosurgery: Pancreas Cryosurgery

Fig. 13.2.7[1]. Pancreas cryosurgery. Postoperative ultrasound monitoring of pancreas cryosurgery (1st postoperative day). No essential changes from intraoperative monitoring

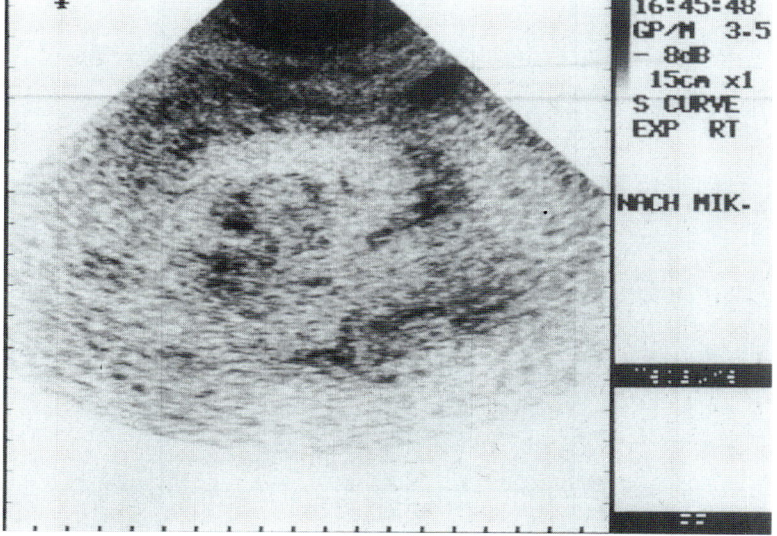

Chapter 13
Abdominal Cryosurgery: Pancreas Cryosurgery

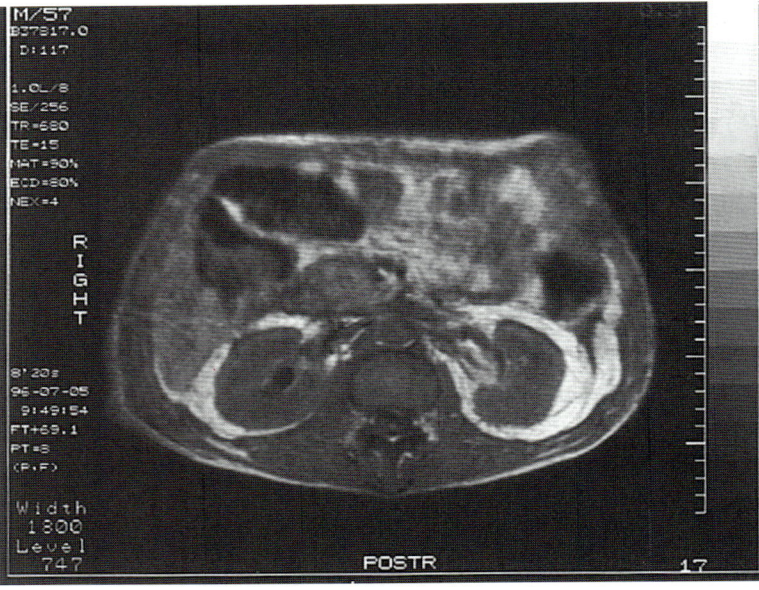

A

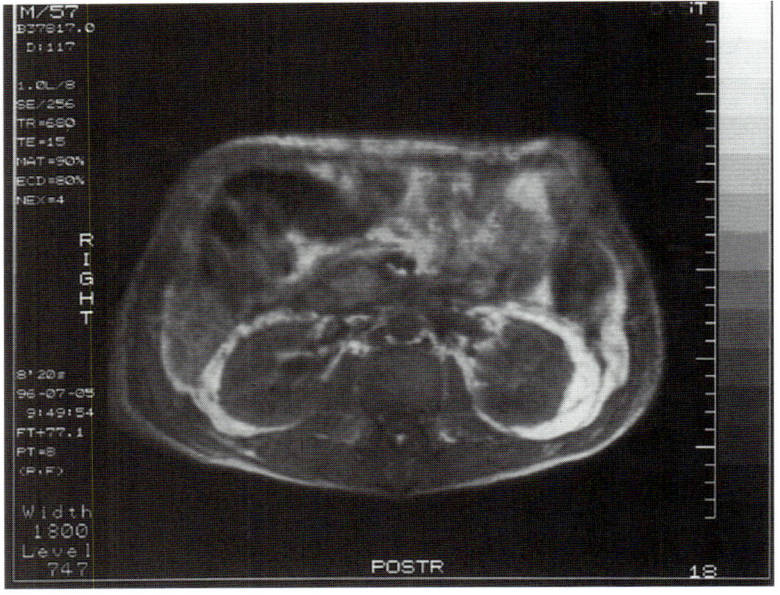

B

Fig. 13.2.8[1] A, B. Pancreas cryosurgery. MRI monitoring on 7th postoperative day. In comparison with the CT examination prior to the operation, the size of the pancreas head tumor has decreased. The head of the pancreas is clearly smaller, above all in the caudal area, and measures roughly 2.5 cm in diameter (in the examination prior to the operation it was approximately 5 cm). Otherwise the pancreas image is normal

Pulmonary Cryosurgery

Jean-Paul Homasson[1], Omar Maiwand[2] and Daniel Luna Sabate[3]

14.0 Introduction

The use of cryosurgery in thoracic medicine is a relatively recent development compared to other medical specialties where the lesions are easily accessible. In fact, thoracic medicine is reliant on endoscopes with a very narrow bore in order to treat tracheal or bronchial lesions. The cryoprobes must be of a sufficiently narrow diameter in order to pass through the lumen of rigid or fibreoptic bronchoscopes.

After initial experimental interest in the technique in the United States between 1975 and 1982 it was discontinued in favor of the laser. In 1986 Scientific researchers in France, Great Britain, Italy and in the former USSR in the field of pulmonary cryosurgery started to use and further develop the technique for the treatment of bronchiogenic tumors and endobronchial metastases, again using European devices. Since then it is being used more frequently in other countries. Tracheobronchial cryosurgery recently underwent a renaissance in the USA after the Food and Drug Administration (FDA) agreed to the use of European materials.

Tracheobronchial cryosurgery may be carried out using either rigid or flexible probes. At present most cryoprobes use nitrous oxide as a cooling agent, according to the Joule Thomson effect. *Nevertheless, very powerful cryoprobes use liquid nitrogen.*

The freeze-thaw procedures are carried out under direct vision via the endoscope. The most suitable type of lesion is polypoid either, benign or malignant. The metallic tip of the cryoprobe is pushed into the tumor, which produces circumferential freezing of maximal volume. After three freeze-thaw cycles the probe is then moved and another three cycles carried out in the adjoining area. The procedure is continued until the entire visible part of the lesion has been frozen. With infiltrating lesions, cryosurgical session can be performed using lateral tangential contact.

Cryosurgery may be used to treat symptoms such as hemoptysis. Freezing has a hemostatic, but not always immediate effect. Dyspnea is also a frequent symptom. However, at present it must be stated that the fact that cryosurgery has a delayed effect in relieving bronchial obstructions means that it should not be used as emergency treatment in acute respiratory distress, especially if due to tracheal obstruction. Most lesions treated are malignant tumors. They may be treated several times and this treatment is clearly indicated for palliation in these cases. Benign tumors are well suited to cryosurgery as good results are generally obtained. Granulation tissues are also excellent indications for cryosurgery.

The results of pulmonary cryosurgery are judged by several means, endoscopic appearance, clinical criteria, radiological changes, changes in respiratory function and histological appearance. Cryosurgery is a palliative treatment of bronchial tumors, and in these cases the overall results are favorable in 70–85% of all cases according to standard criteria used to measure performance.

Cryosurgery is a simple and efficient method, easy to perform, without complications and relatively inexpensive.

Chapter 14
Pulmonary Cryosurgery

14.1 Bronchiogenic Tumors and Endobronchial Metastases

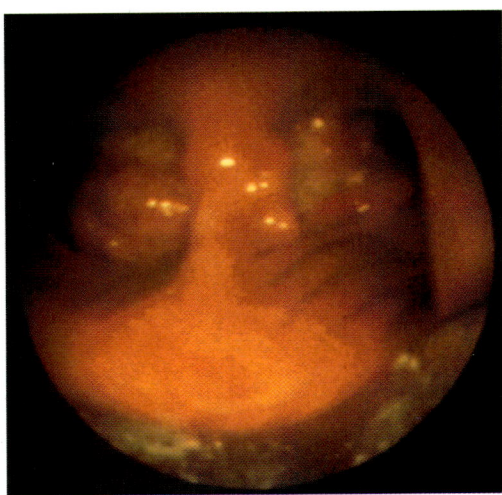

Fig. 14.1.1[1]. Squamous cell carcinoma (carina) partially obstructing both main bronchi. No respiratory distress

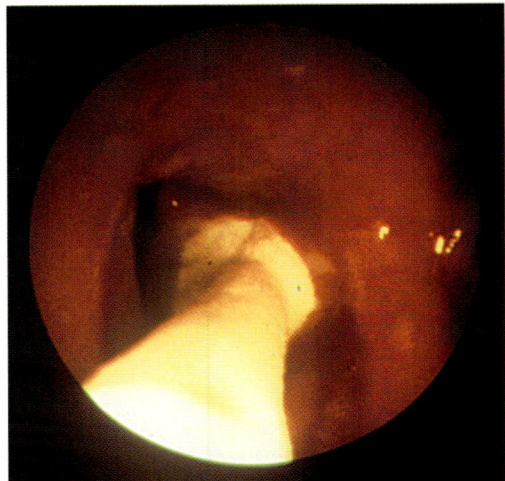

Fig. 14.1.2[1]. Cryosurgery of tumor (left main bronchus)

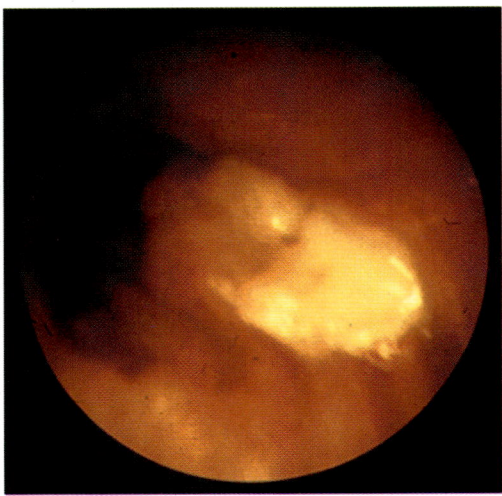

Fig. 14.1.3[1]. Appearance of left main bronchus one week later showing sloughed area and untreated tumor

Section F Clinical Aspects

**Chapter 14
Pulmonary
Cryosurgery**

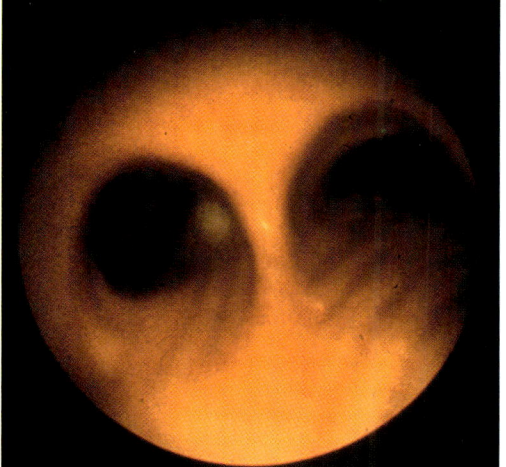

Fig. 14.1.4[1]. Appearance of carina 3 weeks after the last treatment of the two main bronchi

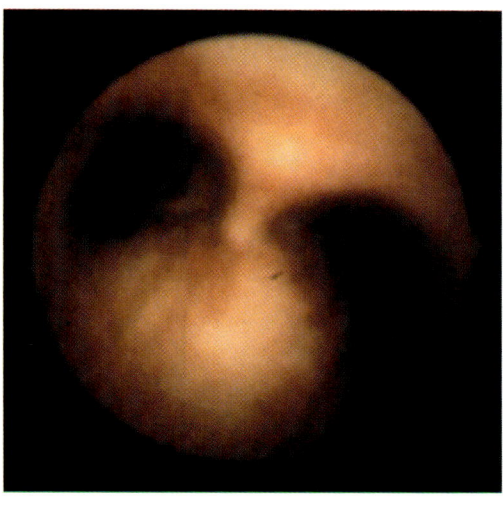

Fig. 14.1.5[1]. Appearance of carina 18 months later, and after additional radiotherapy following cryotherapy. Complete eradication of the tumor histologically confirmed. Unfortunately the patient died of metastatic disease around this time

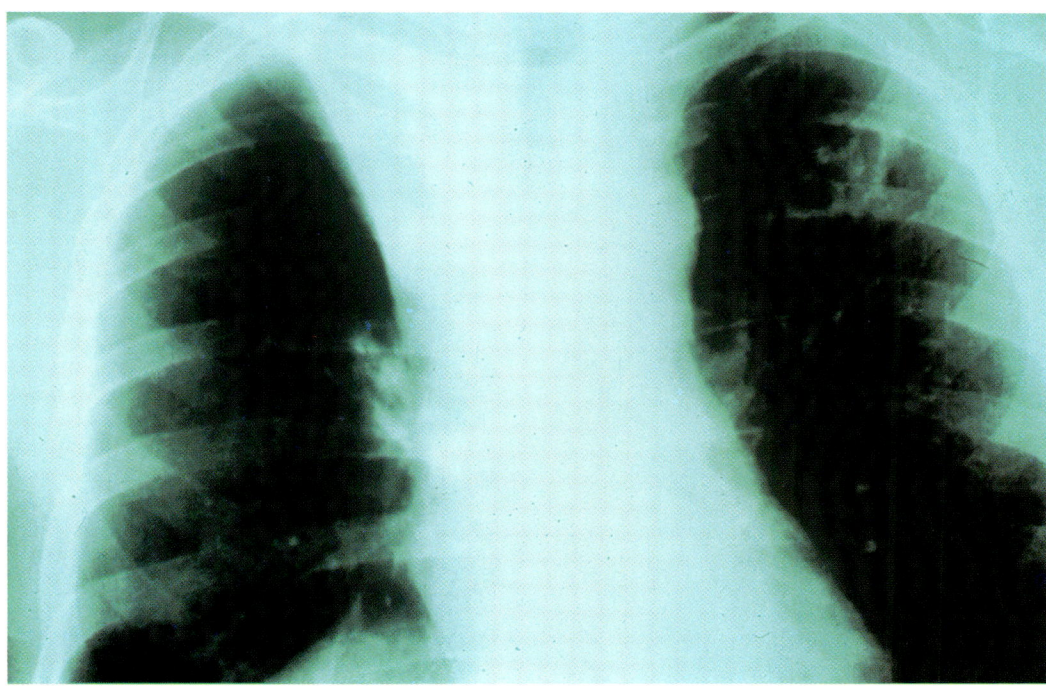

Fig. 14.1.6[1]. Collapse of right upper lobe

**Chapter 14
Pulmonary
Cryosurgery**

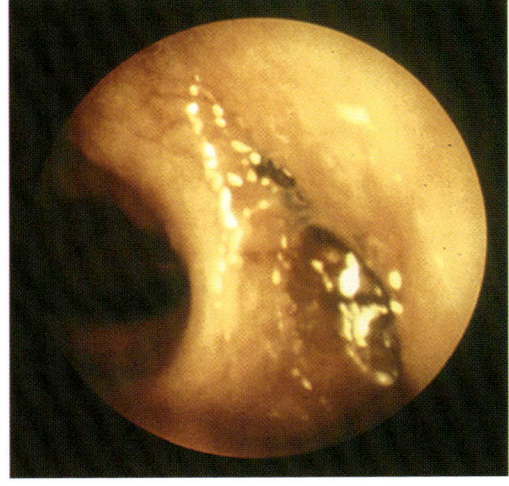

Fig. 14.1.7[1]. Squamous cell carcinoma obstructing the right upper lobe bronchus

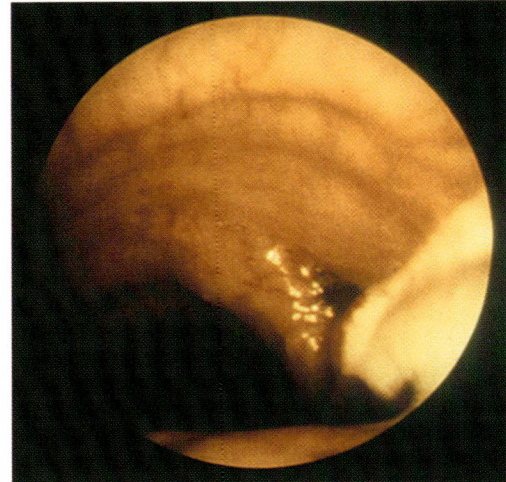

Fig. 14.1.8[1]. Tumor being frozen

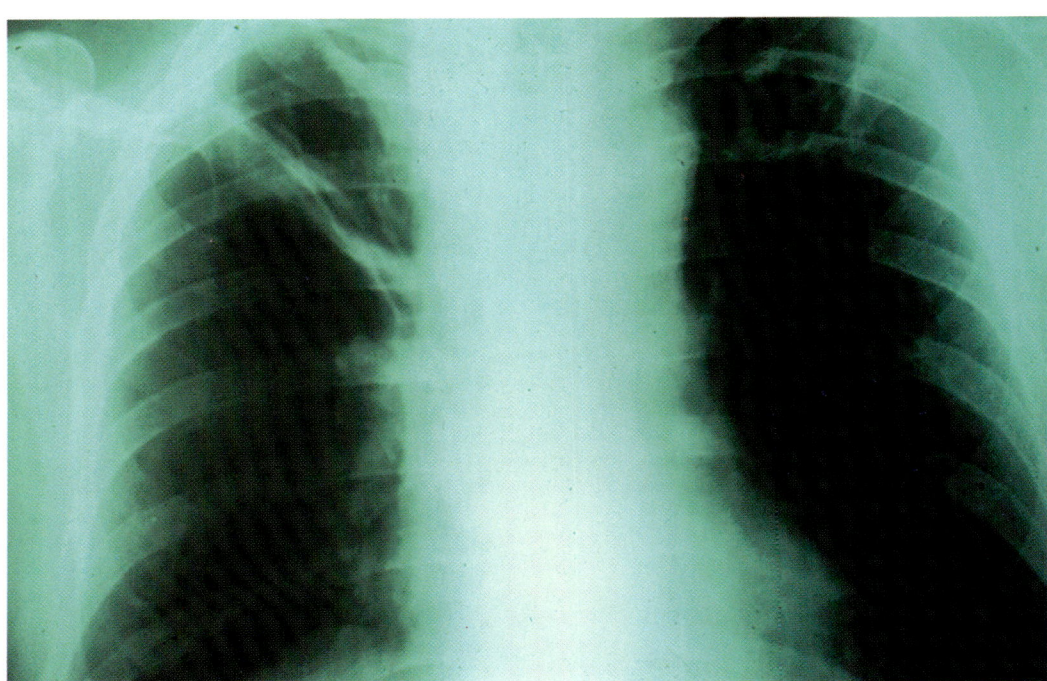

Fig. 14.1.9[1]. Radiological appearance showing reventilation 10 days later

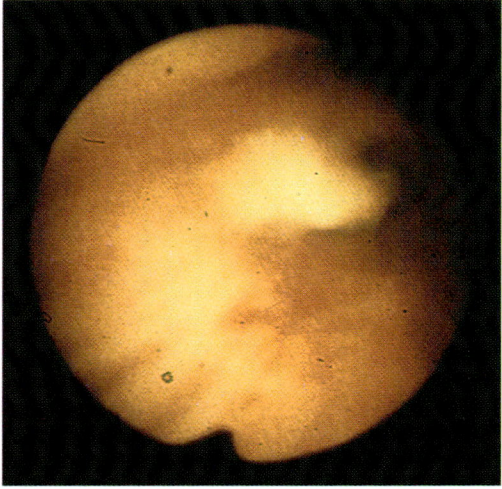

Fig. 14.1.10[1]. Follow-up fiberoptic bronchoscopy ten days later showing small slough

Section F Clinical Aspects

Chapter 14
Pulmonary
Cryosurgery

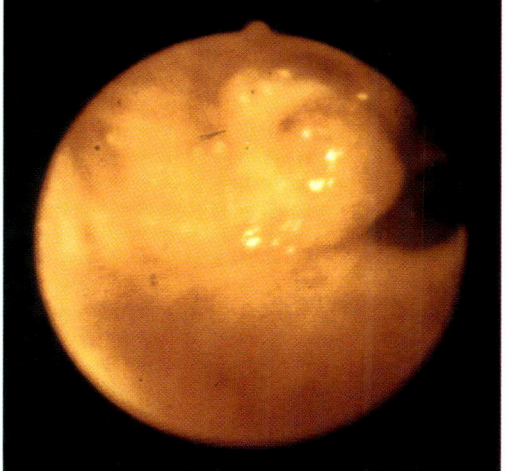

Fig. 14.1.11[1]. Leiomyoma in apical bronchus of right lower lobe

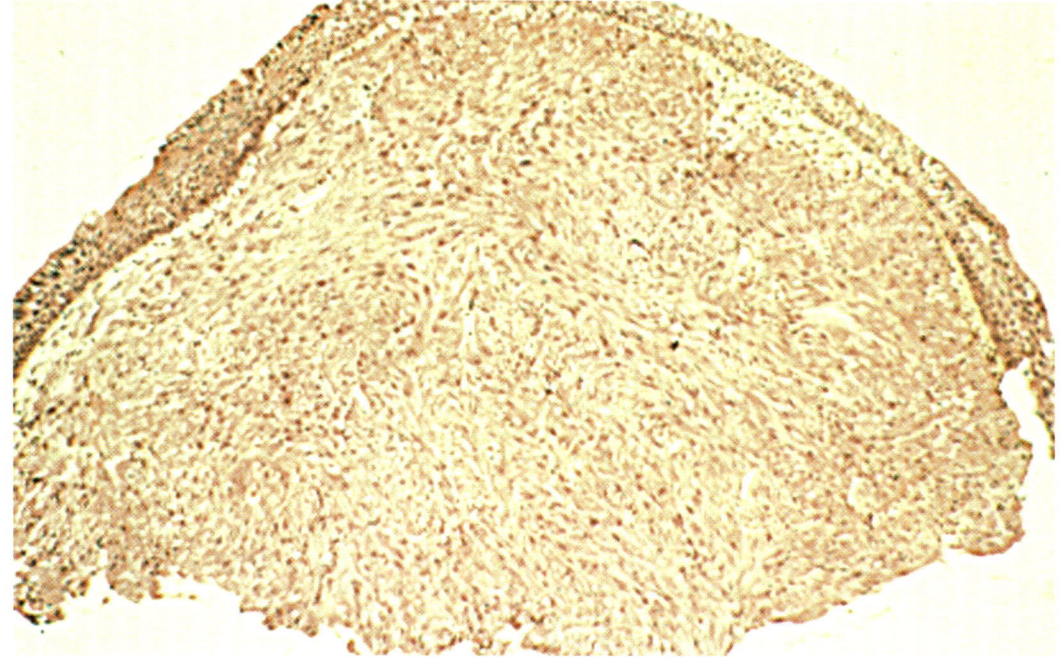

Fig. 14.1.12[1]. Histological appearance of biopsy

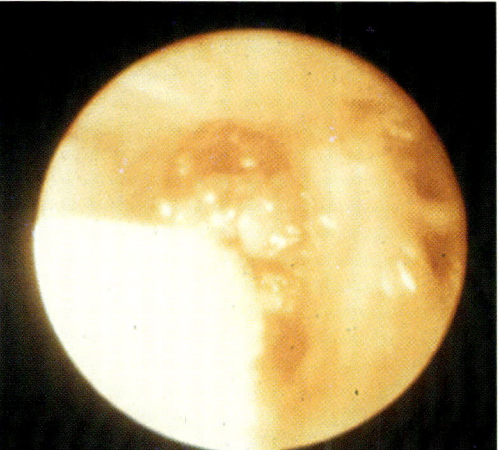

Fig. 14.1.13[1]. The tumor being frozen (flexible probe)

Chapter 14
Pulmonary
Cryosurgery

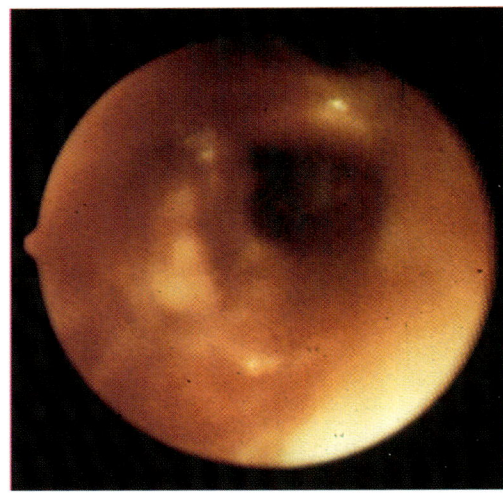

Fig. 14.1.14[1]. Appearance following slough removal, one week later

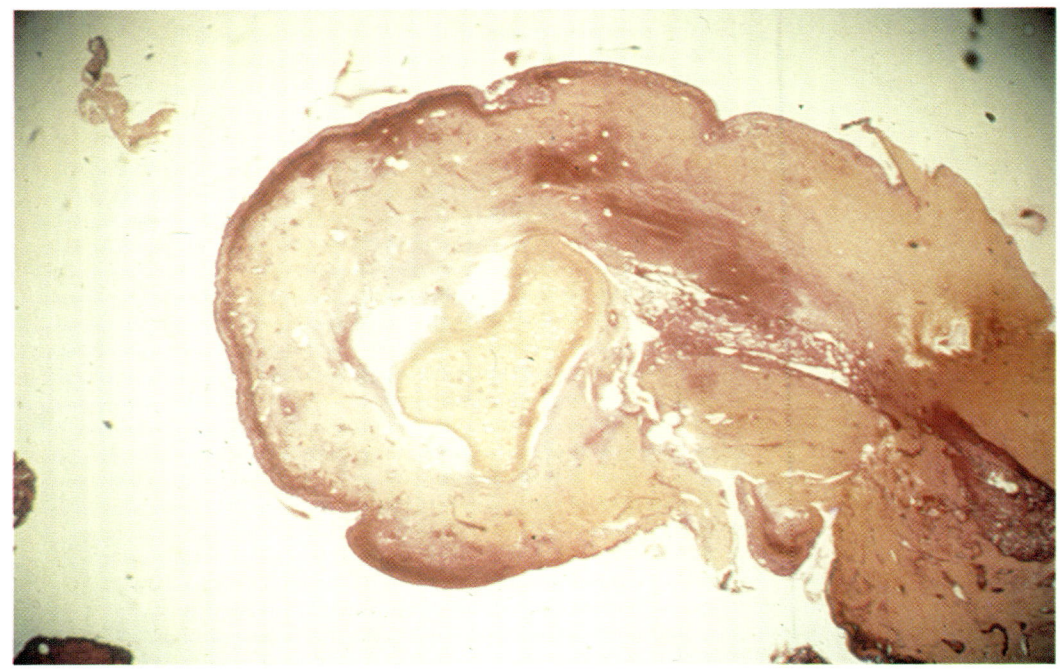

Fig. 14.1.15[1]. Histological appearance of slough. Entire destruction of tissues

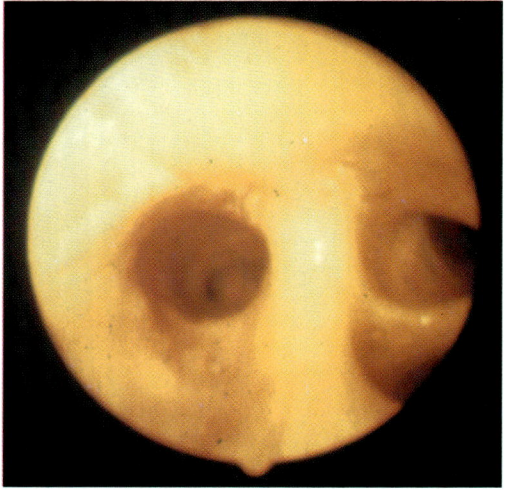

Fig. 14.1.16[1]. Appearance 6 months after treatment. No recurrence

Section F Clinical Aspects

Chapter 14
Pulmonary
Cryosurgery

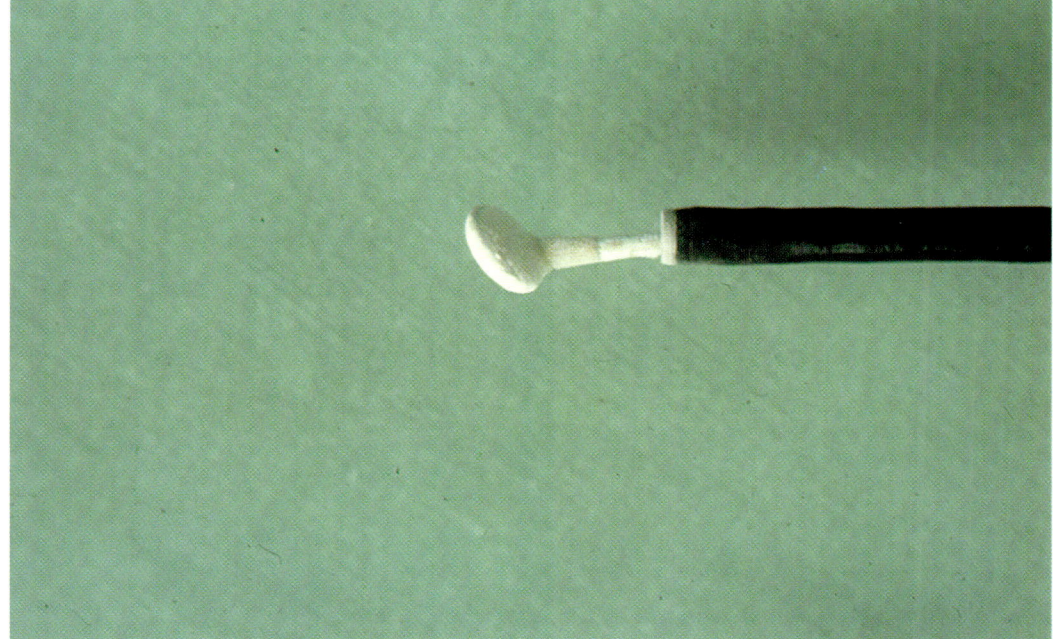

A

Fig. 14.1.17[1]. Extraction of foreign bodies. **A** Retrieval of inhaled pill. **B** Removal of slough using cryoadherence

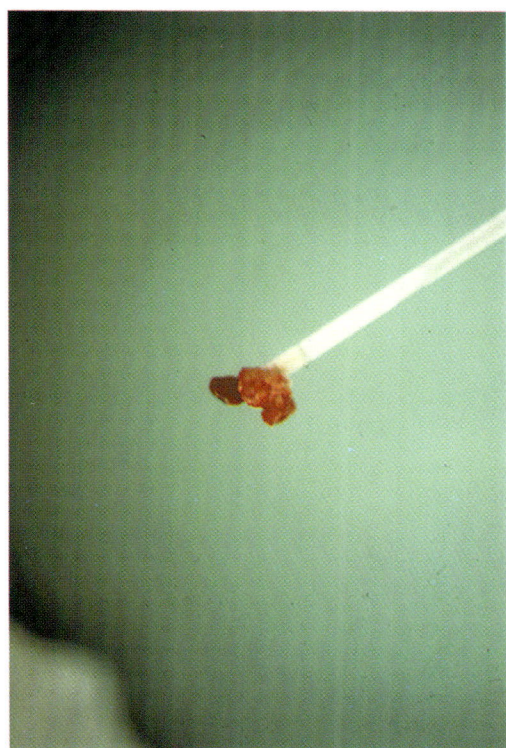

B

Chapter 14
Pulmonary
Cryosurgery

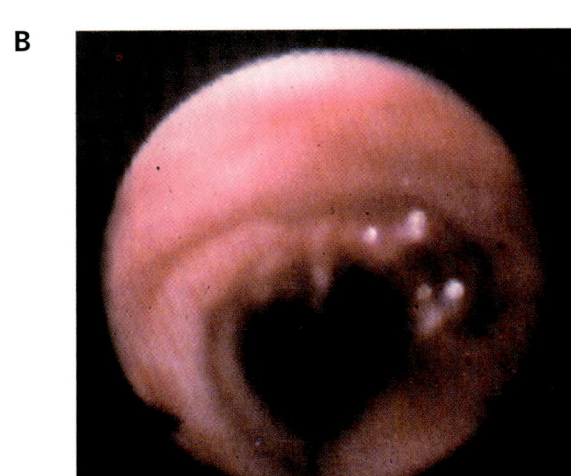

Fig. 14.1.18². Carcinoma of trachea. Before (A) and after (B) cryosurgery

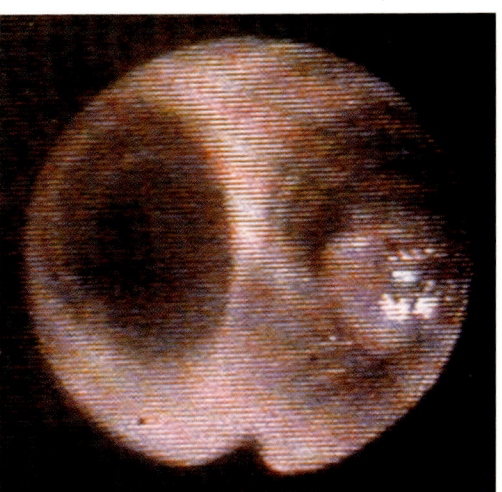

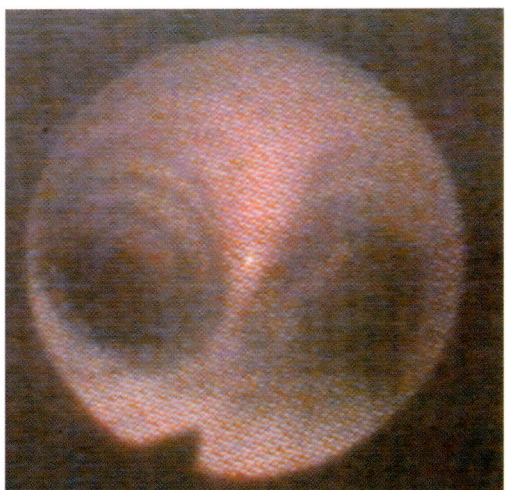

Fig. 14.1.19². Carcinoma of right main bronchus. Before (A) and after (B) cryosurgery

Section F   Clinical Aspects   311

Chapter 14
Pulmonary
Cryosurgery

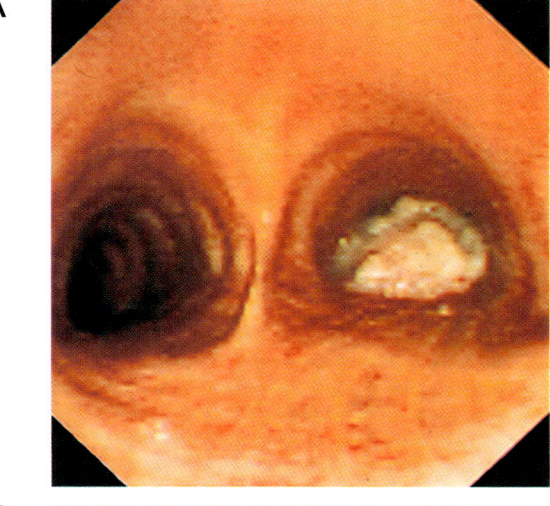

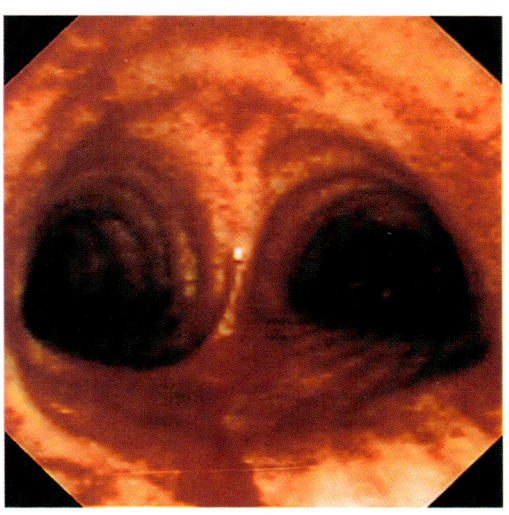

Fig. 14.1.20[2]. Carcinoid tumor of right main bronchus. Before (**A**) and after (**B**) cryosurgery

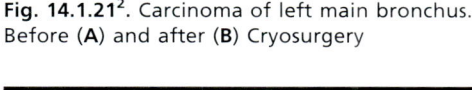

Fig. 14.1.21[2]. Carcinoma of left main bronchus. Before (**A**) and after (**B**) Cryosurgery

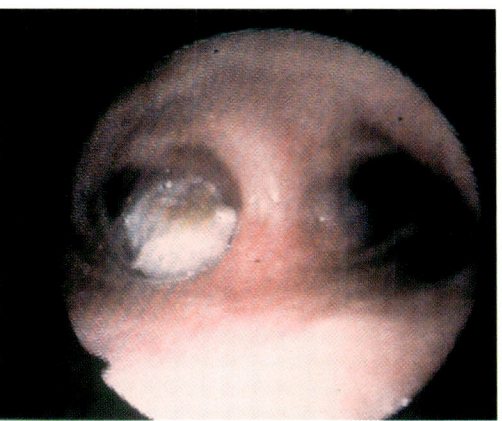

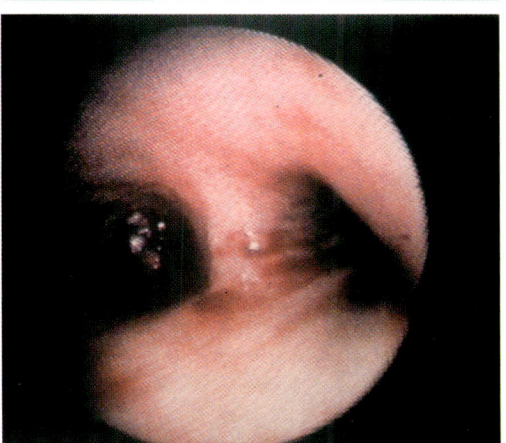

Chapter 14
Pulmonary
Cryosurgery

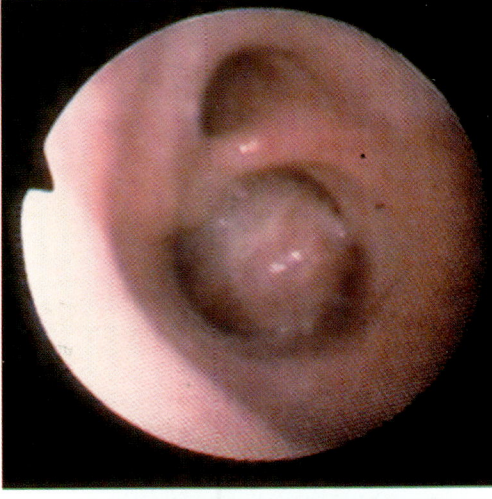

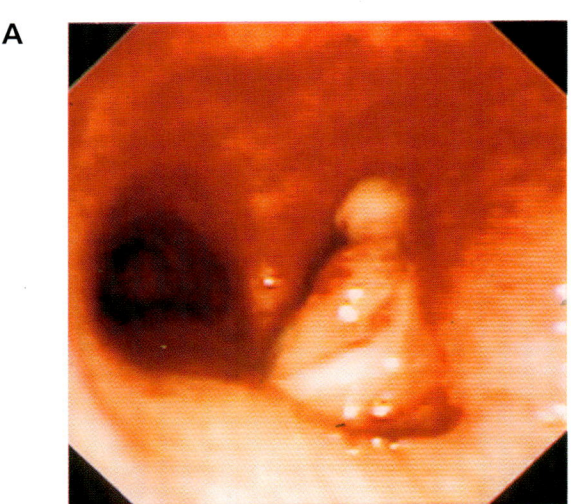

Fig. 14.1.23[2]. Carcinoma of lower end of trachea. Before (**A**) and after (**B**) cryosurgery

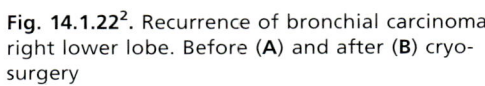

Fig. 14.1.22[2]. Recurrence of bronchial carcinoma right lower lobe. Before (**A**) and after (**B**) cryosurgery

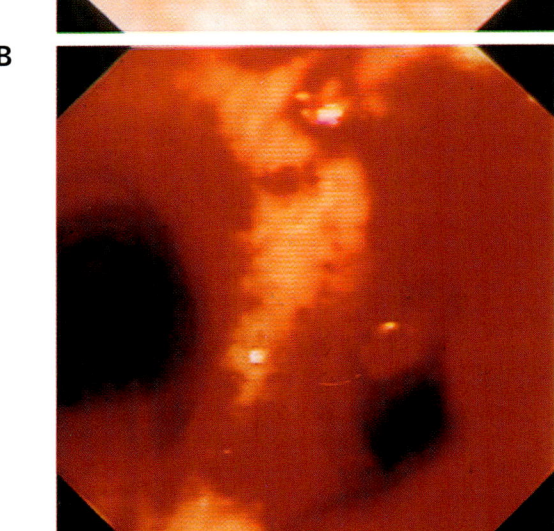

Section F   Clinical Aspects   313

Chapter 14
Pulmonary
Cryosurgery

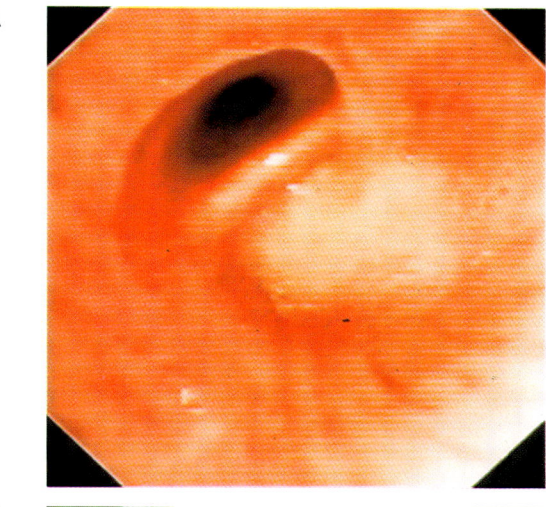

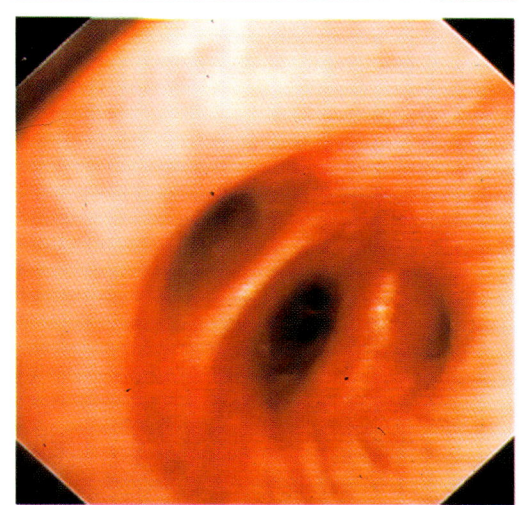

Fig. 14.1.24[2]. Carcinoma of right lower Lobe. Before (**A**) and after (**B**) cryosurgery

Fig. 14.1.25[2]. Carcinoma of right lower lobe. Before (**A**) and after (**B**) cryosurgery

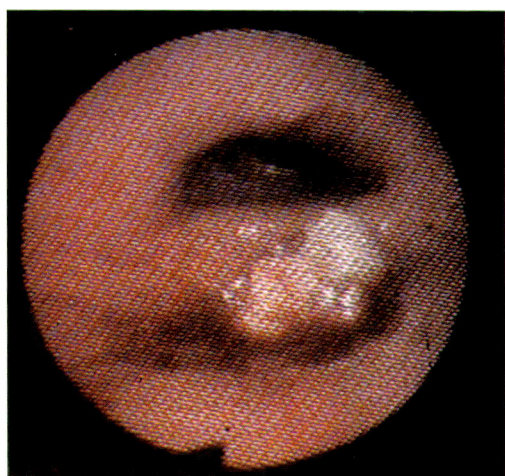

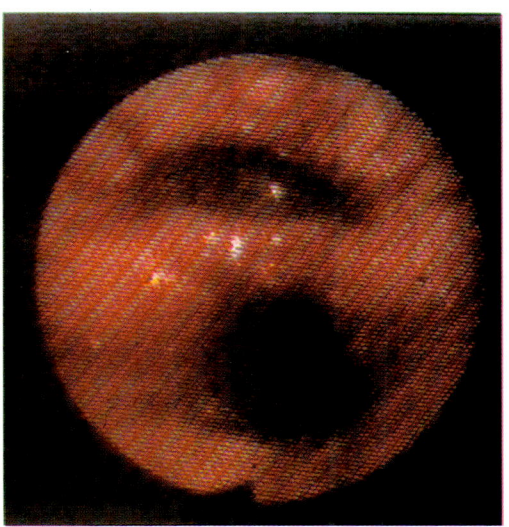

Chapter 14
Pulmonary
Cryosurgery

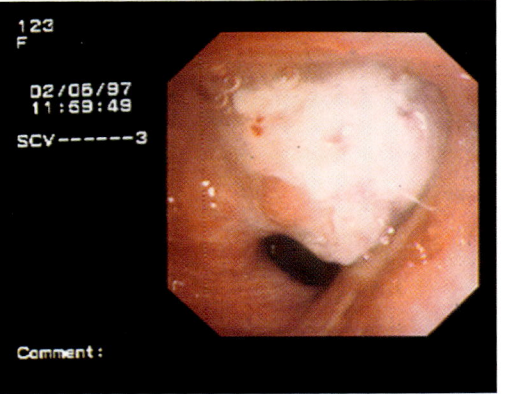

Fig. 14.1.27[2]. Carcinoma, multiple sites: right upper lobe and right intermedius bronchus. Before (A) and after (B) cryosurgery

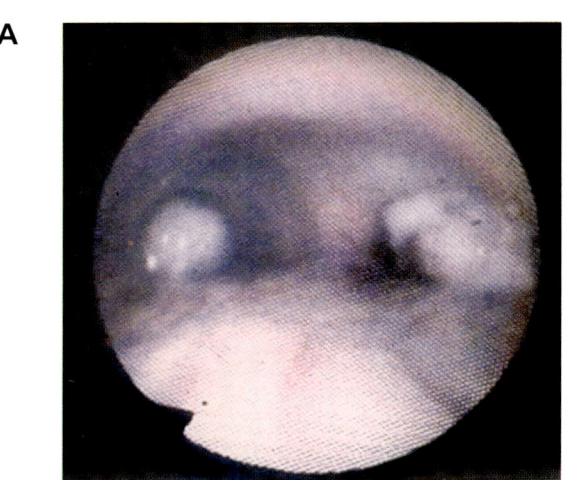

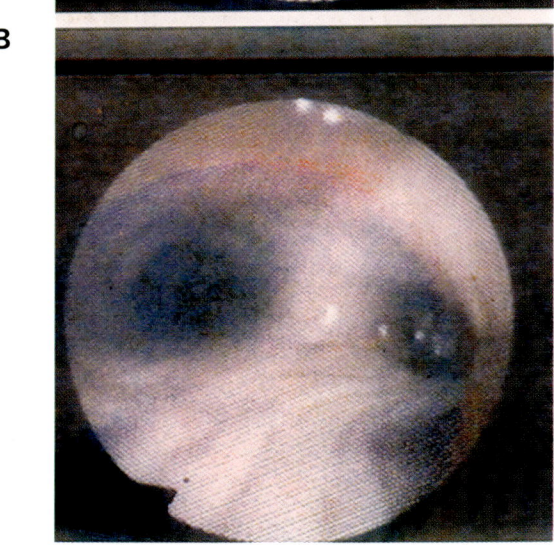

Fig. 14.1.26[2]. Carcinoma of left main bronchus. Before (A) and after (B) cryosurgery

Section F   Clinical Aspects   **315**

Chapter 14
Pulmonary
Cryosurgery

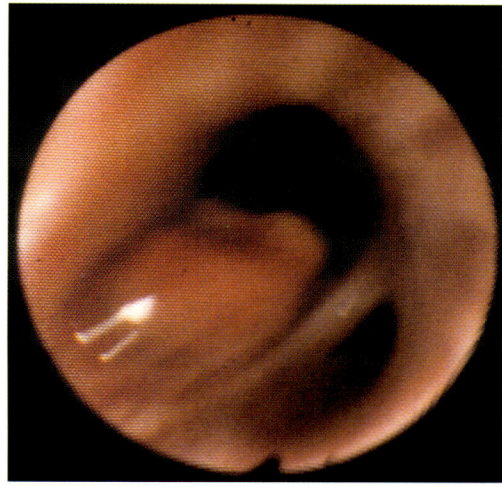

A

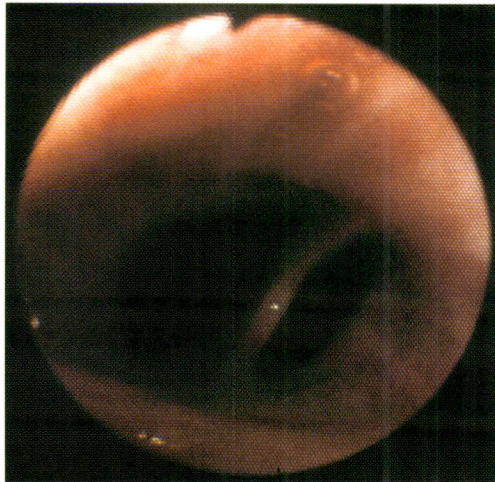

B

Fig. 14.1.28³. Endobronchial metastasis in a 72-year-old woman, who was operated on for adenocarcinoma of rectum 5 years earlier. Bronchoscopy. **A** Partial blocking in the right lower lobe due to tumor. Histological appearance: metastases of adenocarcinoma into the intestinal area. **B** 1 month later after endoscopic cryosurgery

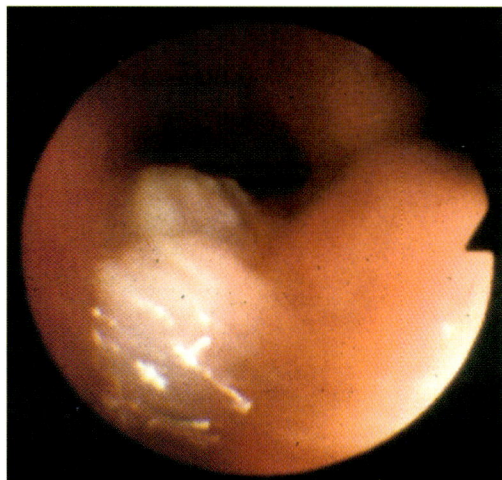

A

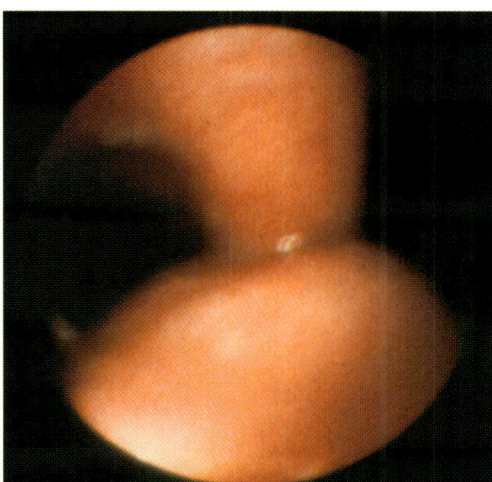

B

Fig. 14.1.29³. Epidermoid tumor in a 75-year-old man. Radiography: right hilar mass, mediastinal lymph nodes, carinal nodes. Emphysema. Inoperable. Bronchoscopy. **A** Necrosing tumor in the right stem bronchus. Biopsy: squamous cell carcinoma poorly differentiated. **B** 3 months after endoscopic cryosurgery

Chapter 14
Pulmonary
Cryosurgery

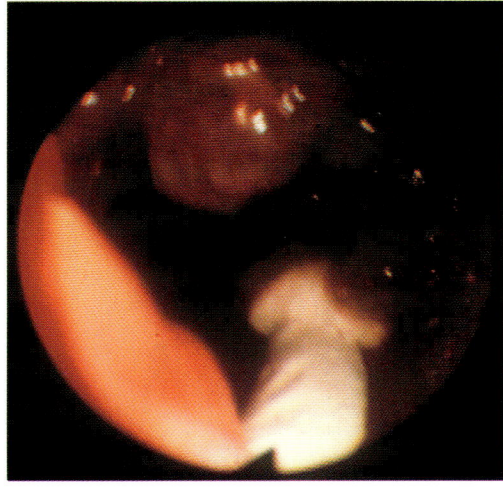
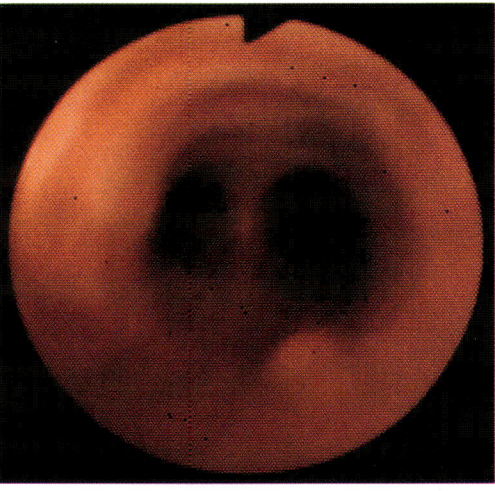

Fig. 14.1.30[3]. Papillomatosis of trachea in a 26-year-old woman. Several tracheotomies. Treatment with Yag-laser. Early recurrence after endoscopic laser treatment. Endoscopic cryosurgical treatment through the tracheal orifice for a period of over two years. Treatment every 4–6 months. **A** Tracheal papillomatosis. Treatment: cryoprobe freezing of a papilloma. Some papillomas were previously treated with the electrocautery. **B** 10 days after the cryosurgical operation

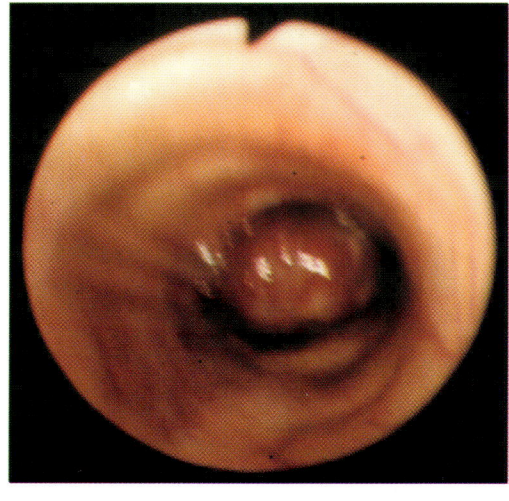

Fig. 14.1.31[3]. Typical tumor carcinoid in a 76-year-old woman. Bronchoscopy: vascularized tumor in the left mainstem bronchus. Indication: cryosurgery before biopsy to avoid bleeding/fatal hemoptysis. **A** Tumor before cryosurgery. After the cryosurgery. Biopsy without bleeding. **B** 10 days after the cryosurgery. **C** Follow-up after 12 months. Bronchoscopy – normal

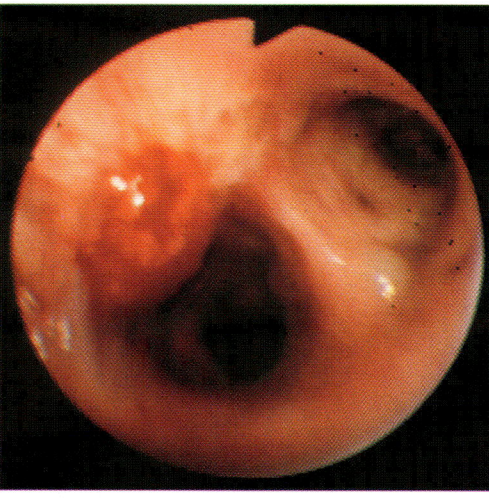
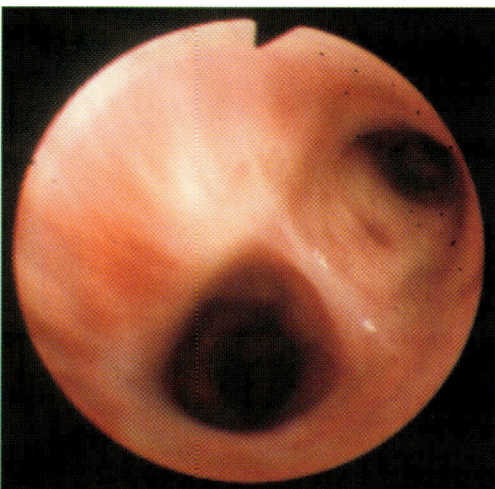

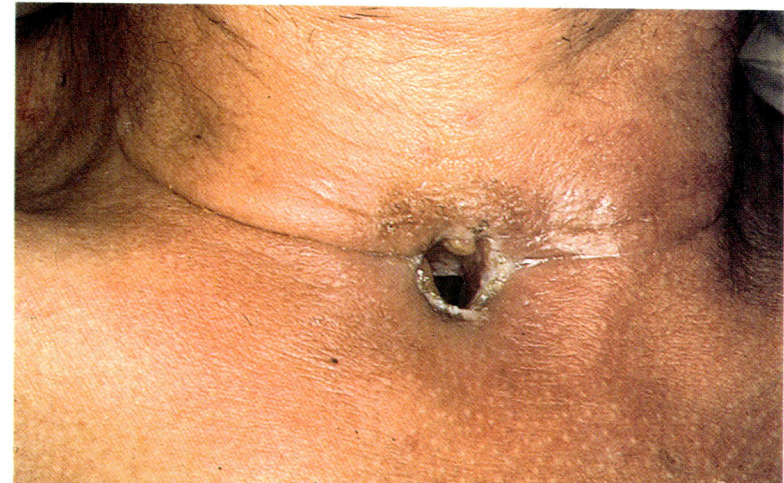

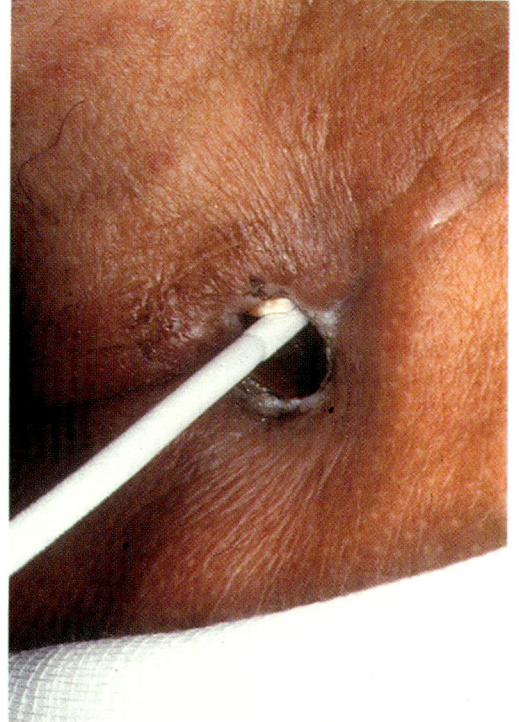

Fig. 14.1.32³. Granulomas post-tracheostomy in a 68-year-old man with cancer of the larynx. Tracheostomy. Stridor. Bronchoscopy: two granulomas, one in the middle of the trachea and another in the entrance of the orifice of tracheostomy. **A** Granuloma in entrance of the orifice of trachea. **B** Cryoprobe demonstration, freezing of the granuloma. **C** 12 days after the cryosurgical treatment

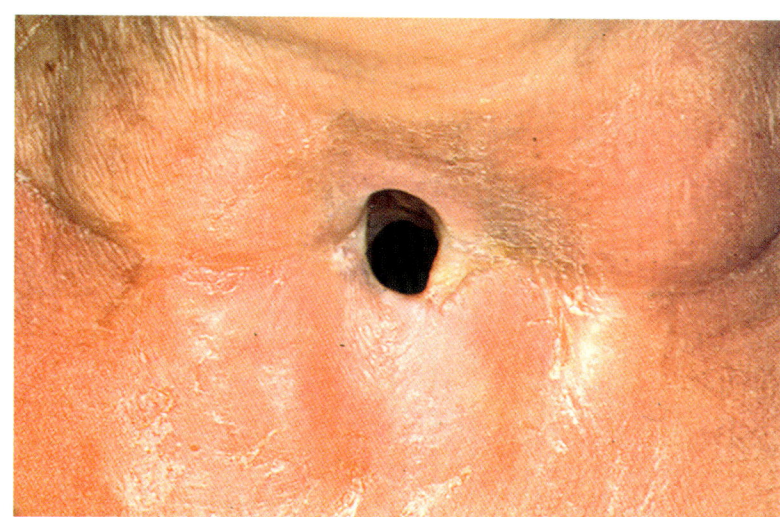

Anorectal Cryosurgery: Curative and Palliative Cryosurgery

Nikolai N. Korpan[1] with contributions by Sybren Meijer[2], Patrick J.M. Le Pivert[3] and Alberto Tajana[4]

15.0 Introduction

Surgery, whether curative or for palliation, remains the "gold standard" treatment for anorectal disorders, especially benign and malignant tumors.

Endoscopic cryosurgery is proposed as the treatment of choice for rectal polyps among other types of nonoperative approaches since it is an easy and safe technique.

Many new surgical and nonsurgical approaches to the treatment of hemorrhoidal disease have been described: sclerotherapy, rubber band ligation, anal dilatation, infrared photocoagulation, bipolar diathermy, electrocoagulation, and cryosurgery. The effectiveness of these treatments depends on the size and degree of hemorrhoids, but also depends on the experience of the individual proctologist. In modern treatment, fast and painless procedures that can be carried out on an ambulatory basis or with only a short stay in hospital will be more frequently indicated.

In the treatment of hemorrhoids all procedures will have good results, if the indications are correct. Cryosurgery for the treatment of hemorrhoidal disease has from the first had extraordinary success, as it treats all symptoms in an office visit, is painless, fast, and free of complications. Cryosurgery as the noninvasive treatment of hemorrhoidal disease is indicated for symptomatic piles of degree I and II and only in few cases for degree III and IV. Cryosurgery is especially suitable for the treatment of internal hemorrhoids in all cases. However, all operations for hemorrhoids must be avoided in Crohn's disease.

Condylomata acuminata (anal and perianal warts) is the most common sexually transmitted disease seen by colorectal surgeons. Many types of therapy have been used to manage anal condylomata. Each method has advantages and disadvantages. Cryosurgery can also be used to destroy condylomata. The procedure is exact because the depth of destruction can be accurately gauged intraoperatively. A special cryogenic applicator may be used to carefully treat individual anal and perianal warts.

In a small proportion of patients, however, advanced anorectal carcinoma, locally unresectable and incurable recurrent rectal cancer, patients' frailties, or refusal to have a stoma – mainly in patients with a high operative risk, with known metastases or with unresectable tumor – requires alternative measures to be considered. Many different local treatment strategies have been used. One type of treatment is not necessarily the best for every patient. Therefore, a variety of approaches may be considered. Endoscopic cryosurgery can be used with some success in the treatment of non-resectable rectal cancer. Palliation is warranted for bleeding, mucous discharge, obstruction or pain. The primary aim of cryosurgical palliation must be to improve patient quality of life with minimum intervention and a low associated morbidity and mortality. Cryosurgery for rectal cancer is a simple and safe treatment.

Chapter 15
Anorectal Cryosurgery: Curative and Palliative Cryosurgery

It should be considered for alleviation of local symptoms in patients with rectal cancer who are unsuitable for radical surgery.

The treatment of epidermoid cancer of the anal region has undergone a major change. Combined modality treatment with cryosurgery has resulted in increased survival and in sphincter preservation for most patients.

Superficial perianal skin carcinomas (i.e., squamous and basal cell) outside the anal verge may be treated with cryosurgery with good results.

Treatment of Bowen's disease is by cryosurgery, with control of the margins. In the absence of invasive cancer, Paget's disease is treated by the cryosurgical method, without skin grafting. Multiple biopsies from the margins are crucial. For early noninvasive lesions local cryosurgery has been successful. Primary abdomino-perineal resection is almost never indicated as the initial treatment of margin lesions.

Patients with recurrent anal canal cancer after conventional surgery may be considered for multimodal therapy with cryosurgery. Multimodal therapy including cryosurgery for locally advanced primary anal canal tumors will yield good palliation and, in some cases, cure.

Cryosurgery will play a more important role in patients with anorectal tumor in the years to come.

Section F Clinical Aspects

15.1 Hemorrhoidal Disease

Chapter 15
Anorectal
Cryosurgery:
Curative and
Palliative
Cryosurgery

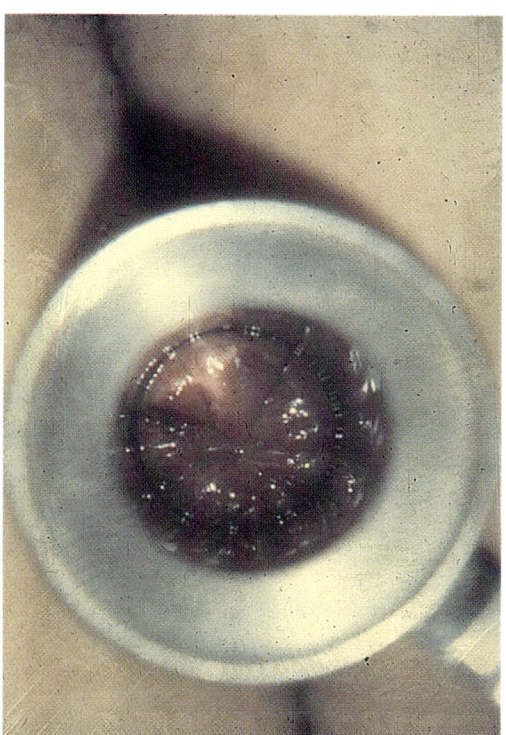

Fig. 15.1.1[4]. Symptomatic first degree hemorrhoids: indication for cryosurgery

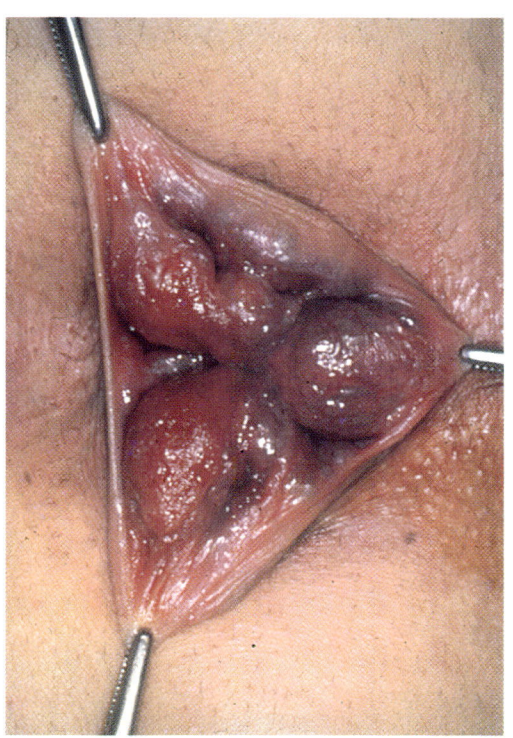

Fig. 15.1.2[4]. Symptomatic second degree hemorrhoids: selected indication for cryosurgery

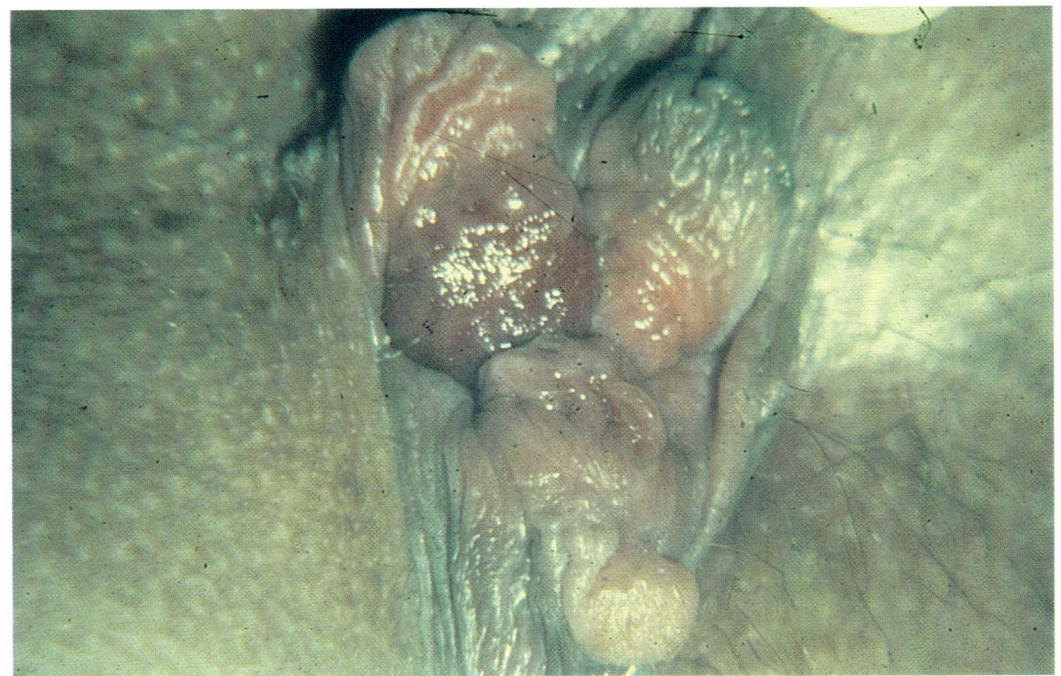

Fig. 15.1.3⁴. Fourth degree hemorrhoids: surgical indication

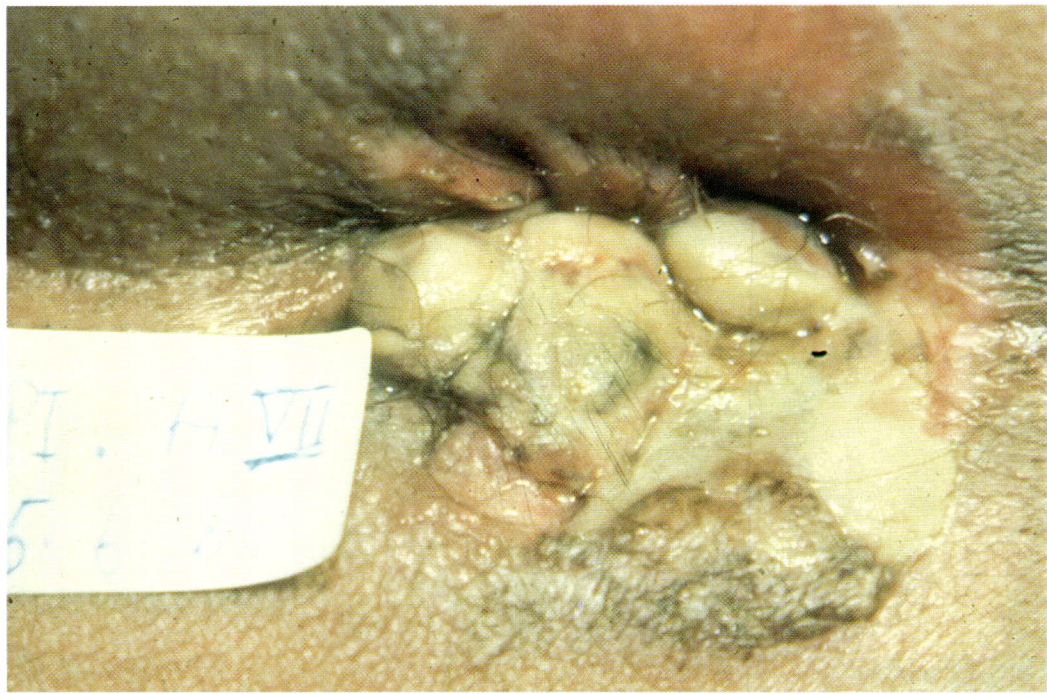

Fig. 15.1.4⁴. Torpid sore due to cryosurgery fourth degree hemorrhoids

Section F　　　　Clinical Aspects

**Chapter 15
Anorectal
Cryosurgery:
Curative and
Palliative
Cryosurgery**

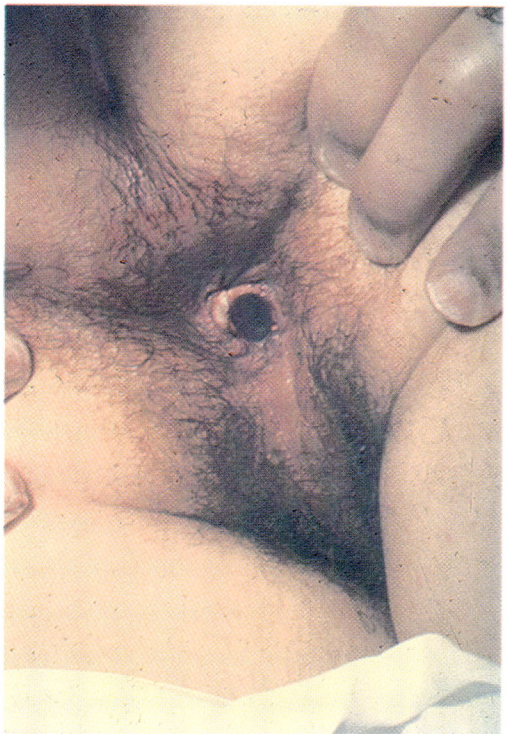

Fig. 15.1.5[4]. Anal stenosis due to incorrect cryotreatment

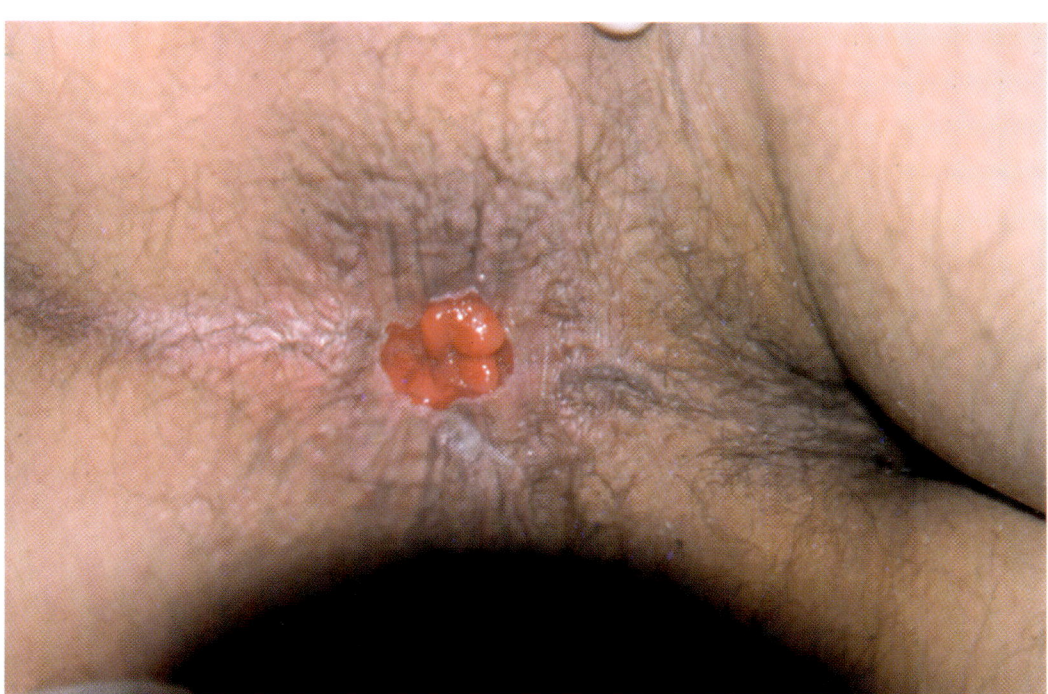

Fig. 15.1.6[4]. Sensorial incontinence due to wrong cryotreatment

Chapter 15
Anorectal
Cryosurgery:
Curative and
Palliative
Cryosurgery

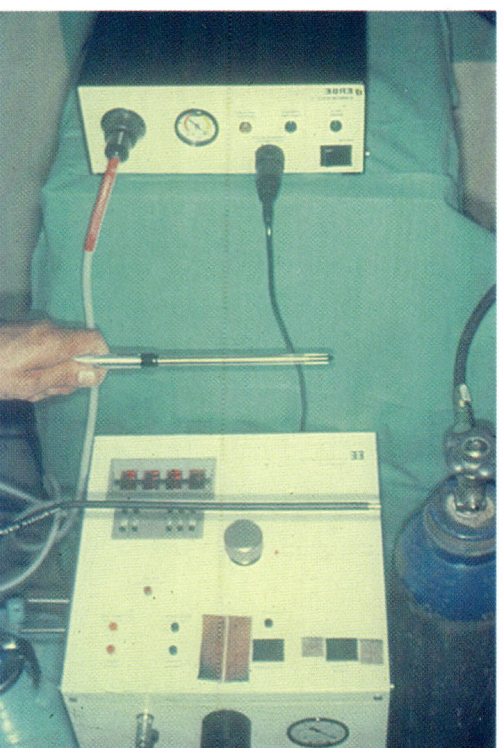

Fig. 15.1.7[4]. Nitrous oxide and liquid nitrogen cryosurgery devices

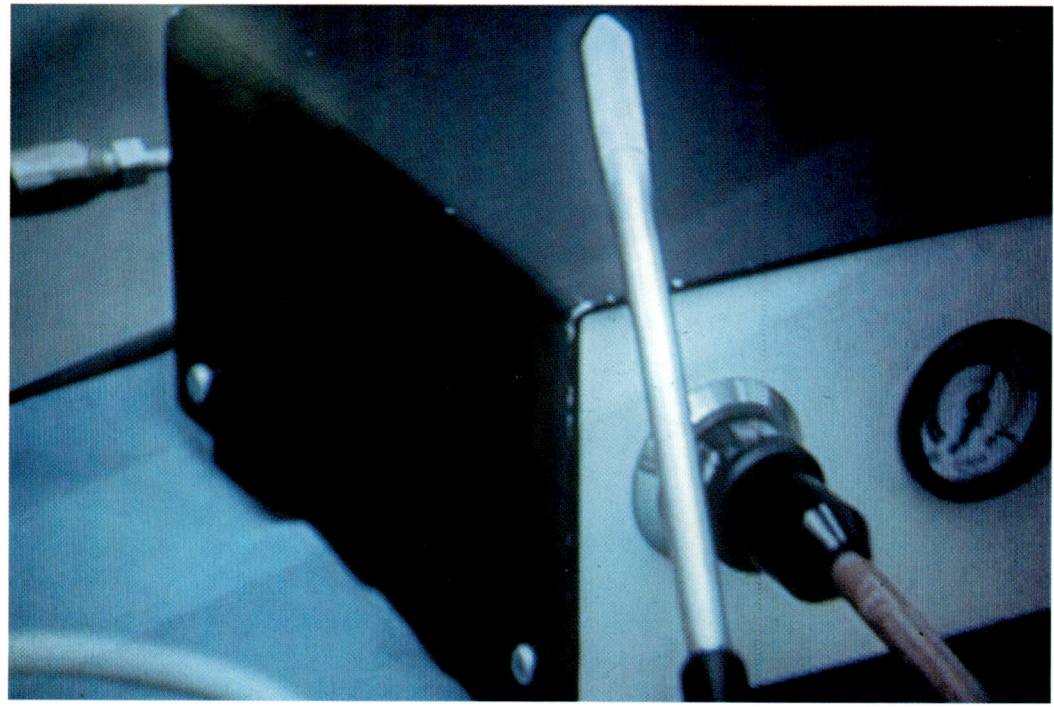

Fig. 15.1.8[4]. Regular cryogenic probe

Chapter 15
Anorectal Cryosurgery: Curative and Palliative Cryosurgery

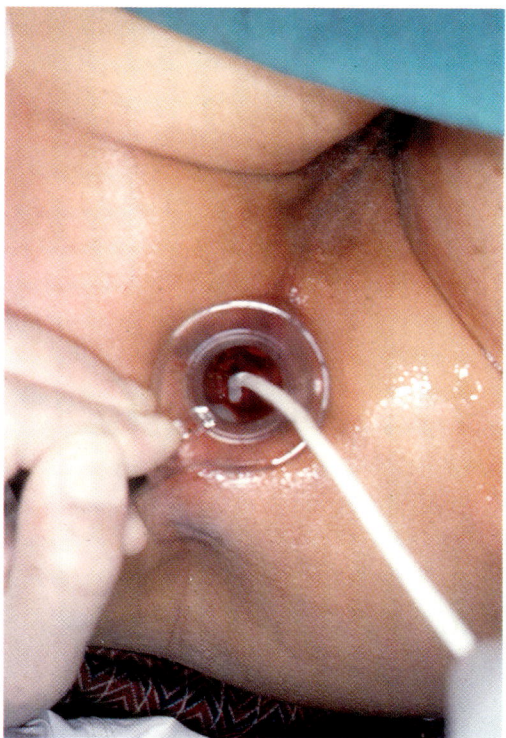

Fig. 15.1.9[4]. Small cryogenic probe

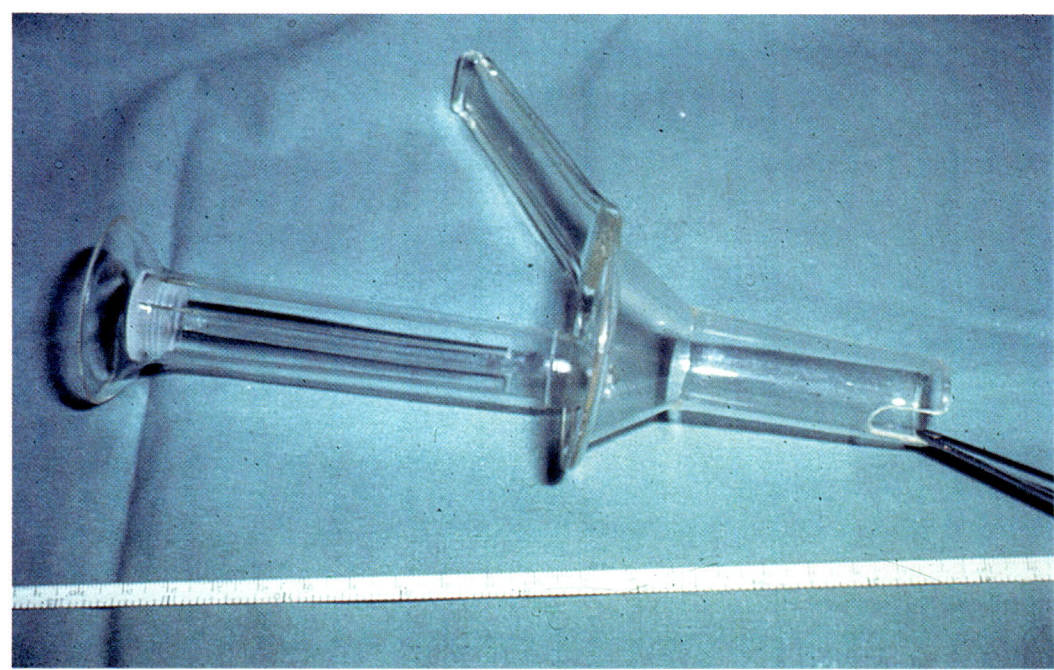

Fig. 15.1.10[4]. Transparent plastic anoscope

Chapter 15
Anorectal Cryosurgery: Curative and Palliative Cryosurgery

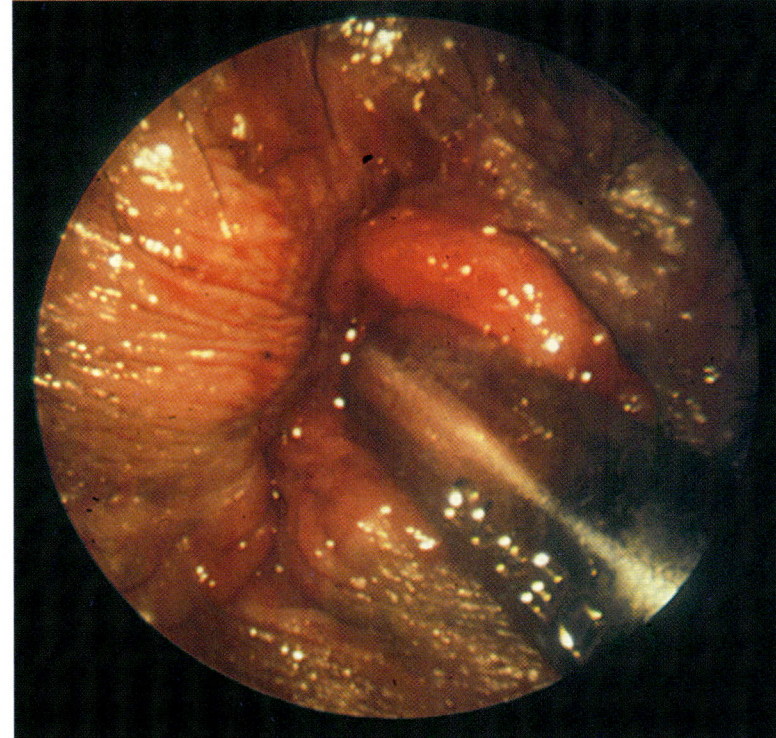

Fig. 15.1.11[4]. Probe pressing hemorrhoidal nodule

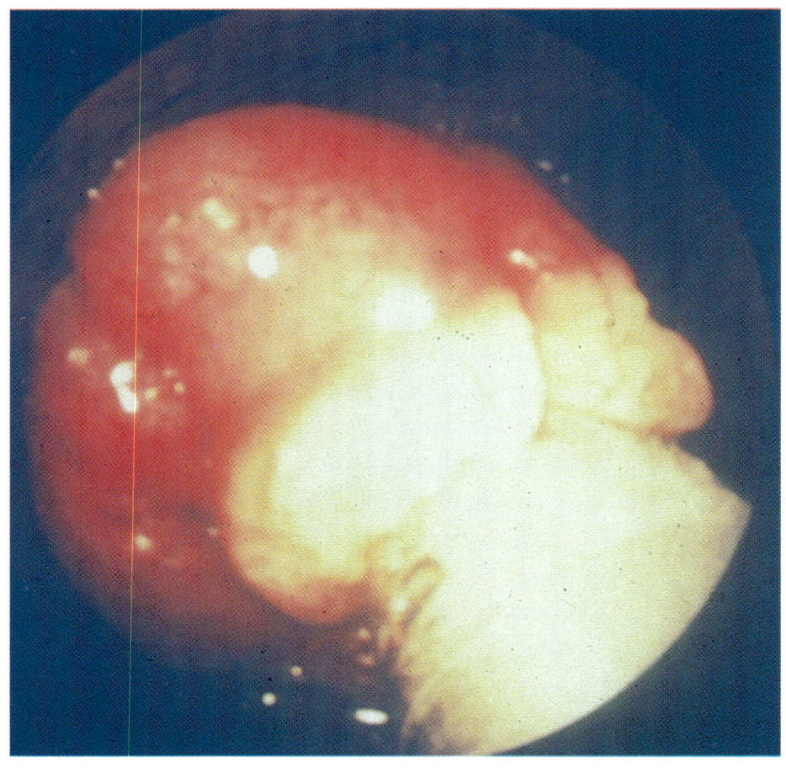

Fig. 15.1.12[4]. Ice ball formation

Section F Clinical Aspects 327

Chapter 15
Anorectal
Cryosurgery:
Curative and
Palliative
Cryosurgery

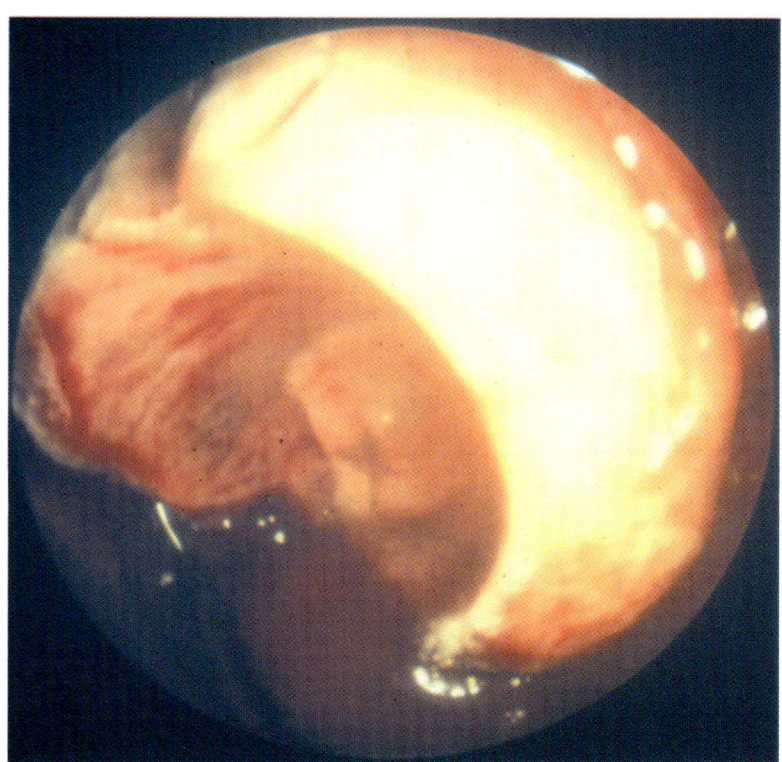

Fig. 15.1.13[4]. Ice ball after probe detachment

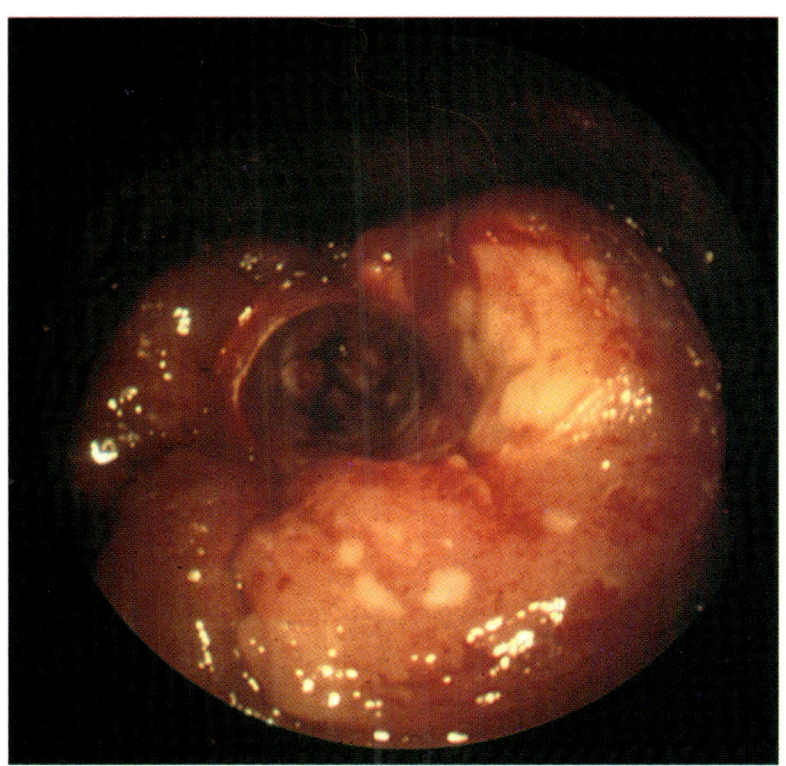

Fig. 15.1.14[4]. Hemorrhoidal edema, ten minutes after ice ball formation

Chapter 15
Anorectal Cryosurgery: Curative and Palliative Cryosurgery

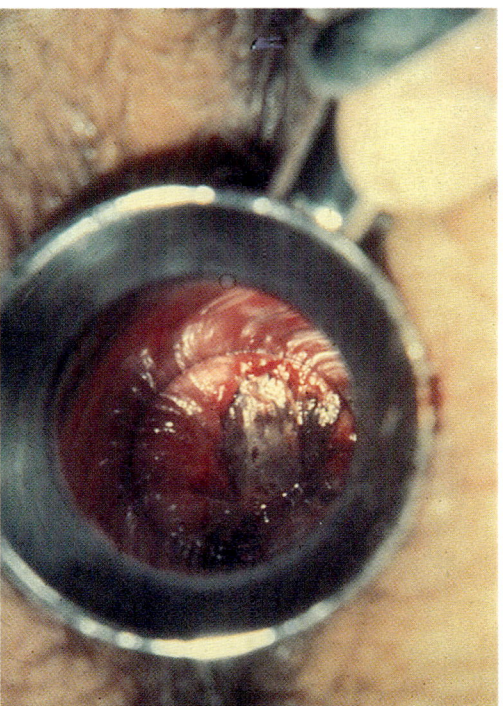

Fig. 15.1.15[4]. Sore after detachment of hemorrhoid

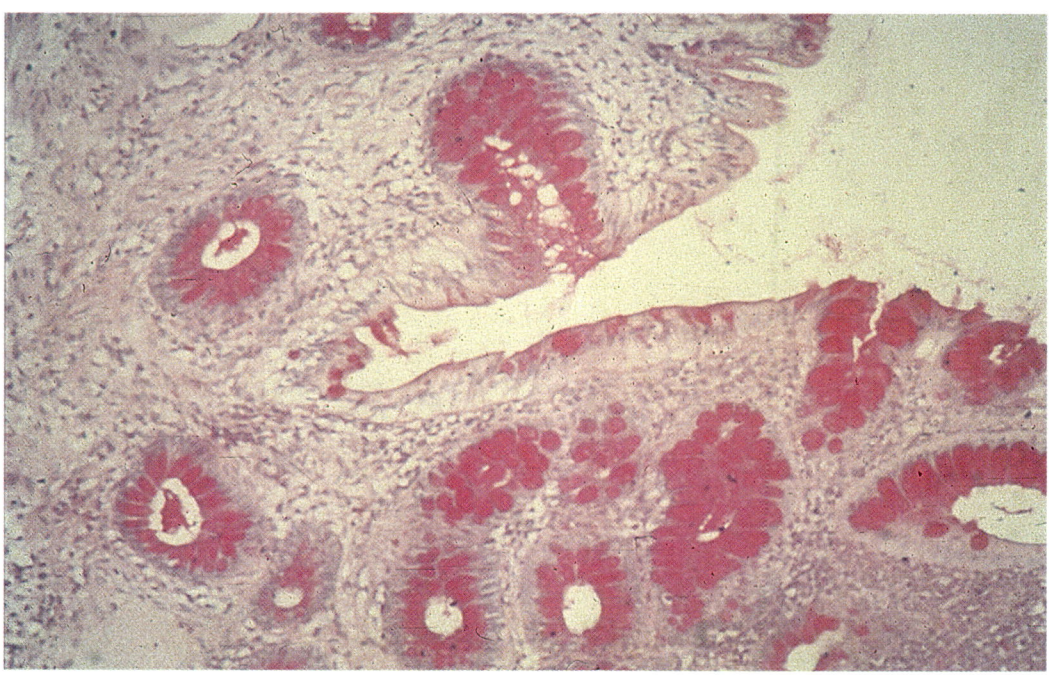

Fig. 15.1.16[4]. Restitutio ad integrum 30 days after cryosurgery

Chapter 15
Anorectal Cryosurgery: Curative and Palliative Cryosurgery

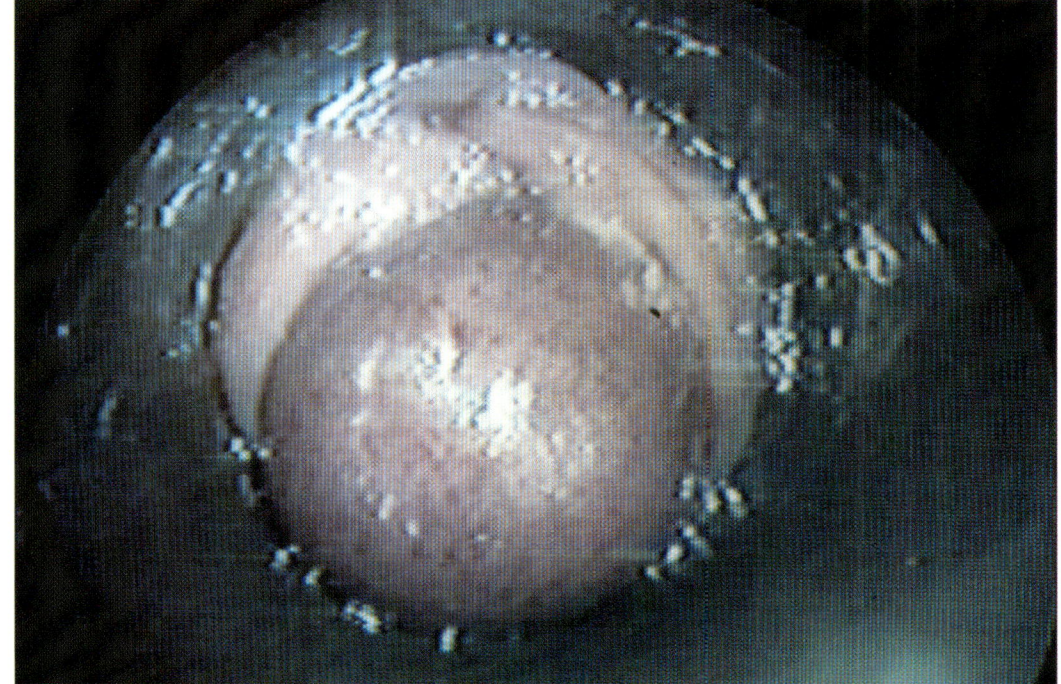

Fig. 15.1.17[4]. Ligated hemorrhoid before cryosurgery

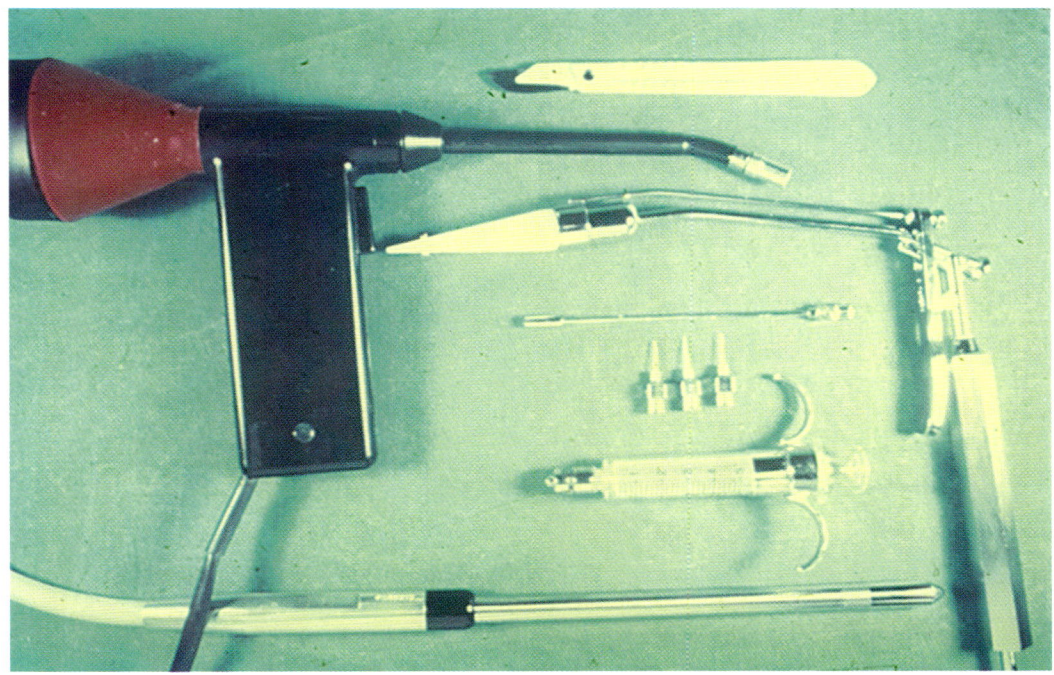

Fig. 15.1.18[4]. Devices for treatment of hemorrhoidal disease

Chapter 15
Anorectal Cryosurgery: Curative and Palliative Cryosurgery

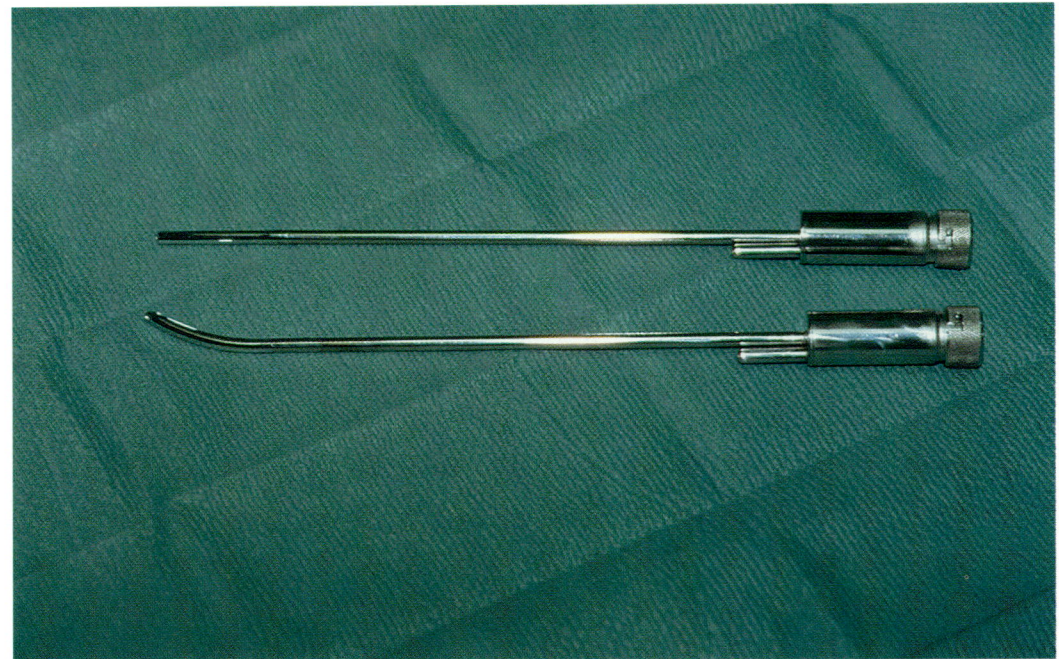

Fig. 15.1.19[1]. Set of cryoinstruments for anorectal cryosurgery

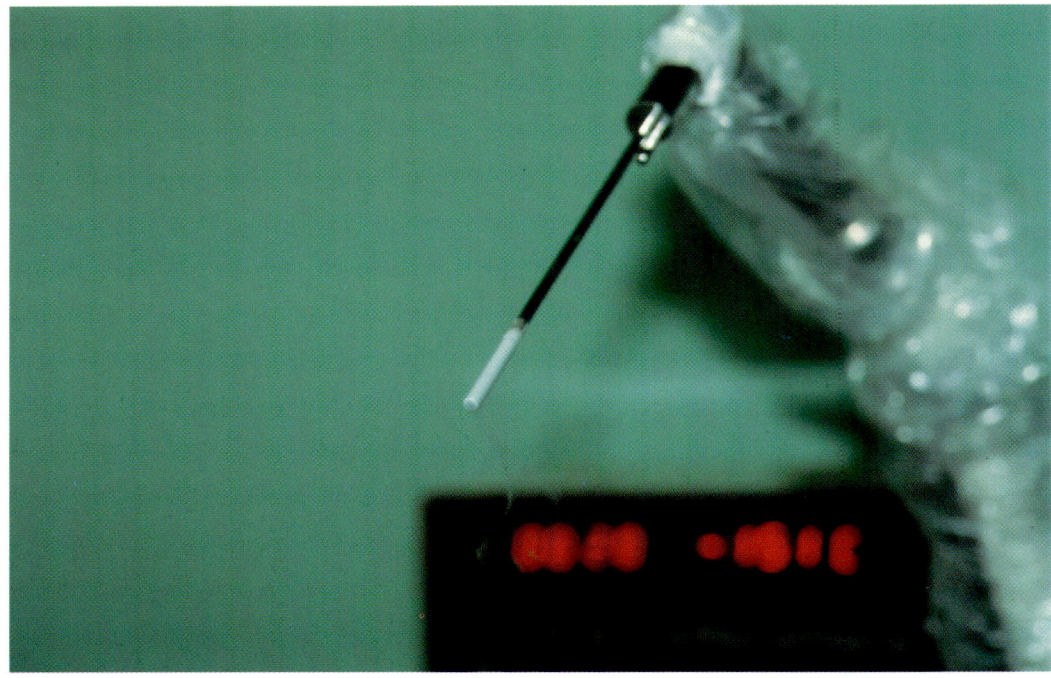

Fig. 15.1.20[1]. Cryoinstrument with straight working tip for anorectal cryosurgery, connected to universal cryosurgical unit

Chapter 15
Anorectal Cryosurgery: Curative and Palliative Cryosurgery

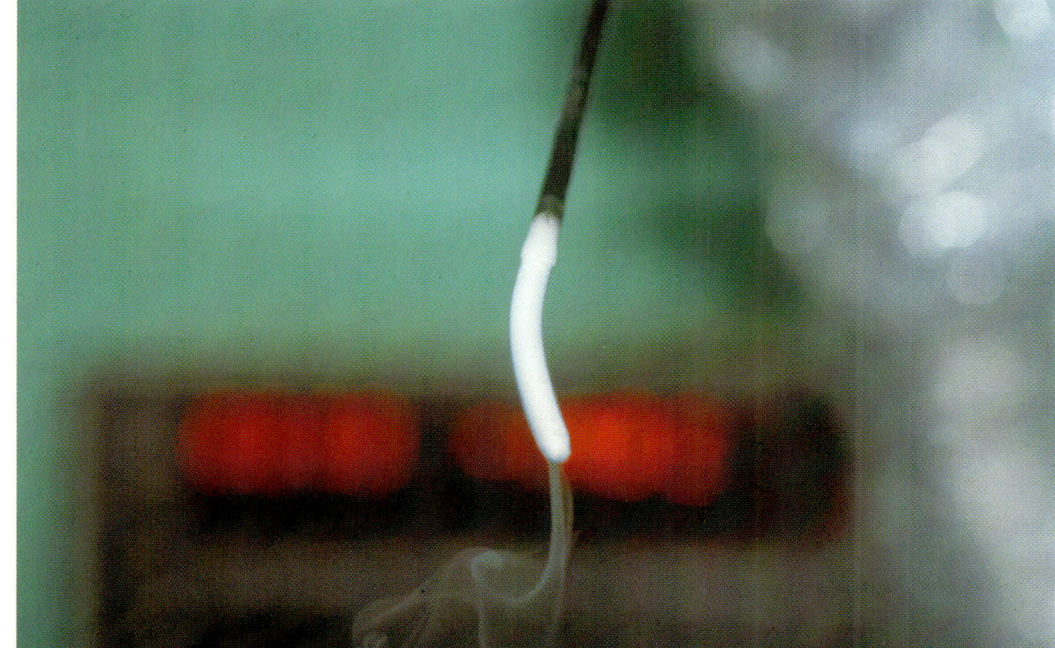

A

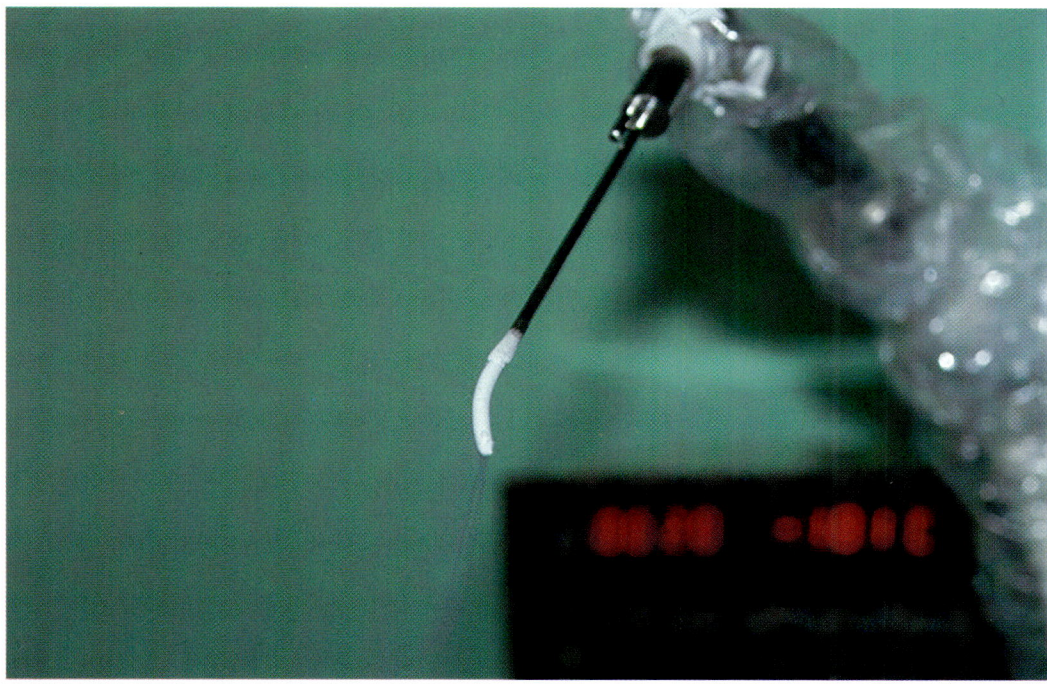

B

Fig. 15.1.21[1] A, B. Curved cryoinstrument for anorectal cryosurgery connected to universal cryosurgical unit

Chapter 15
Anorectal
Cryosurgery:
Curative and
Palliative
Cryosurgery

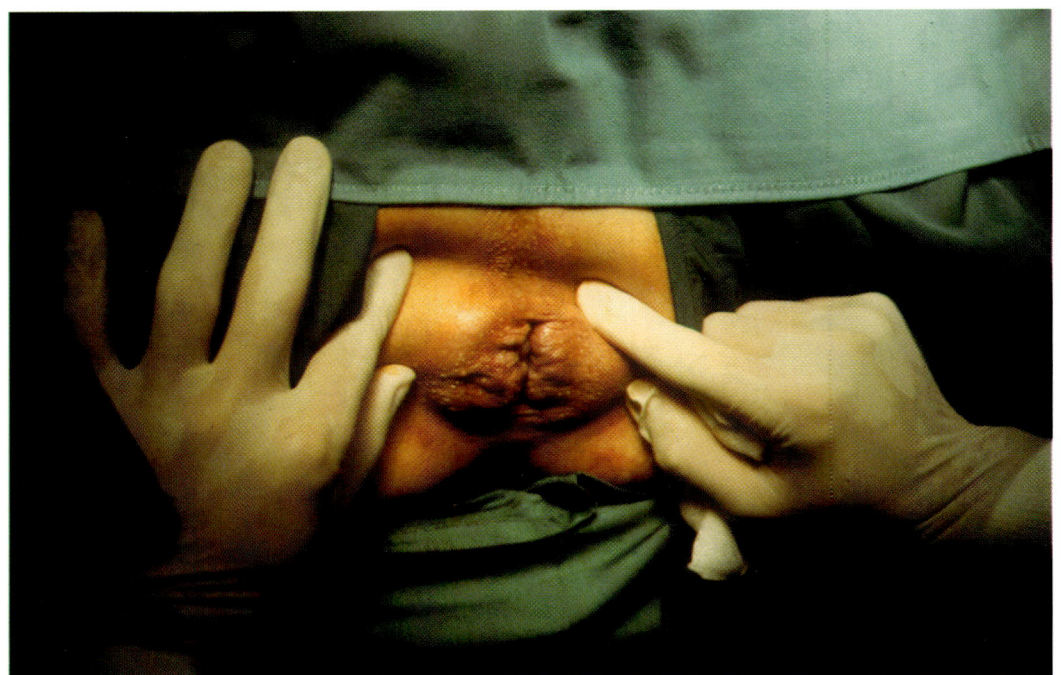

Fig. 15.1.22[1]. Hemorrhoidal disease: preoperative view

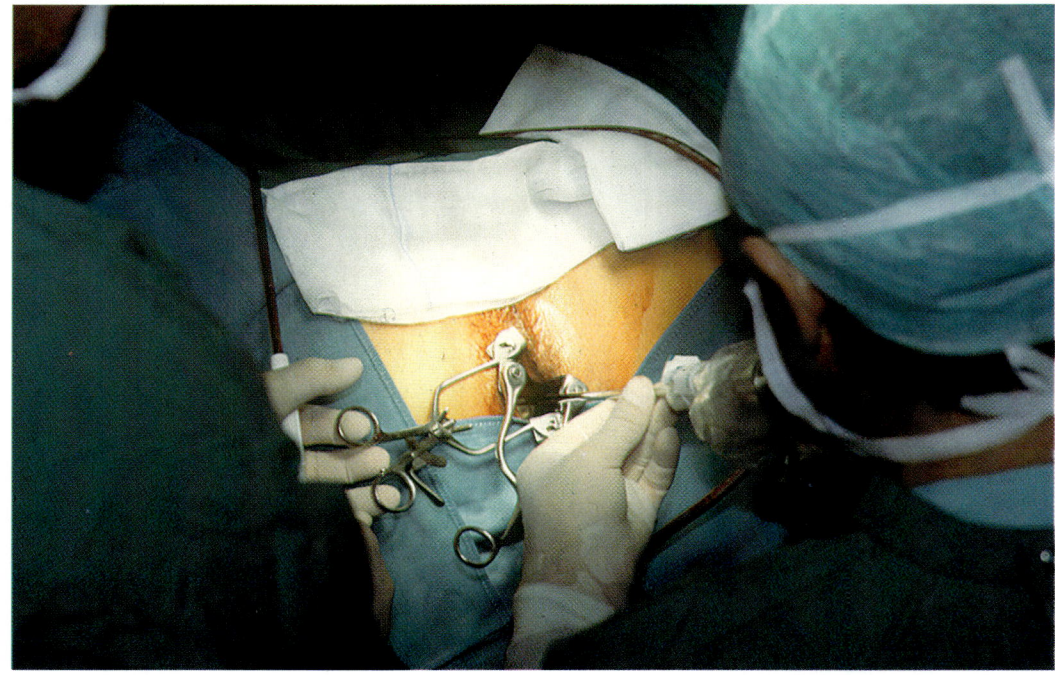

Fig. 15.1.23[1]. Hemorrhoidal disease: view of cryosurgical session intraoperatively

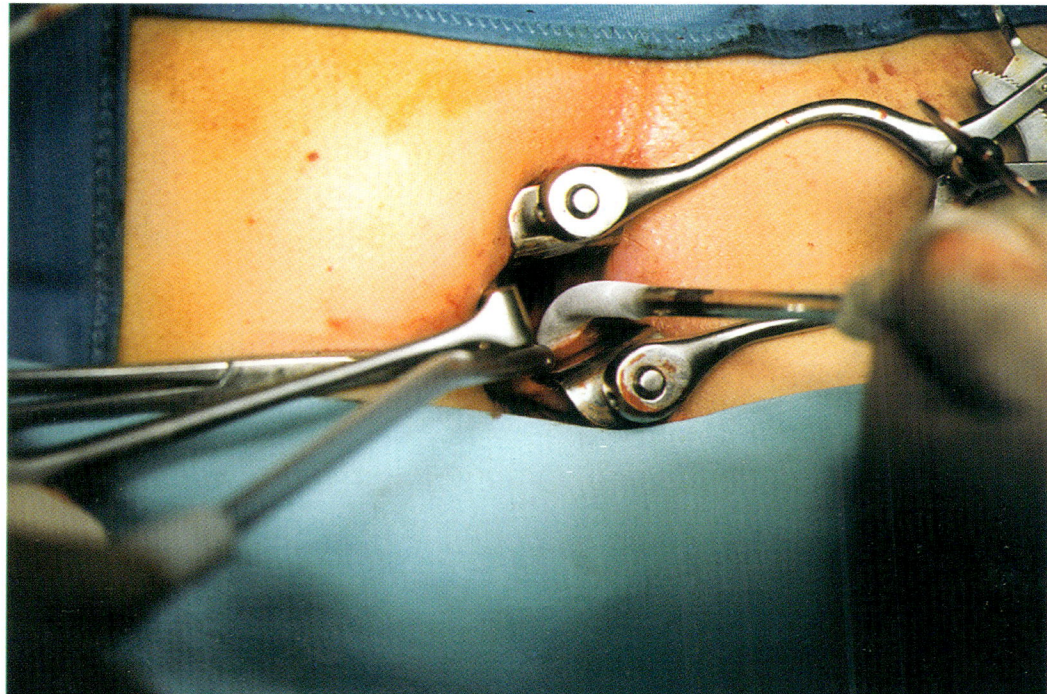

Fig. 15.1.24[1]. Hemorrhoidal disease: a single cryosurgical freeze-thaw cycle using the curved cryo-instrument for anorectal cryosurgery which is connected to the universal cryosurgical unit.
The following cryosurgical parameters are used: a temperature of −80°C, an exposure 10–20 sec

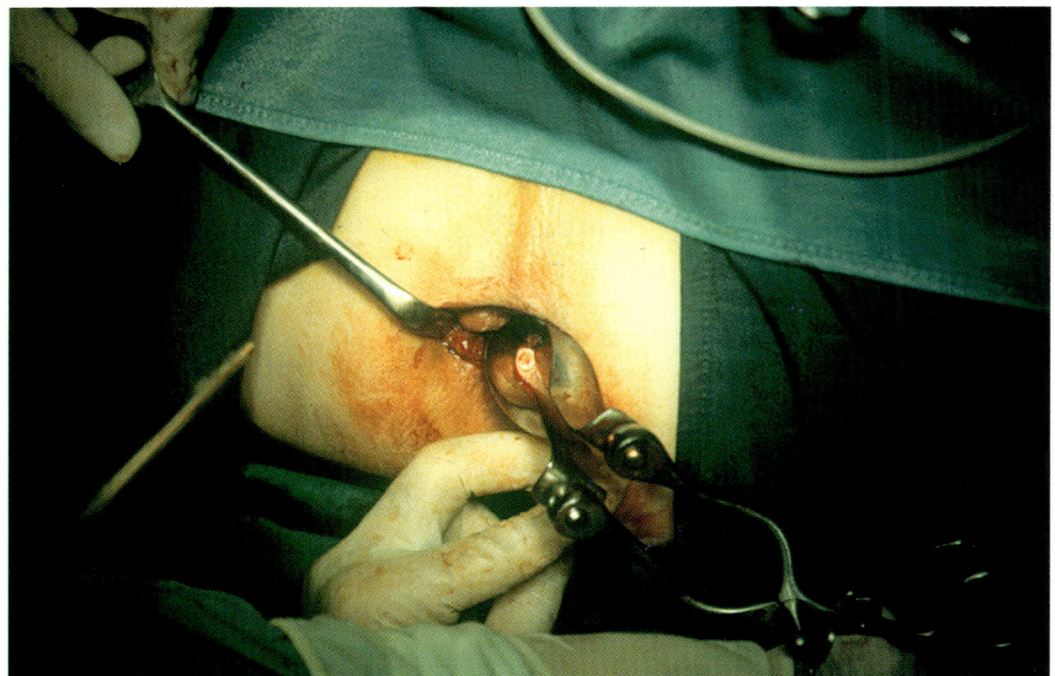

Fig. 15.1.25[1]. Hemorrhoidal disease: post-cryosurgical view of a cryozone with the ice crater in the middle, and of the ice margin with the line of demarcation, immediately after the single cryosurgical session

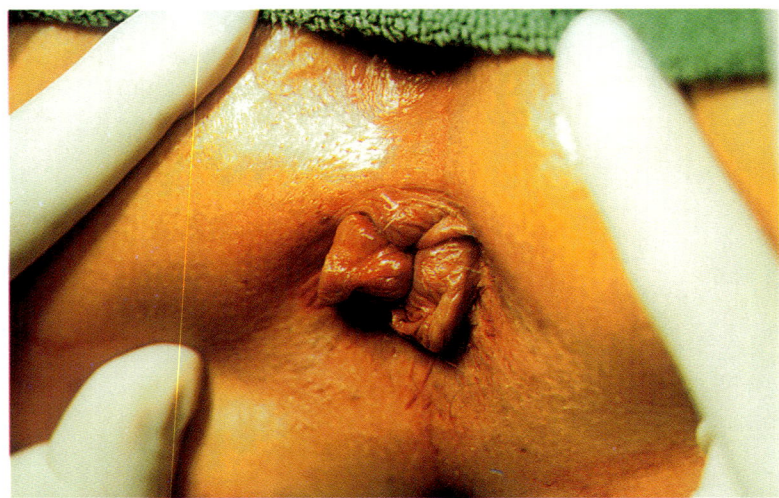

A

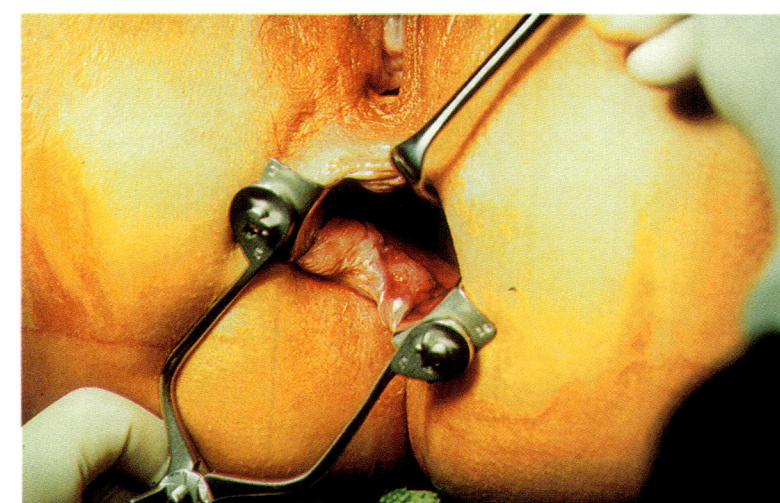

B

Fig. 15.1.26[1]. Hemorrhoidal disease in a 41-year-old female: preoperatively (**A**), intraoperatively (**B**), and postoperatively after cryosurgery (**C**)

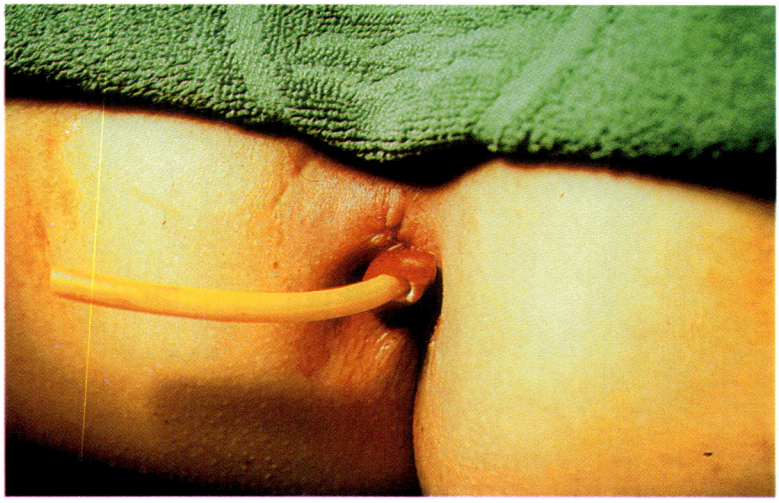

C

Section F   Clinical Aspects

Chapter 15
Anorectal Cryosurgery: Curative and Palliative Cryosurgery

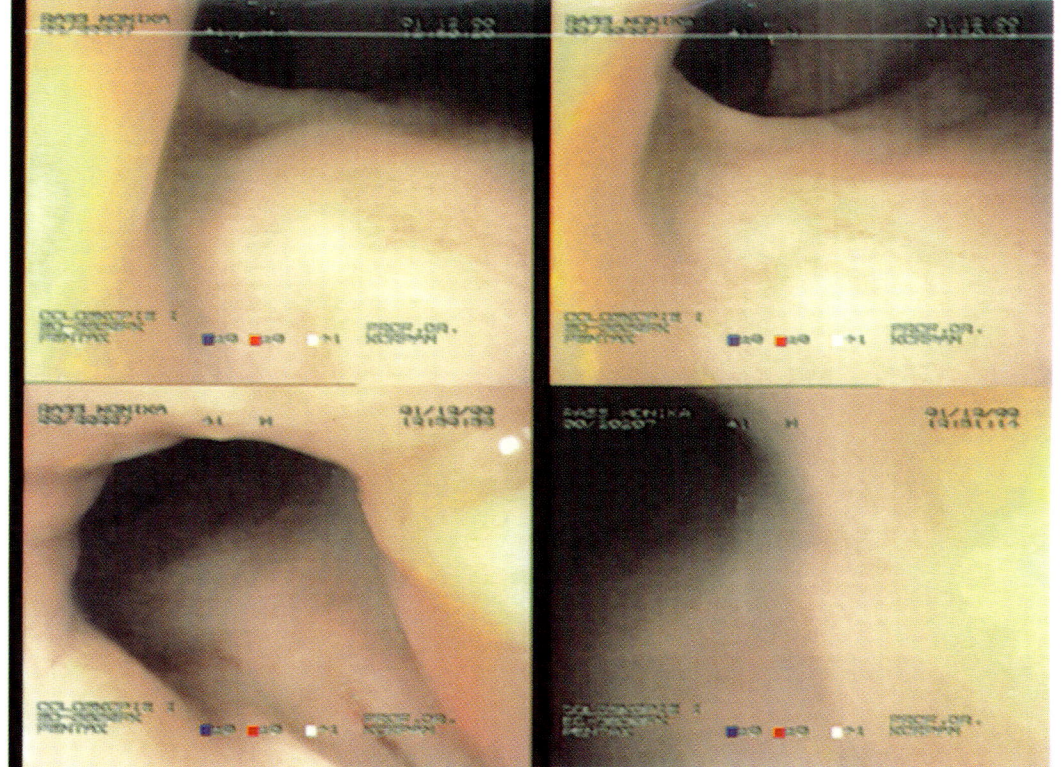

A

Fig. 15.1.27[1]. The same patient. Coloscopy (**A**) and inverted coloscopic examination (**B**) show the excellent results 3 years after cryosurgery (cryosurgical hemorrhoidectomy)

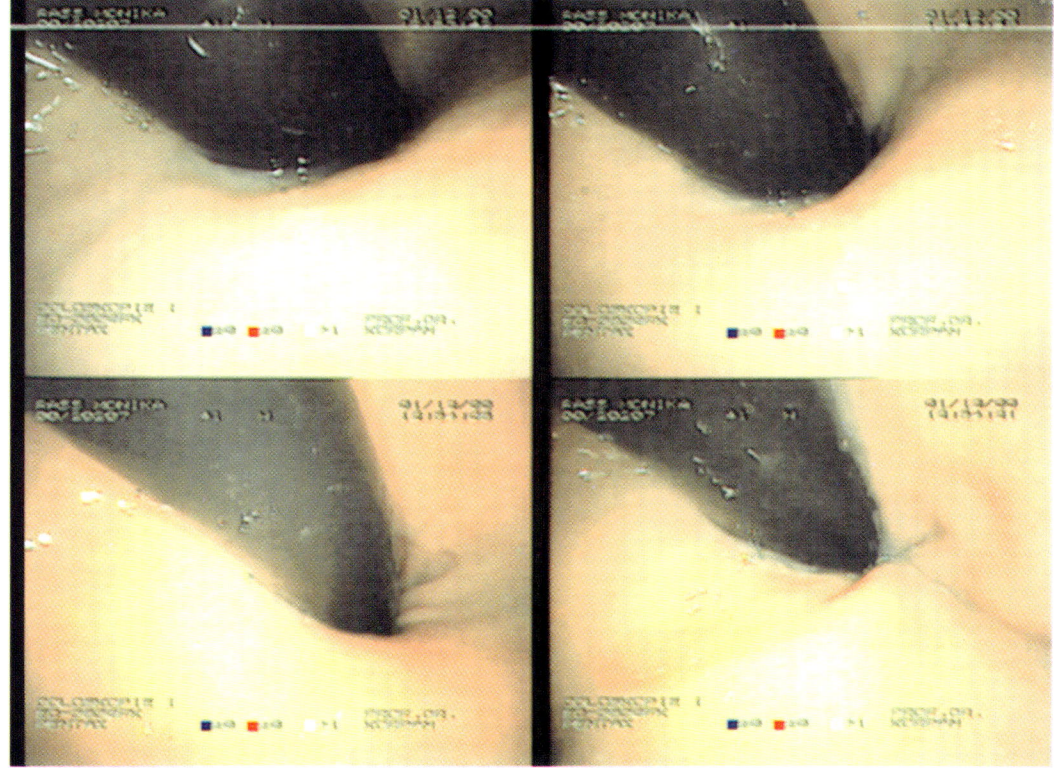

B

15.2 Anorectal Tumors

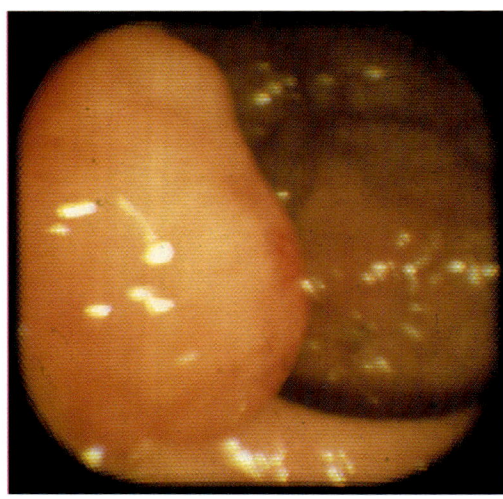

Fig. 15.2.1[2]. Male, 38 years. Adenomatous polyp 2 cm in diameter

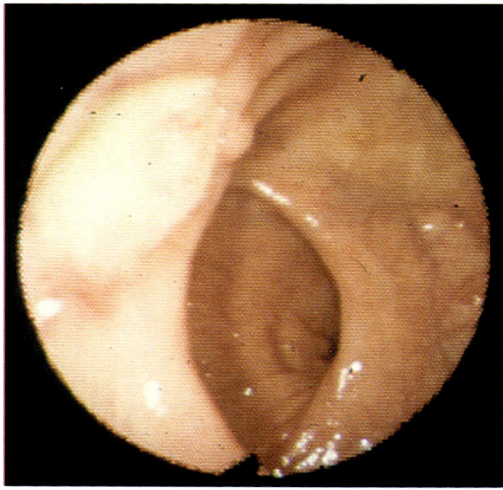

Fig. 15.2.2[2]. After one cryosurgical session the mass has disappeared completely. The focal superficial necrosis will heal within weeks

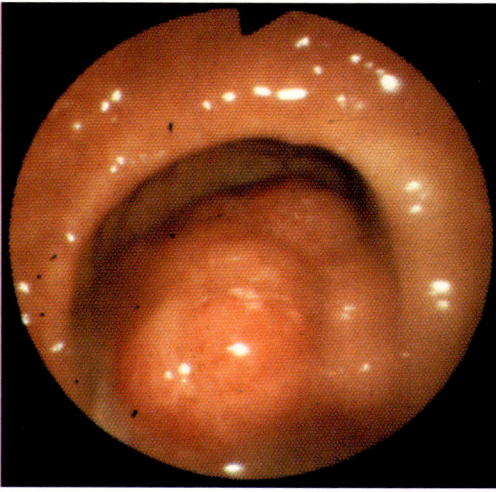 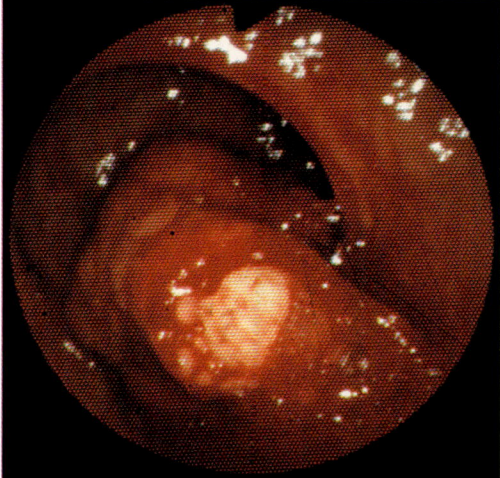

Fig. 15.2.3[2]. Male, 75 years. Polypoid tumor at 10 cm from the anal verge (left). The ice ball resulting from the cryosurgical session is clearly depicted (right)

Section F   Clinical Aspects   337

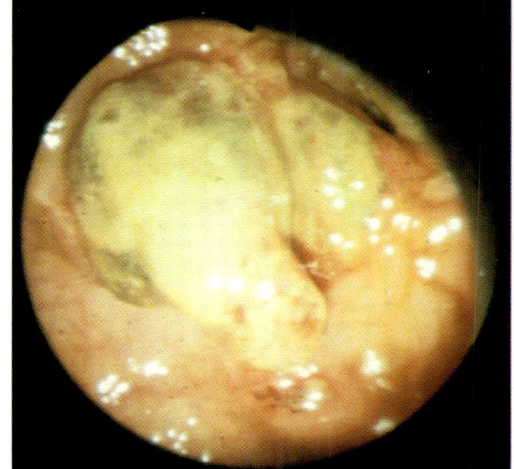

**Chapter 15
Anorectal
Cryosurgery:
Curative and
Palliative
Cryosurgery**

Fig. 15.2.4[2]. After three sessions the tumor is necrotic

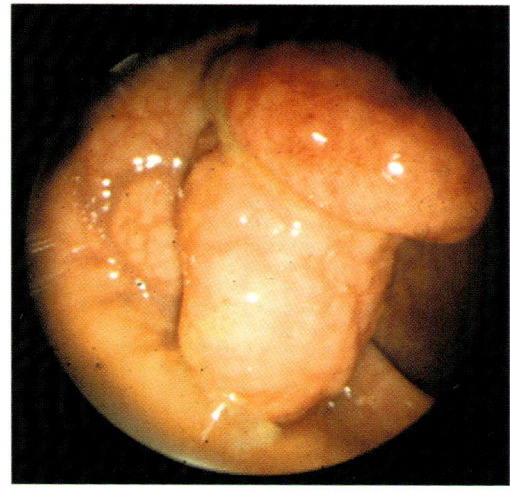

Fig. 15.2.5[2]. Male, 48 years, polyp at 12 cm from the anal verge. Biopsies of this large polypoid tumor revealed a tubulo-villous adenoma, no signs of malignancy. The patient refused conventional surgical resection

Fig. 15.2.6[2]. Four months after a number of cryosurgical sessions a small remnant is seen

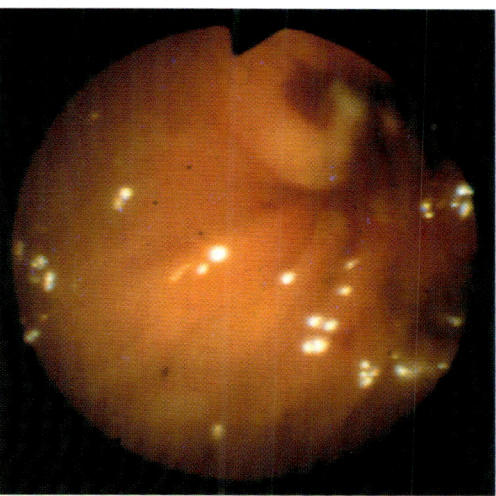

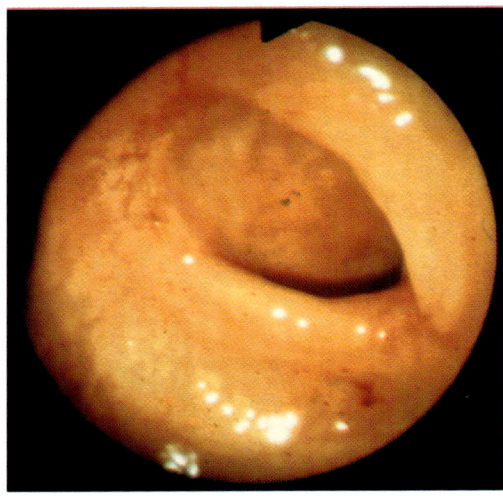

Fig. 15.2.7[2]. After 6 months there is focal atrophy of the rectal mucosa

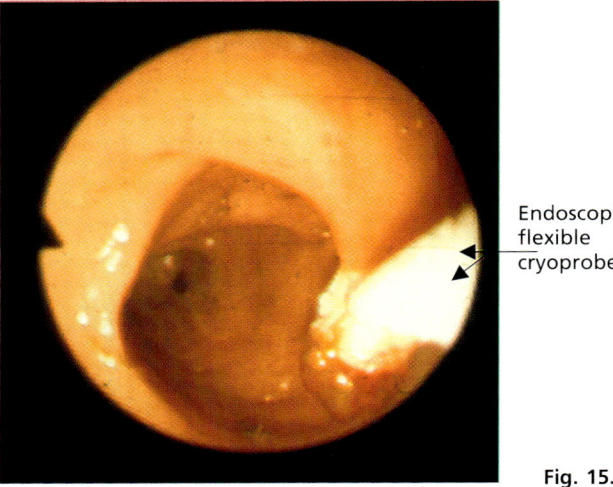

Fig. 15.2.8[3]. Endoscopic cryopolypectomy (1)

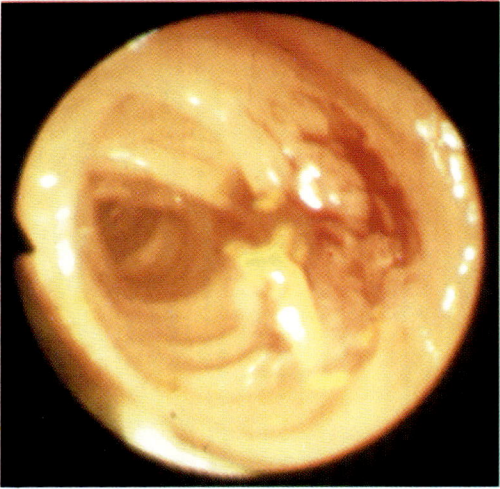

Fig. 15.2.9[3]. Endoscopic cryopolypectomy (2)

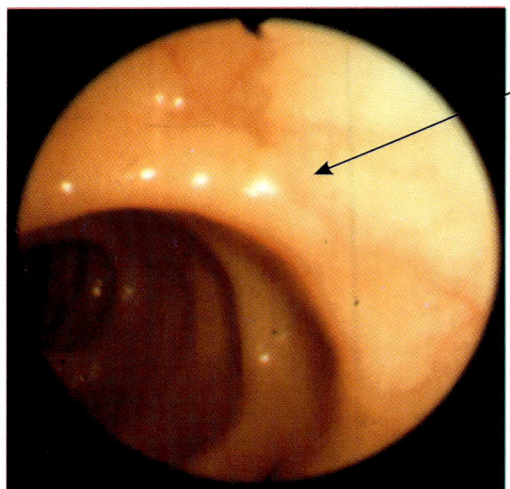

Fig. 15.2.10[3]. Endoscopic cryopolypectomy (3)

Section F Clinical Aspects

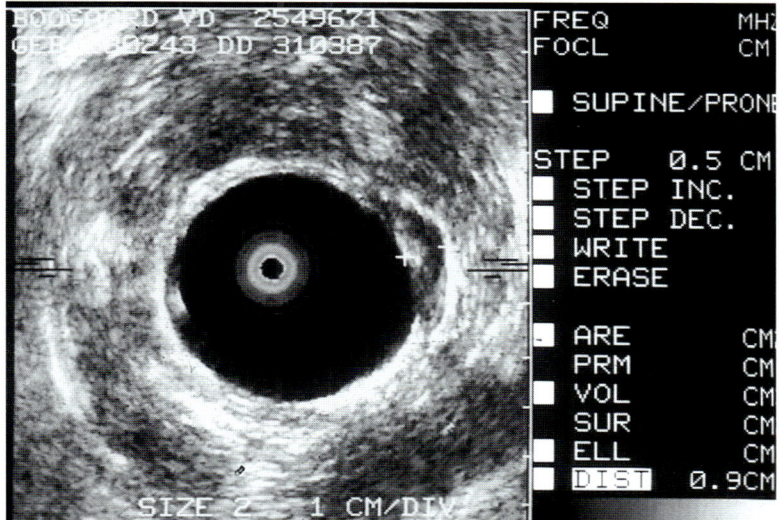

Fig. 15.2.11[2]. Female, 47 years. Intraluminal ultrasound revealed a T1-T2 adenocarcinoma (confirmed by biopsy). Preoperative cryosurgery of rectal cancer to assess the local effects

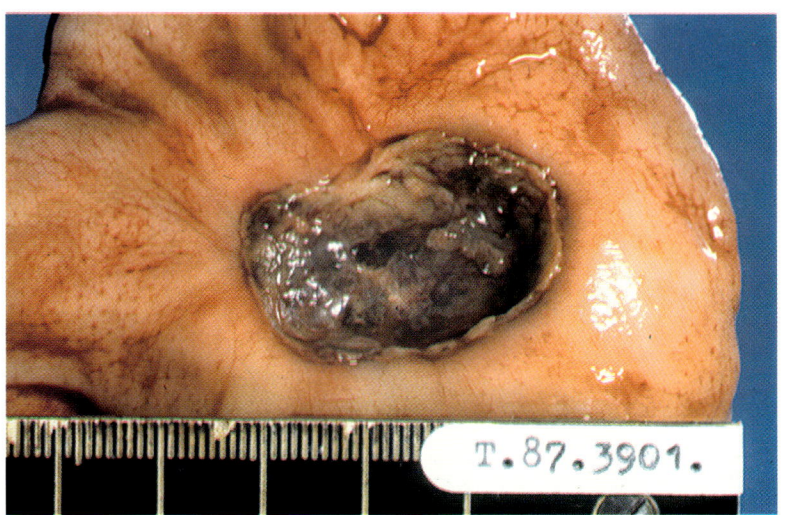

Fig. 15.2.12[2]. After two cryosurgical sessions, the surgical specimen showed a deep, well-demarcated ulcer at the cryoprobe application site

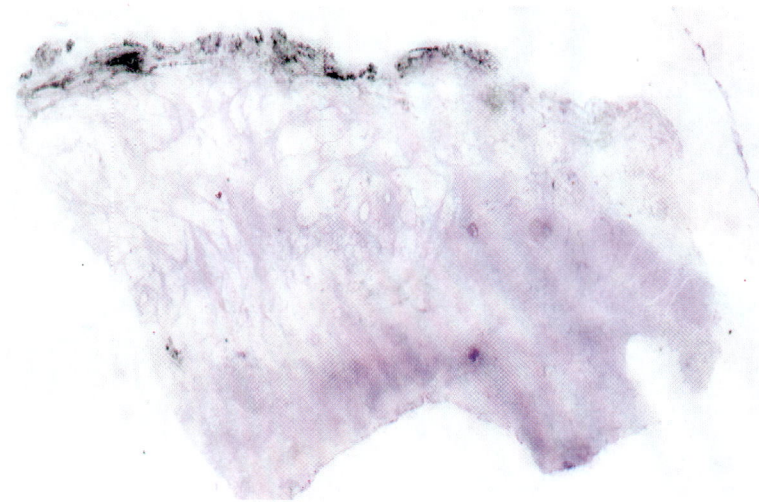

Fig. 15.2.13[2]. On histopathological examination ulceration and transmural fibrosis is seen without tumor

Chapter 15
Anorectal Cryosurgery: Curative and Palliative Cryosurgery

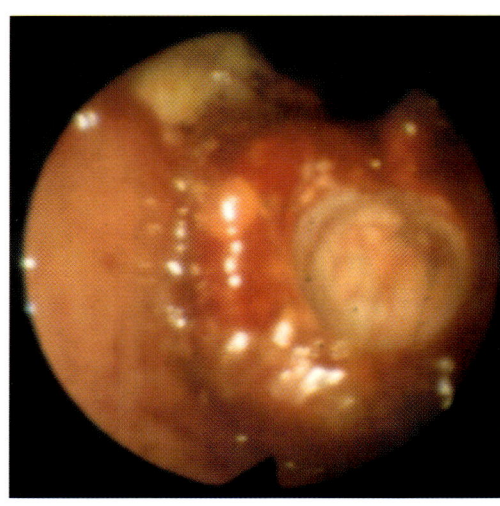

Fig. 15.2.14[2]. Female, 65 years. Preoperative cryosurgery to assess the local response. Rectal cancer during the first treatment. The cryoprobe has been applied centrally on the tumor with resulting ice ball formation

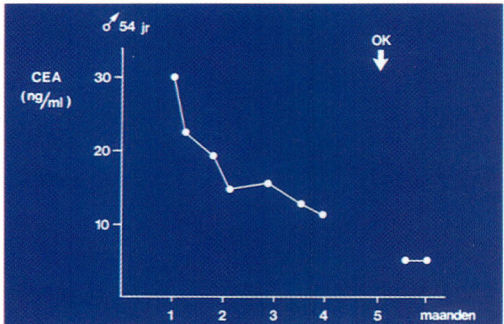

Fig. 15.2.15[2]. After several cryosurgical sessions serum levels of CEA have decreased

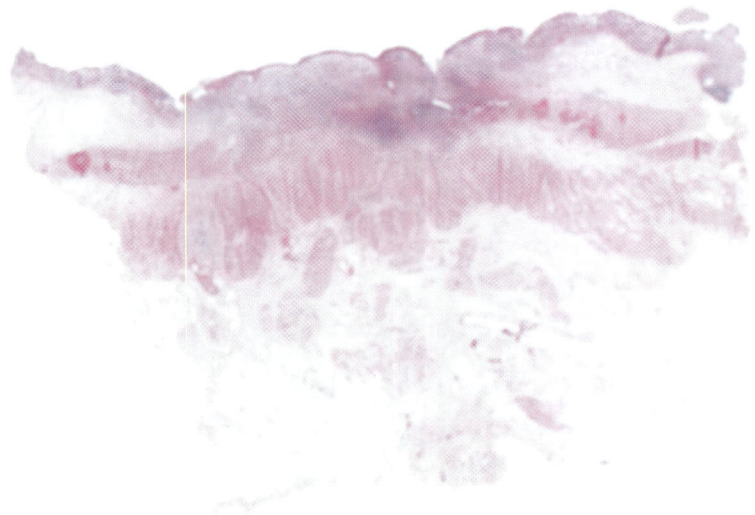

Fig. 15.2.16[2]. In the surgical specimen no intraluminal tumor could be found

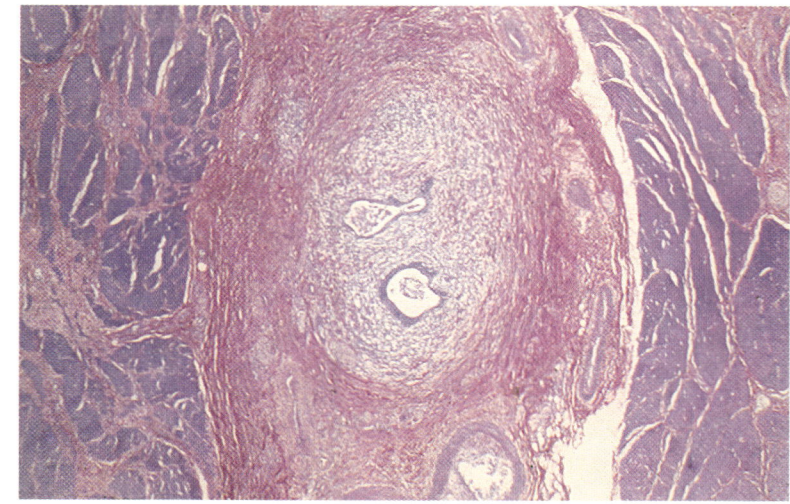

Fig. 15.2.17[2]. However, on microscopic examination tumor deposits between the muscle layers were identified

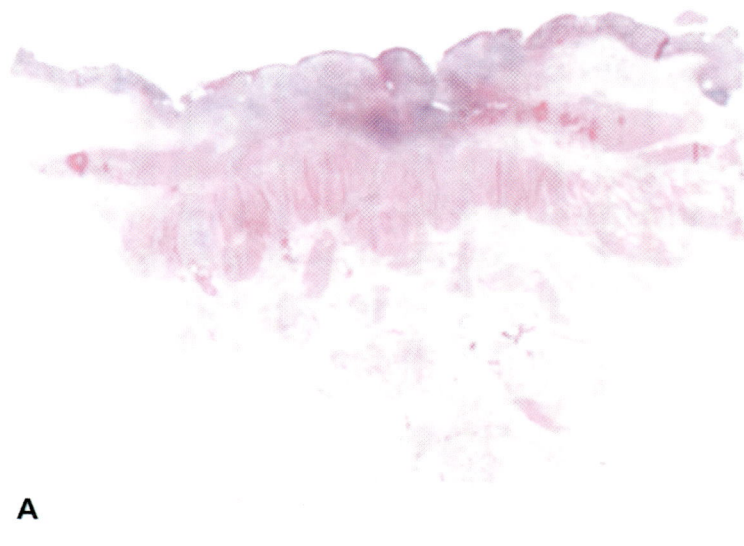
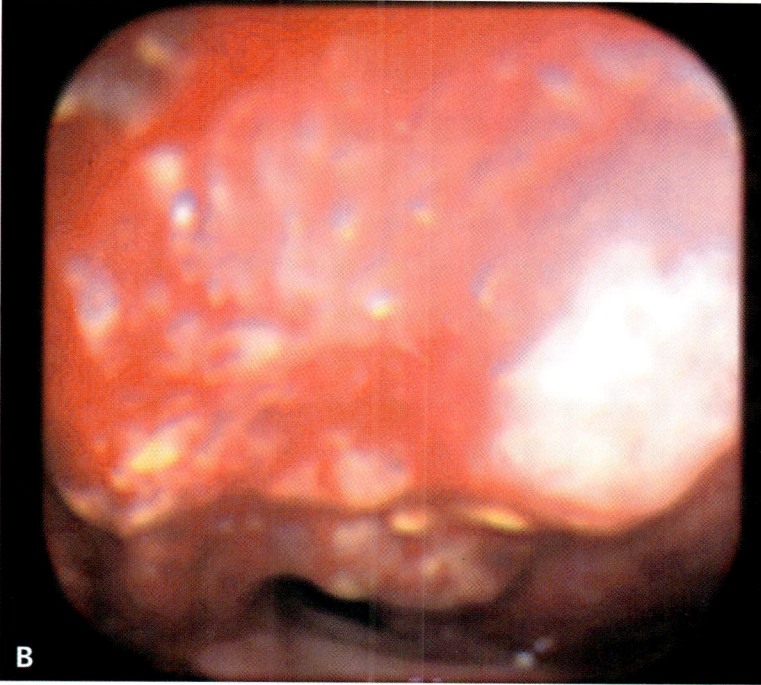

Fig. 15.2.18[1]. Histological findings in sixty-eight-year old patient with inoperable rectal mucosanguineous adenocarcinoma, (**A**) complicated by bleeding (**B**)

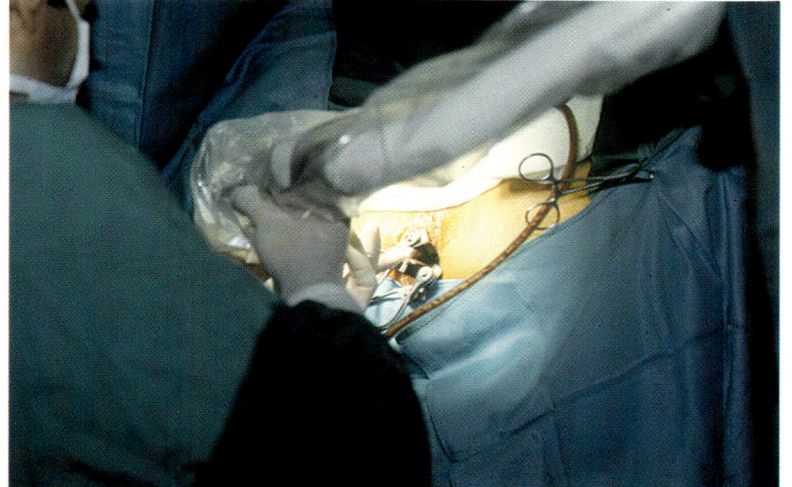
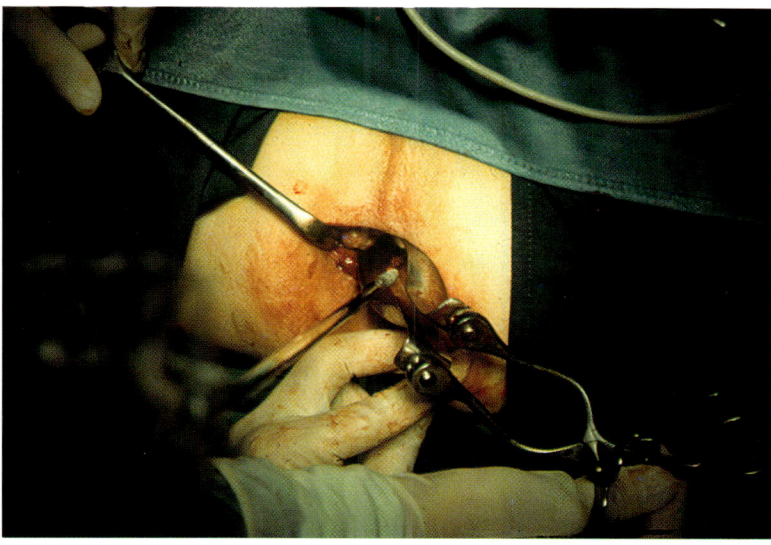

Fig. 15.2.19[1] A, B. Palliative cryosurgical intervention with the aim of stopping a hemorrhage and reducing the tumor mass. Using the cryosurgical approach, the hemostatic action is simple and effective in all patients with advanced anorectal cancer

Breast Cancer Cryosurgery

Nikolai N. Korpan[1] with contributions by Jose Carlos d'Almeida Gonçalves[2], Patrick J.M. Le Pivert[3], Yoed Rabin[4] and Shigeo Tanaka[5]

16.0 Introduction

The number of cases of breast cancer is rising world-wide. Secondary manifestations such as metastases and local recurrences by dissemination of cancer cells in the course of diagnostic interventions or operations spell death for patients with breast cancer.

A new way of thinking should, therefore, direct the future of cancer research and treatment. New methods of cancer diagnosis and therapy are needed to increase the cure rate of this disease.

Modern cryosurgery has today achieved international recognition and is widely practiced. Years of practical experience and many international publications document the good results obtained. It has become clear that successful application of this technique can only be achieved if efficient medico-technical devices are developed.

This high-tech method of surgery could be further developed in the shortest possible time in the field of breast cryosurgery by pooling personal, theoretical, experimental and clinical knowledge that has been gained world-wide.

Cryomastectomy is medically indicated for cancers that are inoperable and resistant to chemotherapy.

Early experience with breast cryosurgery has indicated a new possibility for the treatment of breast cancer. Research toward elucidating the fundamental process of freezing in breast parenchyma must become the focal point of future studies.

Doppler-ultrasound imaging of the "ice ball" formation was demonstrated in a sheep breast model.

Chapter 16 Breast Cancer Cryosurgery

16.1 Imaging of Breast Cryosurgery

16.1.1 Doppler-Ultrasound Imaging of the "Ice Ball" Formation in a Sheep Breast Model[4]

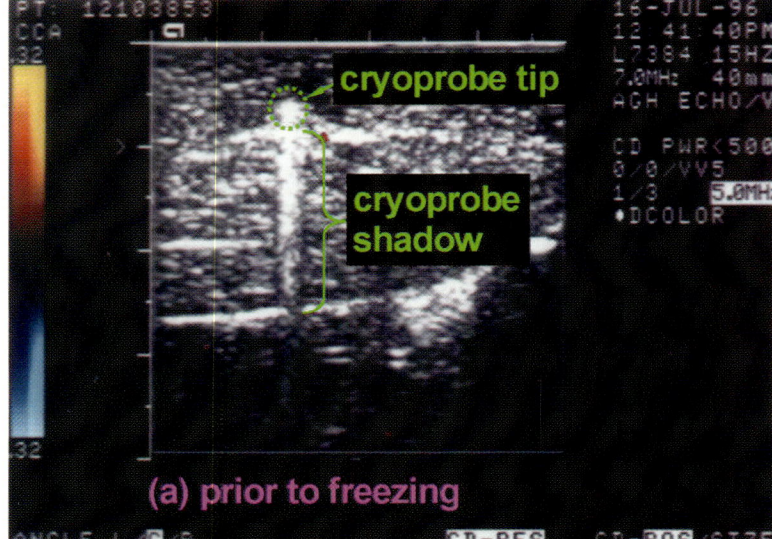

Fig. 16.1.1[4] A. Prior to freezing

Fig. 16.1.1[4]. Ultrasound imaged "ice ball" formation in a sheep breast model using a 7 MHz linear array transducer. The frozen region appears as a dark area in the ultrasound image. The cryoprobe is placed perpendicular to the ultrasound transducer (to the monitor), the ultrasound transducer is applied from above and, therefore, the cryoprobe shadow is projected downwards, as illustrated in **A**. A measurement of the "ice ball" diameter is illustrated in **D**, which appears to be about 2 cm after 3 min of cryo-operation. The cryoprobe applied in this study has been designed specifically for the application of minimally invasive breast cryosurgery and is constructed of hypodermic tubes with a diameter of 1.15 mm (Rabin et al., 1997)

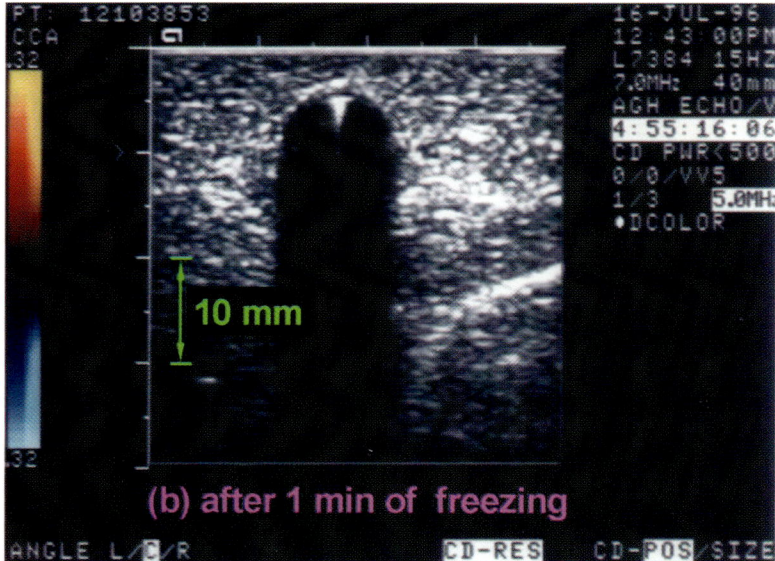

Fig. 16.1.1[4] B. After 1 min of freezing

Section F Clinical Aspects **345**

Chapter 16
Breast Cancer
Cryosurgery

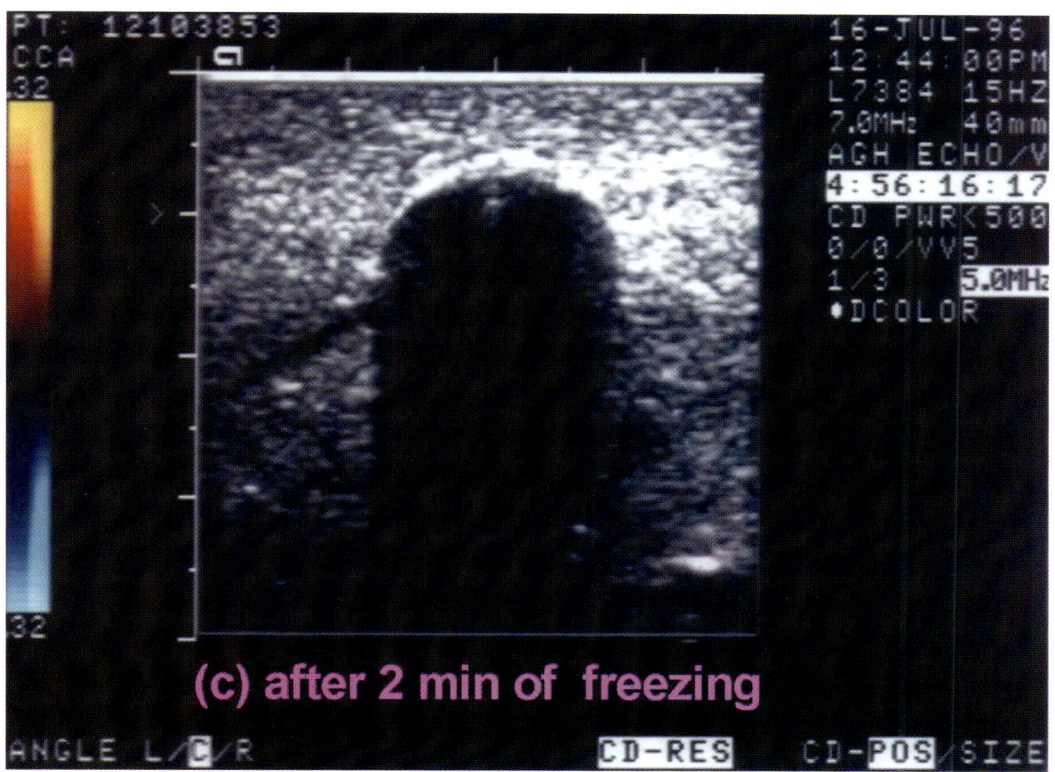

Fig. 16.1.1[4] C. After 2 min of freezing

Fig. 16.1.1[4]. Ultrasound imaged "ice ball" formation in a sheep breast model using a 7 MHz linear array transducer. The frozen region appears as a dark area in the ultrasound image. The cryoprobe is placed perpendicular to the ultrasound transducer (to the monitor), the ultrasound transducer is applied from above and, therefore, the cryoprobe shadow is projected downwards, as illustrated in **A**. A measurement of the "ice ball" diameter is illustrated in **D**, which appears to be about 2 cm after 3 min of cryo-operation. The cryoprobe applied in this study has been designed specifically for the application of minimally invasive breast cryosurgery and is constructed of hypodermic tubes with a diameter of 1.15 mm (Rabin et al., 1997)

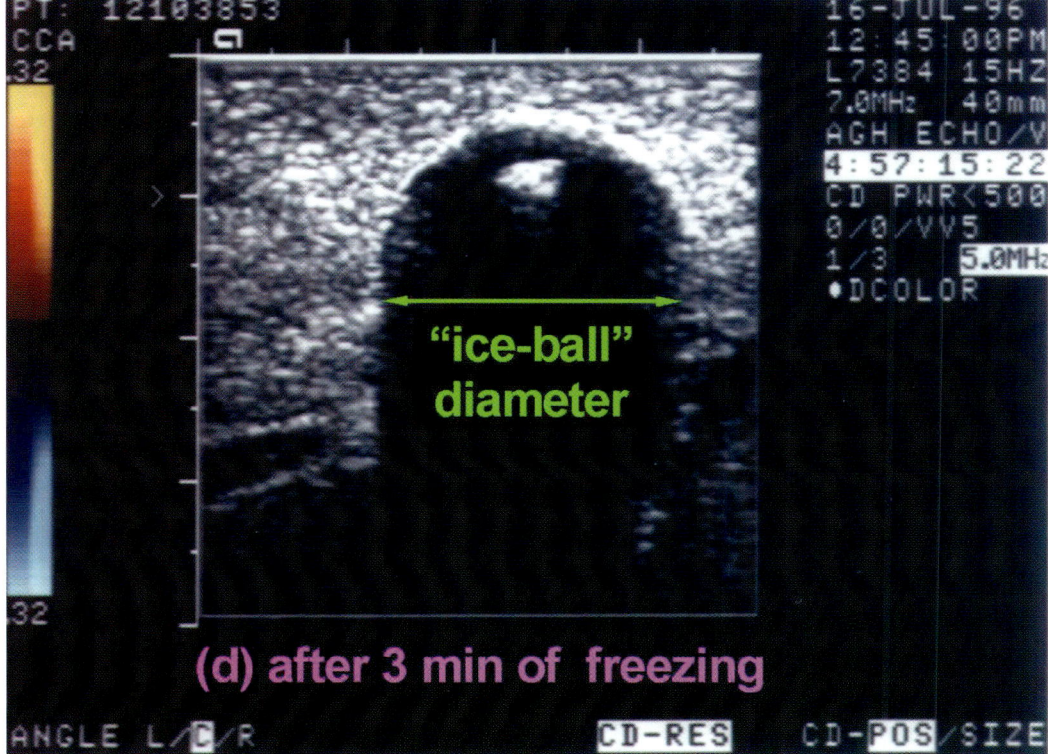

Fig. 16.1.1[4] D. After 3 min of freezing

Chapter 16 Breast Cancer Cryosurgery

16.1.2 Evaluation of Post Cryosurgery Injury in a Sheep Breast Model Using the Vital Stain 2,3,5-Triphenyltetrazolium Chloride[4]

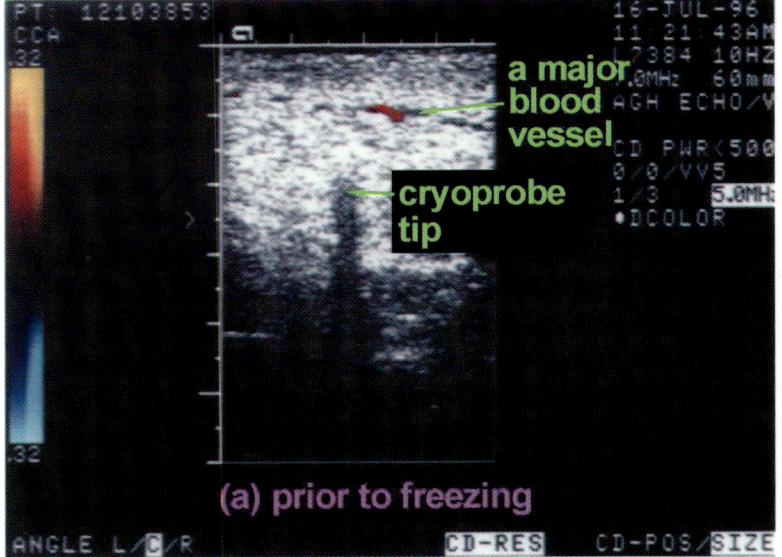

Fig. 16.1.2[4] A. Prior to freezing

Fig. 16.1.2[4]. Ultrasound imaged "ice ball" formation in a sheep breast model using a 7 MHz linear array transducer (Rabin et al., 1997; 1999). The cryoprocedure is performed adjacent to one of the major blood vessels of the breast, where the red and blue colors indicate blood flow in Doppler ultrasound imaging, as indicated in **A** prior to freezing. The non-circular contour of the "ice ball" adjacent to the blood vessel is a result of the heating effect of the blood flow, as can be seen after 3 min of freezing, **D**. The purple dashed line after 7 min of freezing, **H**, indicates the frozen interface that would probably have developed in the absence of the major blood vessel. The blue dashed line after 9.3 min, **I**, represents the location of the already frozen blood vessel. Some blood flow is still shown adjacent to the top-left contour of the frozen region after 9.3 min of freezing, due to the presence of an unfrozen blood vessel branch. Echo measurements at the location of the unfrozen blood vessel branch are shown in **J**

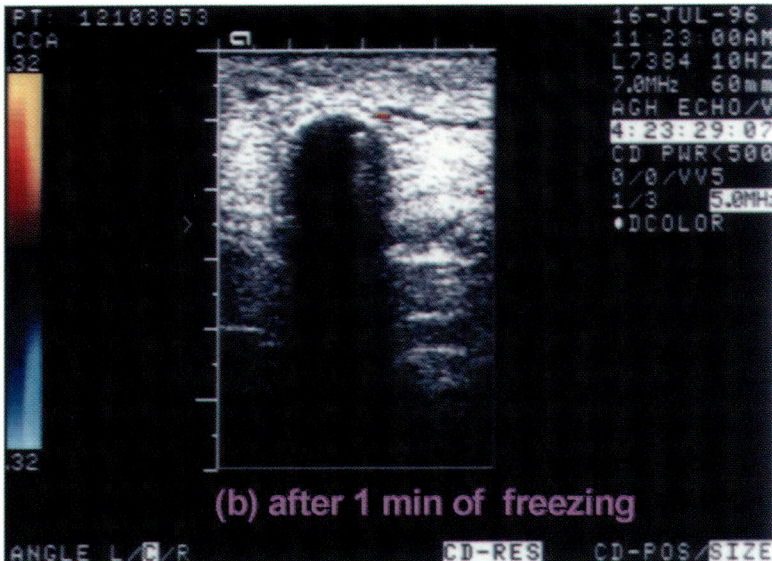

Fig. 16.1.2[4] B. After 1 min of freezing

Section F   Clinical Aspects   **347**

**Chapter 16
Breast Cancer
Cryosurgery**

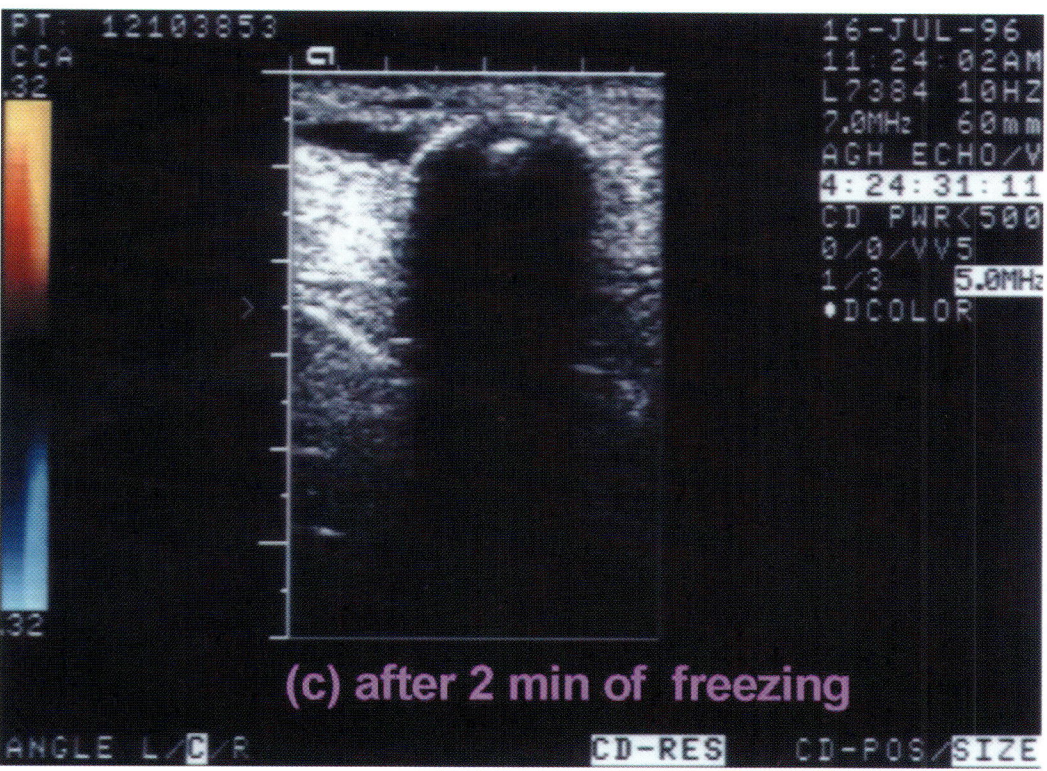

Fig. 16.1.2[4] C. After 2 min of freezing

Fig. 16.1.2[4]. Ultrasound imaged "ice ball" formation in a sheep breast model using a 7 MHz linear array transducer (Rabin et al., 1997; 1999). The cryoprocedure is performed adjacent to one of the major blood vessels of the breast, where the red and blue colors indicate blood flow in Doppler ultrasound imaging, as pointed in **A** prior to freezing. The non-circular contour of the "ice ball" adjacent to the blood vessel is a result of the heating effect of the blood flow, as can be seen after 3 min of freezing, **D**. The purple dashed line after 7 min of freezing, **H**, indicates the frozen interface that would probably have developed in the absence of the major blood vessel. The blue dashed line after 9.3 min, **I**, represents the location of the already frozen blood vessel. Some blood flow is still shown adjacent to the top-left contour of the frozen region after 9.3 min of freezing, due to the presence of an unfrozen blood vessel branch. Echo measurements at the location of the unfrozen blood vessel branch are shown in **J**

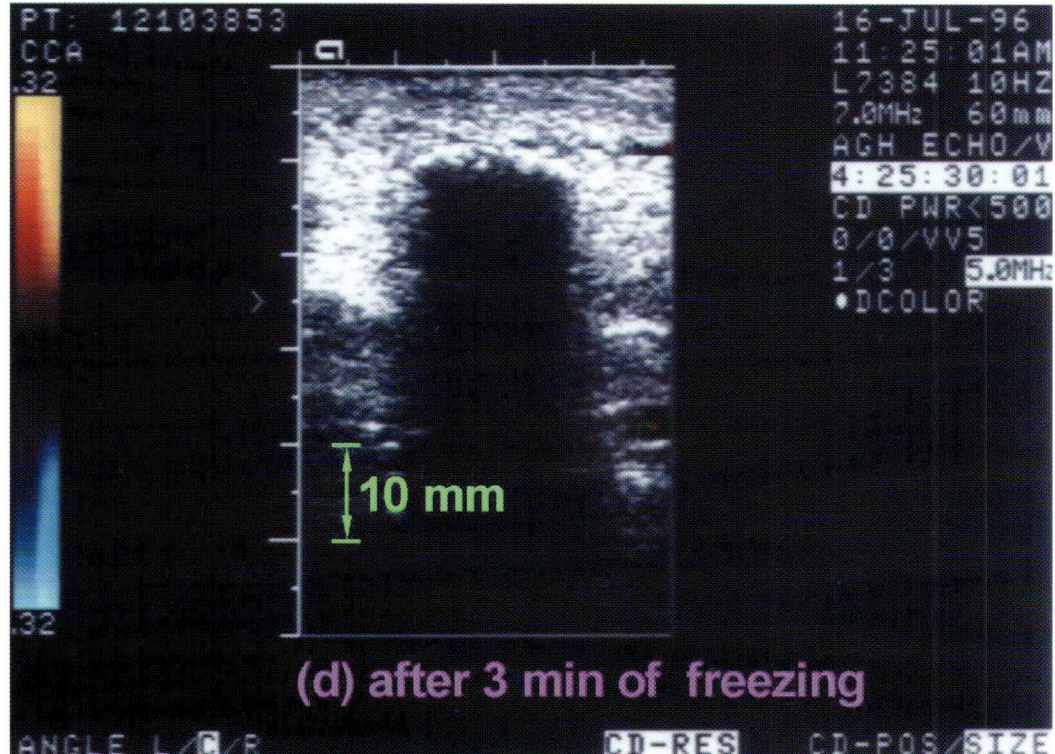

Fig. 16.1.2[4] D. After 3 min of freezing

Chapter 16
Breast Cancer Cryosurgery

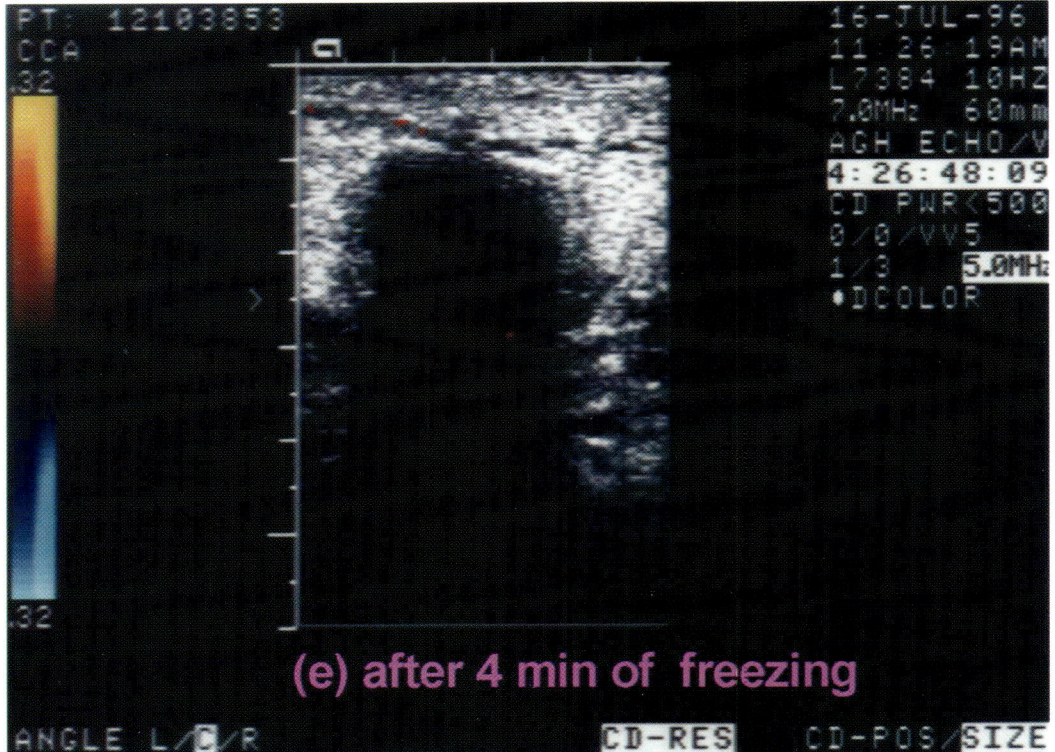

Fig. 16.1.2⁴ E. After 4 min of freezing

Fig. 16.1.2⁴. Ultrasound imaged "ice ball" formation in a sheep breast model using a 7 MHz linear array transducer (Rabin et al., 1997; 1999). The cryoprocedure is performed adjacent to one of the major blood vessels of the breast, where the red and blue colors indicate blood flow in Doppler ultrasound imaging, as pointed in **A** prior to freezing. The non-circular contour of the "ice ball" adjacent to the blood vessel is a result of the heating effect of the blood flow, as can be seen after 3 min of freezing, **D**. The purple dashed line after 7 min of freezing, **H**, indicates the frozen interface that would probably have developed in the absence of the major blood vessel. The blue dashed line after 9.3 min, **I**, represents the location of the already frozen blood vessel. Some blood flow is still shown adjacent to the top-left contour of the frozen region after 9.3 min of freezing, due to the presence of an unfrozen blood vessel branch. Echo measurements at the location of the unfrozen blood vessel branch are shown in **J**

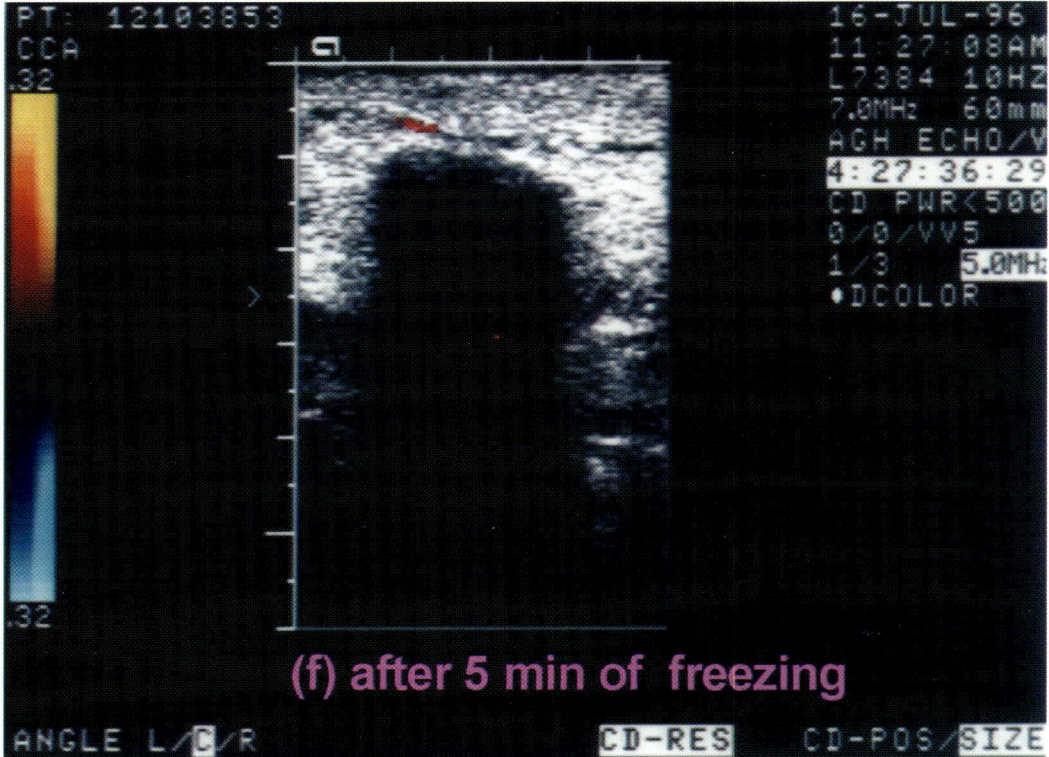

Fig. 16.1.2⁴ F. After 5 min of freezing

Section F Clinical Aspects **349**

**Chapter 16
Breast Cancer
Cryosurgery**

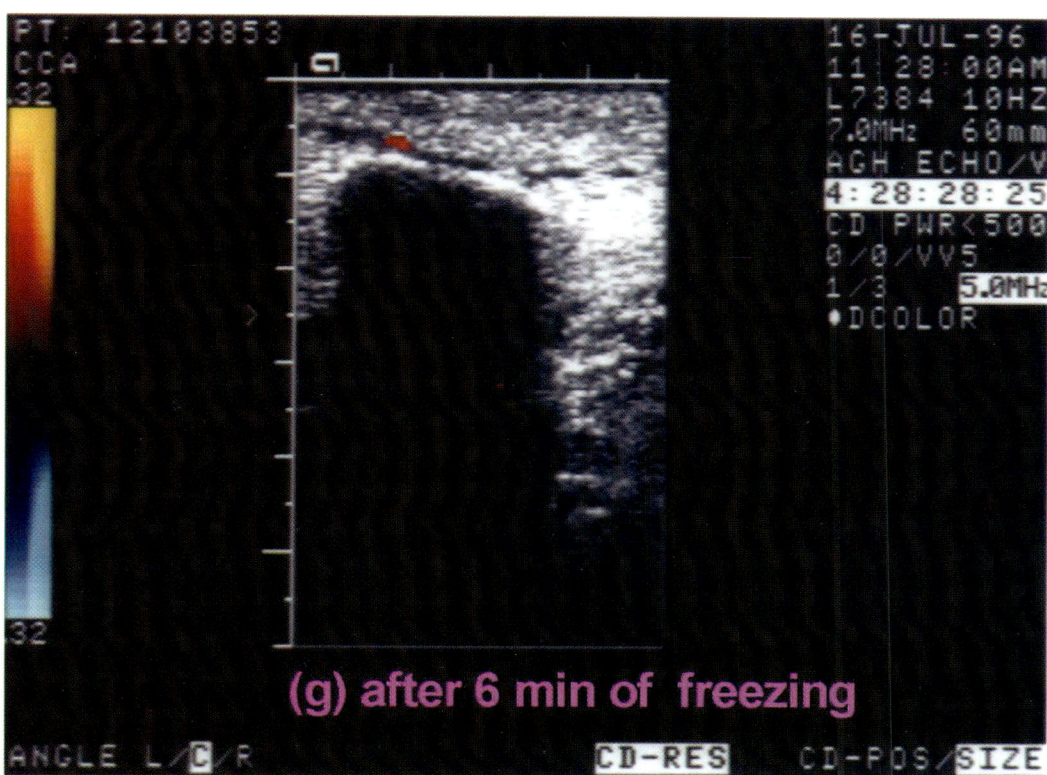

Fig. 16.1.2⁴ G. After 6 min of freezing

Fig. 16.1.2⁴. Ultrasound imaged "ice ball" formation in a sheep breast model using a 7 MHz linear array transducer (Rabin et al., 1997; 1999). The cryoprocedure is performed adjacent to one of the major blood vessels of the breast, where the red and blue colors indicate blood flow in Doppler ultrasound imaging, as pointed in **A** prior to freezing. The non-circular contour of the "ice ball" adjacent to the blood vessel is a result of the heating effect of the blood flow, as can be seen after 3 min of freezing, **D**. The purple dashed line after 7 min of freezing, **H**, indicates the frozen interface that would probably have developed in the absence of the major blood vessel. The blue dashed line after 9.3 min, **I**, represents the location of the already frozen blood vessel. Some blood flow is still shown adjacent to the top-left contour of the frozen region after 9.3 min of freezing, due to the presence of an unfrozen blood vessel branch. Echo measurements at the location of the unfrozen blood vessel branch are shown in **J**

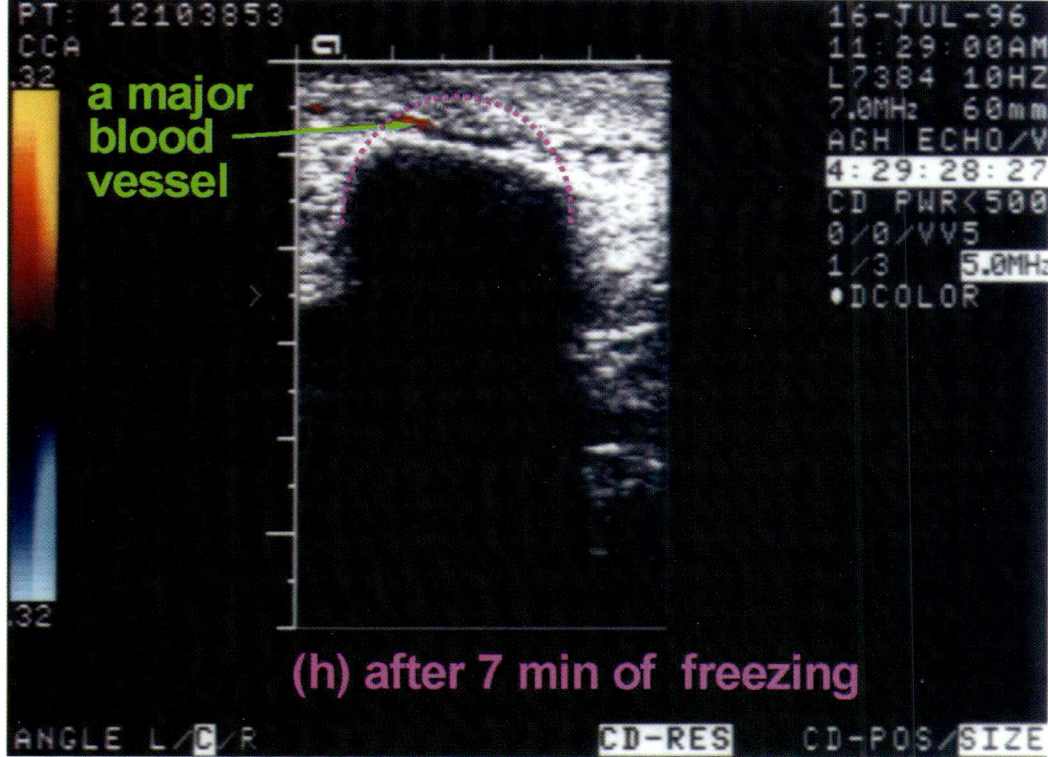

Fig. 16.1.2⁴ H. After 7 min of freezing

Chapter 16
Breast Cancer Cryosurgery

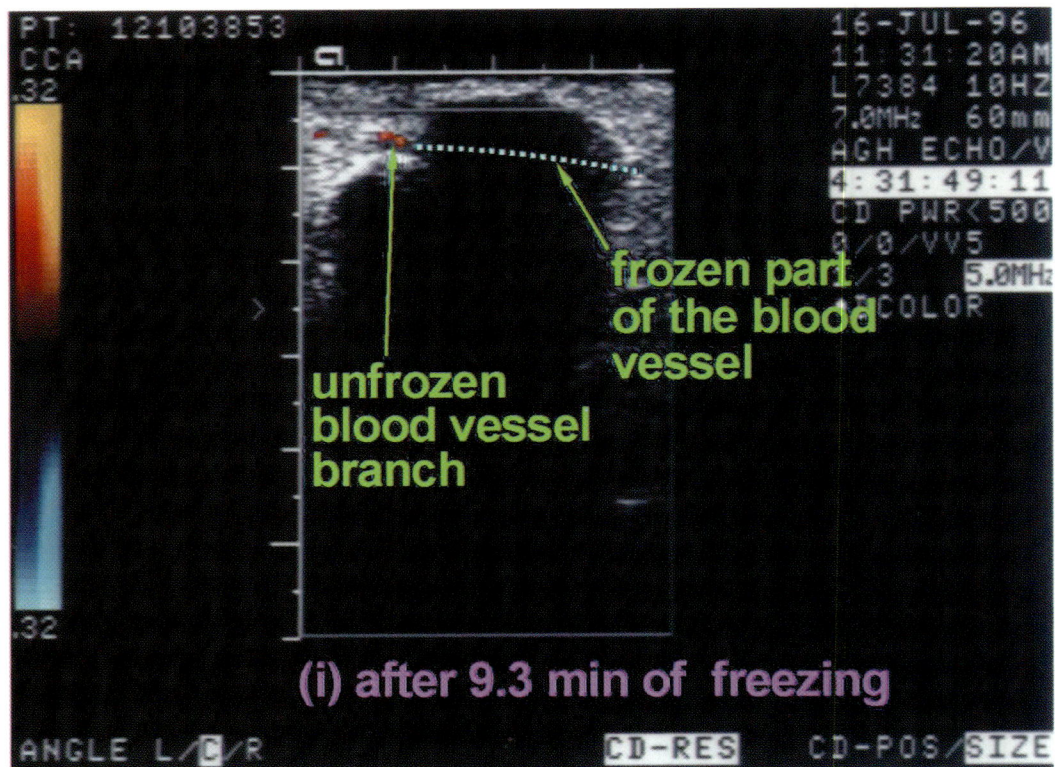

Fig. 16.1.2⁴ I. After 9.3 min of freezing

Fig. 16.1.2⁴. Ultrasound imaged "ice ball" formation in a sheep breast model using a 7 MHz linear array transducer (Rabin et al., 1997; 1999). The cryoprocedure is performed adjacent to one of the major blood vessels of the breast, where the red and blue colors indicate blood flow in Doppler ultrasound imaging, as pointed in **A** prior to freezing. The non-circular contour of the "ice ball" adjacent to the blood vessel is a result of the heating effect of the blood flow, as can be seen after 3 min of freezing, **D**. The purple dashed line after 7 min of freezing, **H**, indicates the frozen interface that would probably have developed in the absence of the major blood vessel. The blue dashed line after 9.3 min, **I**, represents the location of the already frozen blood vessel. Some blood flow is still shown adjacent to the top-left contour of the frozen region after 9.3 min of freezing, due to the presence of an unfrozen blood vessel branch. Echo measurements at the location of the unfrozen blood vessel branch are shown in **J**

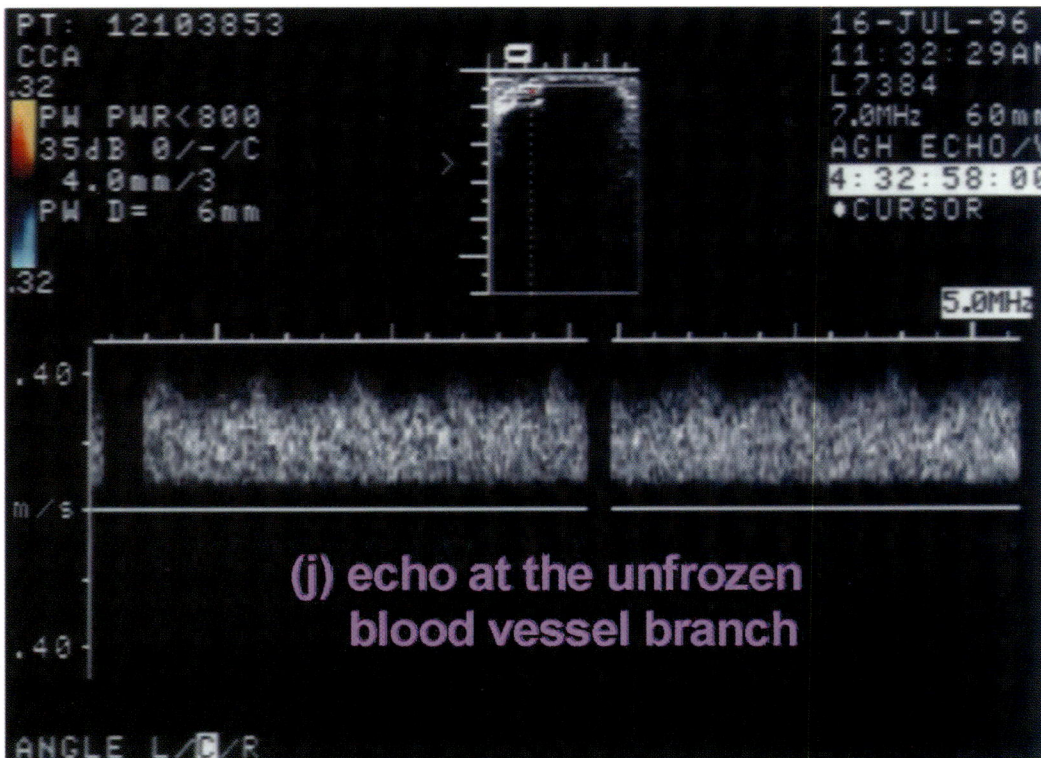

Fig. 16.1.2⁴ J. Echo at the unfrozen blood vessel branch

16.1.3 Long-Term Follow-Up Post-Cryosurgery in a Sheep Breast Model[4]

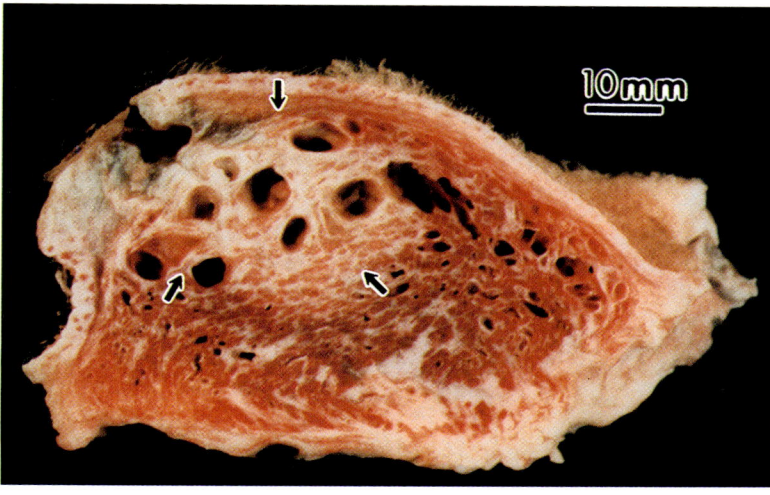

Fig. 16.1.3[4]. Macro cross-section view of a cryotreated sheep breast specimen, which was perfused by 2,3,5-triphenyltetrazolium chloride (TTC) stain and 10% buffered formaldehyde. The TTC is an oxidation-reduction indicator that has been used effectively for histochemical analysis of infarct volume in ischemically injured tissues. TTC, as a water soluble salt is not a dye, but is reduced by certain mitochondrial respiratory enzymes in normal tissue to a deep red, fat soluble, light sensitive compound (formazan) that turns normal tissue brick red and thereby delineates abnormal areas. TTC has been used extensively to stain tissues from human and experimental animals and has been shown to reflect accurately the extent of irreversible ischemic damage. The cryotreated region appears white (indicated by arrows), while the surrounding healthy tissues have a dark-red color due to the staining of viable cells by the TTC. Note the large duct of the recently lactating animal (8 weeks post lambing)

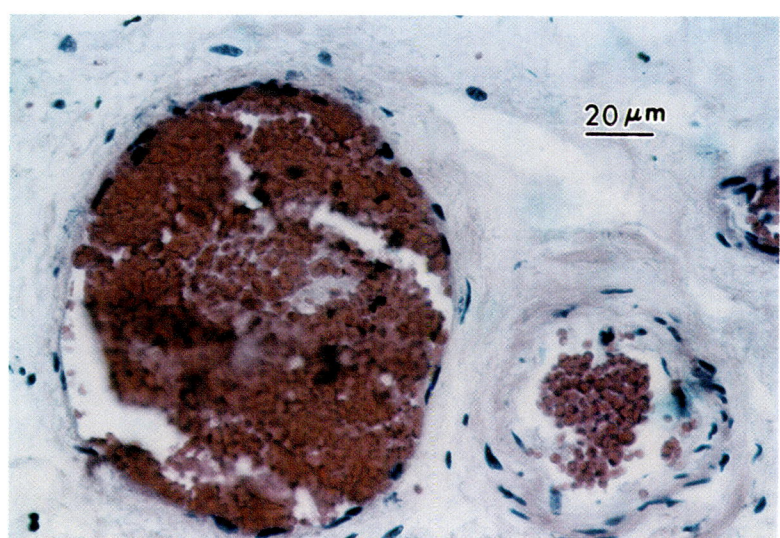

Fig. 16.1.4[4]. Central area of the cryotreated region presented in Fig. 17.5.3[3], stained with H and E, which shows a vein (left) and an artery (right) congested with red blood cells and thrombosis. The blood vessels appear intact 15 min after thawing, however the congestion with red blood cells and thrombosis indicates vascular damage

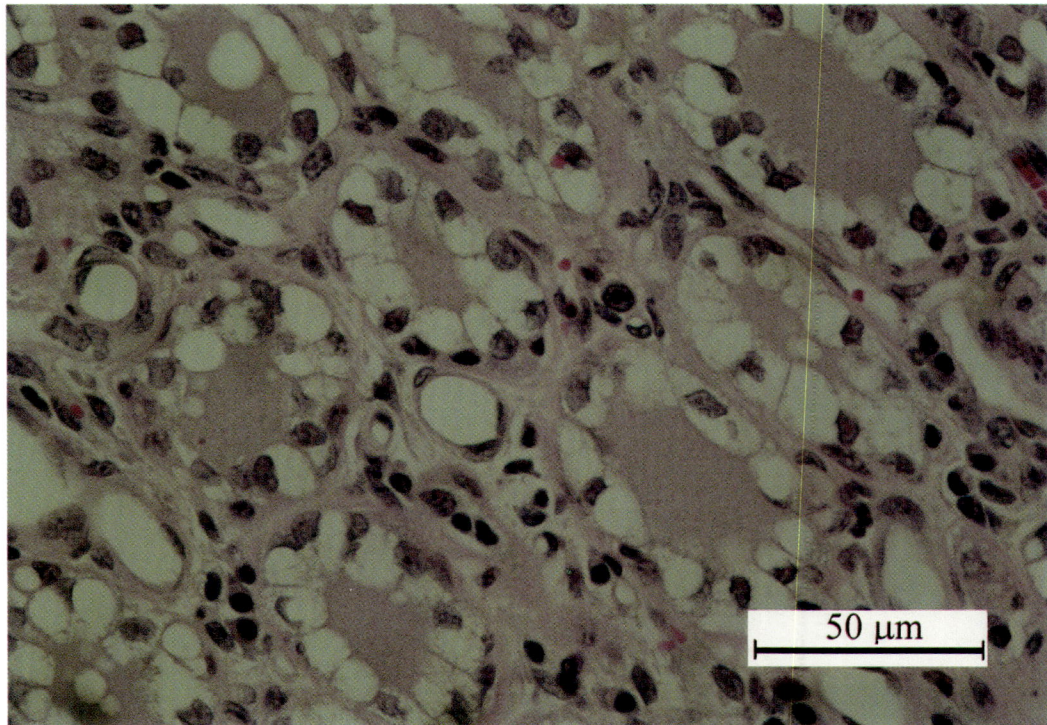

Fig. 16.1.5[4]. Control cross-section showing the normal breast glands in a recently-pregnant sheep breast model stained with H & E (12 weeks post lambing and 8 weeks post lactation). The recently-pregnant sheep breast model is simulative to the human breast for long-term follow-up post-cryosurgery, and makes MRI, mammography, and ultrasound imaging practicable

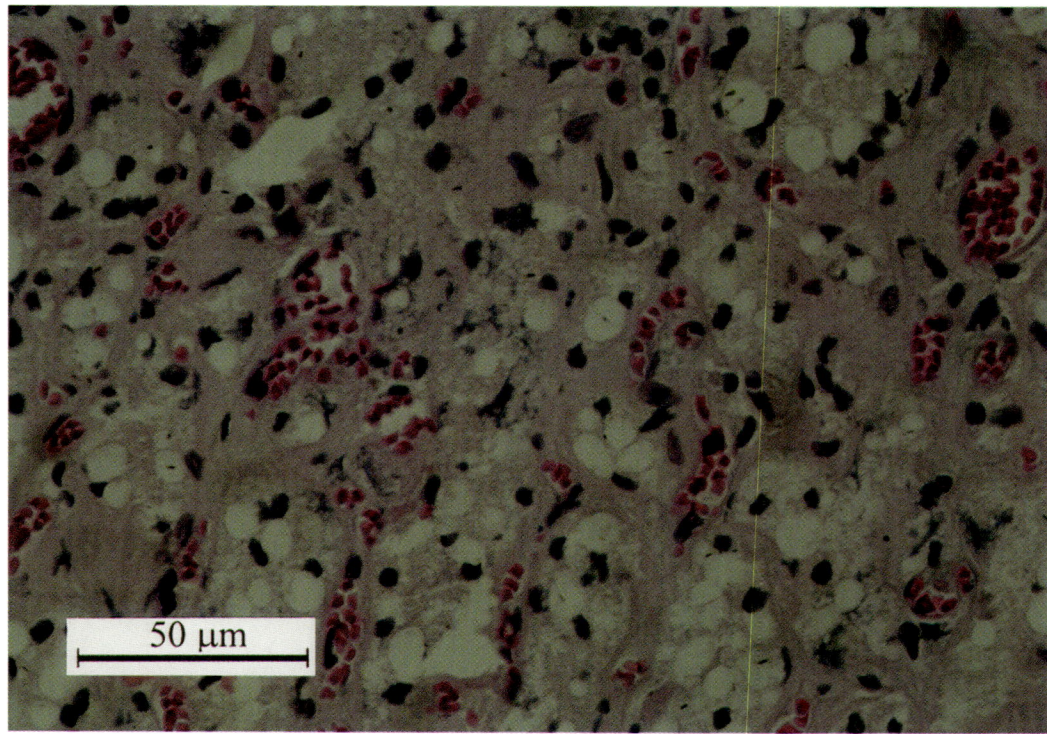

Fig. 16.1.6[4]. Cryoinjured region at 1 day post-cryosurgery stained with H & E. Microscopic findings immediately post-cryosurgery show edema of the interstitial tissue with vascular congestion by red blood cells. The epithelial cells of glands and ducts show swelling and vacuolation of the cytoplasm and nuclear changes consisting of hyperchromasia and irregular shapes

Section F Clinical Aspects

Chapter 16
Breast Cancer
Cryosurgery

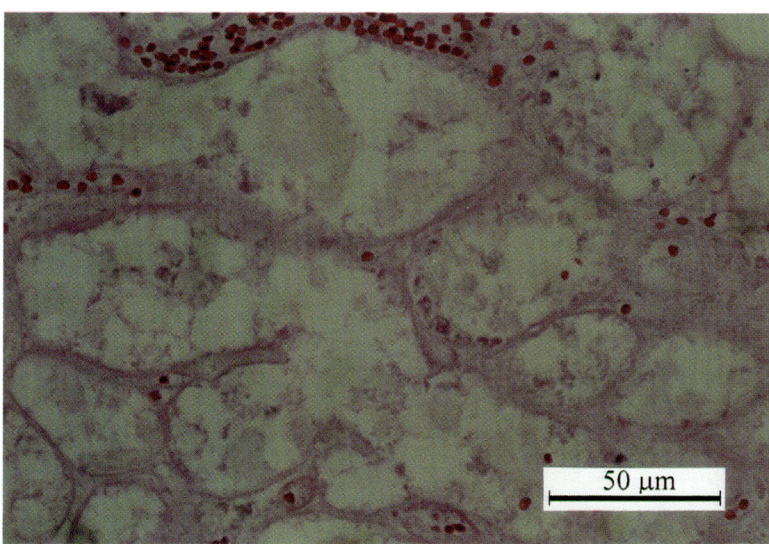

Fig. 16.1.7[4]. Cryoinjured region at 1 week post-cryosurgery stained with H and E. Microscopic findings at 1 week post-cryosurgery show extensive ischemic necrosis, vascular congestion with red blood cells, scattered thrombosed blood vessels of varying size, and extensive intestitial edema. In the areas of ischemic necrosis there was no viable glandular or ductal epithelium, which are the sources of human breast cancer. Very little inflammation with scattered neutrophils in the necrotic debris and damaged breast lobules were found

Fig. 16.1.8[4]. Cryoinjured region at 5 months post-cryosurgery stained with H and E. The cut surface of specimens at 5 months showed a soft white main cryoinjured region surrounded by a light brown peripheral zone. The cryoinjured region was ill-defined and sometimes difficult to characterize. The scar (the main cryoinjured region) showed increased fibrous tissue with collagen. Some fibroblast and capillaries were found in the main cryoinjured region. The ducts showed complex branching but still no acinar development. The diameter of the cryoinjured region at 5 months post-cryosurgery was found to be about 50% of the frozen region diameter

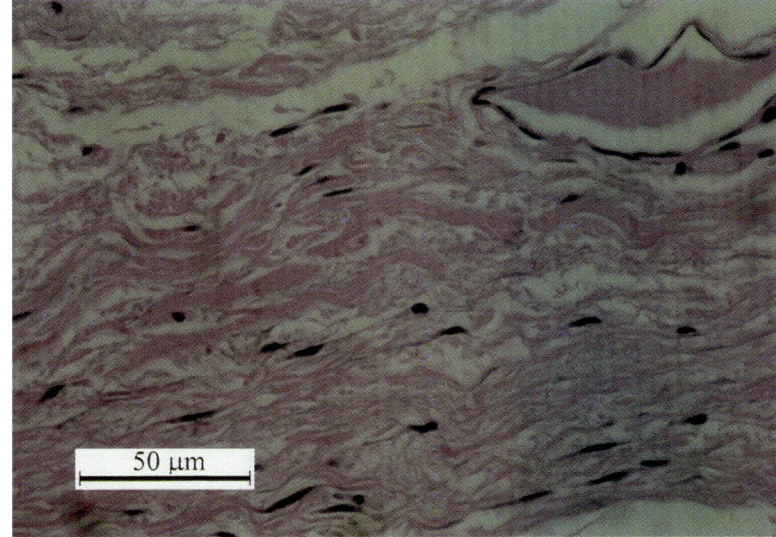

Chapter 16 Breast Cancer Cryosurgery

16.2 Locally Advanced Breast Cancer (LABC)

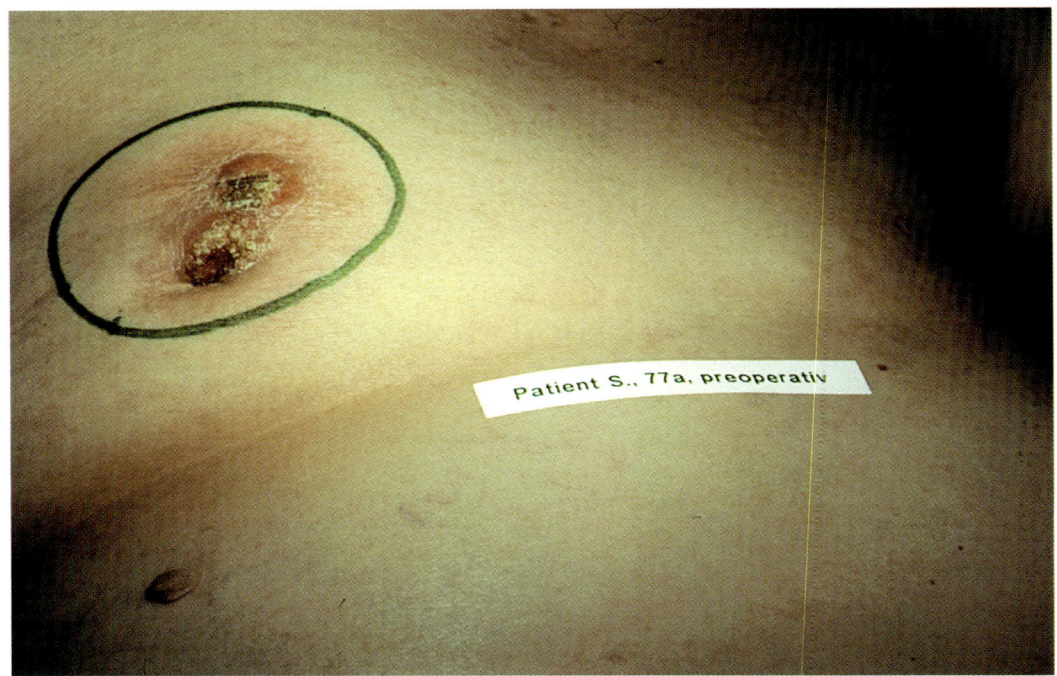

Fig. 16.2.1[1]. LABC. Ulcerated cancer on the right breast of a 77-year-old woman. Preoperative view. This patient neglected to have her second breast removed, as she feared the amputation

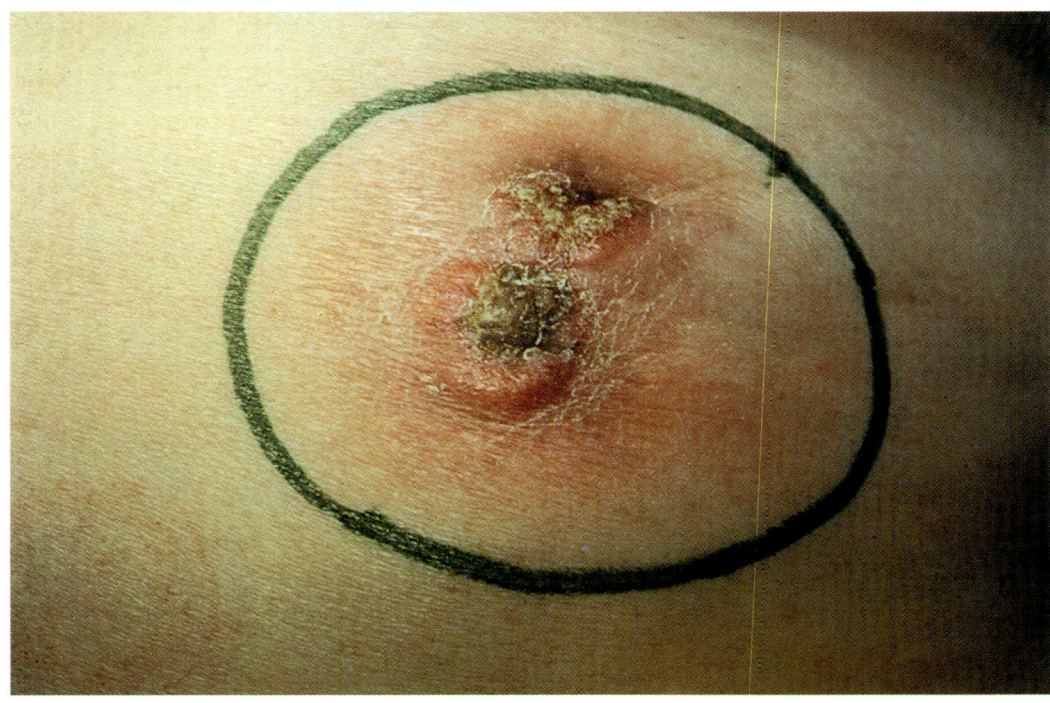

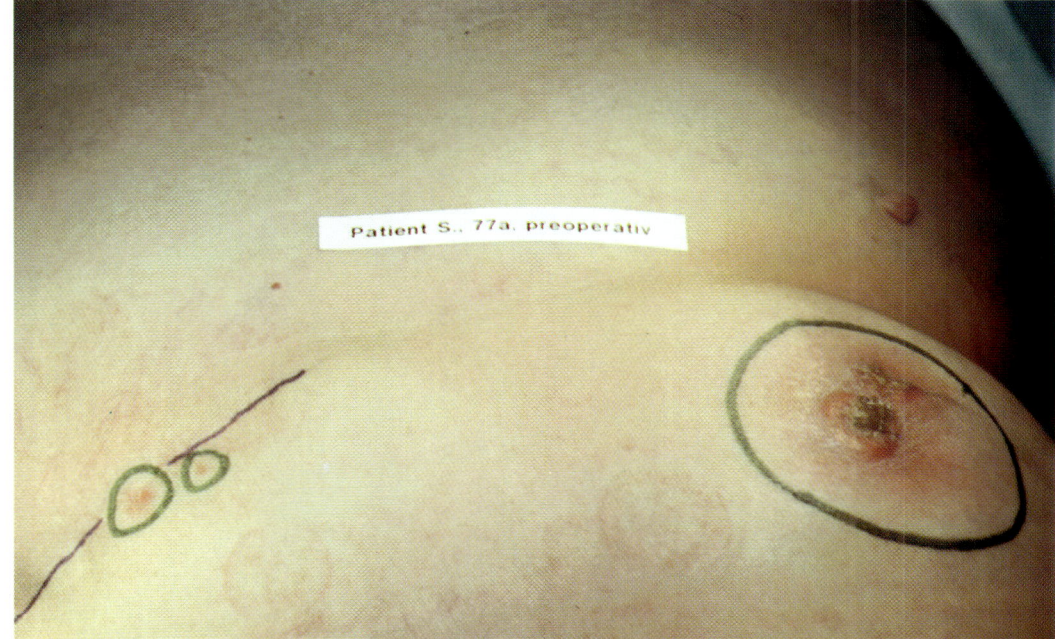

Fig. 16.2.2¹. Local-Regional Disease Recurrence. Ulcerated, primary inflammatory breast carcinoma right (**A**) with skin metastases on the left-hand side of the breast after mastectomy (**B**) in the same patient. Caudal view

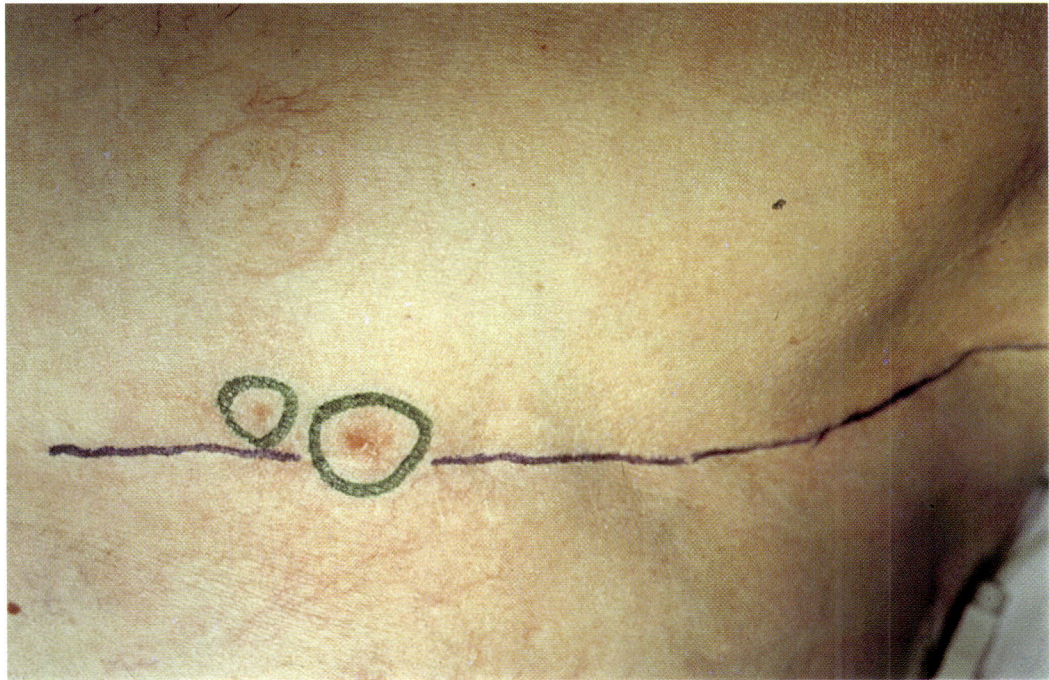

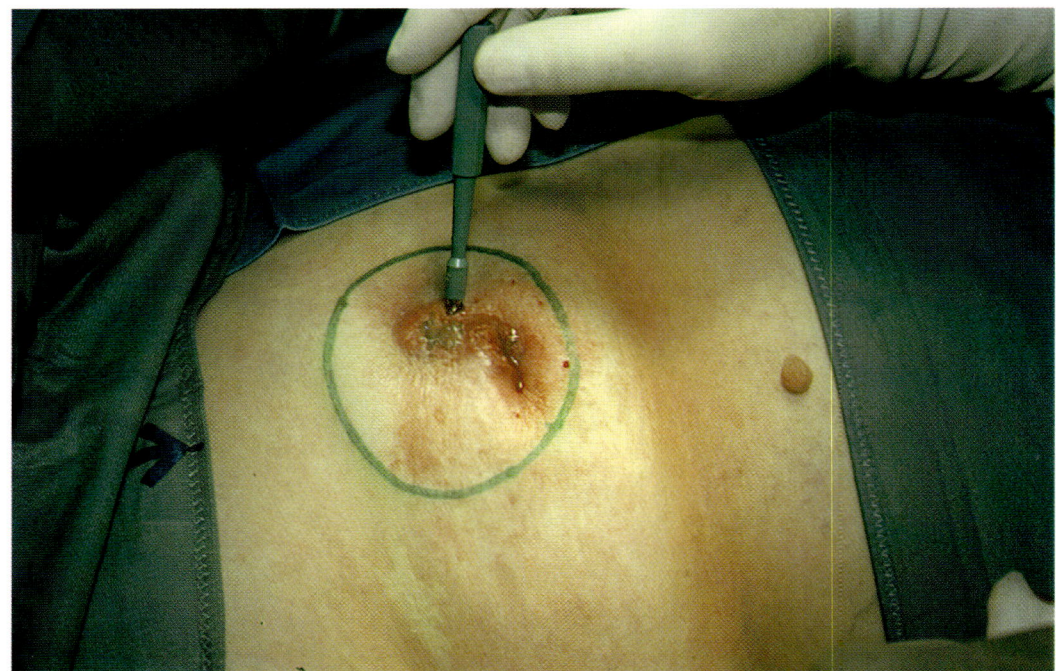

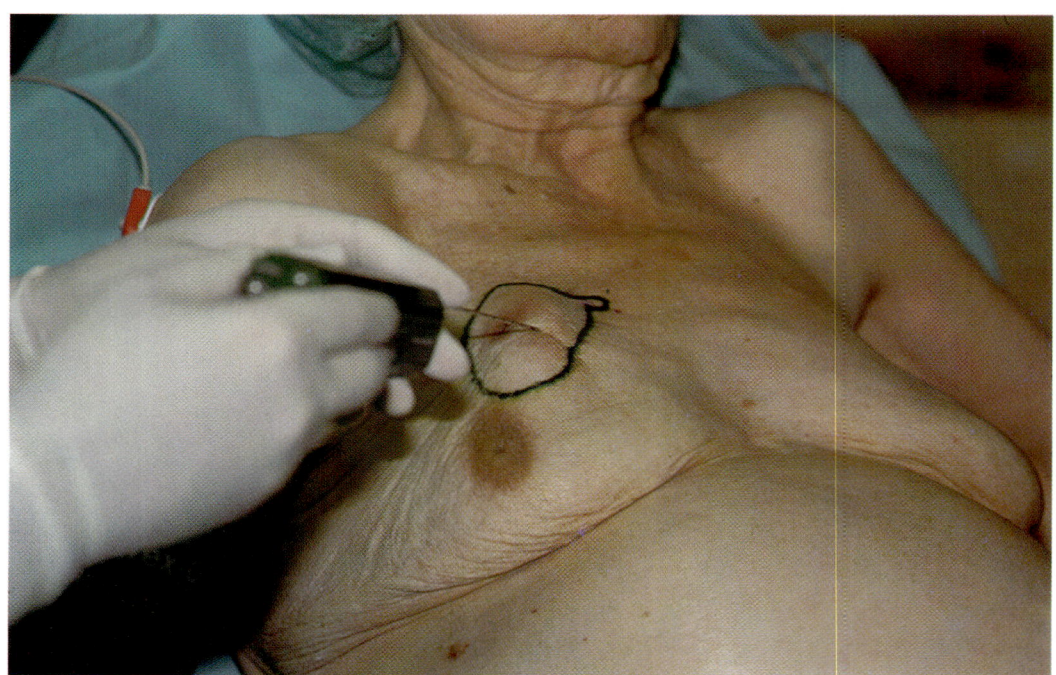

Fig. 16.2.3[1]. LABC. Preoperative biopsy for histological examination is performed under local anesthesia to evaluate and verify the breast tumor by means of a disposable punch (**A**) or with disposable needles such as the Tru-Cut (**B**)

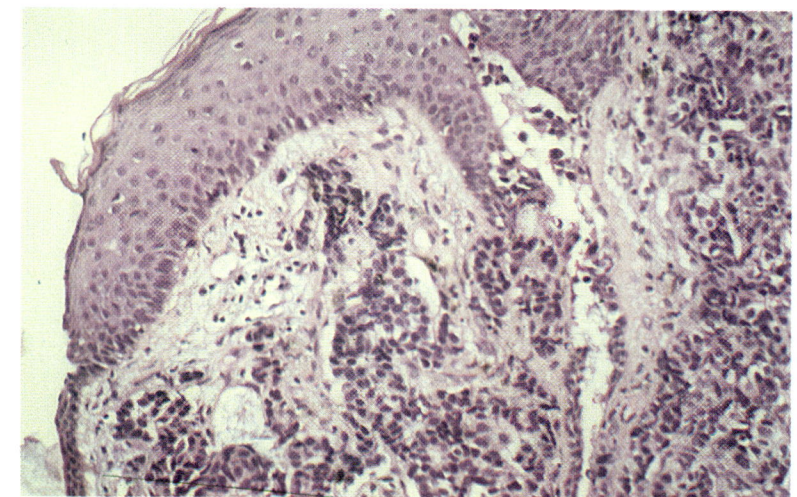

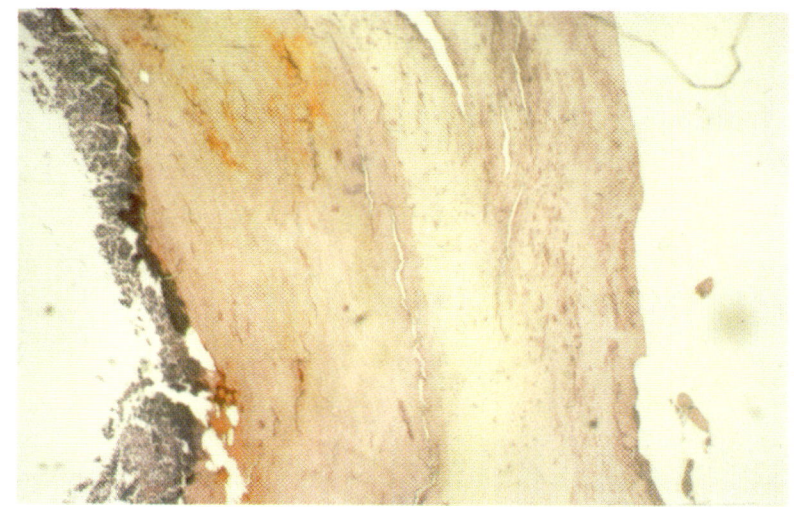

Fig. 16.2.4[1] A–C. LABC. Histological diagnosis: invasive lobular breast cancer: mixed type, degree 1/2, tumor stage: pT4b, pNX

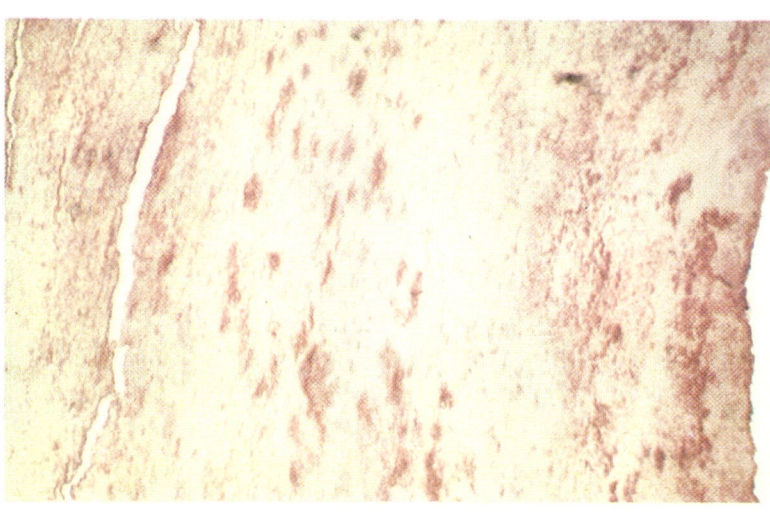

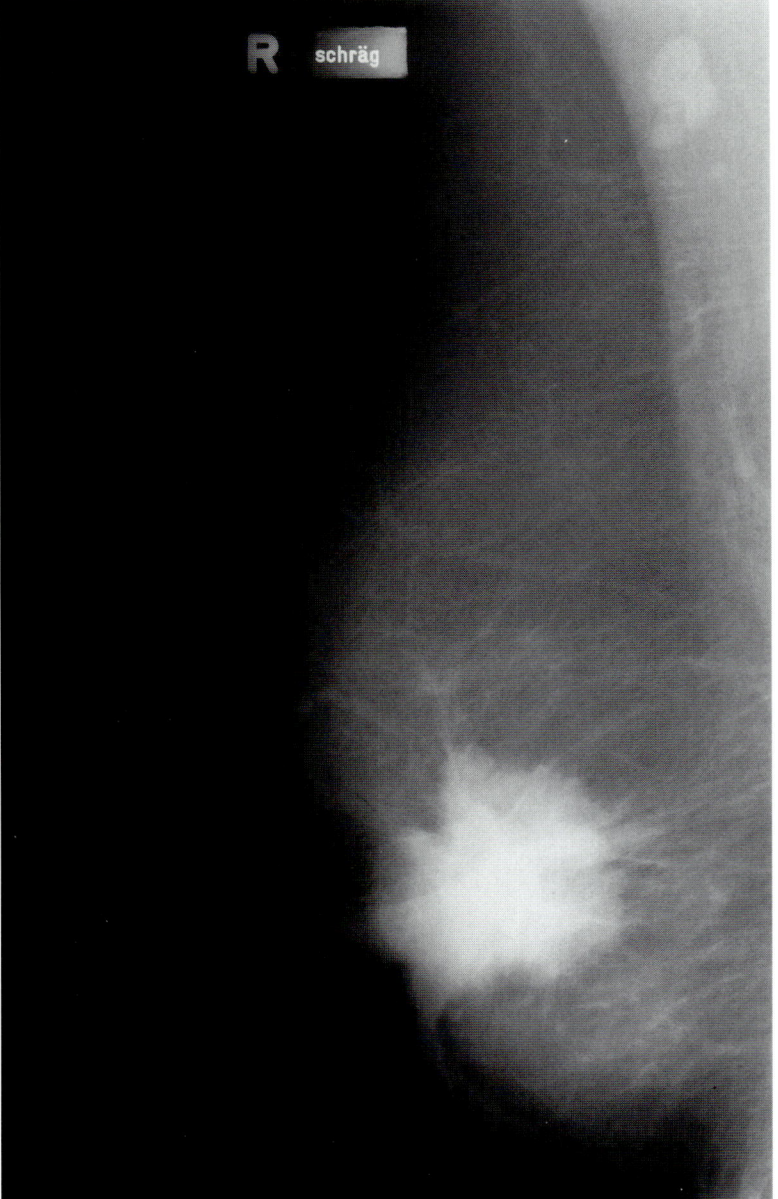

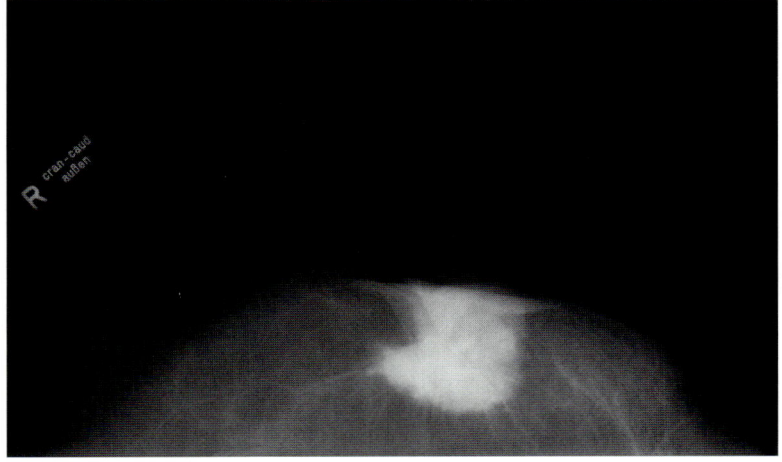

Fig. 16.2.5[1]. Preoperative mammography in the same patient: oblique (A), mediolateral and cranial (B), craniocaudal and external (C) views

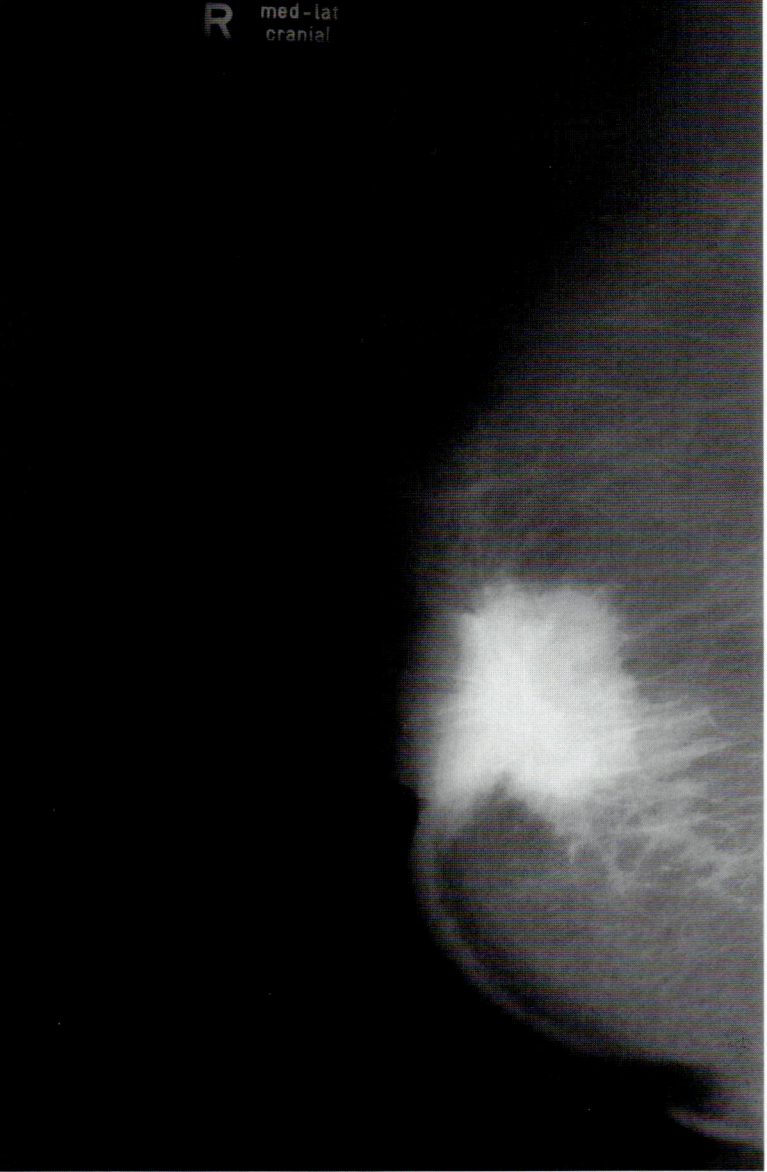

Section F   Clinical Aspects   **359**

**Chapter 16
Breast Cancer
Cryosurgery**

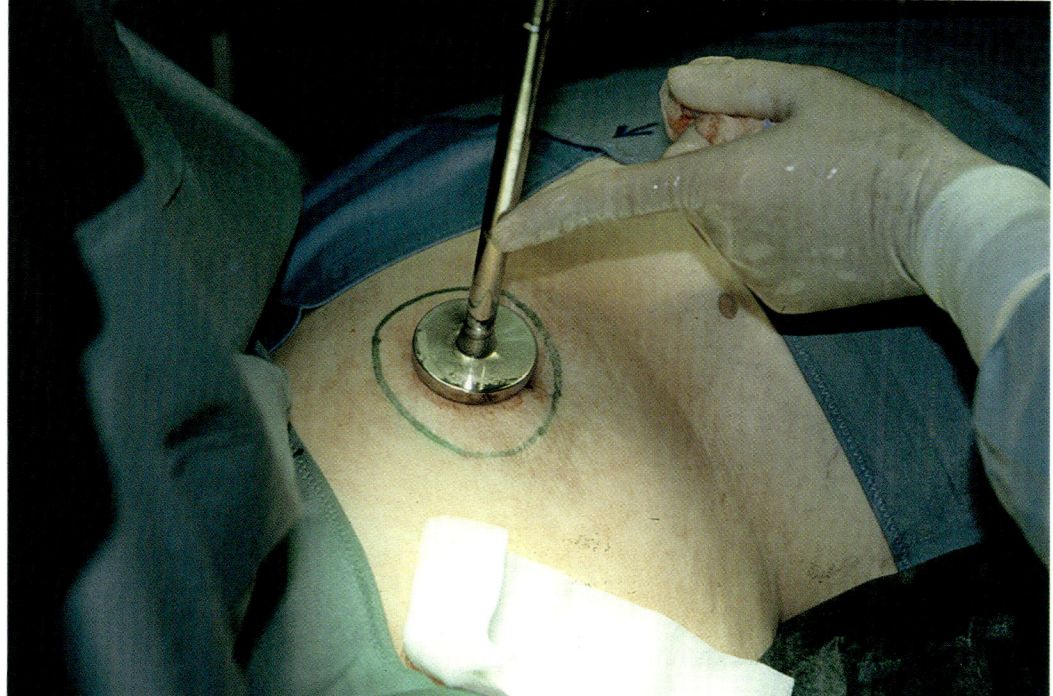

A

Fig. 16.2.6[1]. LABC. Breast Cancer Cryosurgery (BCC): A multiply occurring freeze-thaw cycle using a cryoprobe of 55 mm which is placed on the breast tumor mass (**A**) at a temperature of $-130\,^\circ$C for 3 min using a universal cryosurgical unit (**B**)

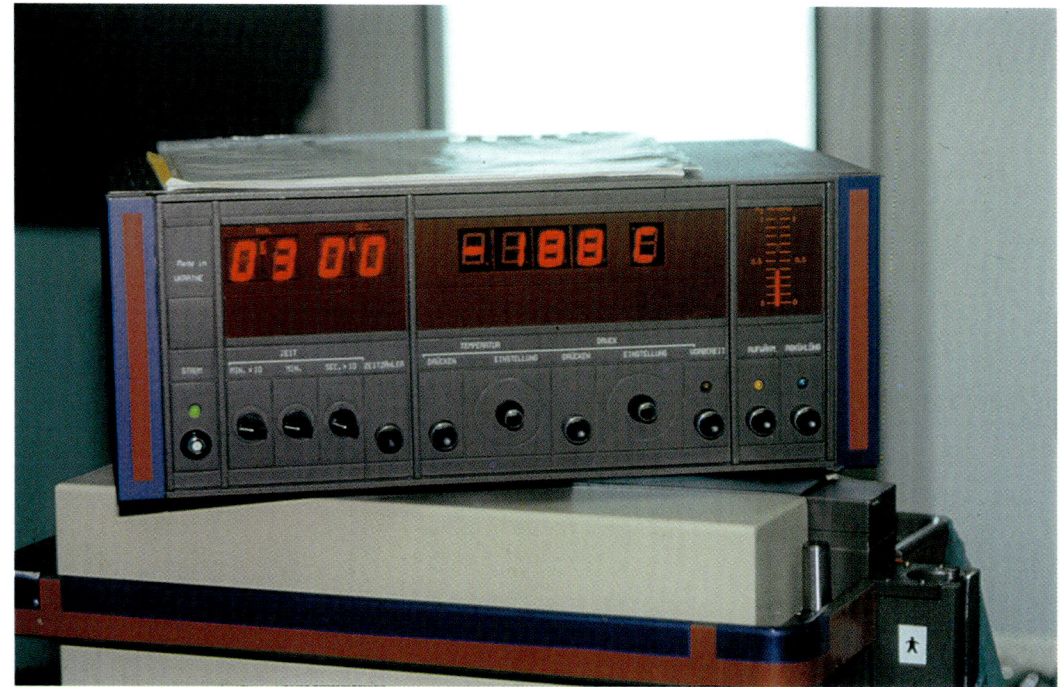

B

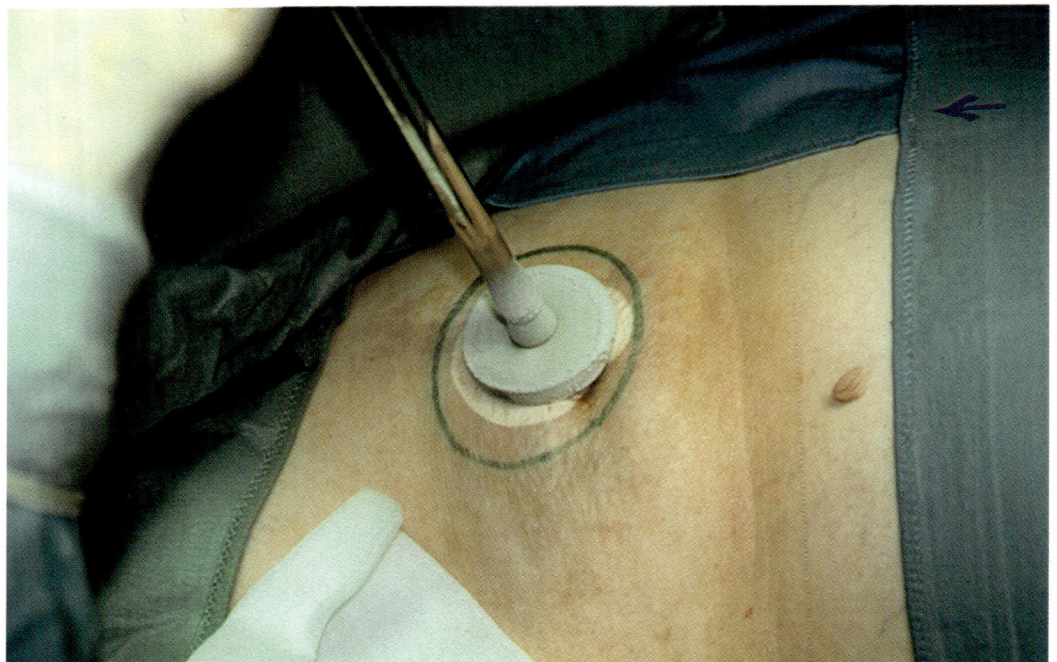

Fig. 16.2.7¹. LABC. The technique of breast cancer cryosurgery, showing a disc probe (**A**) and the cryosurgical rim of the cryozone (**B**), which forms the demarcation line between cryonecrosis and the healthy breast tissue

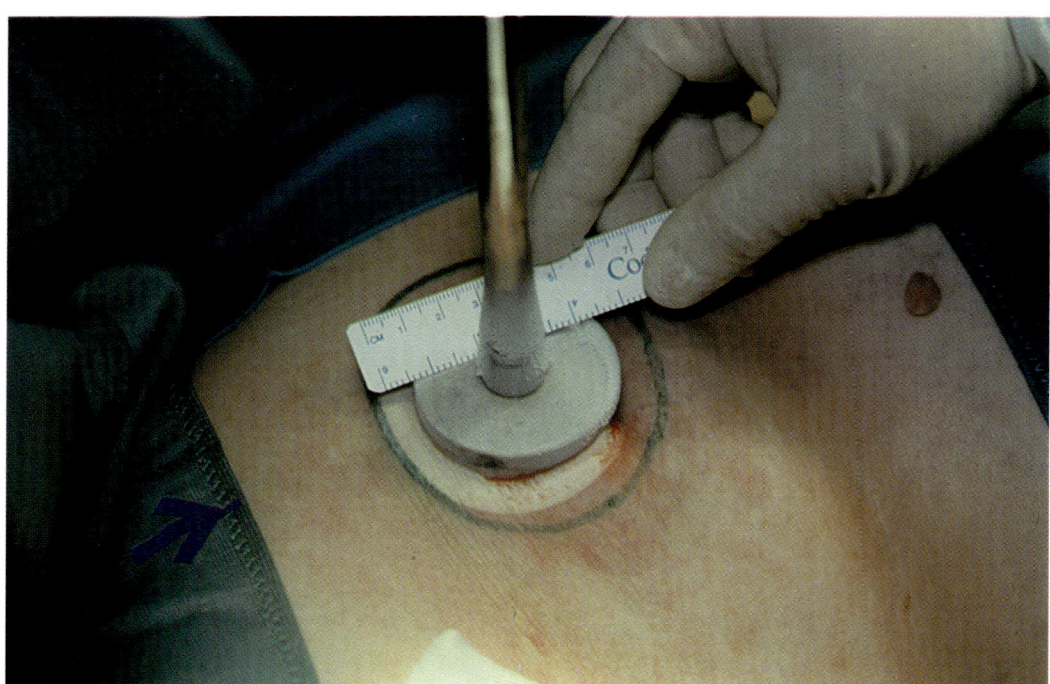

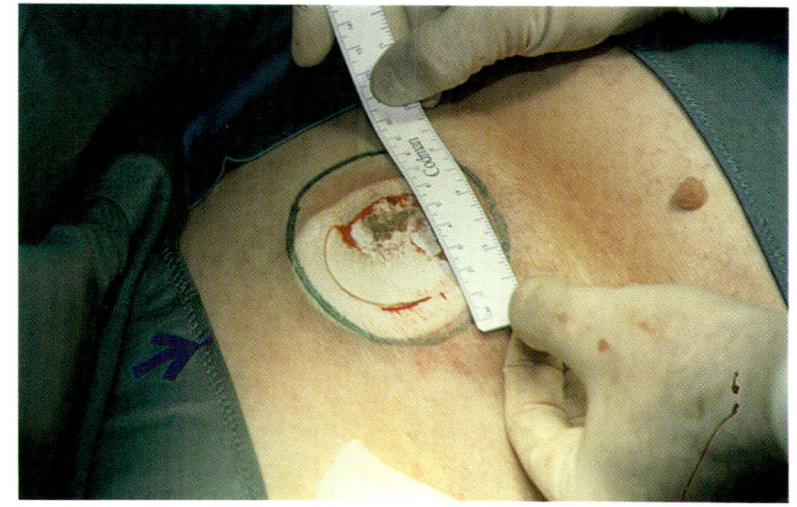

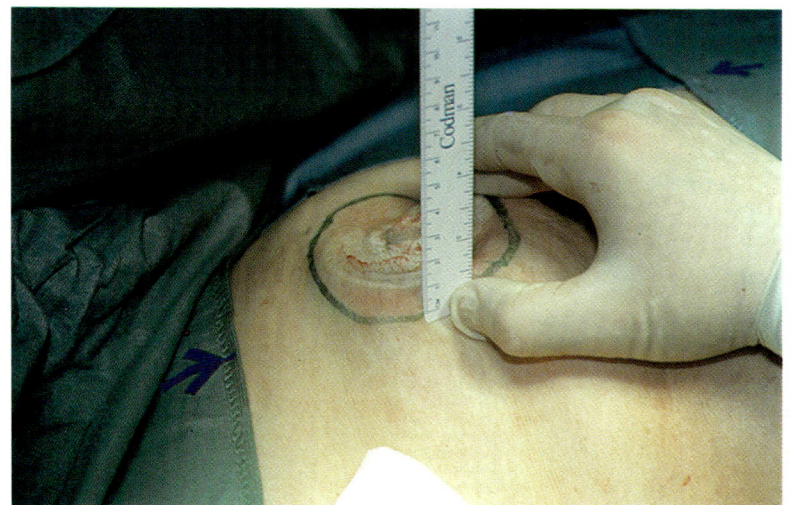

Fig. 16.2.8¹. LABC. Breast Cancer Cryosurgery: The post-cryosurgical zone is clearly outlined by a demarcation line, measures 63 mm in diameter (**A**) and 18 mm in depth (**B, C**)

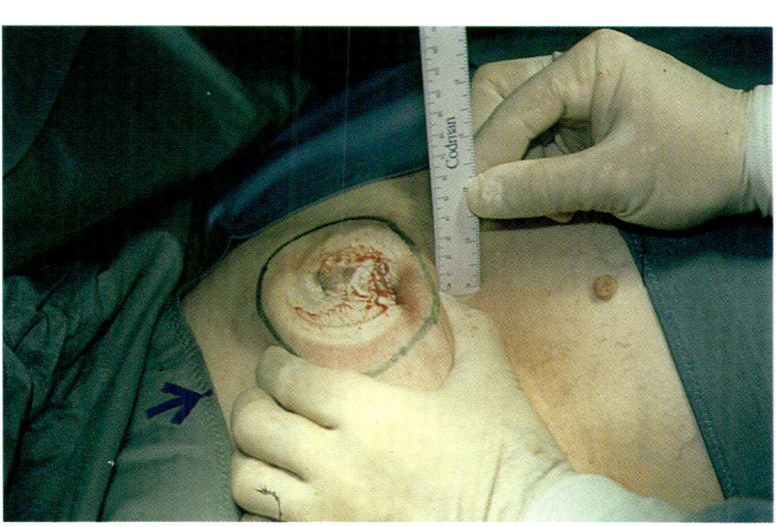

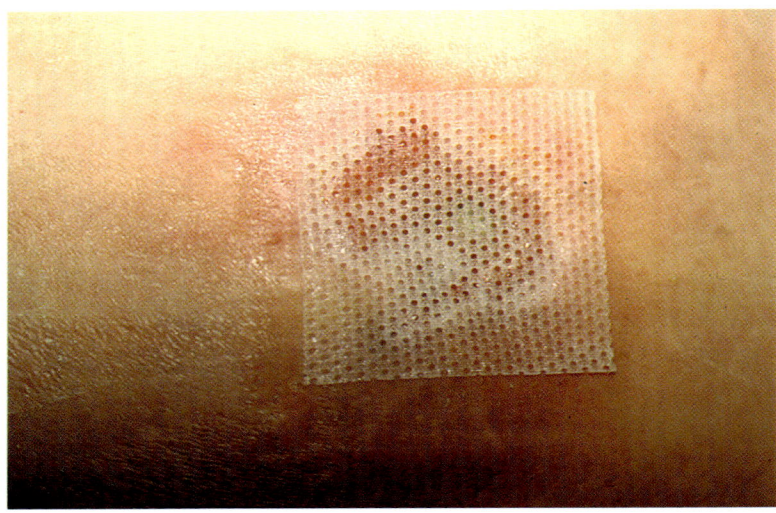

Fig. 16.2.9[1]. A layer of ointment is usually put over the cryozone between the surface of the dressing and the wound after each cryosurgical operation on the breast

A

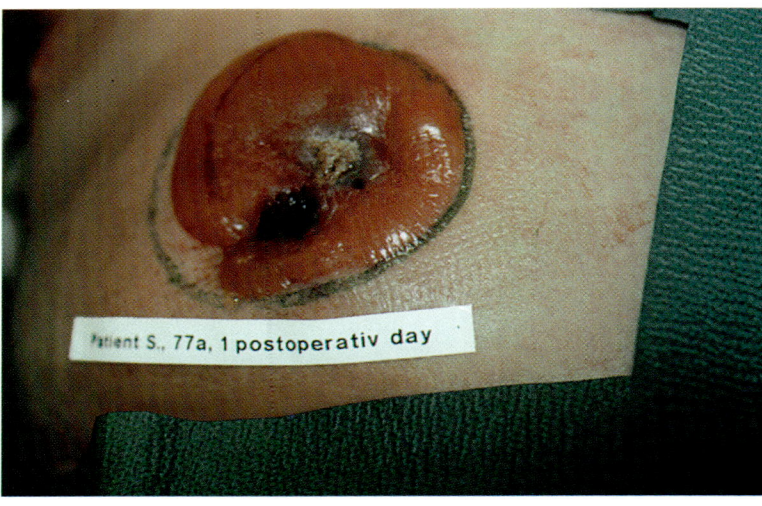

B

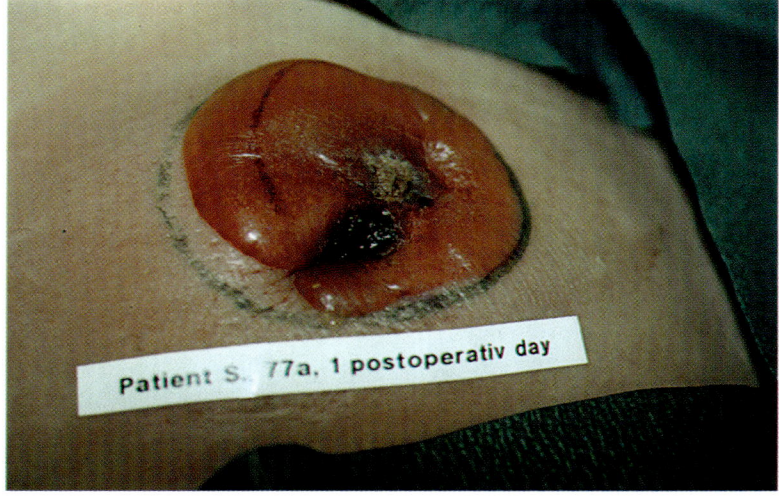

Fig. 16.2.10[1]. LABC. Breast Cancer Cryosurgery: 1st postoperative day after the first cryosurgical session. View of the post-cryosurgical wound (A, B). No pain

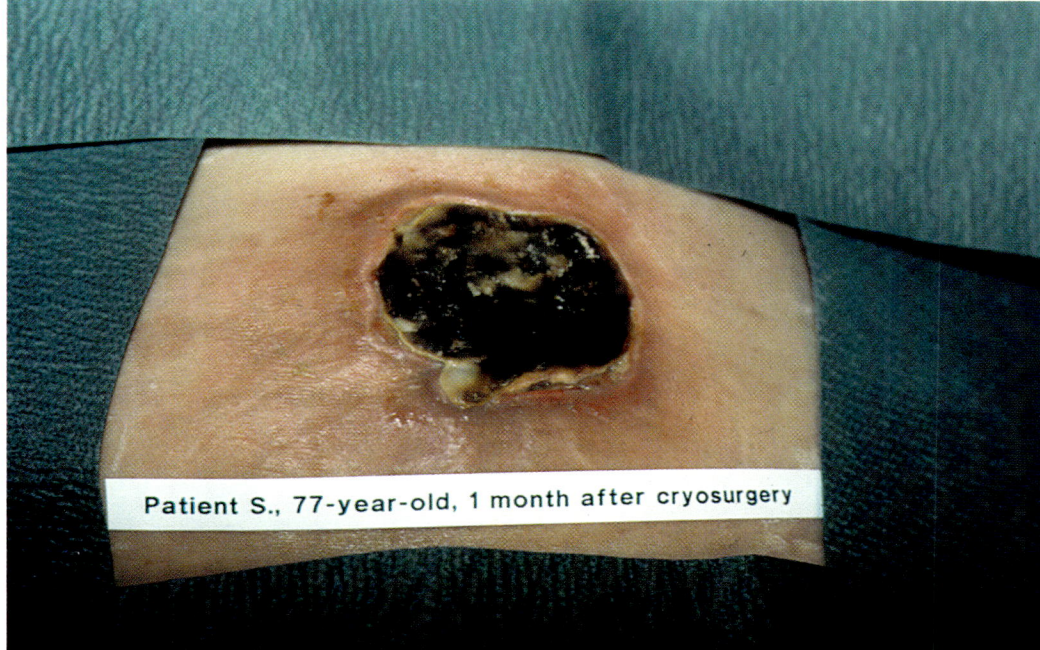

Fig. 16.2.11[1]. LABC. Breast Cancer Cryosurgery: 30 days after the first cryosurgical session. View of the post-cryosurgical wound with the crust (**A, B**). No pain

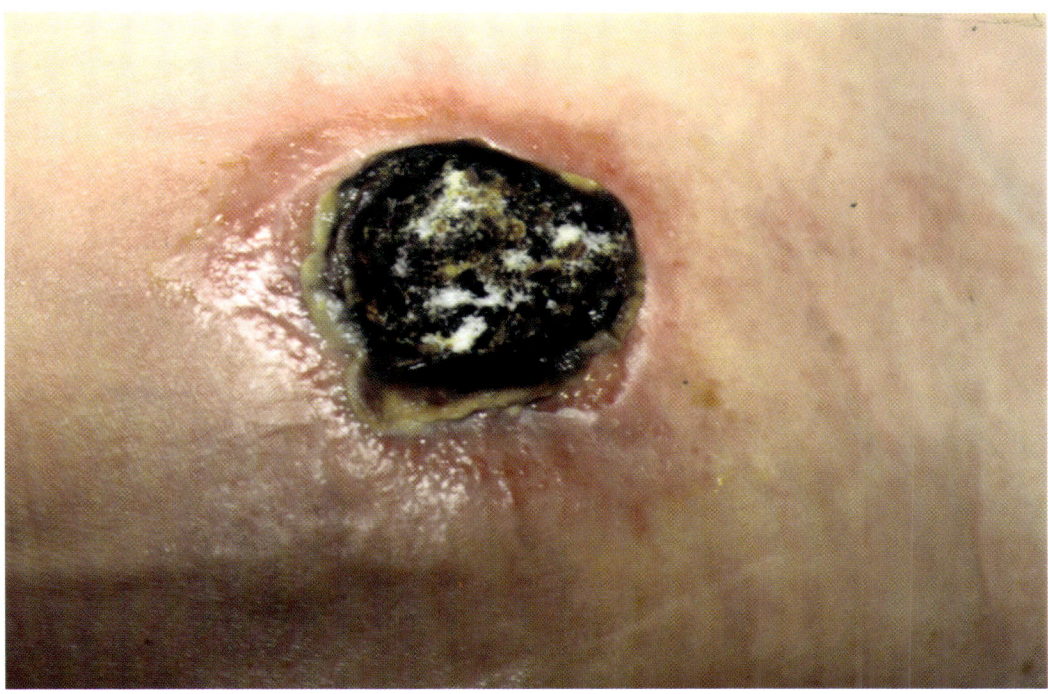

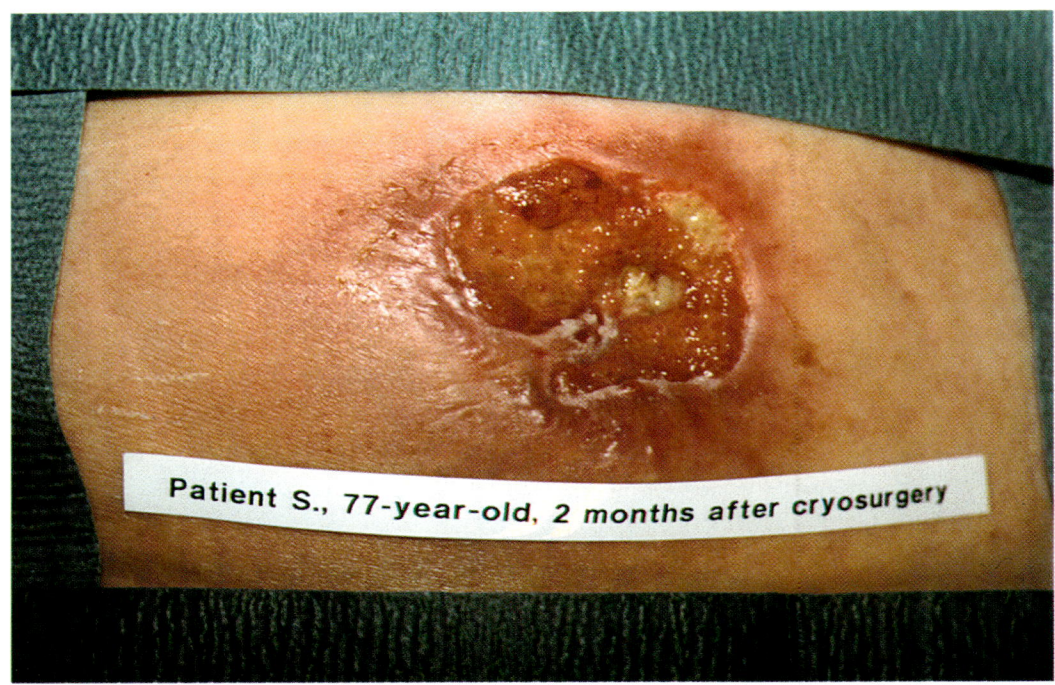

Fig. 16.2.12[1]. LABC. Breast Cancer Cryosurgery: 2 months after the first cryosurgical session. View of the post-cryosurgical wound (**A**) with the sloughed crust (**B**). No pain

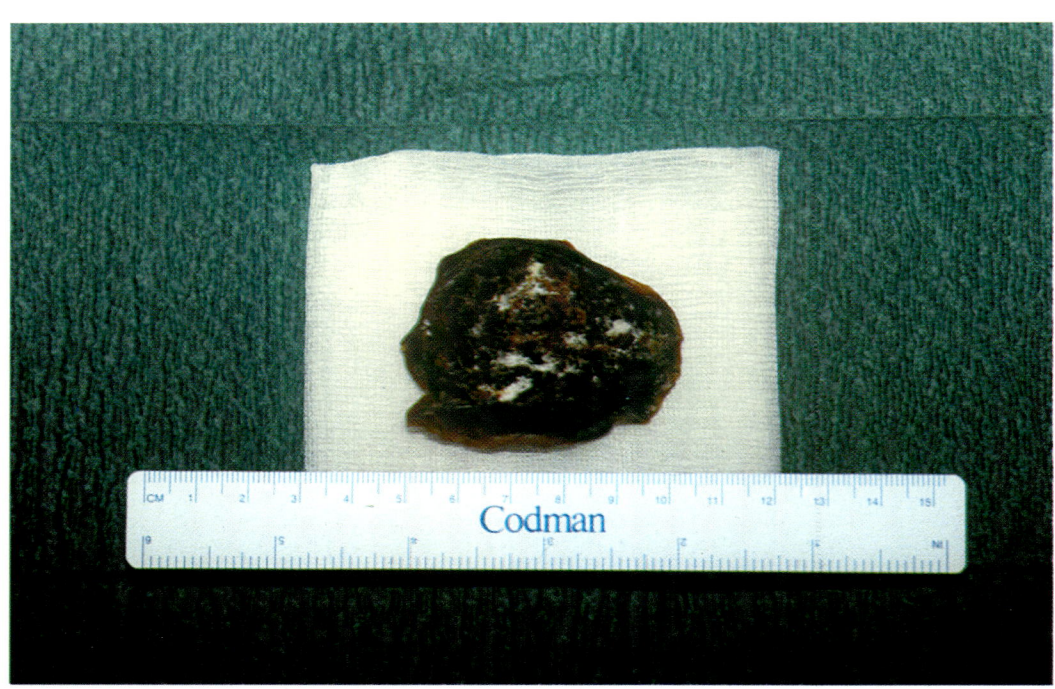

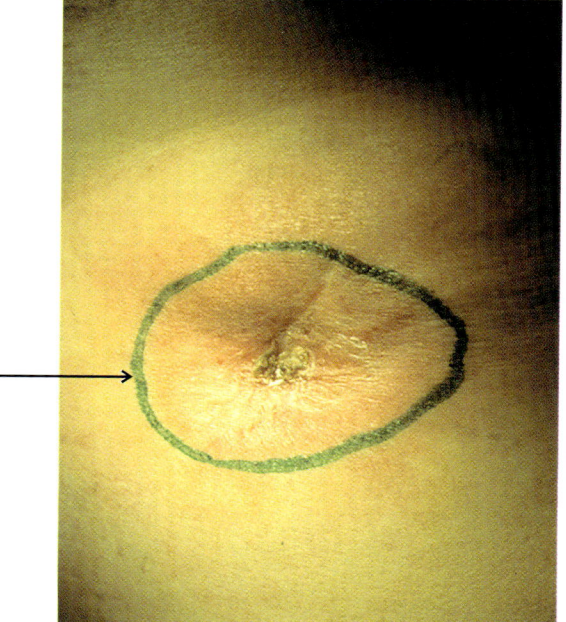

Fig. 16.2.13[1]. LABC. Breast Cancer Cryosurgery: 3 months after the first cryosurgical session. View of the post-cryosurgical wound with external demarcation line (**A**) which surrounds the area of the previous breast cancer and internal demarcation line (**B**) surrounding the remainder of the previous primary breast tumor

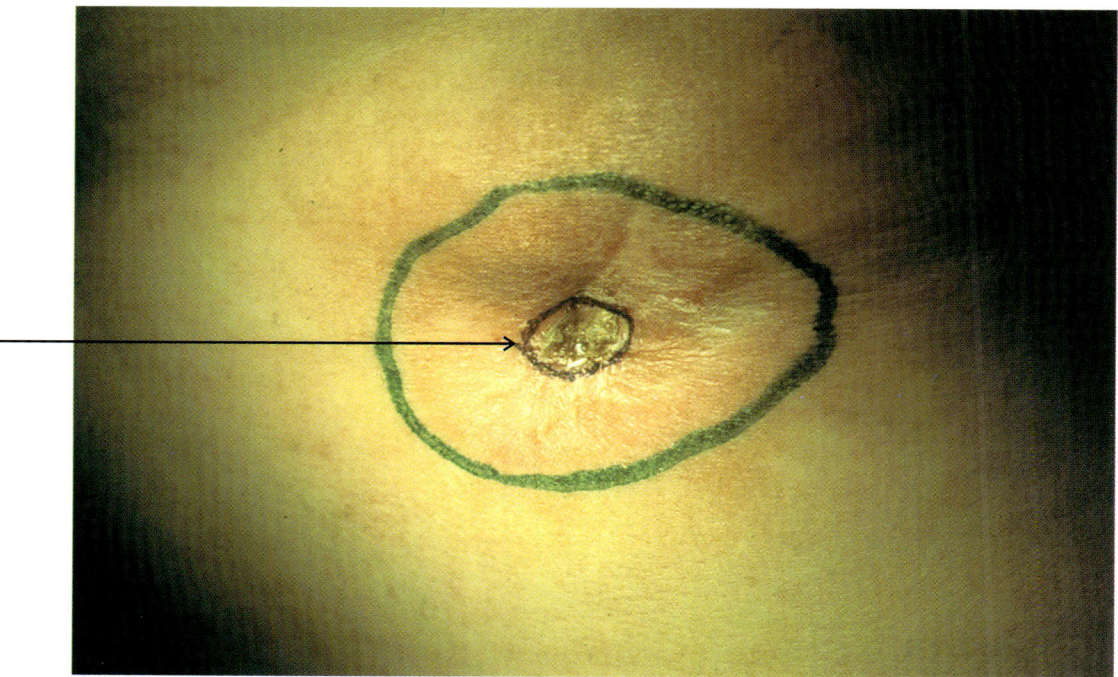

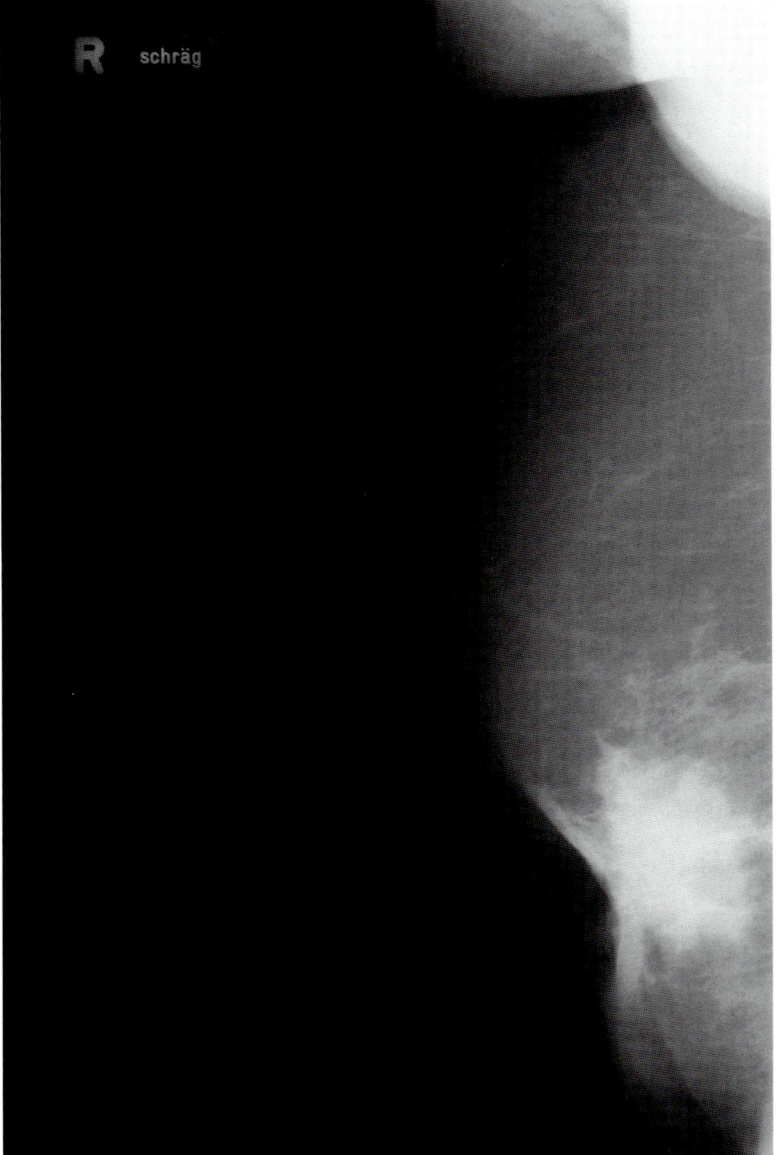

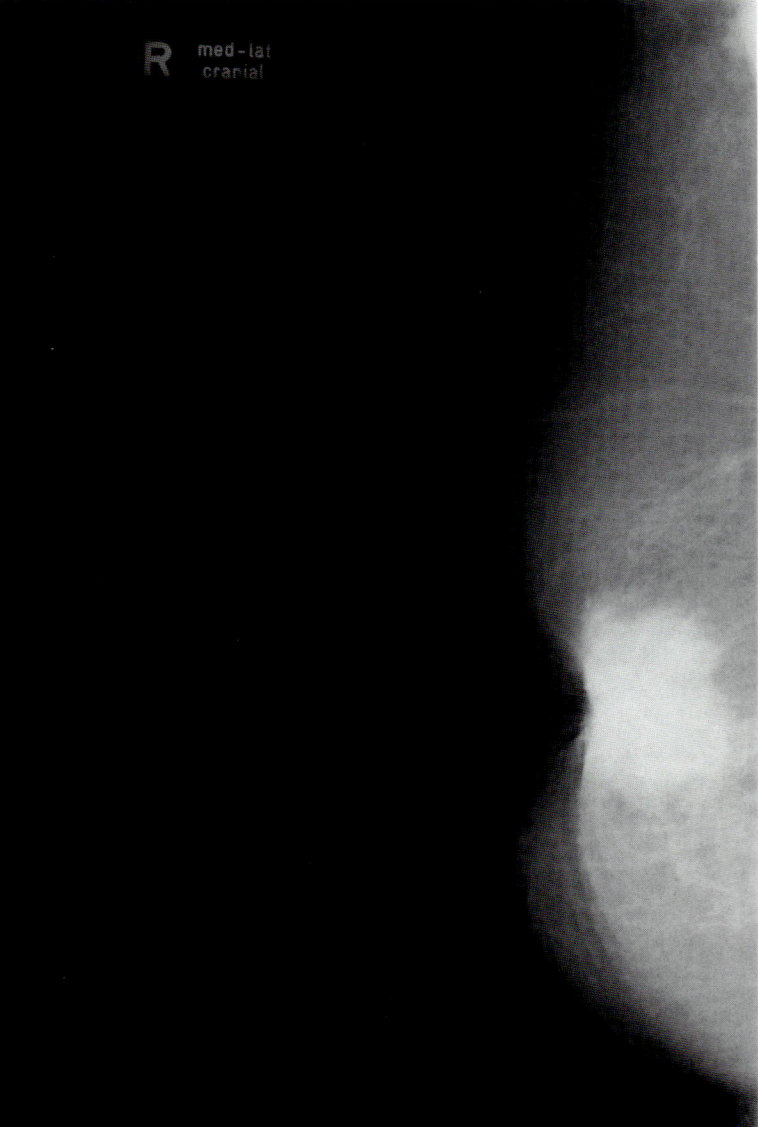

Fig. 16.2.14[1]. LABC. Breast Cancer Cryosurgery: Mammography in the same patient 3 months after the first cryosurgical session: oblique (**A**), mediolateral and cranial (**B**), craniocaudal and external (**C**) views, which point to the remainder of the primary breast tumor

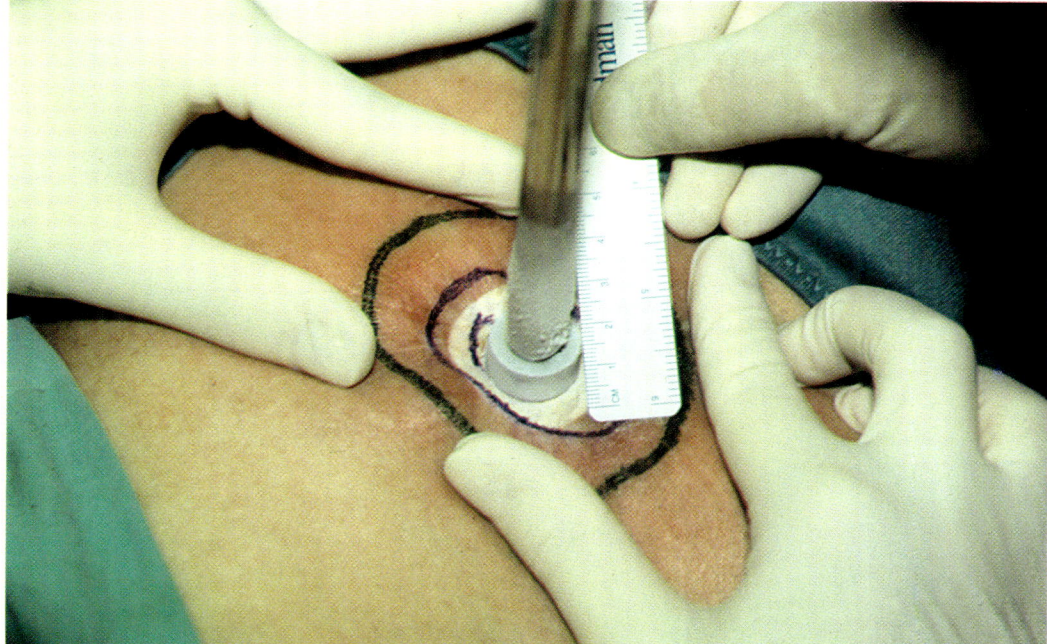

Fig. 16.2.15[1]. LABC. Breast Cancer Cryosurgery: The second cryosurgical session in the same patient. A double freeze-thaw cycle using a cryoprobe of 20 mm which is placed on the remainder of the breast tumor mass (A) at a temperature of −180°C for 3 min. View of the post-cryosurgical zone after the second cryosurgical session (B)

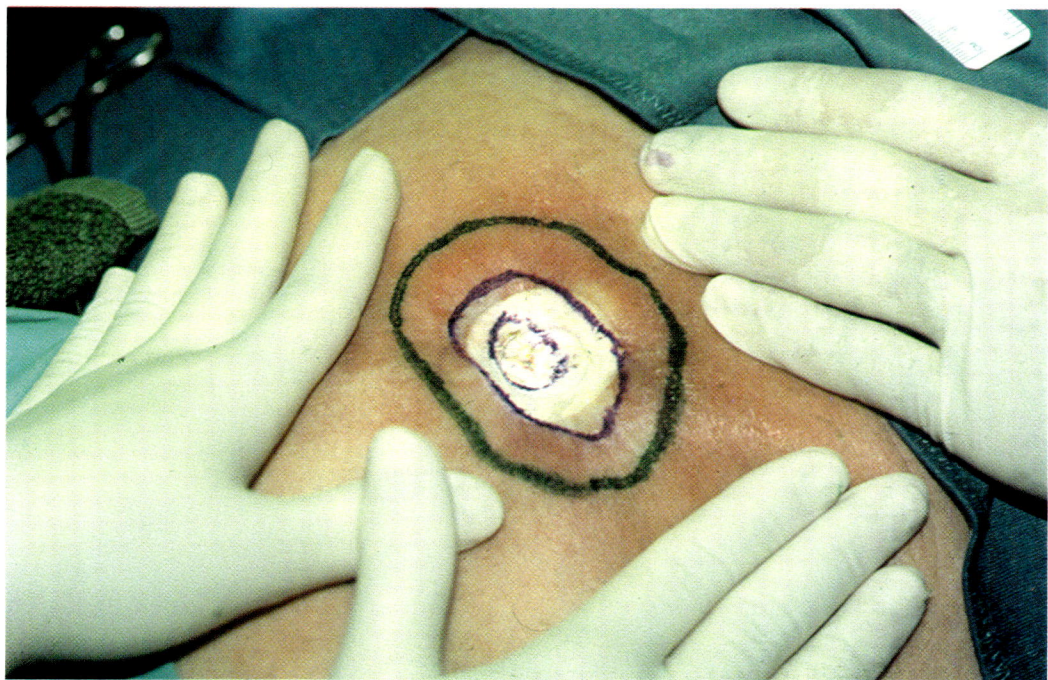

Chapter 16
Breast Cancer Cryosurgery

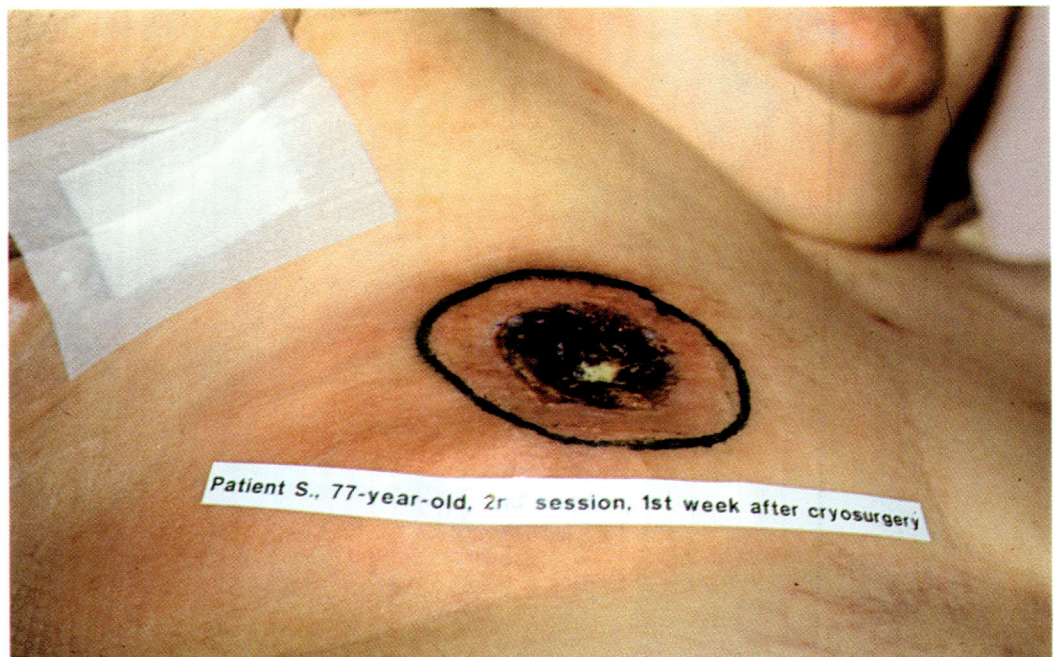

A

Fig. 16.2.16¹ A, B. LABC. Breast Cancer Cryosurgery: 1 week after the second cryosurgical session. View of the wound healing process

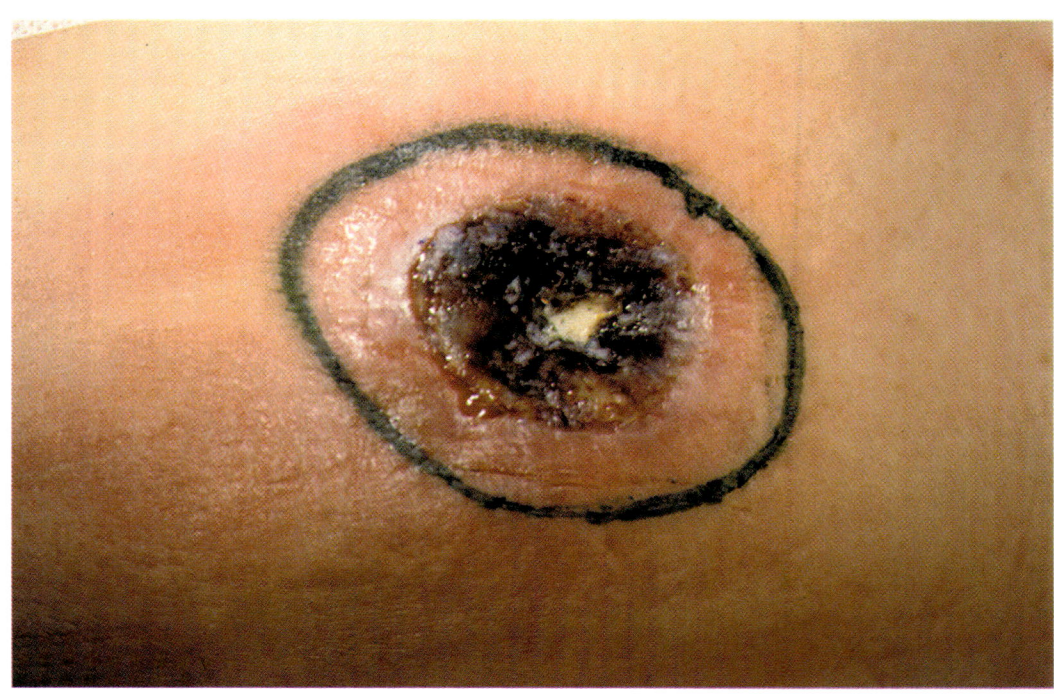

B

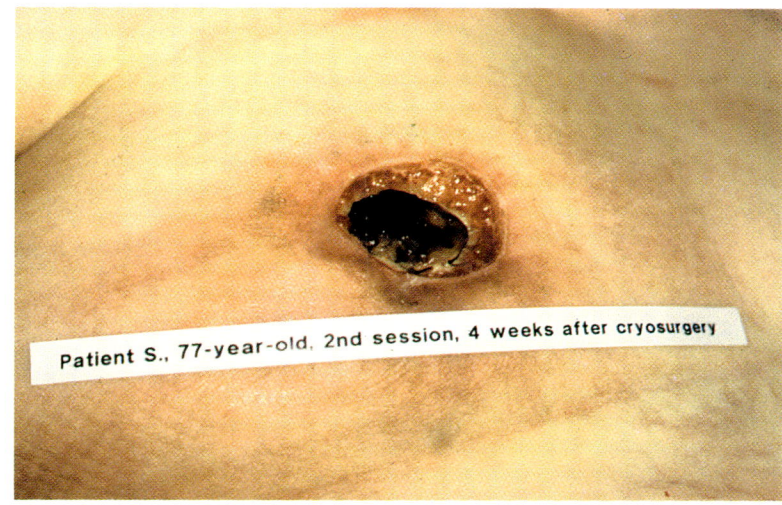

A

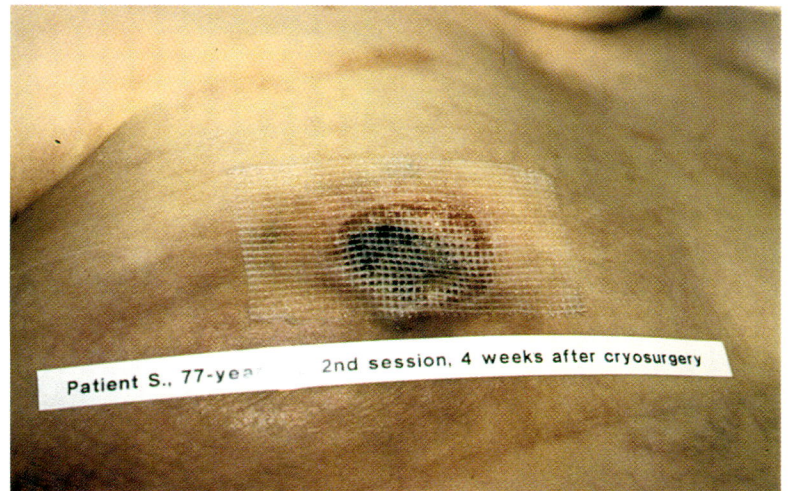

B

Fig. 16.2.17[1] A–C. LABC. Breast Cancer Cryosurgery: 4 weeks after the second cryosurgical session. View of the wound healing process

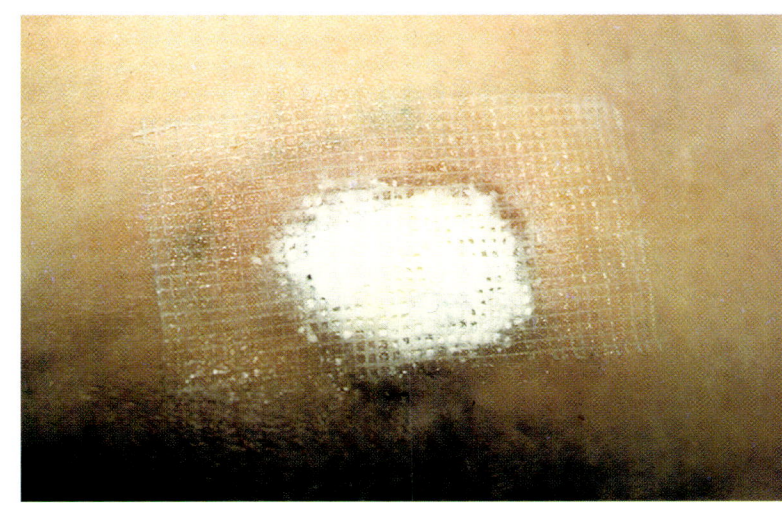

C

Chapter 16
Breast Cancer Cryosurgery

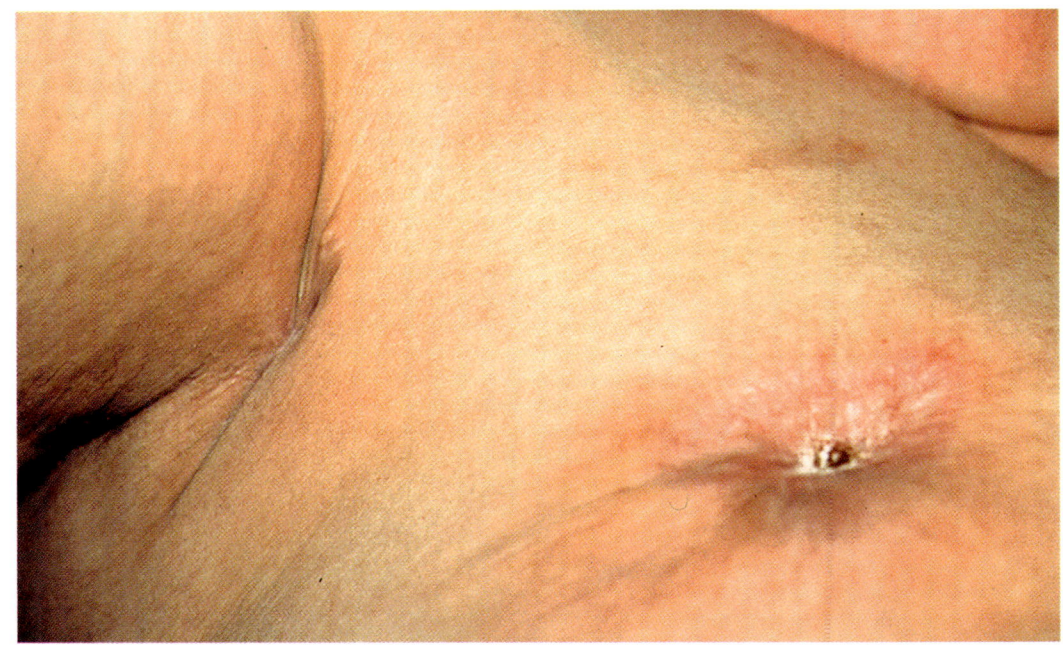

Fig. 16.2.18[1] A, B. LABC. Breast Cancer Cryosurgery: 8 weeks after the second cryosurgical session. View of the wound healing process

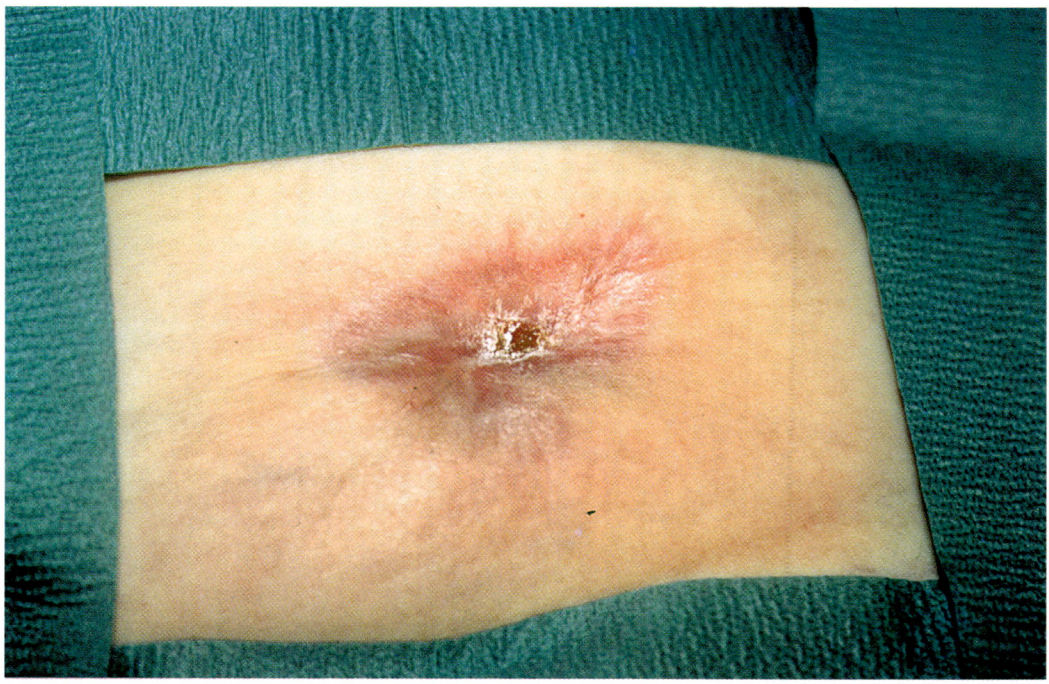

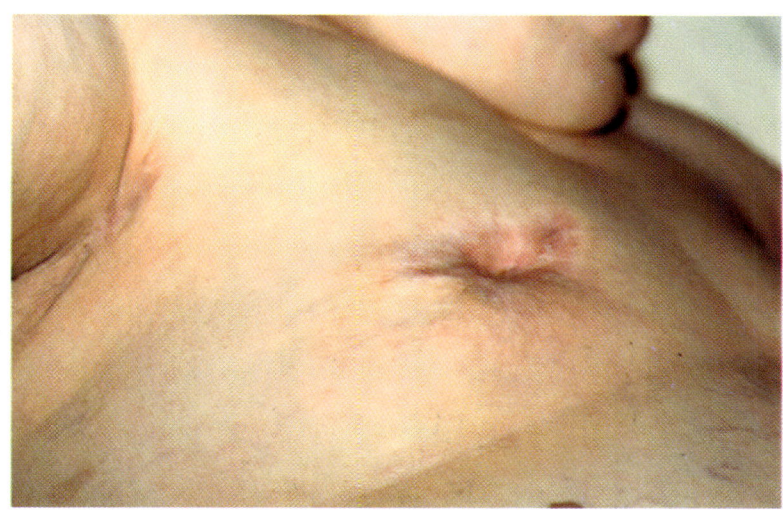

A

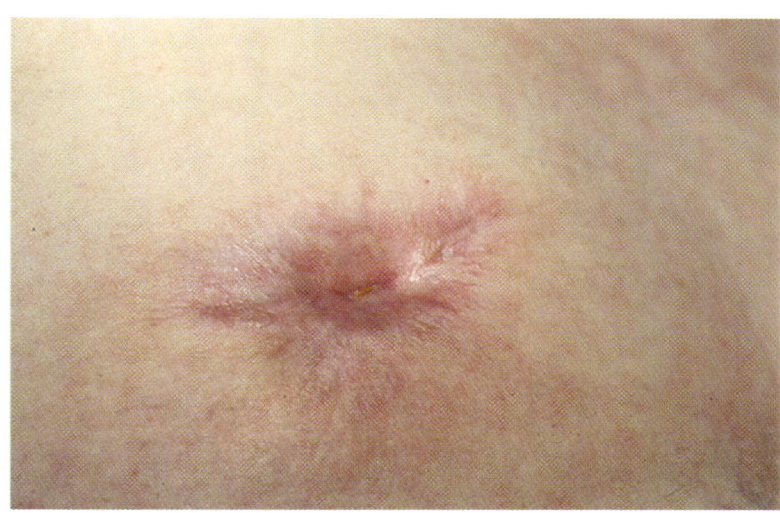

B

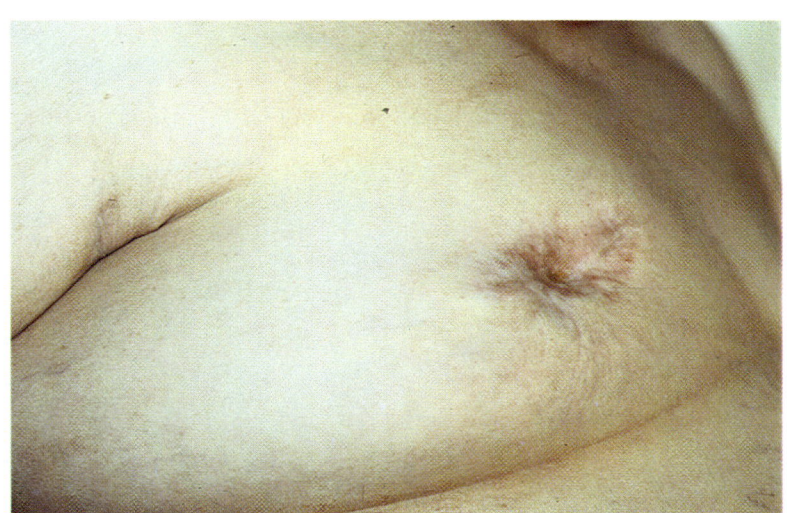

C

Fig. 16.2.19[1]. LABC. Breast Cancer Cryosurgery: Excellent curative and cosmetic results 12 weeks after the second breast cancer cryosurgical session. View of the wound healing process (**A, B**). No reccurence after 1 year (**C, D**)

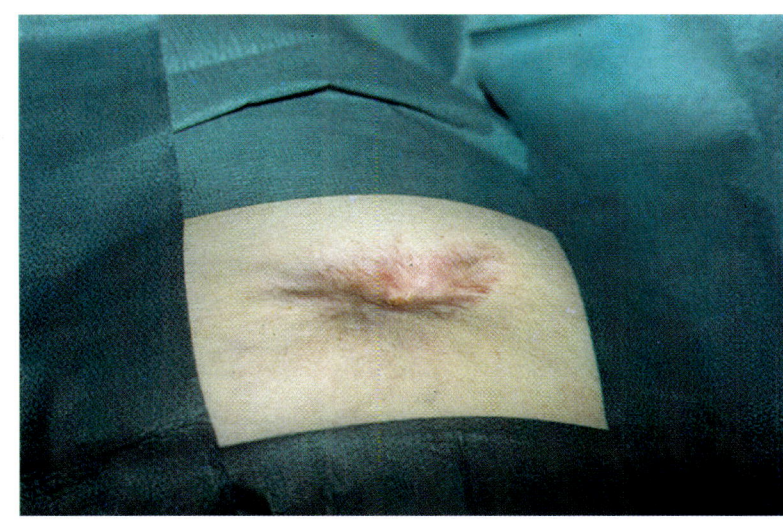

D

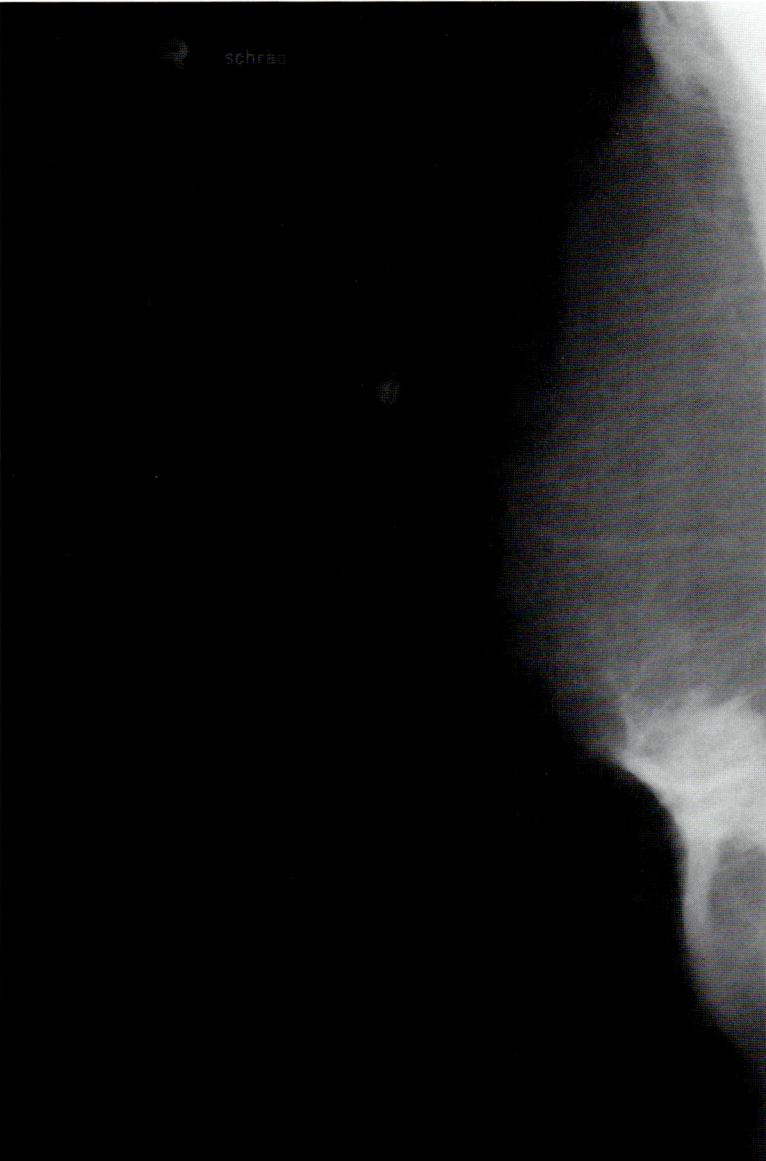

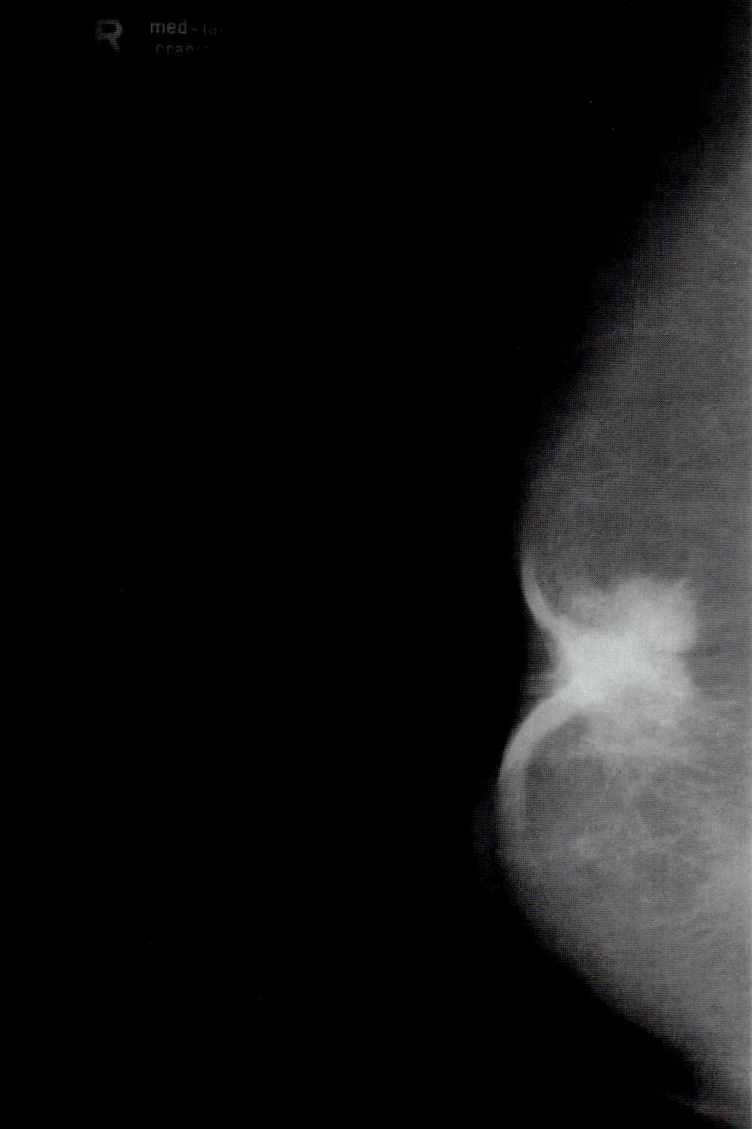

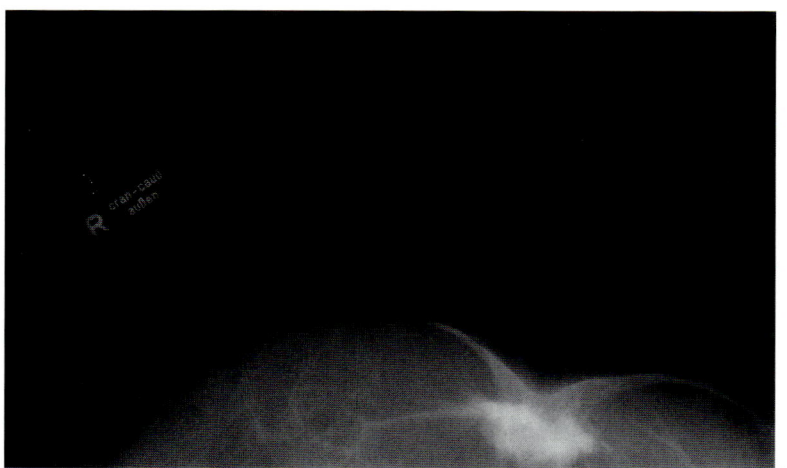

Fig. 16.2.20[1]. LABC. Breast Cancer Cryosurgery: Mammography in the same patient 12 weeks after the second breast cancer cryosurgical session: oblique (**A**), mediolateral and cranial (**B**), craniocaudal and external (**C**) views. The radiological findings point to the newly formed connective tissue which replaced the ulcerated, primary inflammatory breast carcinoma

Section F Clinical Aspects 373

Chapter 16
Breast Cancer
Cryosurgery

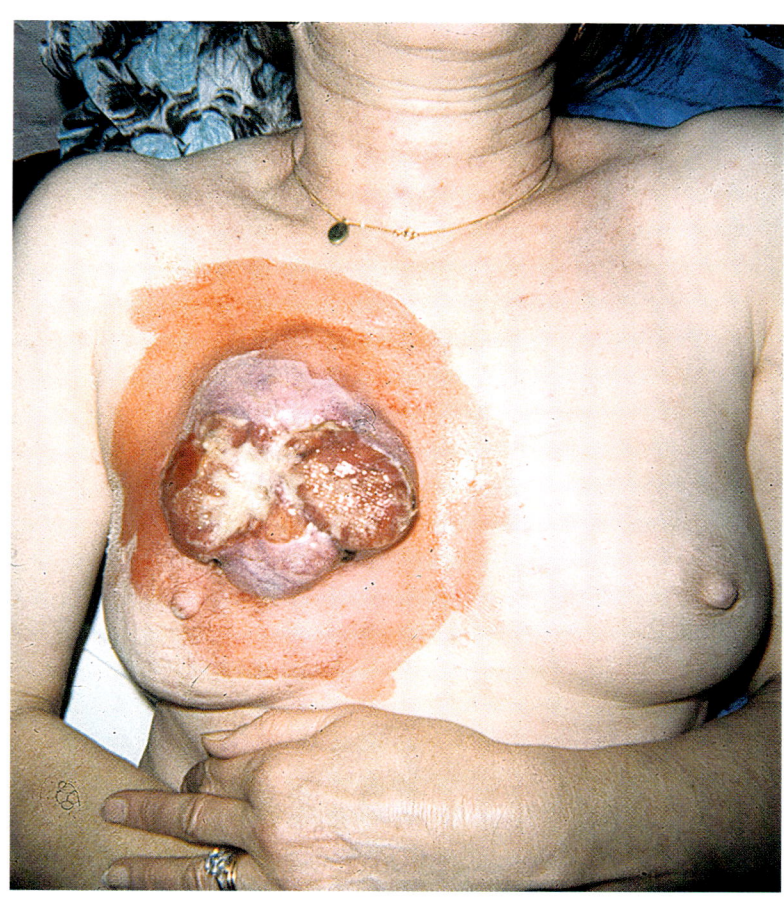

Fig. 16.2.21[3]. Breast cancer: preoperatively

Fig. 16.2.22[3]. Breast cancer: freezing with liquid nitrogen

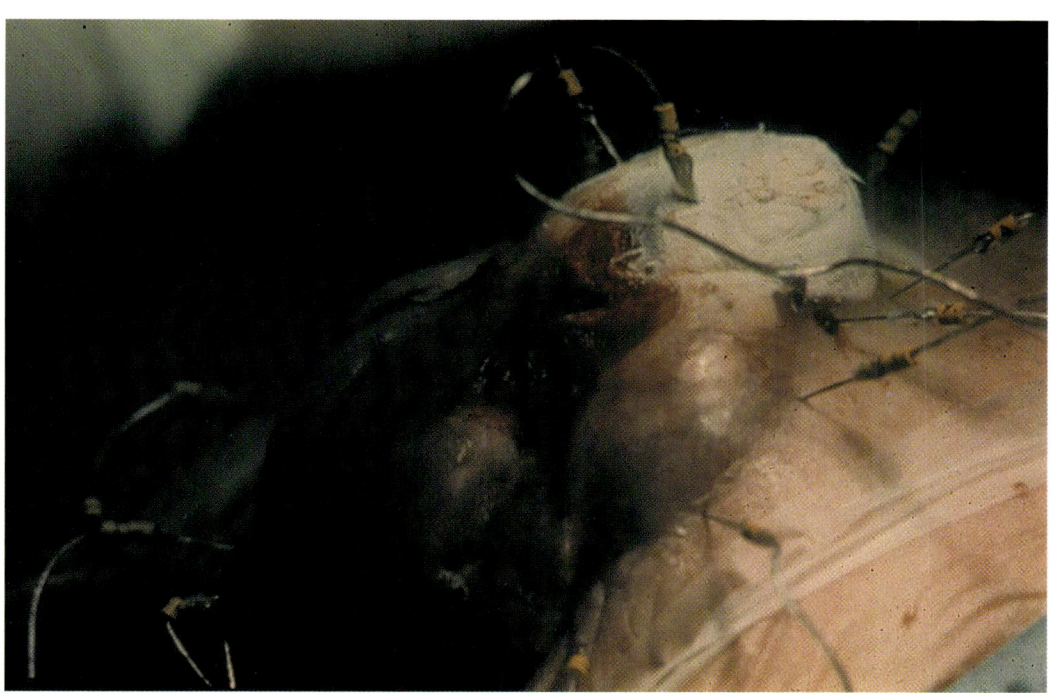

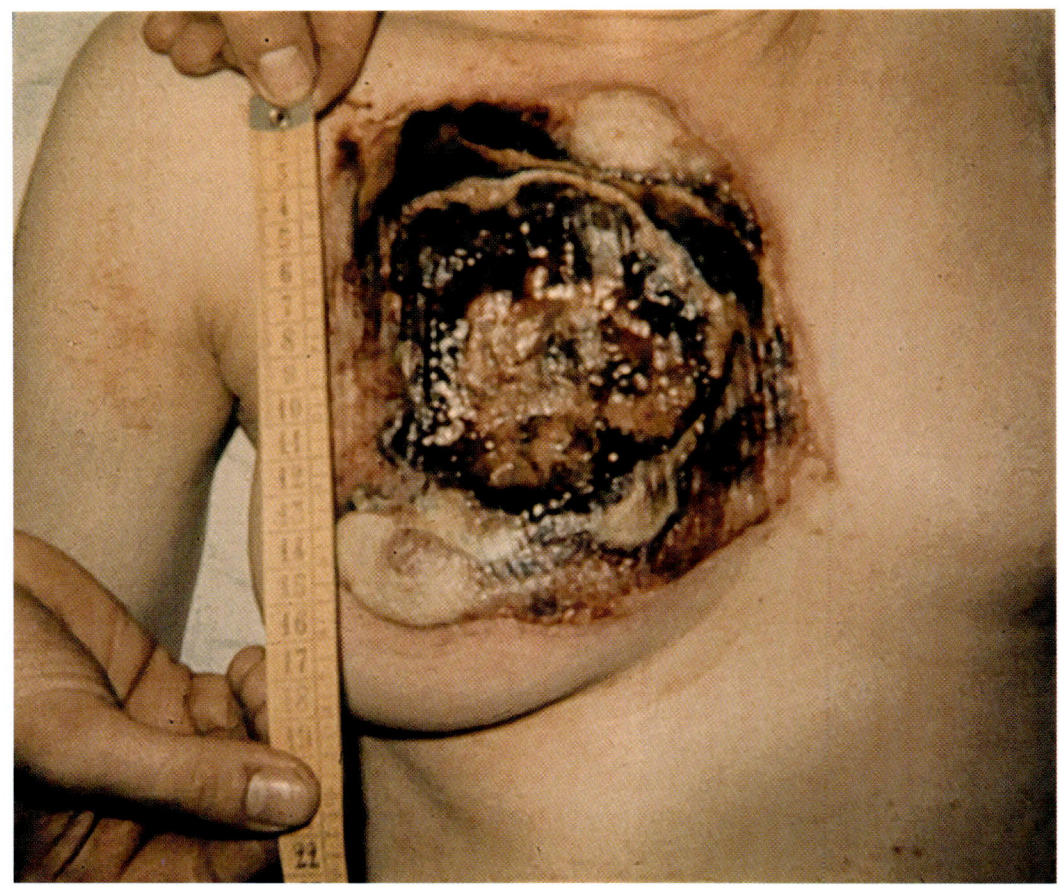

Fig. 16.2.23[3]. Breast cancer: cryonecrosis, occurring between 3 to 5 weeks after cryosurgical session

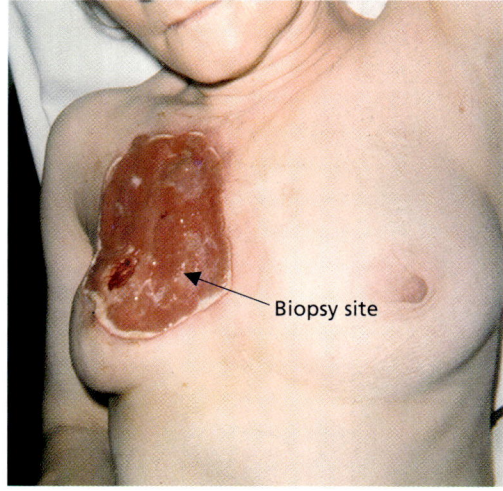

Fig. 16.2.24[3]. Breast cancer: granulated tissue after sloughing, occurring between 4 and 6 weeks after cryosurgery and with the wound being cleaned on a day basis

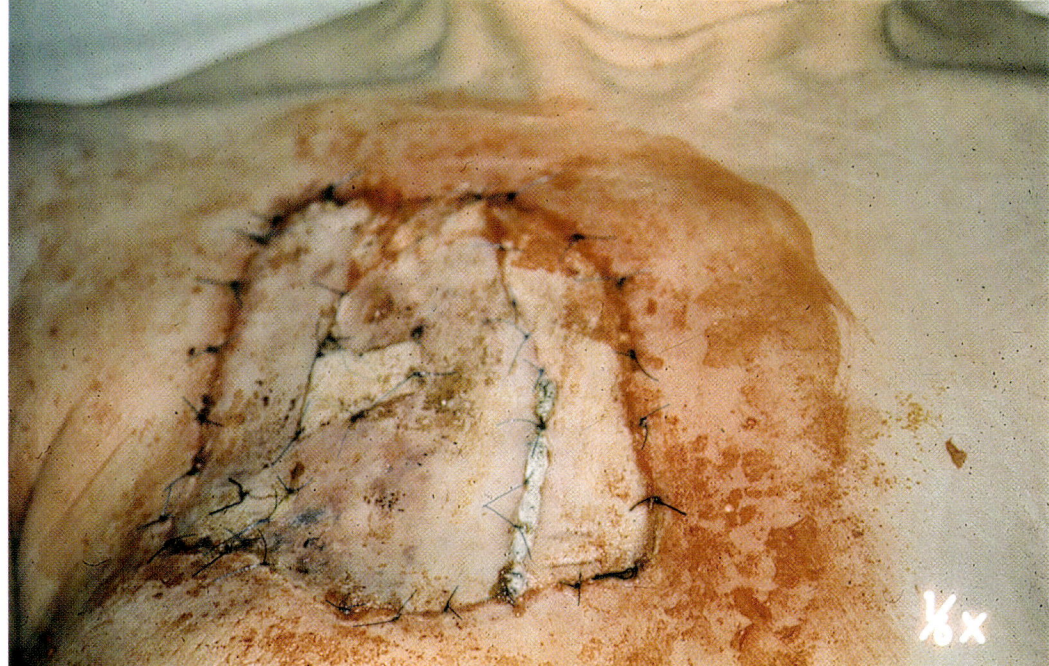

Fig. 16.2.25[3]. Breast cancer: epidermal graft to cover the area. This procedure was performed 8 weeks after cryosurgery and after ascertaining the abscence of any remnants of diseased tissue

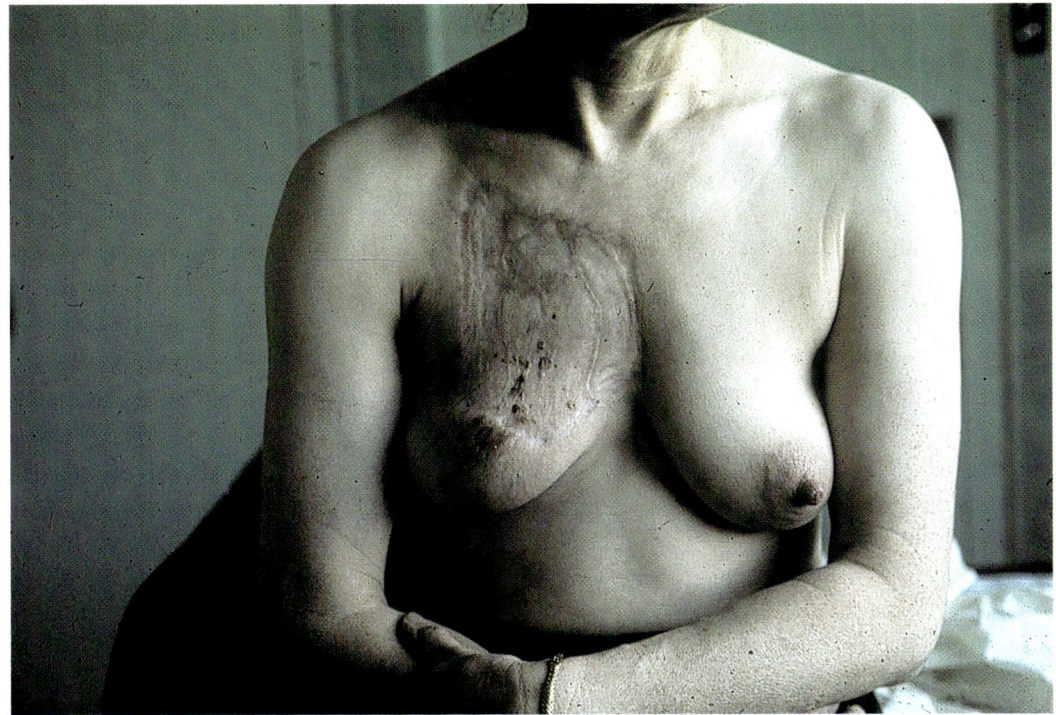

Fig. 16.2.26[3]. Breast cancer: result 1 year after the first cryosurgical application

16.2.1 Cryosurgery by Combined Penetration, Contact and LN$_2$-spraying Methods

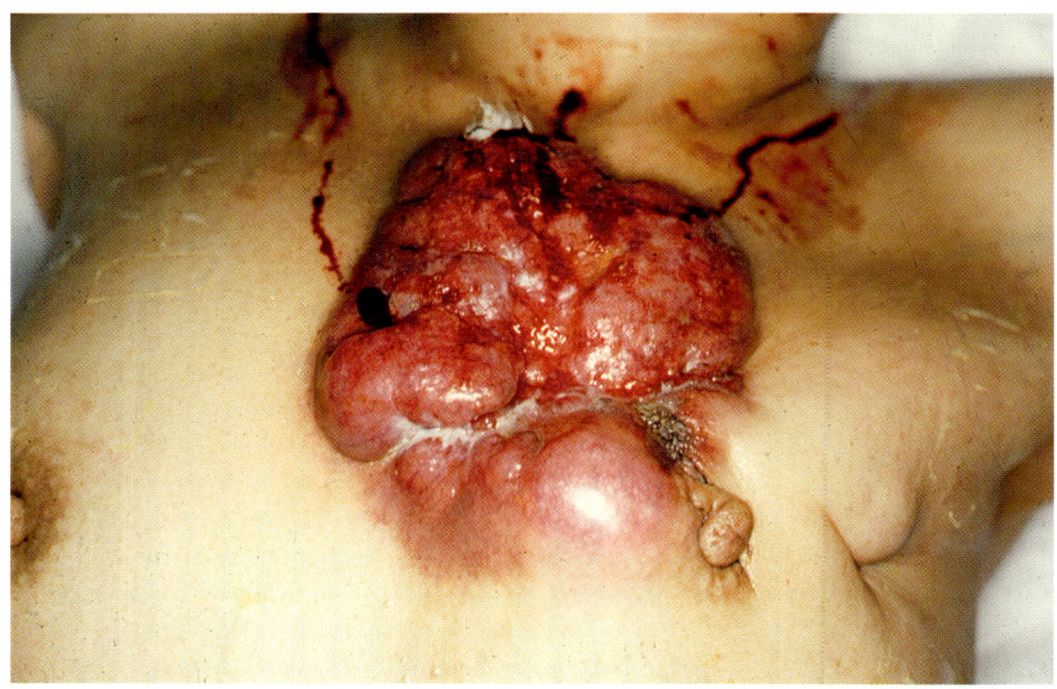

Fig. 16.2.27[5]. 67/F, Primary advanced bilateral breast cancer, T4cN$_2$MX, stage IIIB (UICC 1997), ductal carcinoma with scirrhous pattern. The left main tumor, solid, ulcerated and bleeding

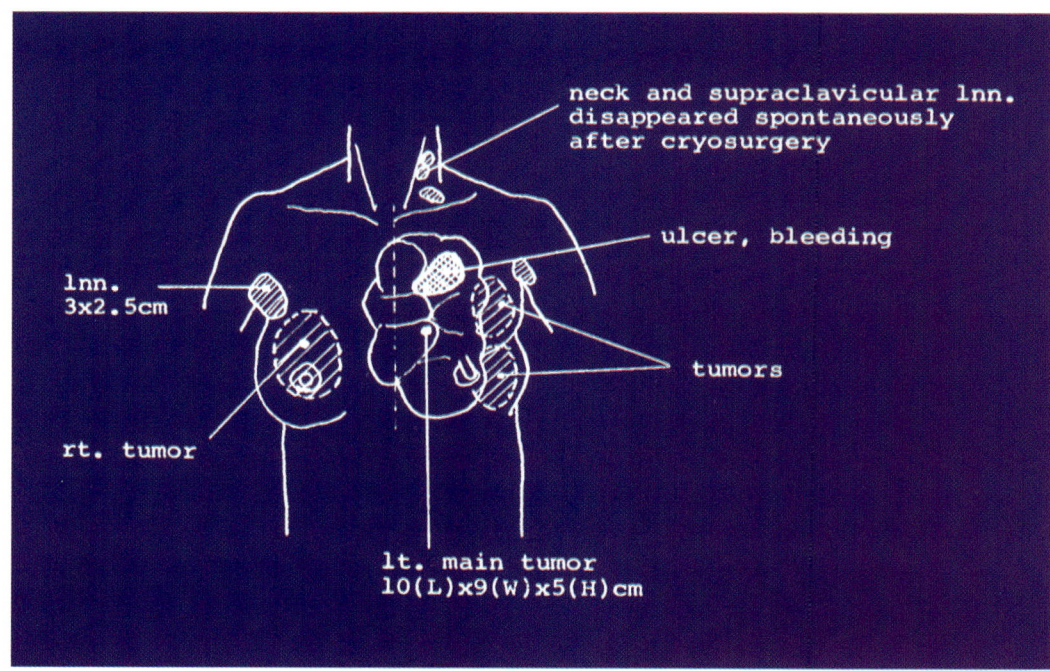

Fig. 16.2.28[5]. A schematic view of the patient at the out-patient clinic

Section F　　　　　　　　　　　Clinical Aspects　　　　　　　　　　　377

Chapter 16
Breast Cancer
Cryosurgery

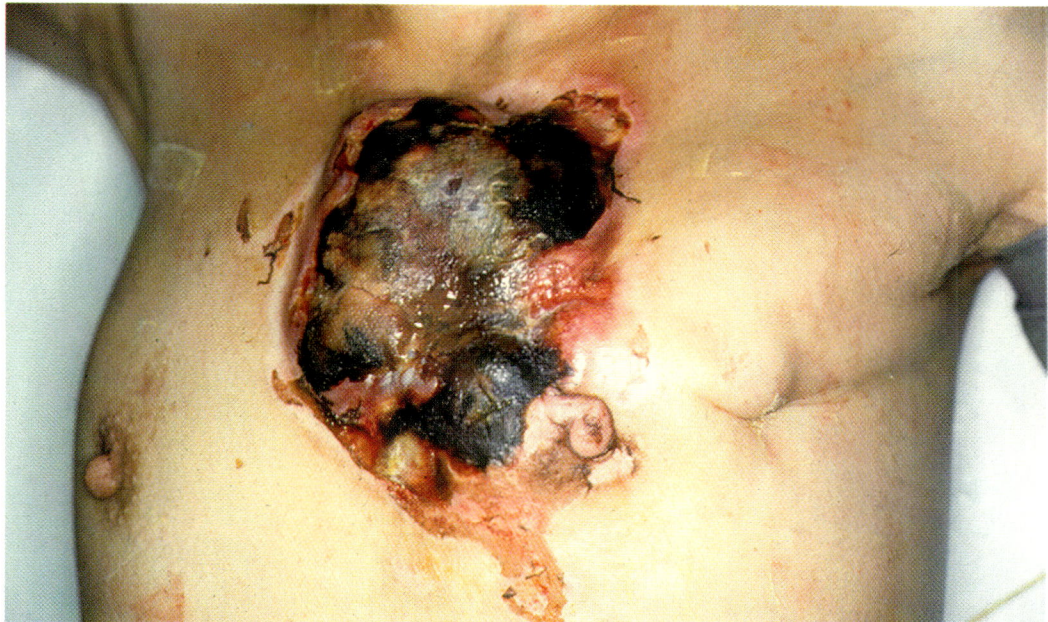

Fig. 16.2.29[5]. Cryonecrotized tumor, 3 weeks after the first cryosurgical operation. Linde CE-4G (USA), a liquid nitrogen-driven device for heavy-duty use, with a PR-6 standard cryoprobe, 7.92 mm in outer diameter and 25.4 mm straight freezing tip, were used for penetration freezing. For contact freezing, the probe was equipped with a round copper probe-tip adaptor, 25 mm in diameter. Two CS-76 (USA) portable probes were used simultaneously for the spraying method. Freezing sites were fractionated and overlapped. A vaseline embankment was prepared to protect juxtatumor normal skin, and small incisions with an electric knife were made deep into the tumor at several points of the tumor to allow insertion of a PR-6 cryoprobe into the tumor, which was frozen at −180°C for 5 min, in two cycles. After thawing, the penetrated holes were packed with oxycellulose cotton as a hemostatic agent

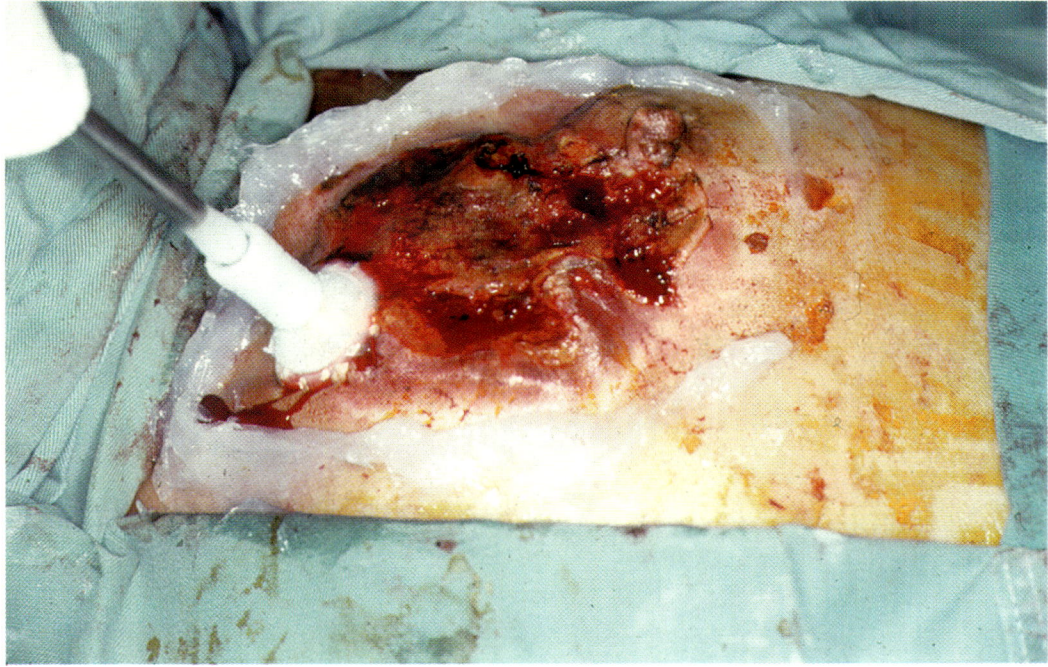

Fig. 16.2.30[5]. Necrotomy, followed by a second cryosurgical operation on the tumor remnants

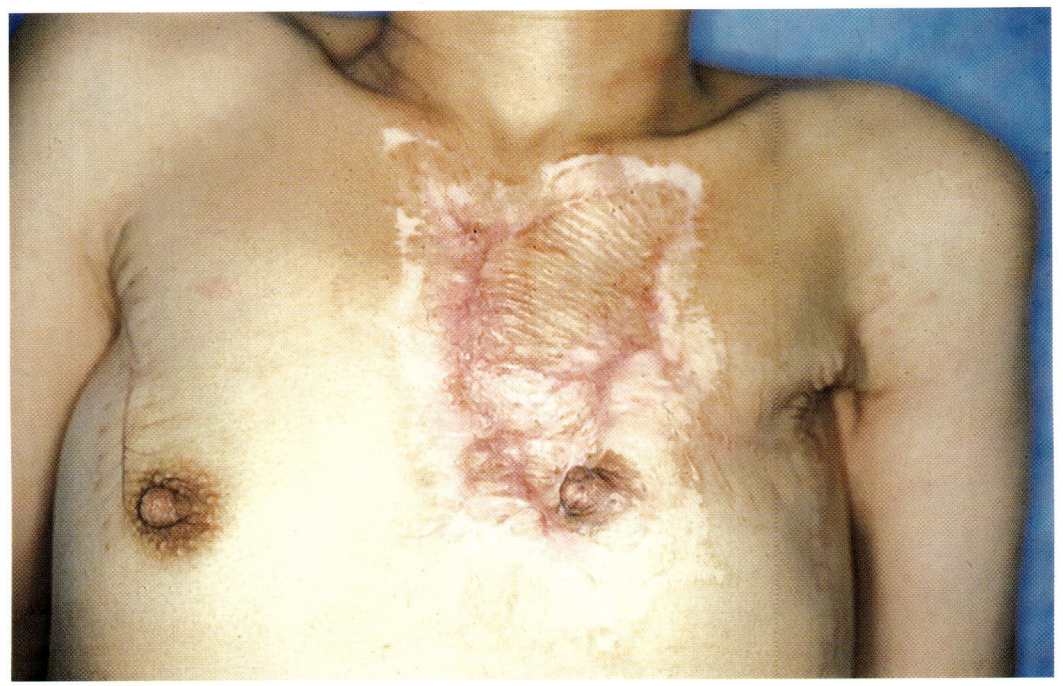

Fig. 16.2.31[5]. Final local appearance, one year after the first treatment. The mesh skin graft has taken well, and bilateral lumpectomy with axillary lymph node dissection was performed

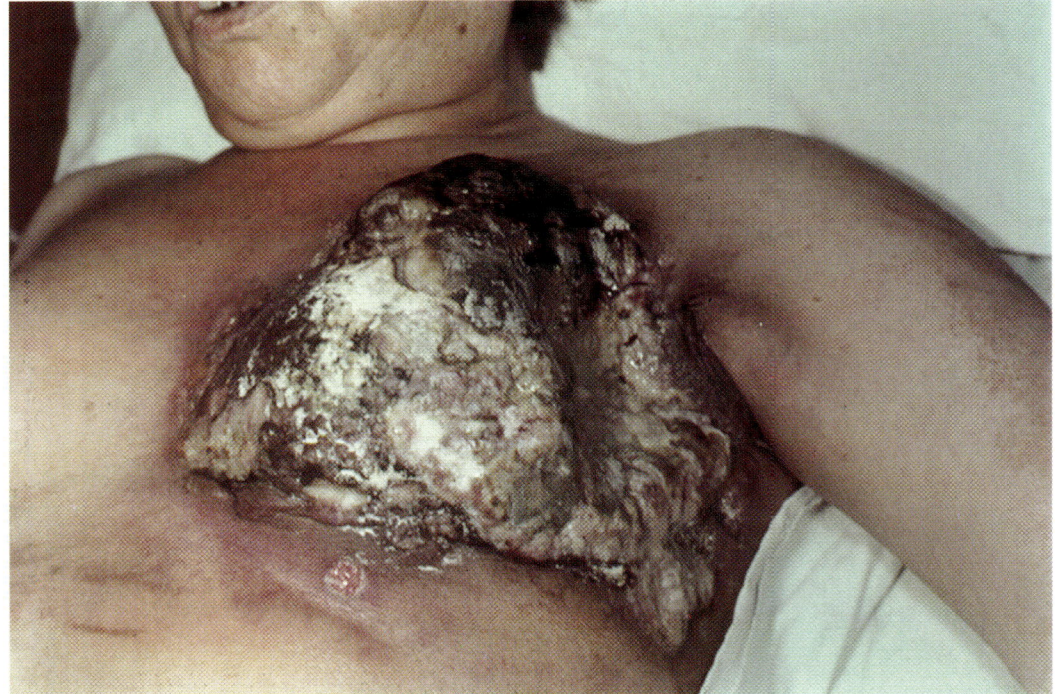

Fig. 16.2.32[5]. 59/F, T4cN$_2$M$_1$, stage IV, medullo-tubular adenocarcinoma. Solid, ulcerating, bleeding and malodorous

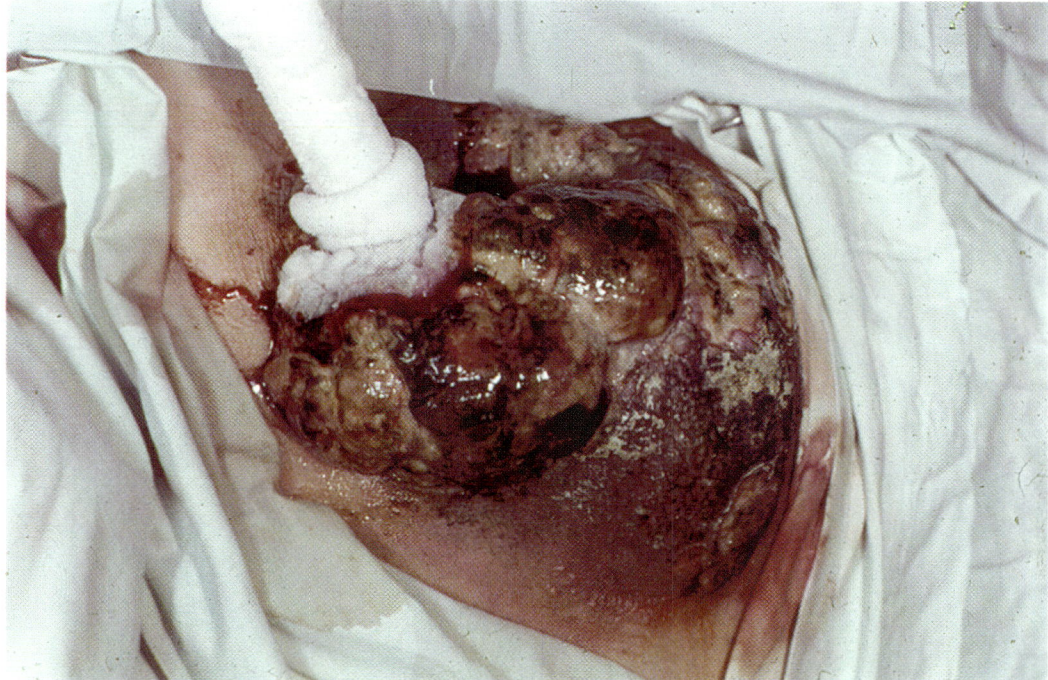

Fig. 16.2.33[5]. Cryosurgery was performed by the contact method for the fractionated, multiple, overlapping sites. Linde CE-2B with an SK-51865-1 (USA) probe equipped with a 4 cm diameter cylindrical probe-tip adaptor for the large tumor

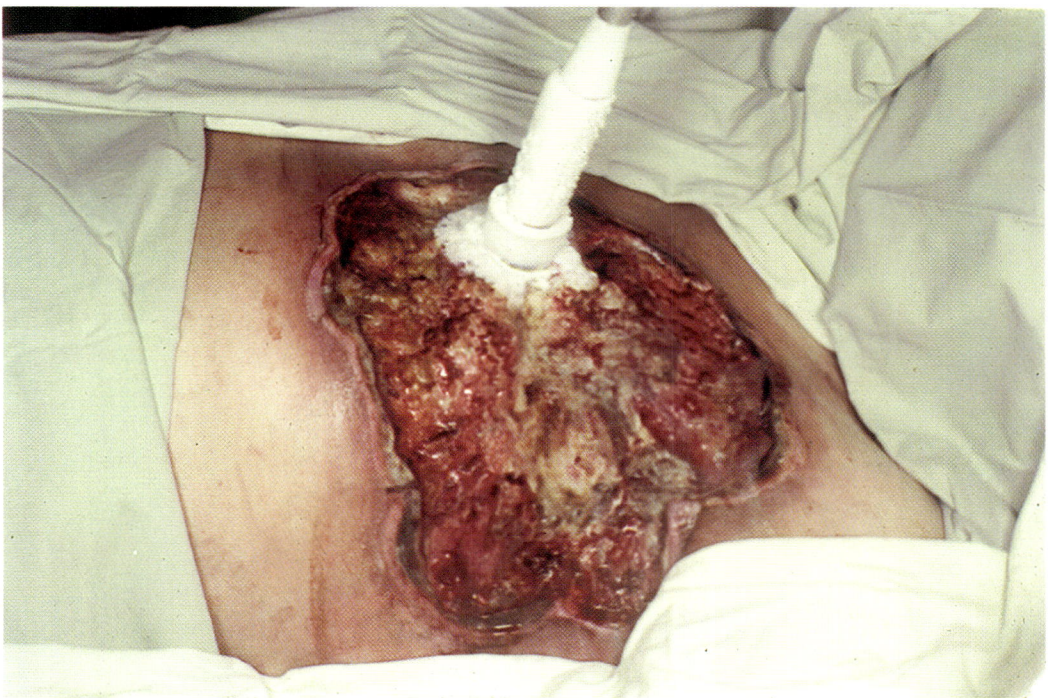

Fig. 16.2.34[5]. 3 weeks later. After necrotomy, suspicious tumor remnants were frozen

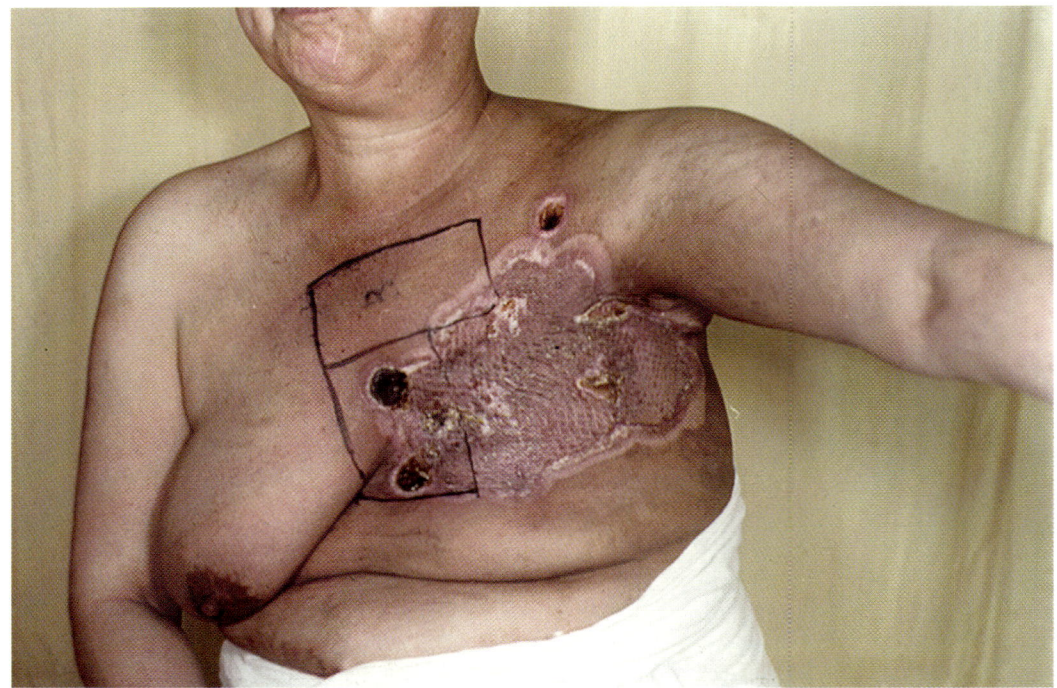

Fig. 16.2.35⁵. 3 months after cryosurgery, at the time of discharge. No palpable lymph nodes in the supraclavicular region and axilla. Irradiation to the parasternal and supraclavicular regions in combination with chemo-endocrine therapy had been performed

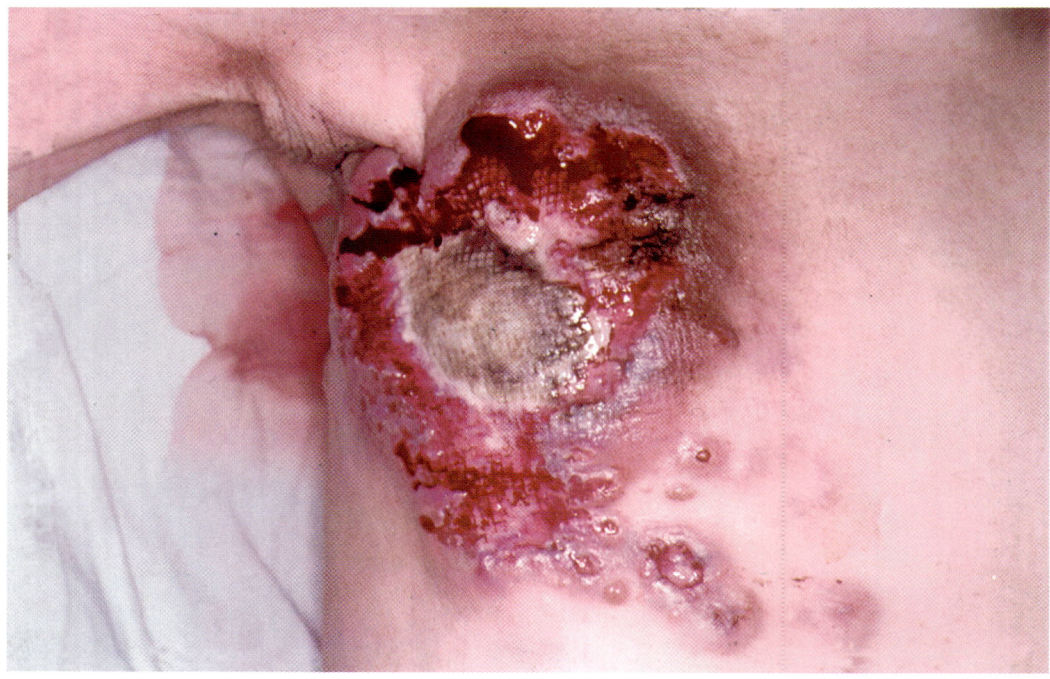

Fig. 16.2.36⁵. 66/F, T$_4$cN$_2$MX, stage IIIB, with an infiltrating tumor, anaplastic medullary carcinoma

Section F Clinical Aspects **381**

**Chapter 16
Breast Cancer
Cryosurgery**

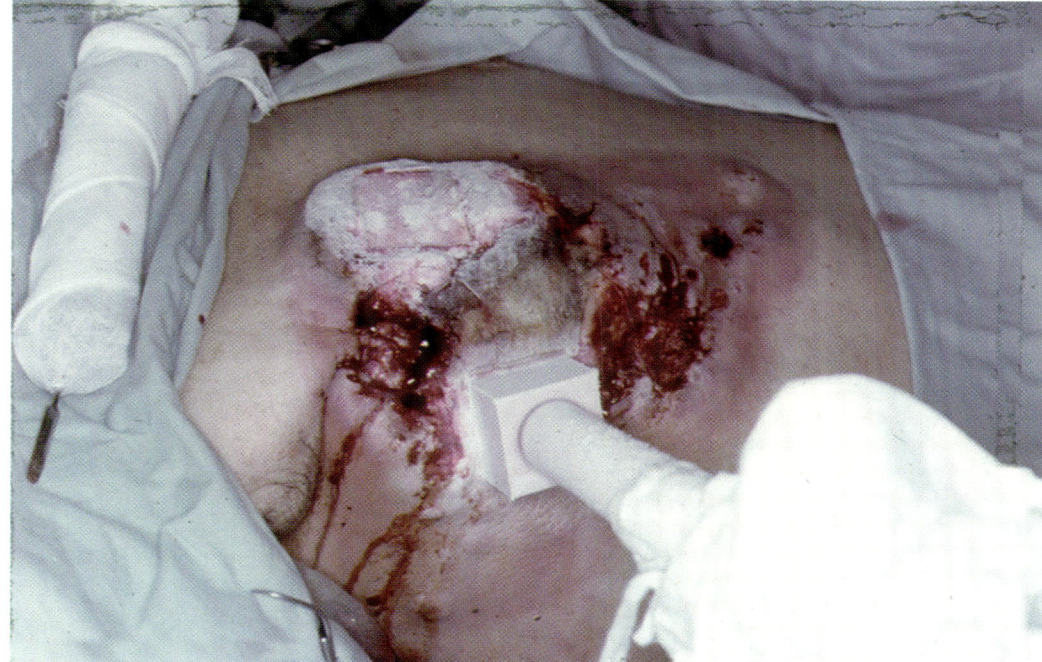

Fig. 16.2.37[5]. Contact freezing with Linde CE-2B, cryoprobe SK-51865-1 and 4 cm square probe-tip adaptor

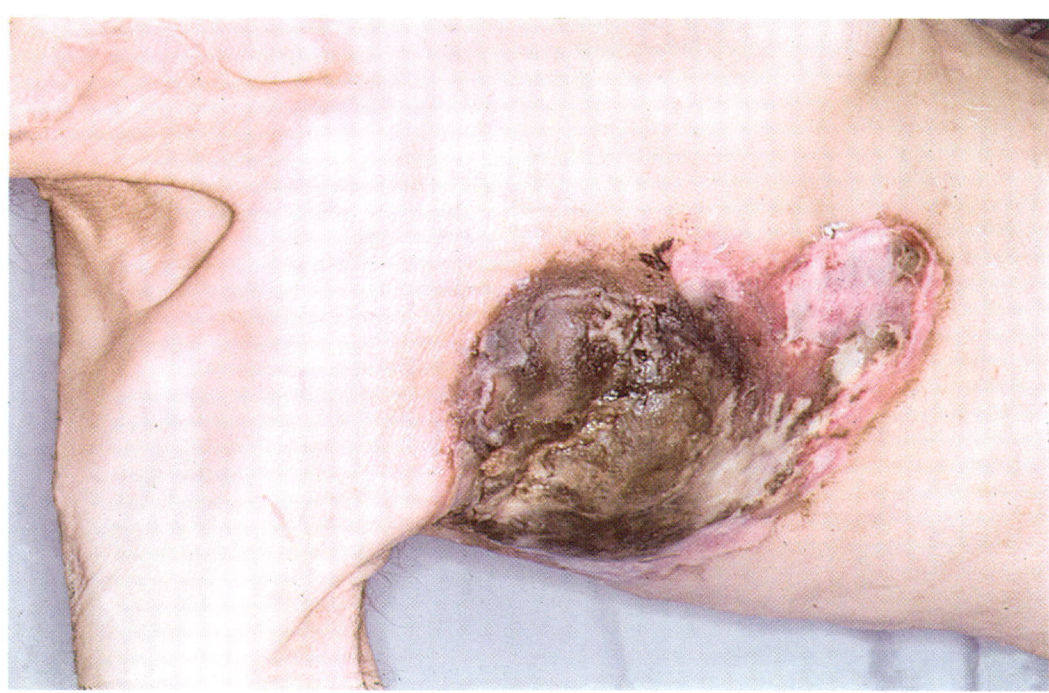

Fig. 16.2.38[5]. 3 weeks later. Cryonecrotized tumor

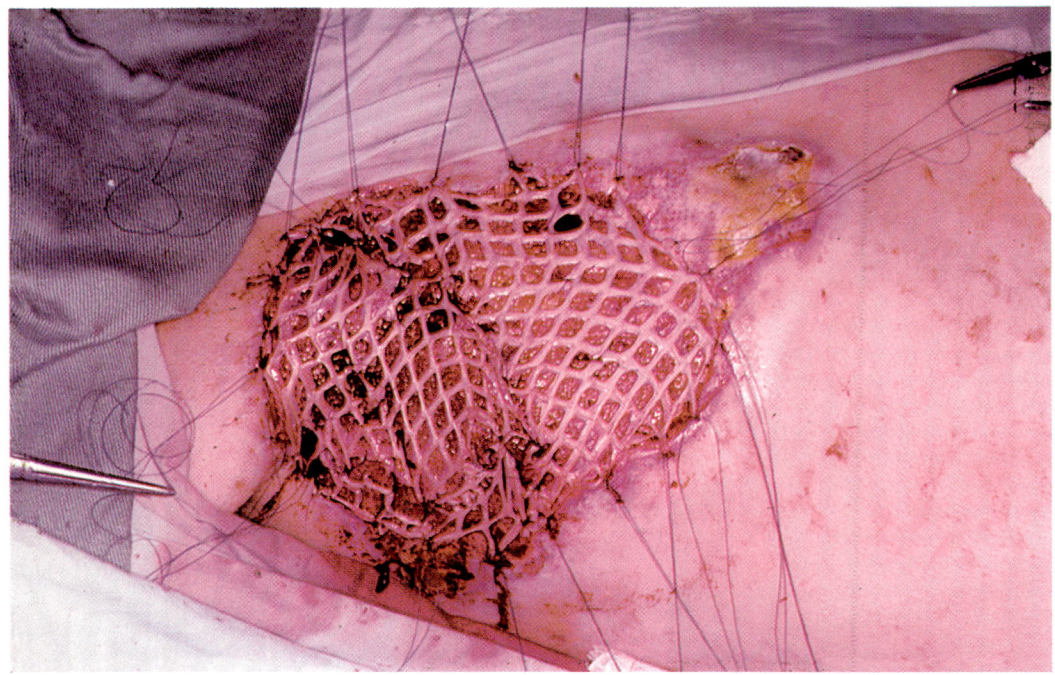

Fig. 16.2.39[5]. After necrotomy, a mesh skin graft was performed

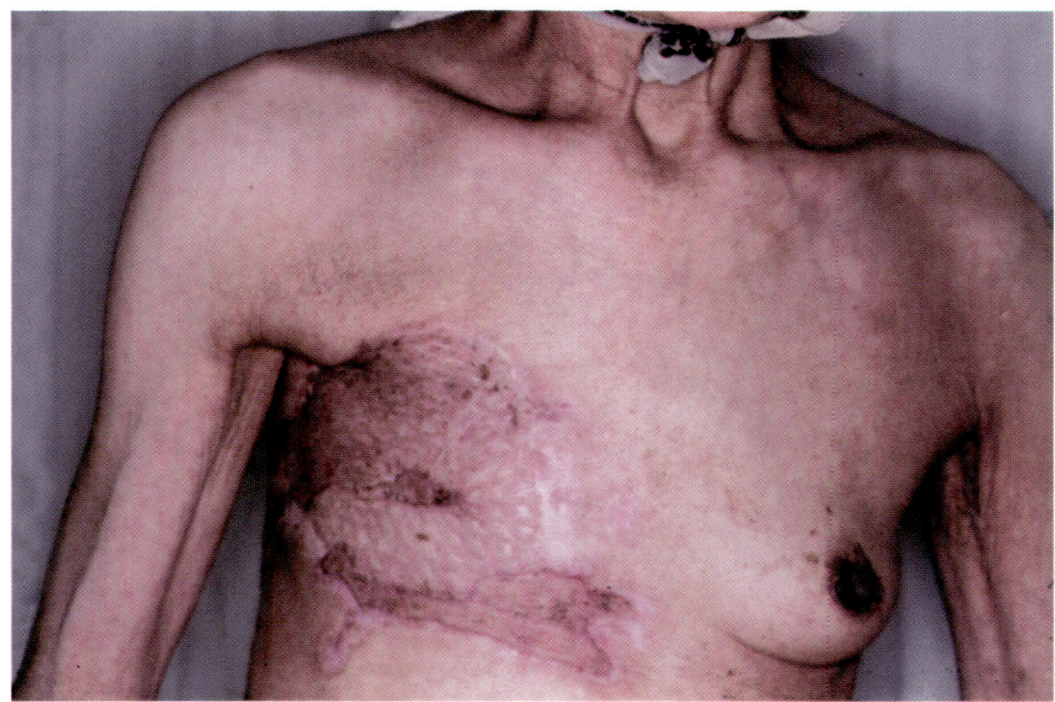

Fig. 16.2.40[5]. 3 months later. The mesh skin graft took well and healed

Section F Clinical Aspects 383

Chapter 16
Breast Cancer
Cryosurgery

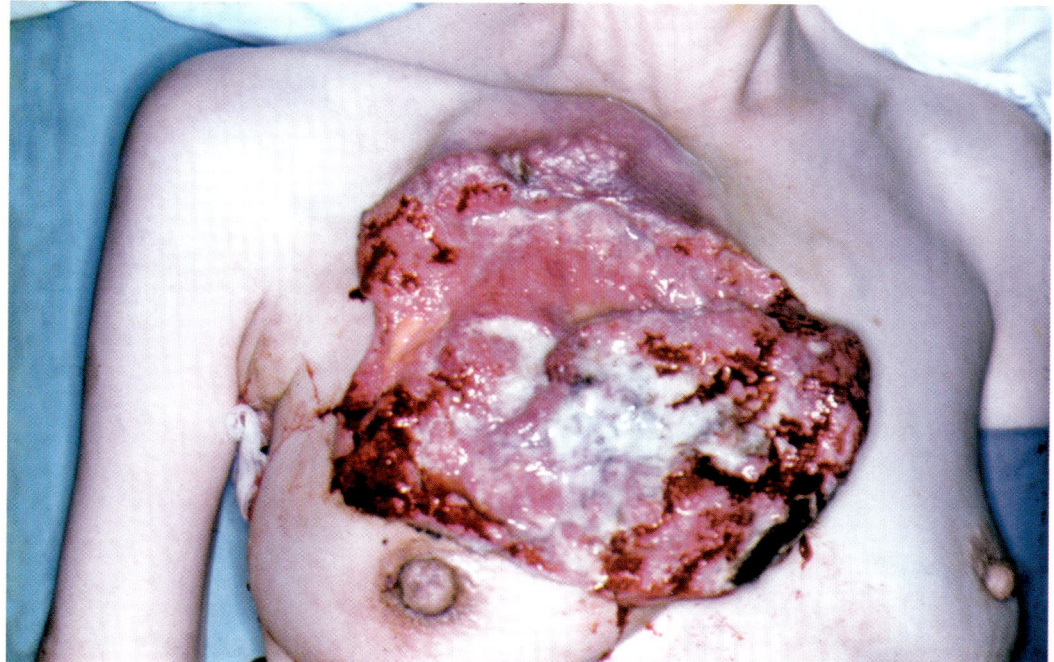

Fig. 16.2.41[5]. 53/F, T_4cN_2MX, stage IIIB, medullary tubular adenocarcinoma, wide-spread, rapidly invasive, ulcerating and bleeding, before cryosurgery

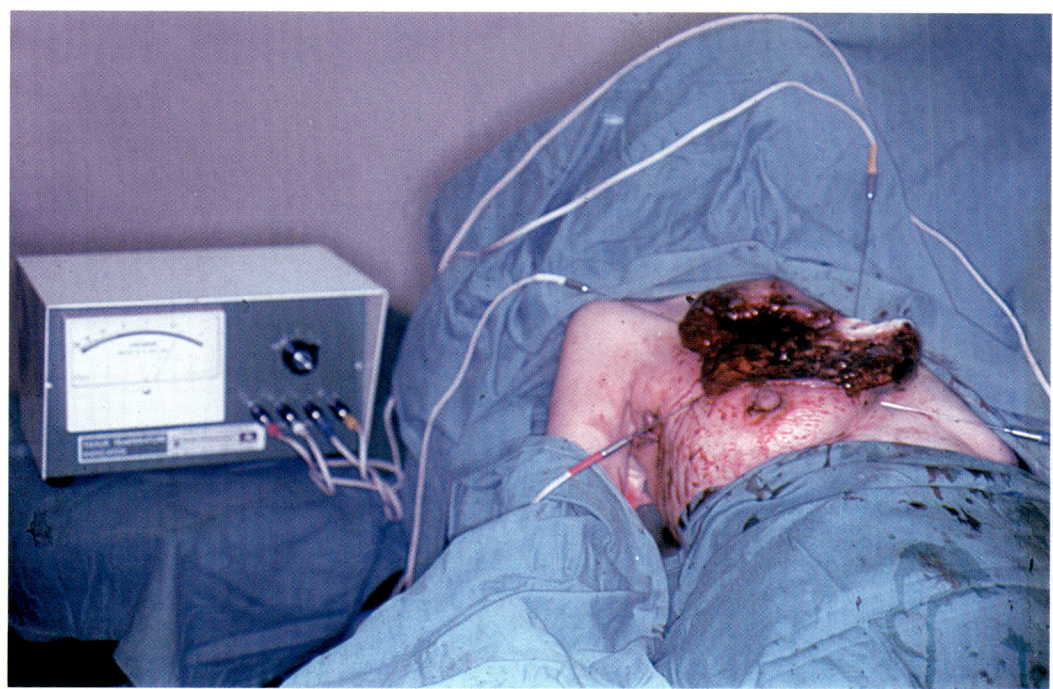

Fig. 16.2.42[5]. Temperature monitoring needles are in position before cryosurgery

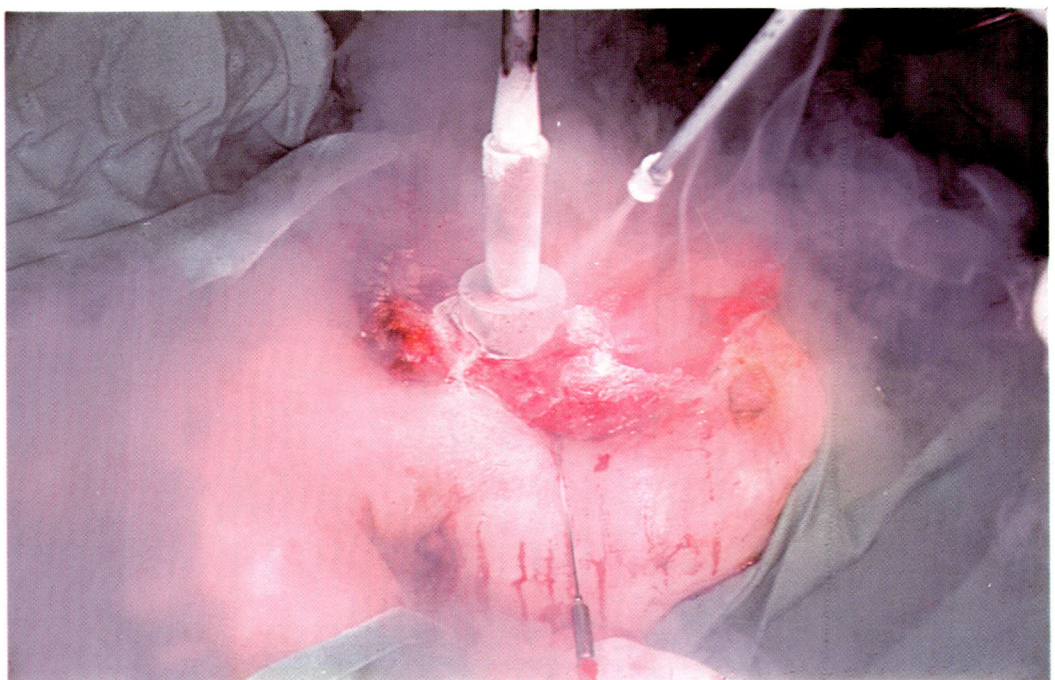

Fig. 16.2.43[5]. Cryosurgery with combined contact and LH_2-spraying method. Linde CE-2B, SK-51865-1 with a 4 cm cylindrical probe-tip adaptor, −160°C, 3 min to 8 min, and spray with Spray Cryomatic (Japan) for 10 min

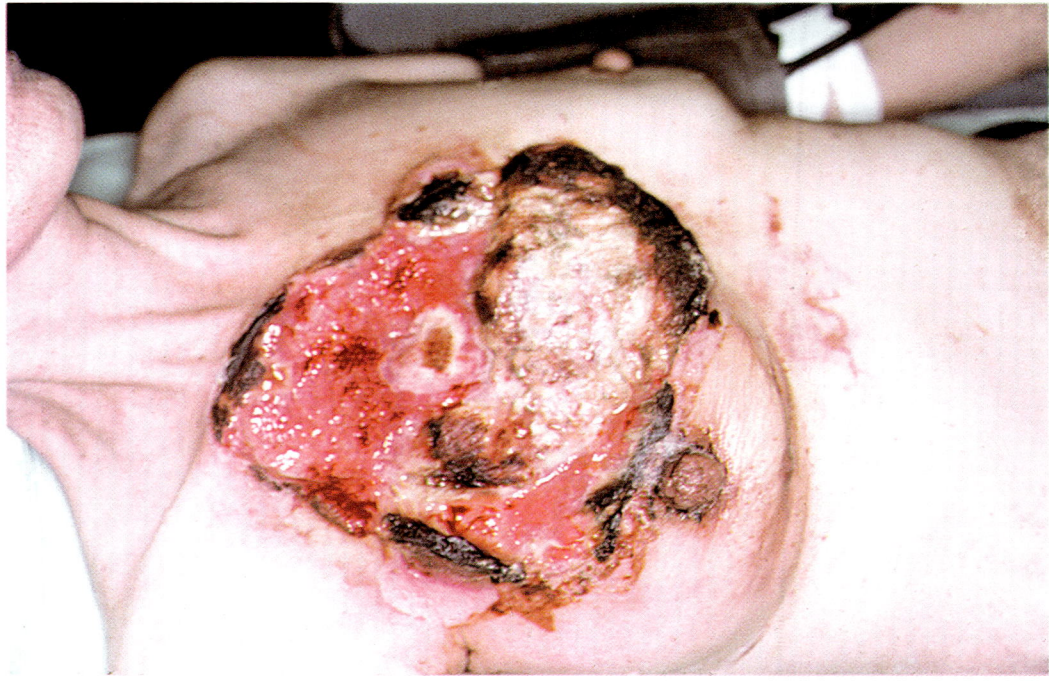

Fig. 16.2.44[5]. 2 weeks later. Necrotized tissue was sloughed off

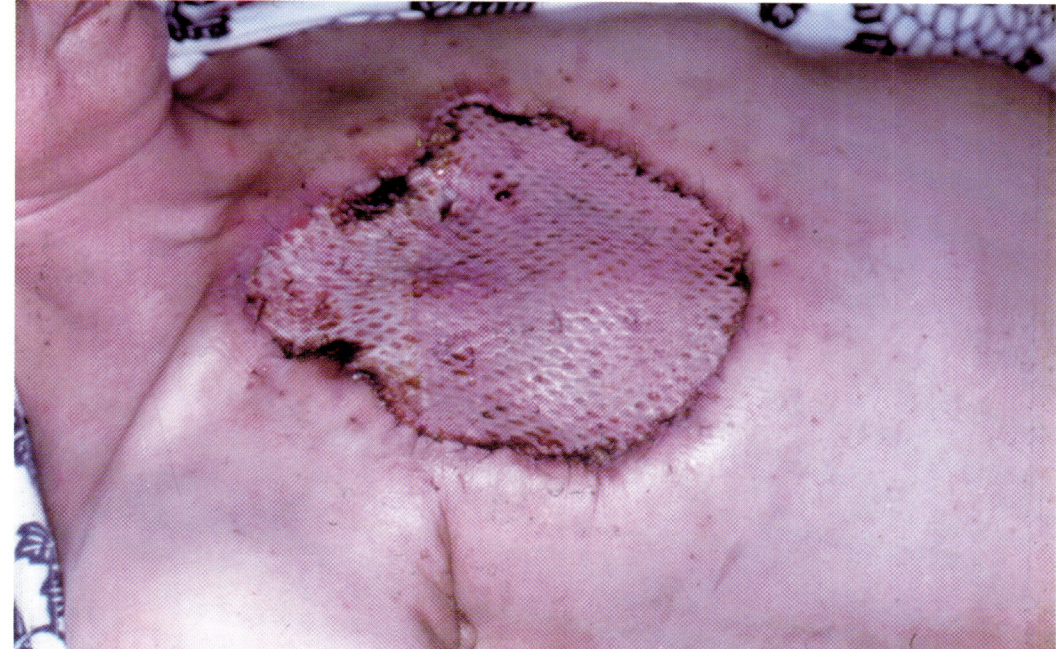

Fig. 16.2.45[5]. 3 weeks later, after necrotomy and simple mastectomy, a mesh skin graft was performed and took well

16.2.2 Combined Contact and Spraying Methods

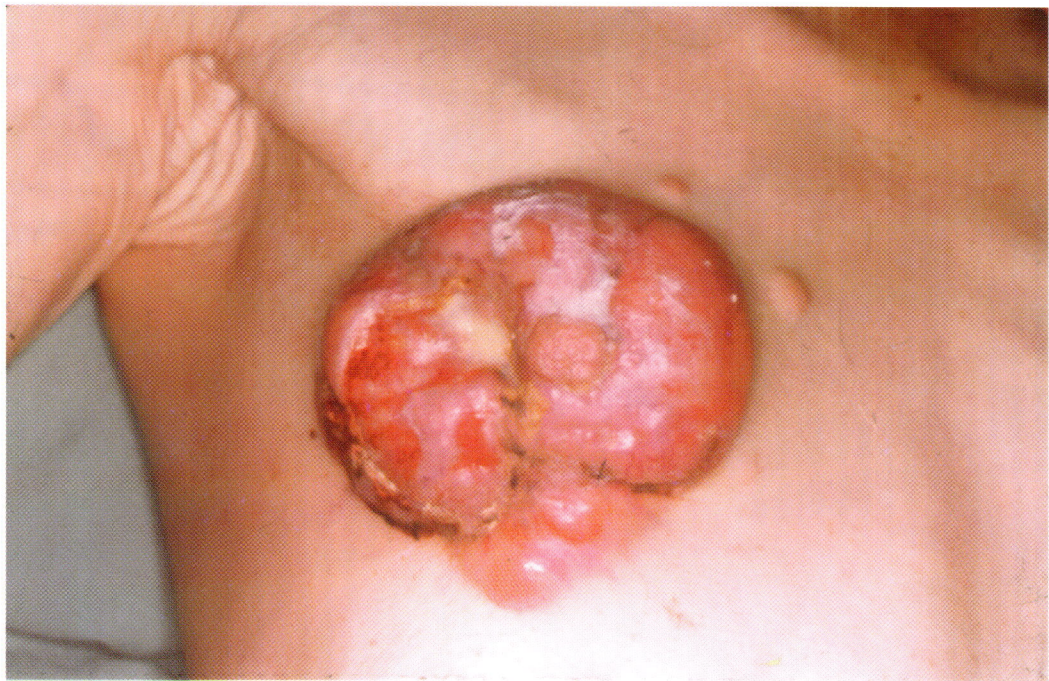

Fig. 16.2.46[5]. 76/F, T4cN2MX, stage IIIB, medullo-tubular carcinoma. A sold and satellite tumors, before cryosurgery

Chapter 16
Breast Cancer Cryosurgery

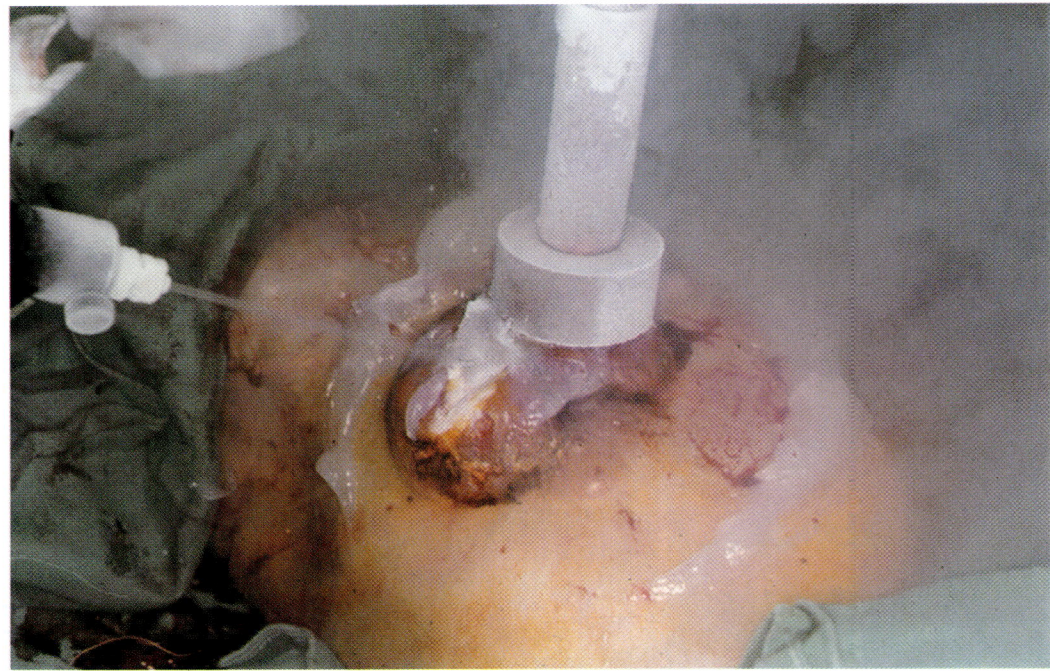

Fig. 16.2.47[5]. Contact and spray freezing, Linde CE-2B, SK-51865-1, with a 4 cm cylindrical probe-tip adaptor, −140°C, 5 min + 10 min LN_2-spray with CS-76 for 10 min

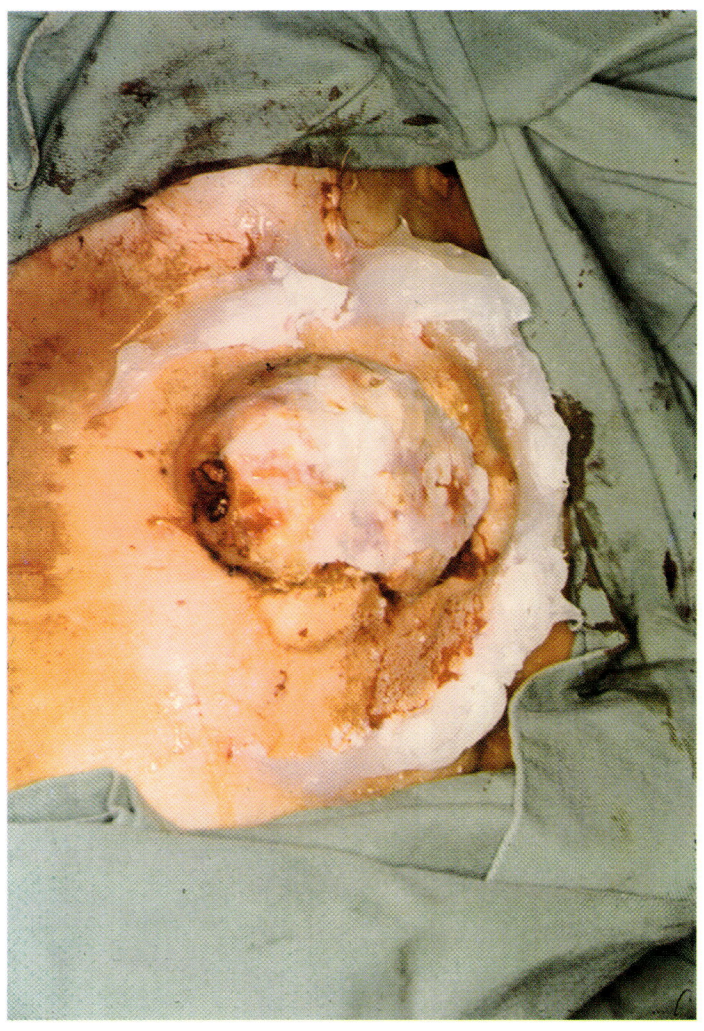

Fig. 16.2.48[5]. After termination of the freezing process. An ice ball, and a vaseline embankment, prepared to protect adjacent normal skin, is shown

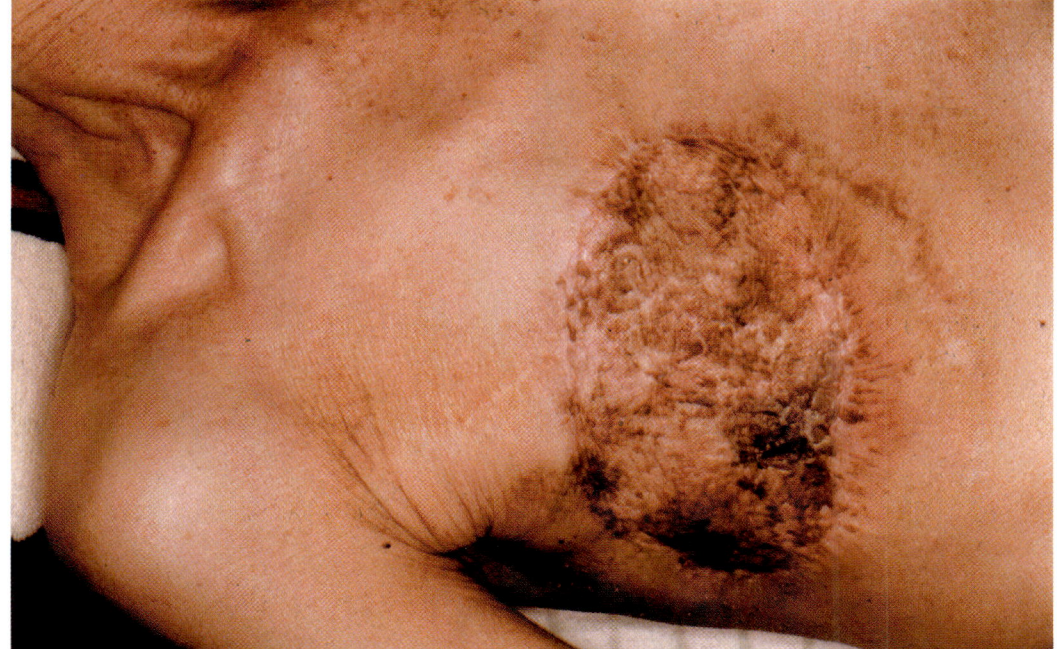

Fig. 16.2.49[5]. Axillary lymph node dissection and a mesh skin graft were performed

16.2.3 Spraying Method

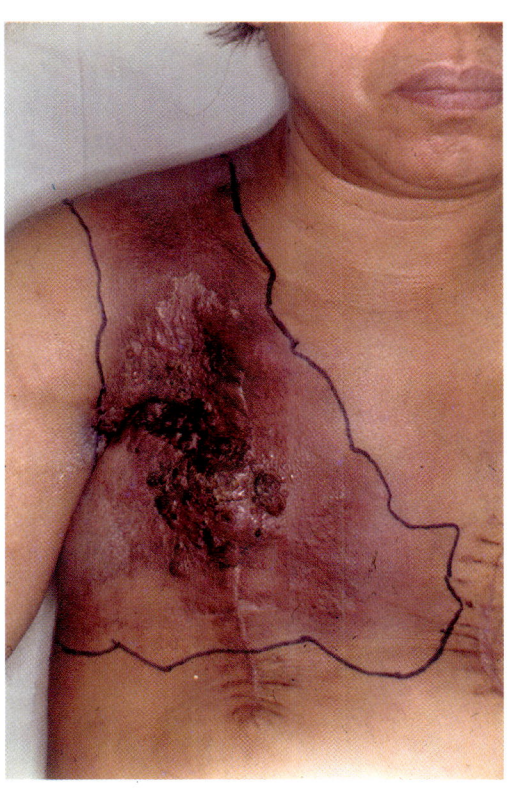

Fig. 16.2.50[5]. 49/F, bilateral recurrent breast cancer, carcinoma erysipelatodes (inflammatory cancer). Shows right side lesion, spreading widely and rapidly

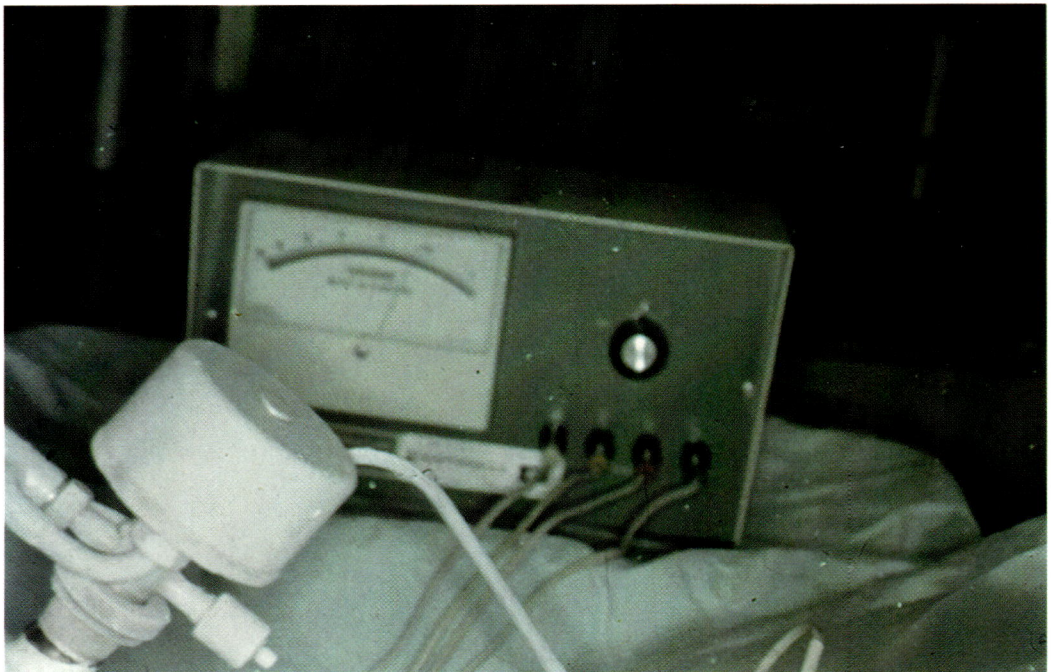

Fig. 16.2.51[5]. Cryosurgery by LN_2-spraying method, subcutaneous temperature monitored at multiple sites, using Spray Cryomatic (Japan)

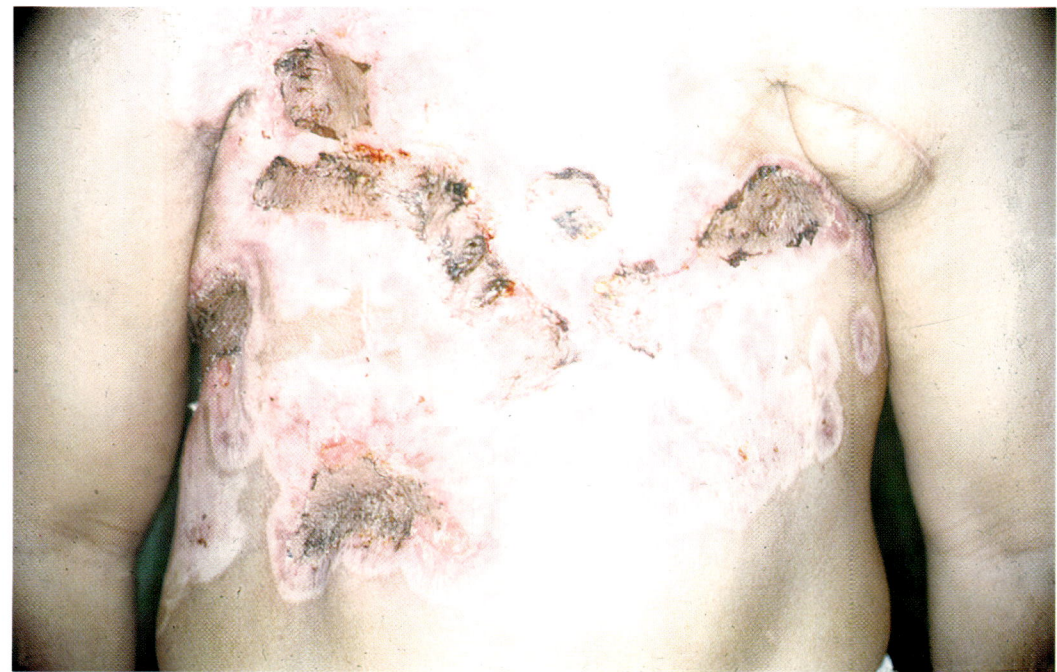

Fig. 16.2.52[5]. 3 months later, wound has healed leaving scars. Cryospray successfully stopped progression of the disease and saved the patient

Section F Clinical Aspects

Chapter 16
Breast Cancer
Cryosurgery

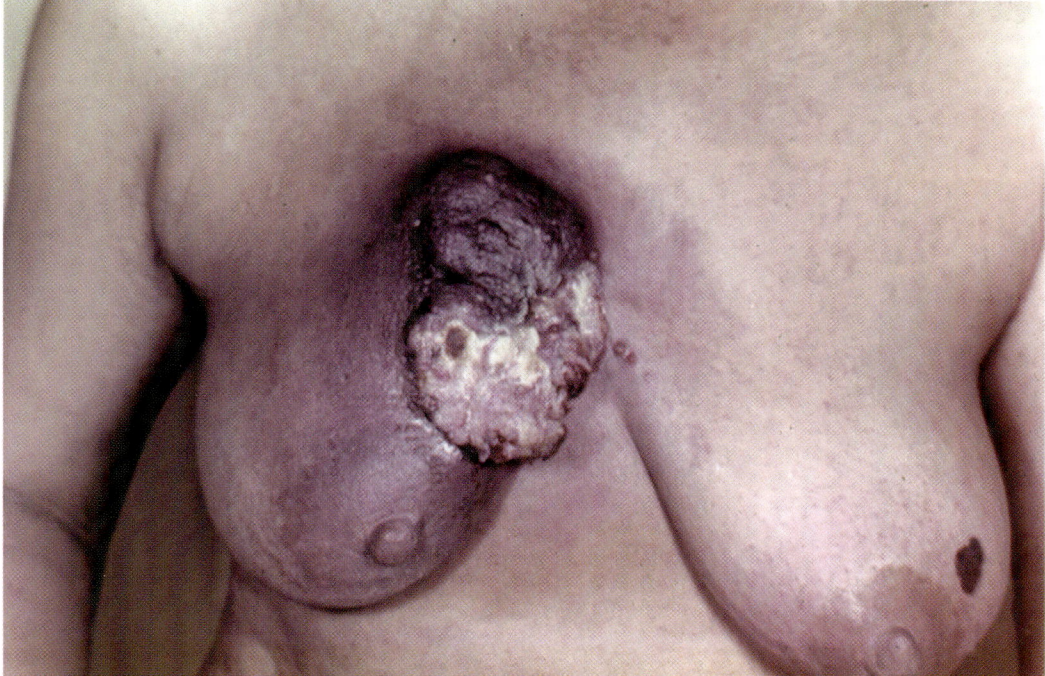

Fig. 16.2.53[5]. 58/F, a Paget's cancer of the right breast. T4cN$_2$MX, stage IIIB. Anticancer chemotherapy was impossible due to a drug allergy, and radiation therapy had failed

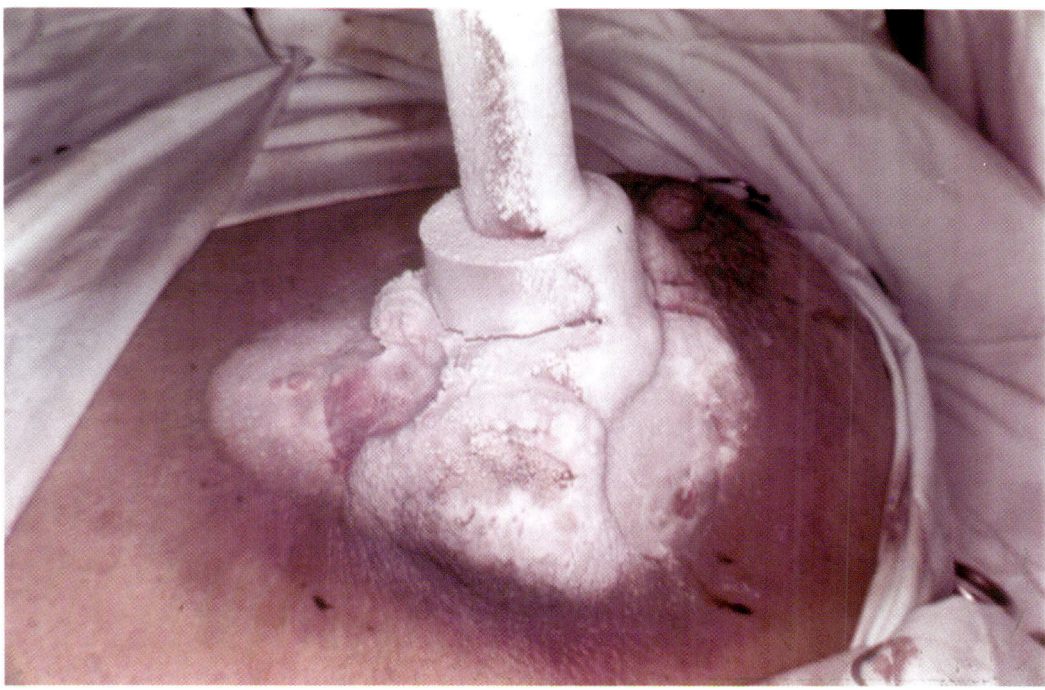

Fig. 16.2.54[5]. Cryosurgery by contact and spraying method, with Linde CE-2B and SK-51865-1 with 4 cm cylindrical and 3 cm hemispherical probe-tip adaptors, −170°C 10 min × 6, and LN$_2$-spray for 10 min well beyond the tumor margin

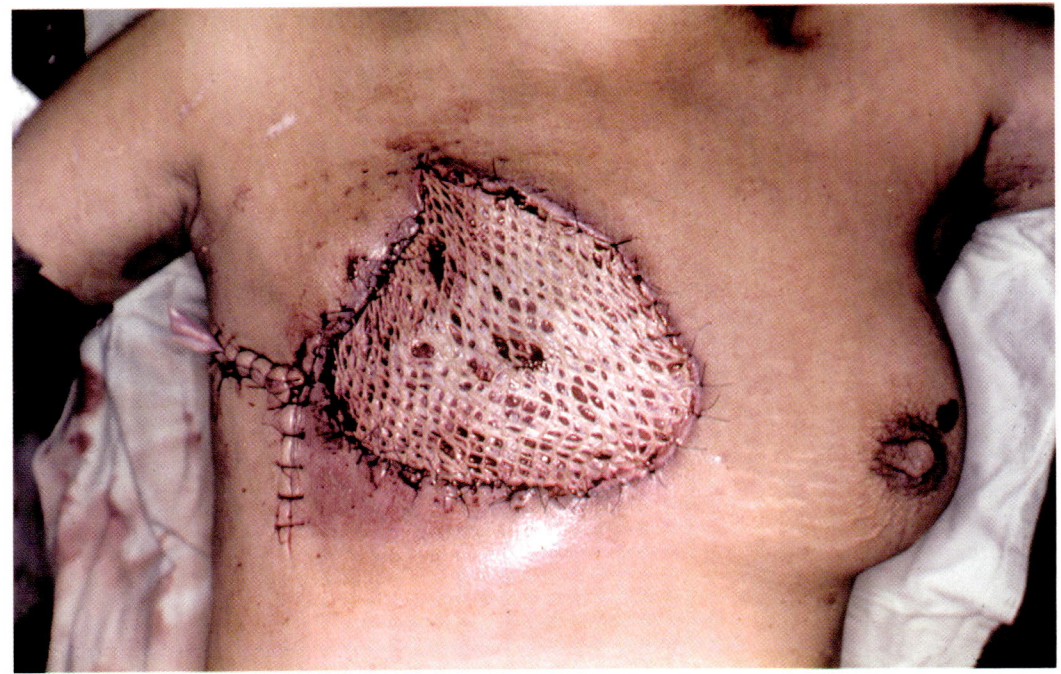

Fig. 16.2.55[5]. After necrotomy and simple mastectomy, a mesh skin graft was performed

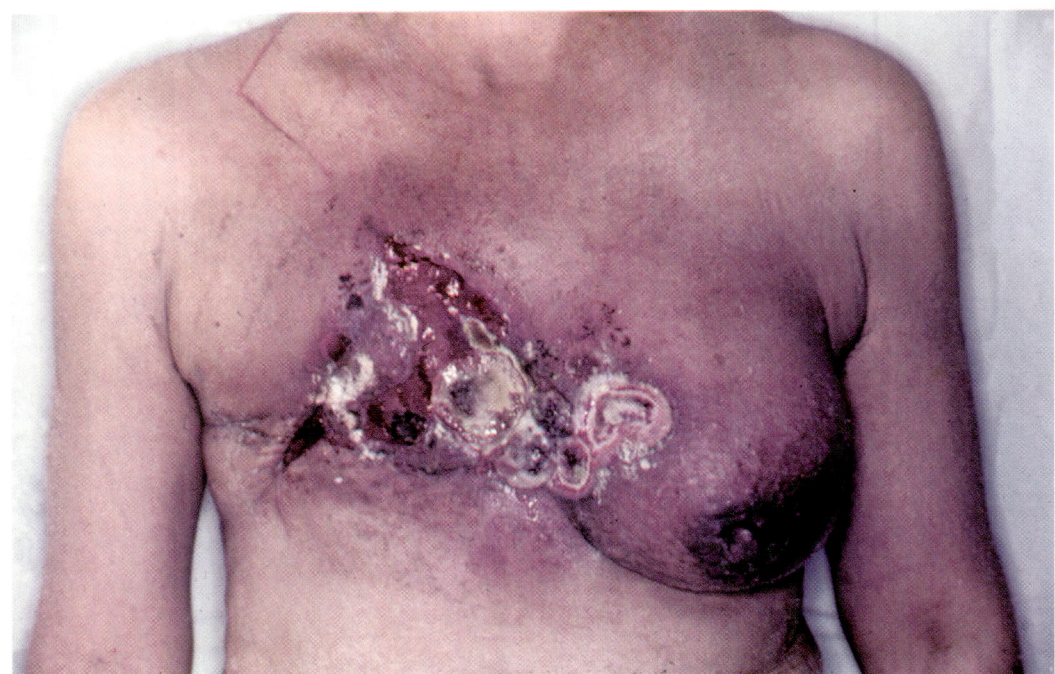

Fig. 16.2.56[5]. 2 months later, local recurrence and inflammatory invasion to the contralateral side was observed. A biopsy performed by cryosurgery revealed an anaplastic cancer, suggestive of anaplastic conversion of the primary cancer, ductal adenocarcinoma

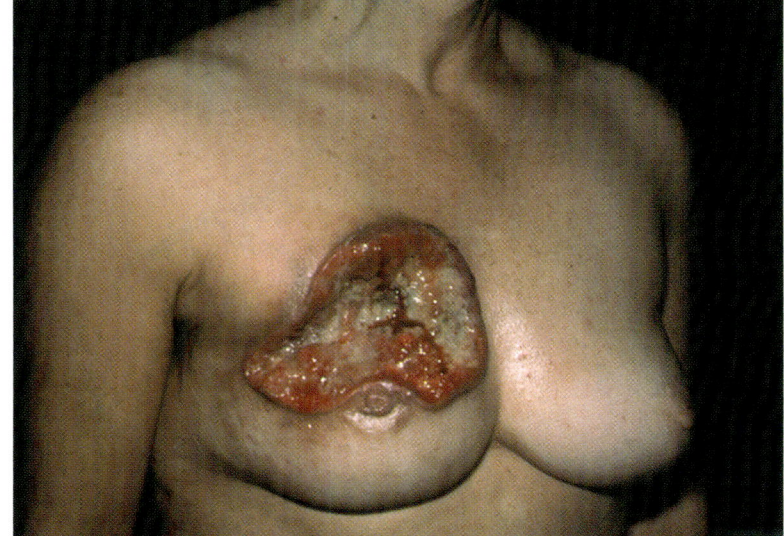

Fig. 16.2.57[2]. The author has devised a protocol for cryomastectomy in which a large, twelve times folded paraffinated bandage is stitched to the skin around the contour of the breast; some 12 thermocouples are strategically placed inside the breast. This is divided into four quadrants. Each quadrant is successively frozen to $(-80)–(-90)°C$, except near the ribs to avoid destroying them due to the excessively low temperature. After thawing, a second freezing is carried out. This young woman neglected her breast cancer for fear of amputation

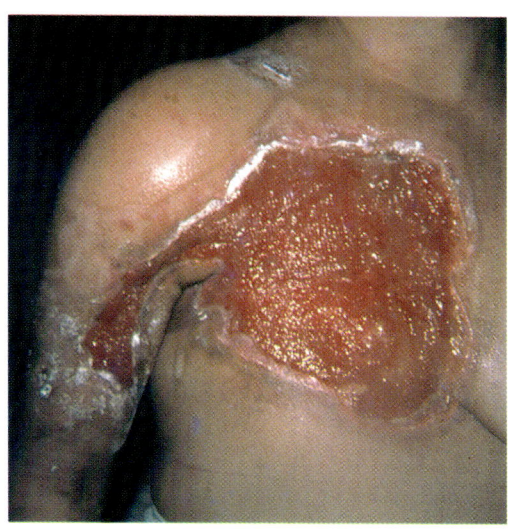

Fig. 16.2.58[2]. The elimination of the necrosed breast tissue began in the second week and was completely removed three weeks after the cryomastectomy, leaving a clean ulceration that healed by second intention

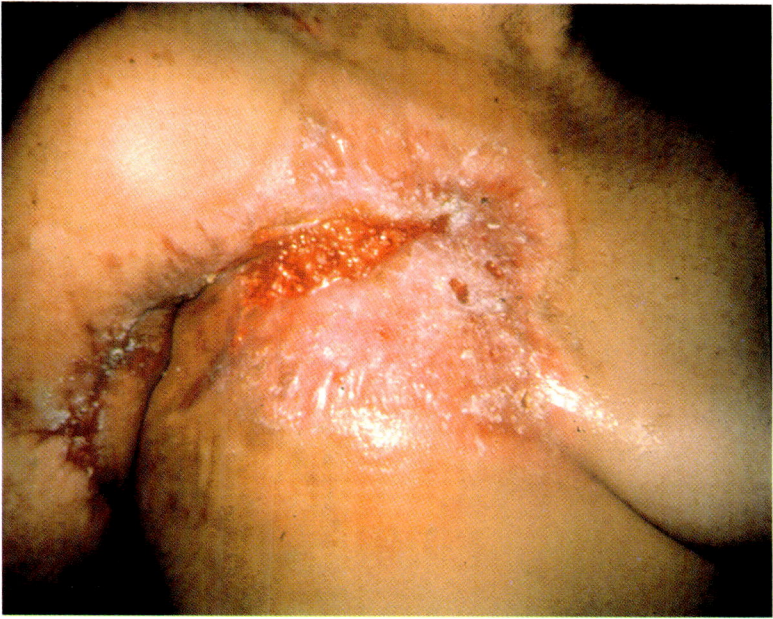

Fig. 16.2.59[2]. There was no local recurrence but the patient died three years later of metastatic disease. Cryomastectomy is medically indicated for the cancers that are inoperable and resistant to chemotherapy

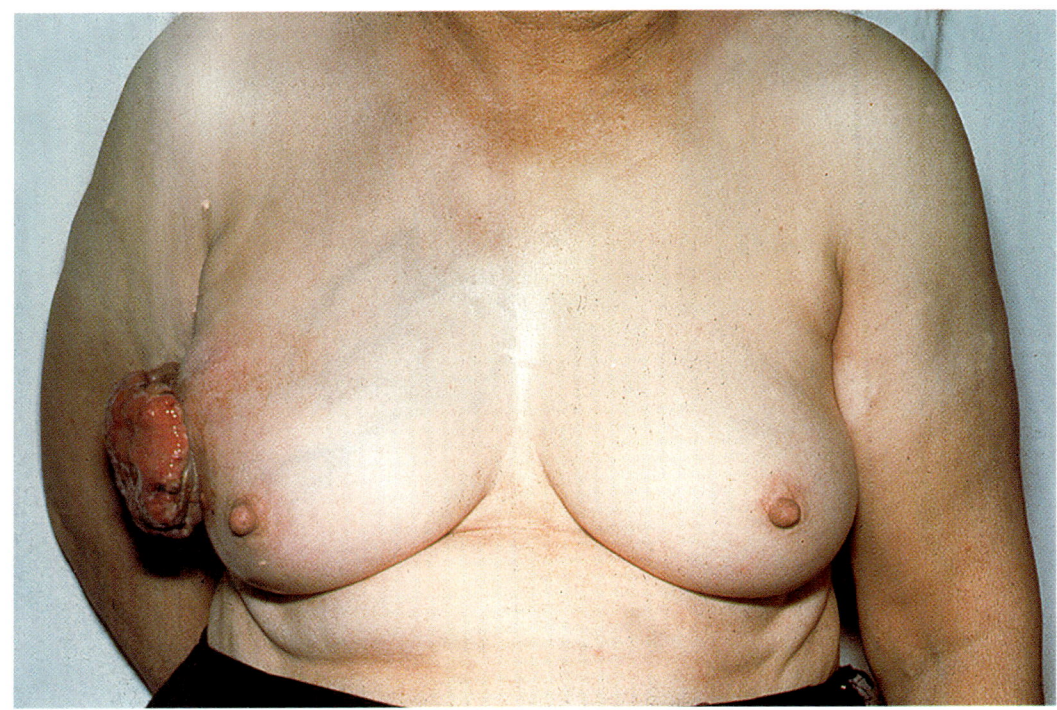

Fig. 16.2.60². An inoperable breast cancer with a bleeding and fungating external tumoral mass. The patient had severe anemia

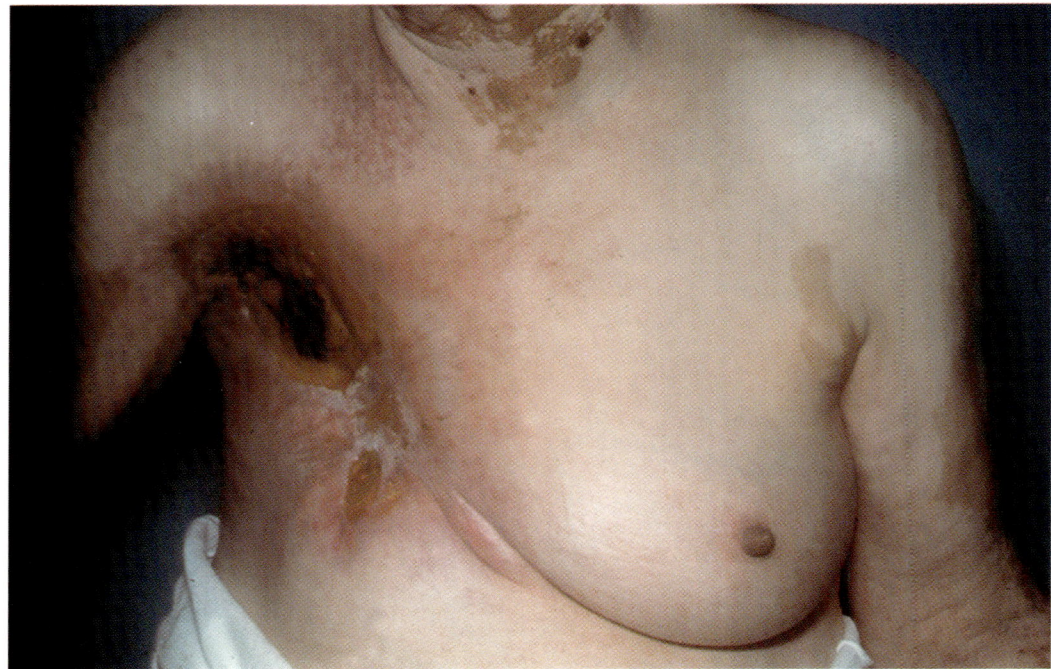

Fig. 16.2.61². Two years later, after the breast had been removed by cryomastectomy. The patient benefited from a good quality of life for four years. She refused chemotherapy. She had no local recurrence but eventually died of metastatic disease

16.3 Local-Regional Disease Recurrence

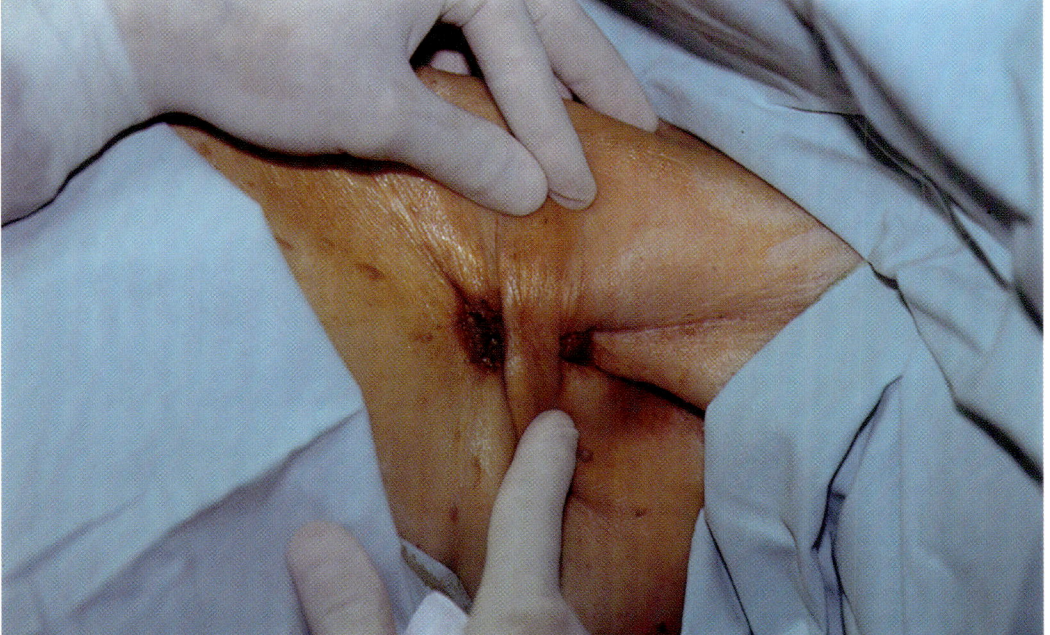

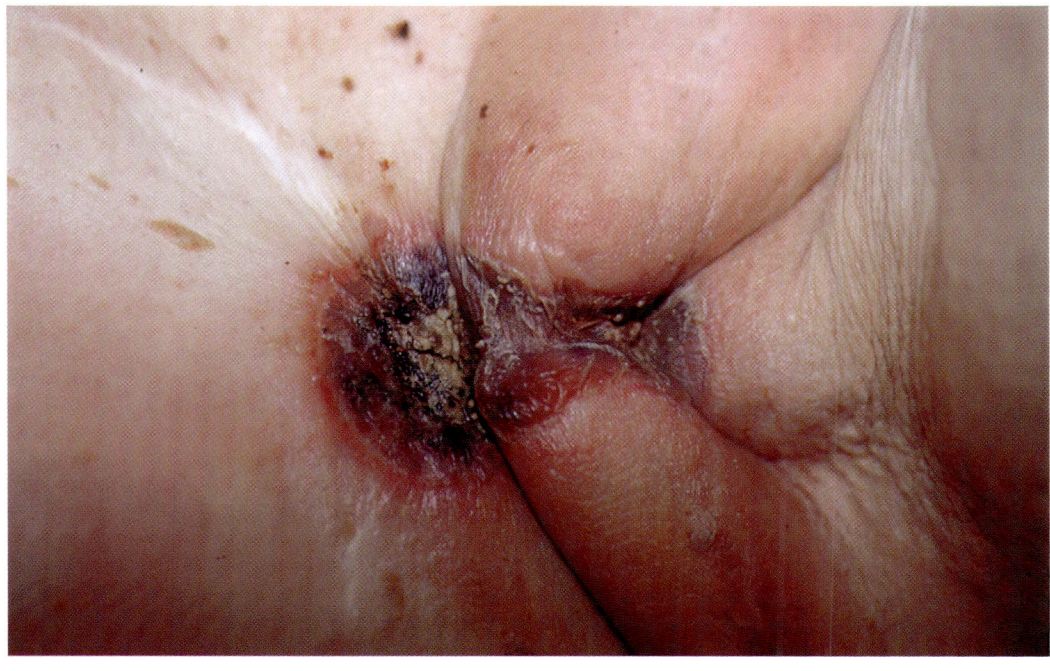

Fig. 16.3.1[1] A, B. Local-regional recurrence of breast cancer in the ipsilateral breast, chest wall and skin overlying the chest wall involving the ipsilateral axillary lymph nodes after mastectomy in a 64-year-old woman. Preoperative view

Chapter 16
Breast Cancer Cryosurgery

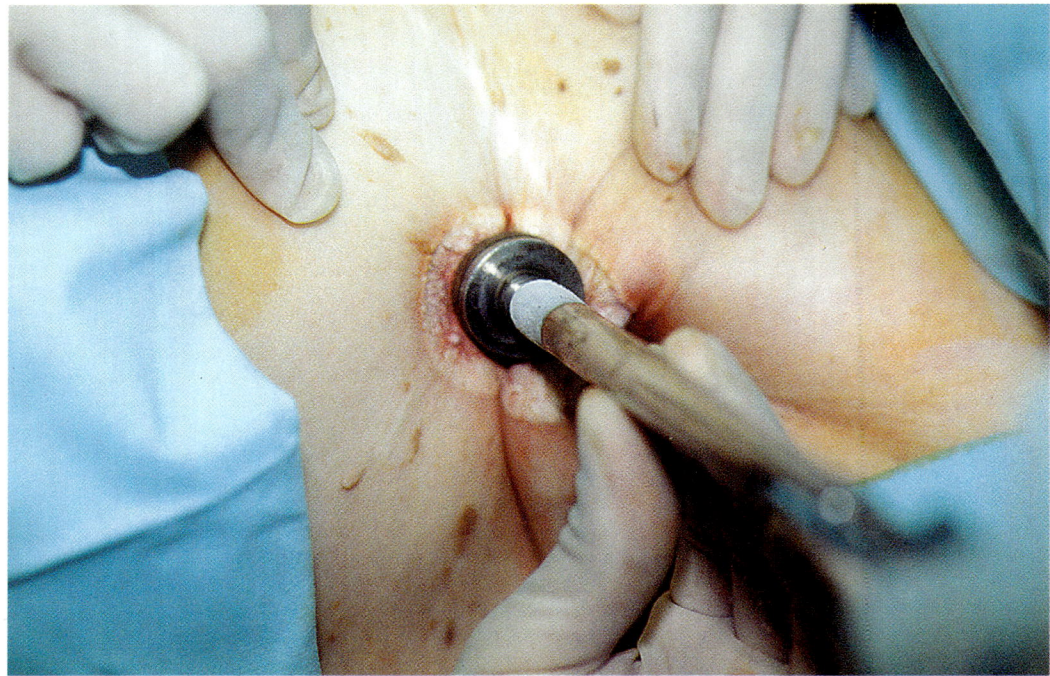

Fig. 16.3.2¹. Local-regional recurrence of breast cancer after mastectomy. A double cryosurgical session by means of a disc cryoprobe with a diameter of 20 mm which is placed on the tumor mass at a temperature of −180°C without local anesthesia (**A**). The post-cryosurgical zone is clearly indicated by a demarcation line when the cryoprobe is removed (**B**)

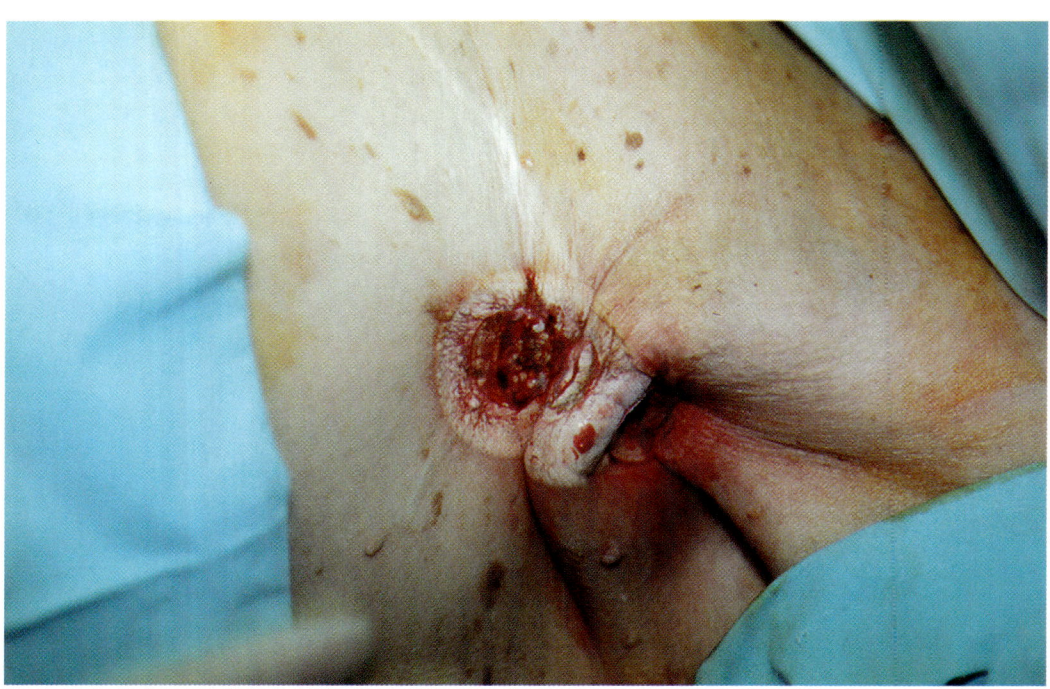

Section F Clinical Aspects 395

Chapter 16
Breast Cancer
Cryosurgery

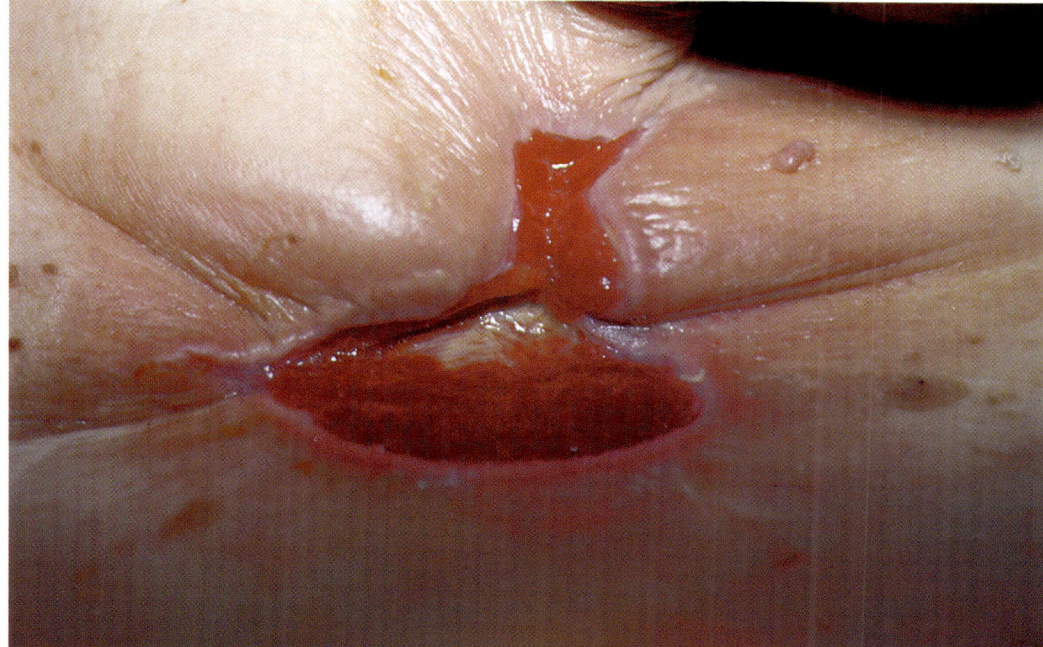

A

Fig. 16.3.3¹. Local-regional recurrence of breast cancer after mastectomy. Breast cancer cryosurgery: 8 weeks (**A**) and 12 weeks (**B**) after the breast cancer cryosurgical session. View of the post-cryosurgical wound

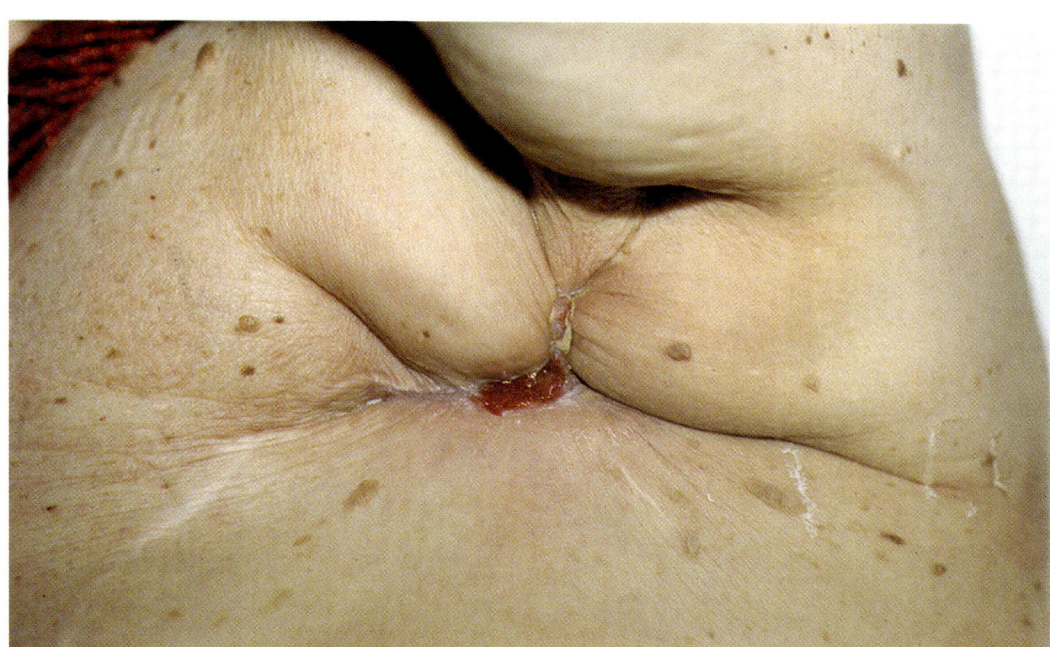

B

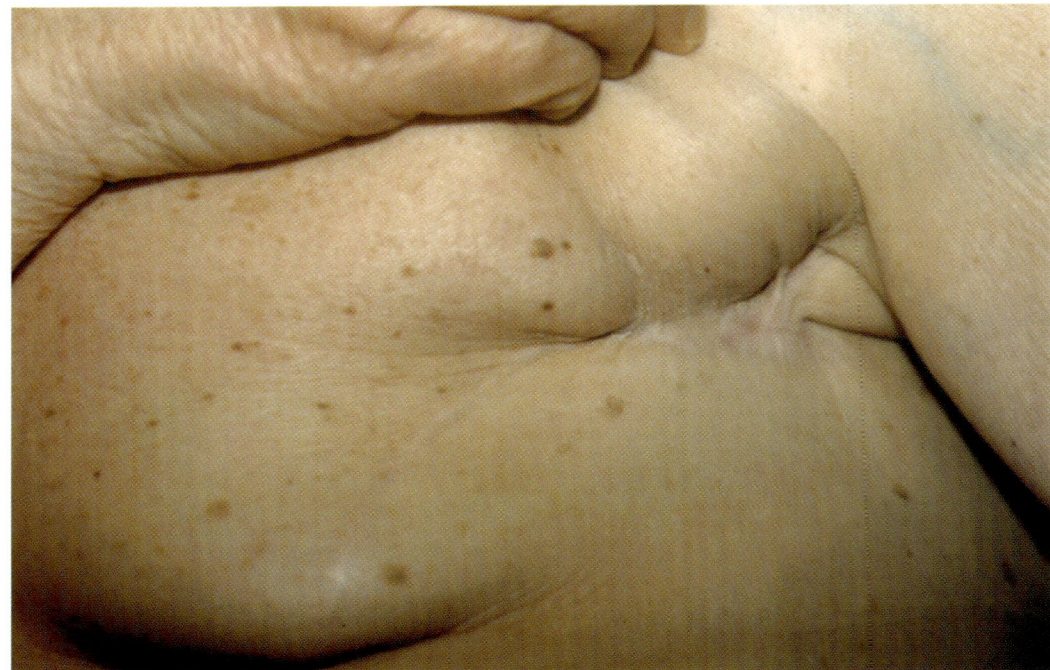

Fig. 16.3.4[1]. Local-regional recurrence of breast cancer after mastectomy. Breast cancer cryosurgery: 3 years after the cryosurgical session. The patient is disease-free 4 years after the breast cryosurgery

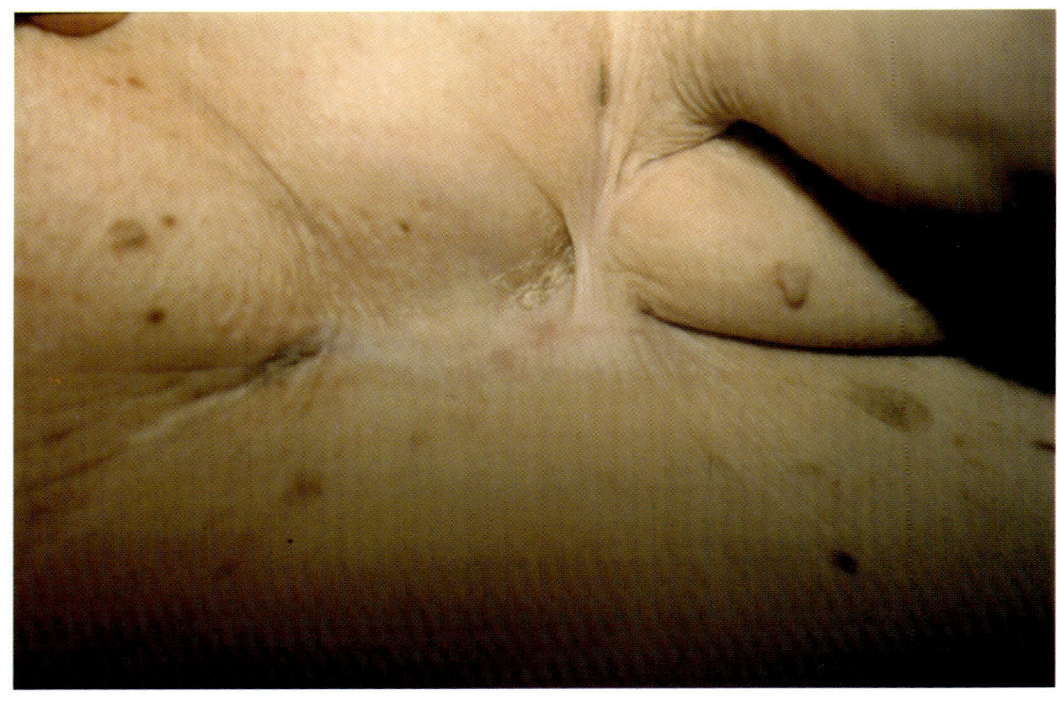

16.4 Skin Metastases

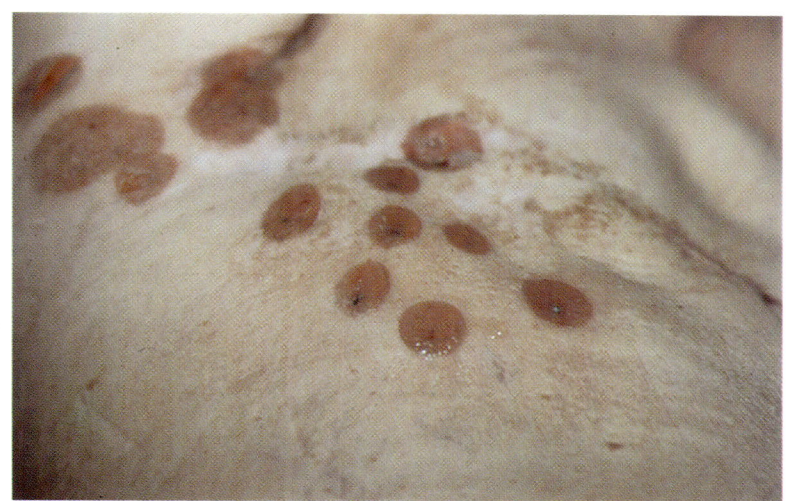

Fig. 16.4.1[1]. A 69-year-old woman with multiple skin metastases after mastectomy. Post-cryosurgical view: 1st postoperative day

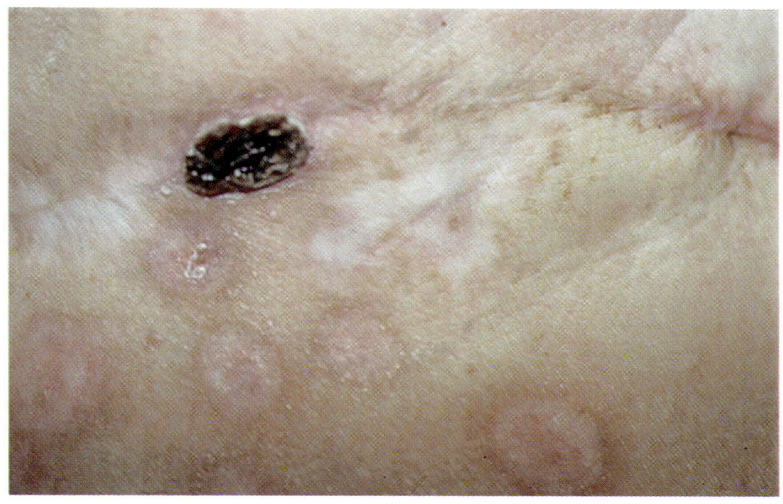

A

B

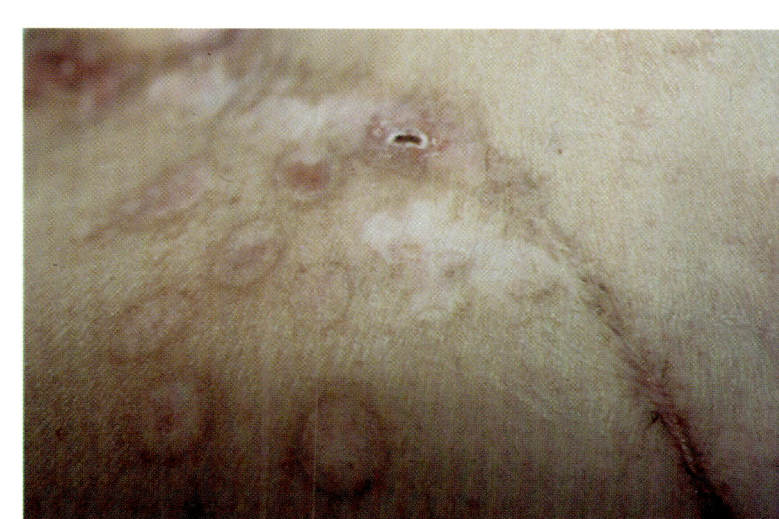

Fig. 16.4.2[1]. Multiple skin metastases in the same patient. Post-cryosurgical view of the wound healing. (**A**) 8 weeks after the cryosurgical session (**B**)

Chapter 16
Breast Cancer Cryosurgery

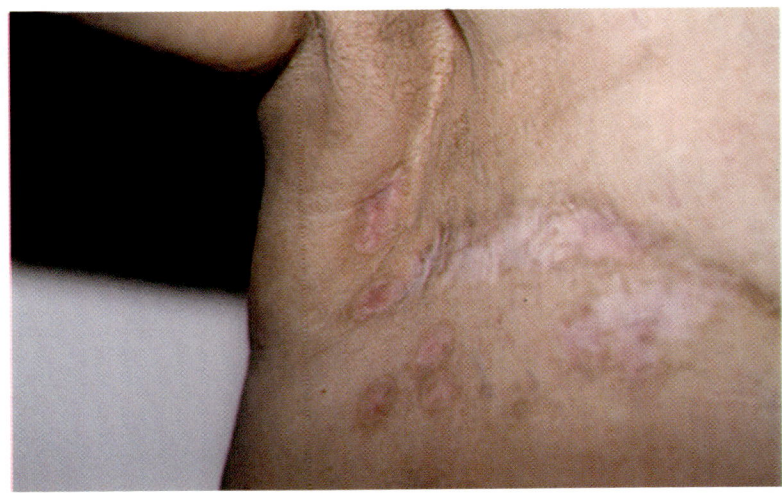

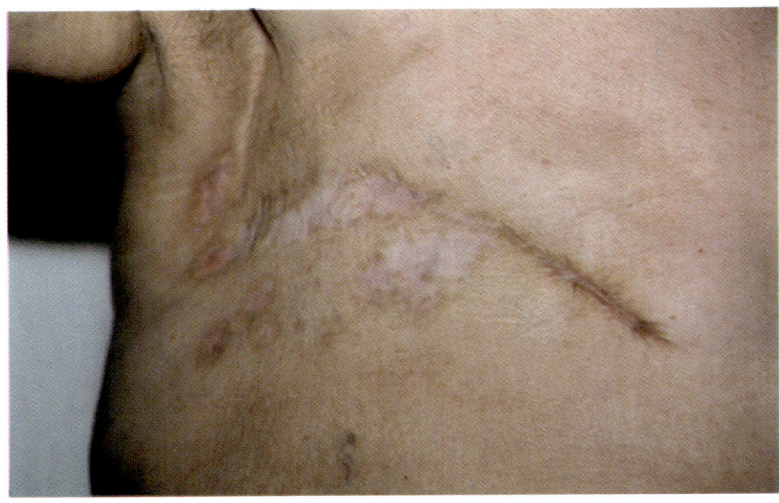

Fig. 16.4.3¹. Multiple skin metastases in the same patient. Post-cryosurgical view of the wound healing. Excellent curative and cosmetic results 6 months after the cryosurgical session. After cryosurgery, no recurrence or metastases during a 5-year observation period

Chapter 17

Breast Cryosurgery: Benign Disorders
Nikolai N. Korpan

17.1 Papillary Lesions

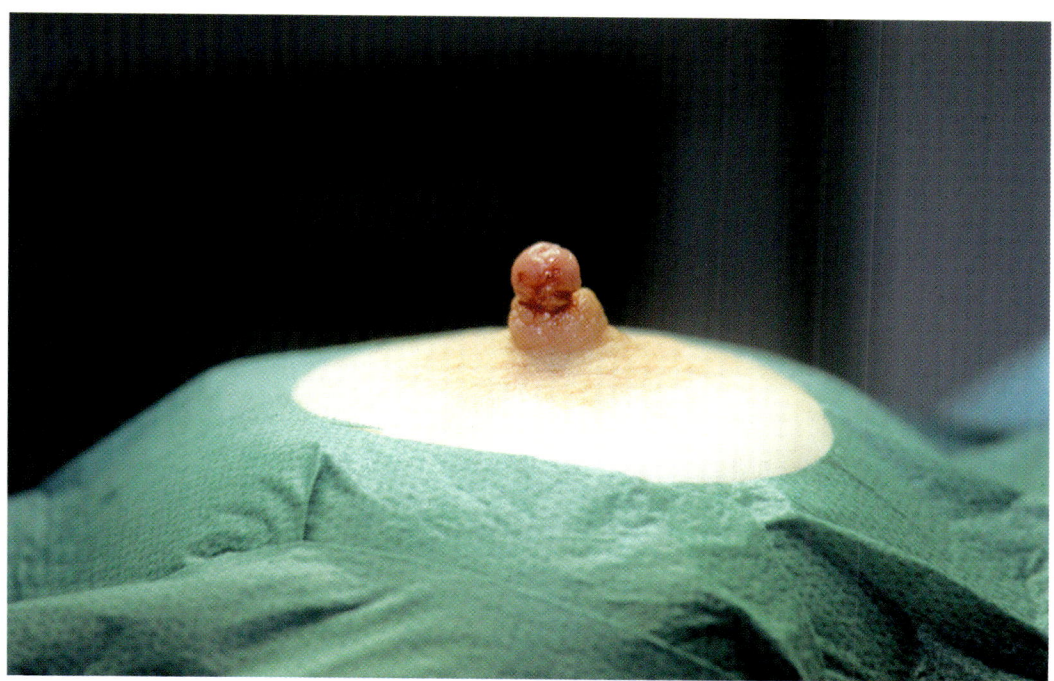

Fig. 17.1.1 A, B. Papillary lesion of the nipple in a 57-year-old woman. Occasional, minimal external bleeding. Preoperative view

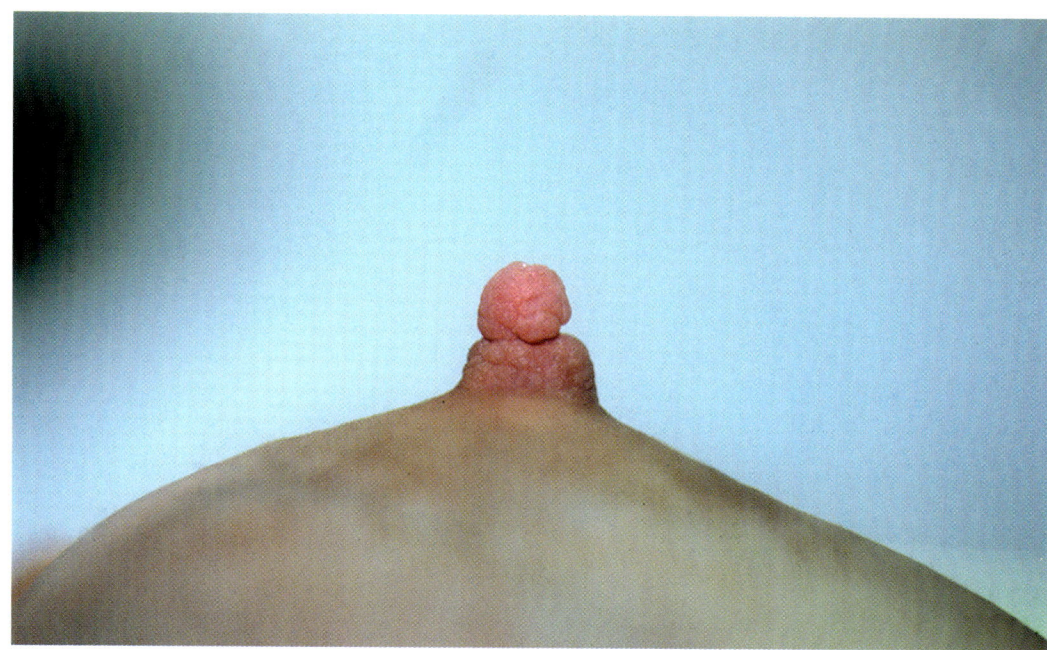

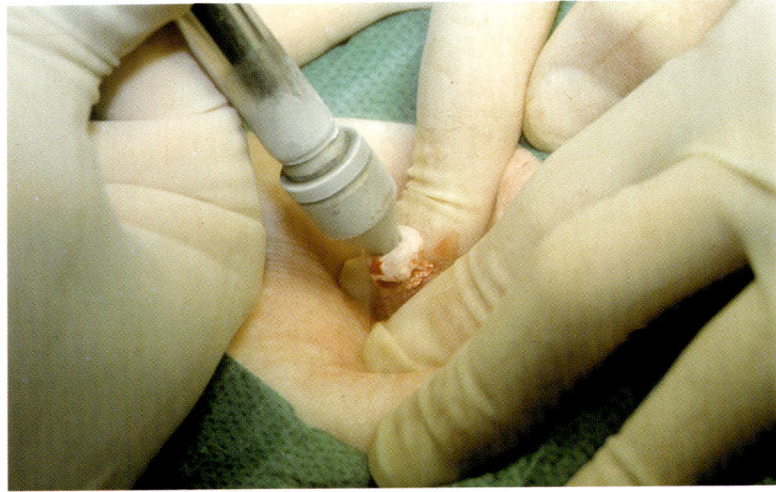

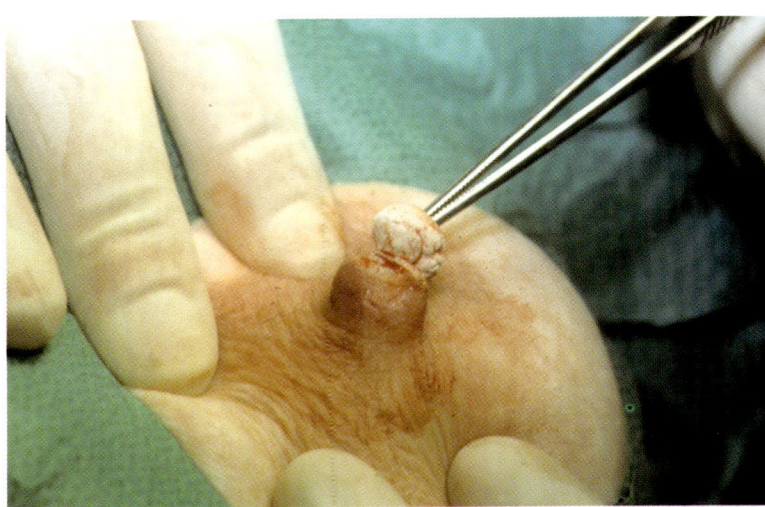

Fig. 17.1.2. Papillary lesion of the nipple. A simple cryosurgical session by means of a disc cryoprobe with a diameter of 5 mm which is placed on the papillary lesion of the nipple at a temperature of −180°C. Exposure time 30 sec

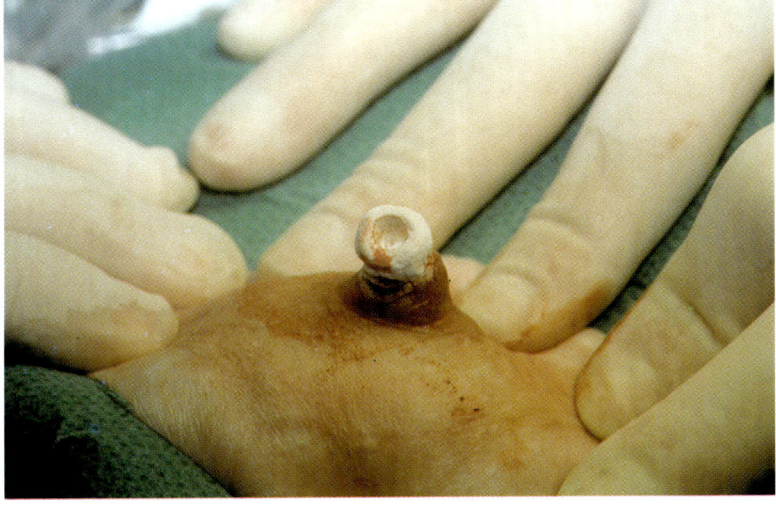

Fig. 17.1.3 A, B. Typical post-cryosurgical appearance of the nipple immediately after the cryosurgical session in the same patient

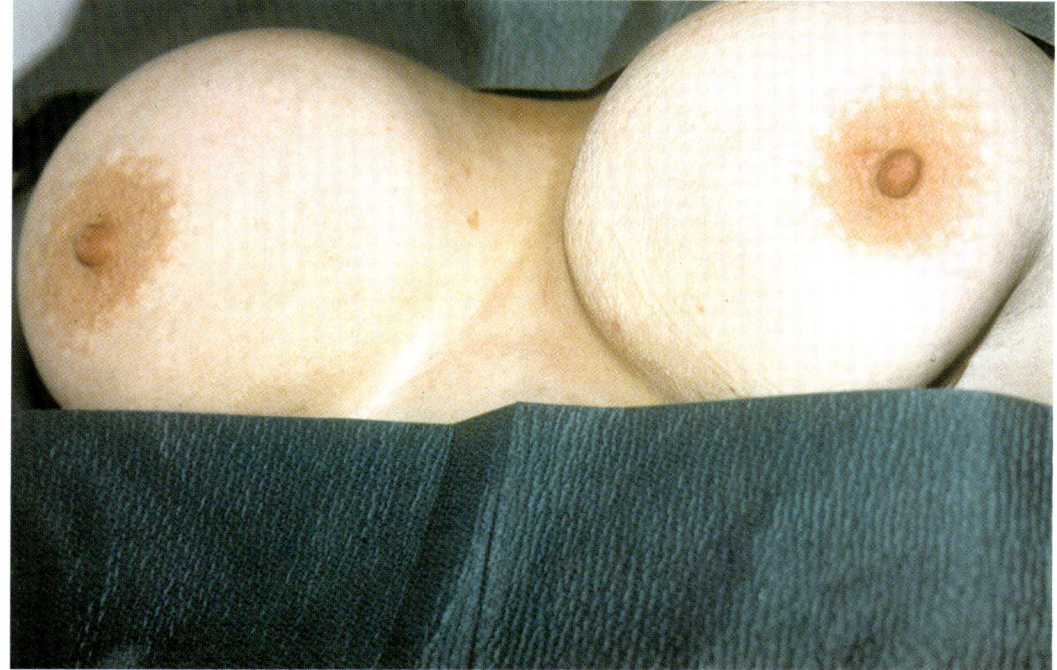

A

Fig. 17.1.4 A, B. Excellent curative and cosmetic results six weeks after cryosurgical treatment. After cryosurgery, no recurrence during a 3-year observation period

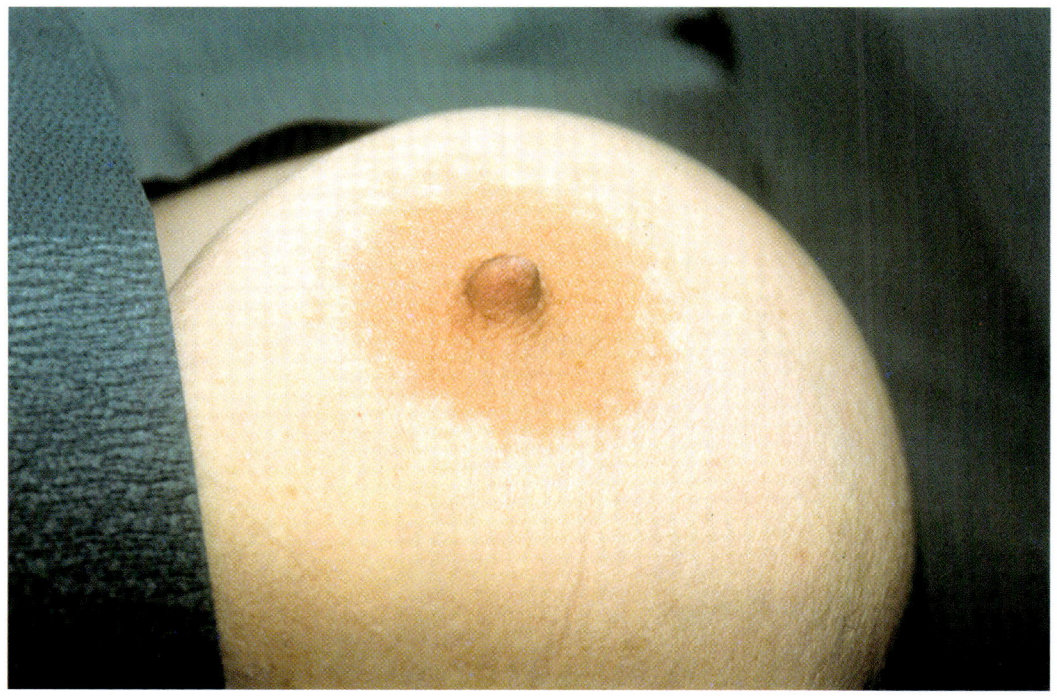

B

Cryosurgical Urology

Inderbir S. Gill[1]

18.0 Introduction

"Renal mass" is today, more often than not, a radiologic diagnosis. The increasing use of abdominal ultrasonography and CT scanning has led to a 5-fold increase in the serendipitous detection of small renal masses over the past 2 decades. This advance has contributed, in part, to a decrease in the incidence of metastatic renal cell carcinoma.

For the practicing urologist, the term 'incidental renal mass' has progressed from being an occasional diagnostic curiosity to being a day-to-day management dilemma. The differential diagnosis of a small, solid or complex cystic, enhancing renal mass includes a variety of benign and malignant conditions. Because of the risk, albeit low, for metastatic dissemination of these small renal cell carcinomas, current opinion has tended to favor surgical excision over watchful waiting, especially for the younger patient. Thus, small (≤ 4 cm) renal tumors can be efficaciously treated with either partial or radical nephrectomy, with comparable crude and cause-specific survival. Select patients with a localized, unilateral, small (≤ 4 cm) renal cell carcinoma can be successfully treated with a nephron-sparing partial nephrectomy, even when the contralateral kidney is normal.

Laparoscopy has made considerable inroads into modern day urology. Minimally invasive techniques are being employed in the management of benign and malignant conditions of the kidney. Clinical laparoscopic cryosurgery has emerged as a method for targeted destruction of a selected, small renal tumor, in lieu of open partial nephrectomy.

The aim of cryosurgery is to ablate the same predetermined volume of tissue that would have been removed had a conventional surgical excision been performed. Established critical prerequisites for successful cryosurgery include rapid freezing, gradual thawing, and a repetition of the freeze-thaw cycle. The targeted diseased tissue, with a surrounding margin of healthy parenchyma is rapidly frozen *in situ*. This devitalized tissue is then allowed to spontaneously slough over time, with healing by secondary granulation.

Potential complications of renal cryosurgery include urine leakage secondary to calyceal cryoinjury with resultant fistula formation, and post-thaw hemorrhage. Careful selection of patients with peripherally-located tumors, and meticulous intraoperative ultrasonographic monitoring of the evolving cryolesion in order to protect the calyceal system are important in this regard. Post-thaw parenchymal hemorrhage from the renal puncture site is routinely controllable with laparoscopic manual hemostatic compression with Surgicel. Nevertheless, postoperative hemorrhage remains a concern. Technical safeguards to minimize post-thaw hemorrhage include gentle insertion of the cryoprobe without any torquing, and removal of the cryoprobe only when the ice ball has melted and 'released' the cryoprobe. Hemostatic pressure with a piece of Surgicel should be maintained for at least 5–10 min, followed by observation under reduced CO_2 pneumatic pressure for another 5–10 min.

Close surveillance following laparoscopic renal cryoablation is critical to rule out local recurrence. Renal cryolesions are radiologically characterized and followed up with magnetic resonance imaging (MRI) with and without gadolinium enhancement. Furthermore, at 6 months postoperatively, CT-directed needle biopsy of the cryoablated tumor site is also obtained.

This atlas provides an understanding of the techniques of laparoscopic renal cryoablation, the equipment utilized and explicit images of post-cryoablation imaging and biopsy findings, with the aim of outlining the basic features of the procedure for the reader. Many important questions remain about cryoablation for renal cancer. Currently, the primary criticism is the lack of histologic data about the completeness of tumor destruction and the adequacy of negative surgical margins. In addition to experimental work, critical long-term radiologic and clinical follow-up data regarding local recurrence and cancer-free survival will be necessary to address this important issue.

Section F   Clinical Aspects

18.1 Laparoscopic Renal Cryoablation

Chapter 18 Cryosurgical Urology

18.1.1 Schematic Representation of the Technique of Laparoscopic Retroperitoneal Renal Cryoablation

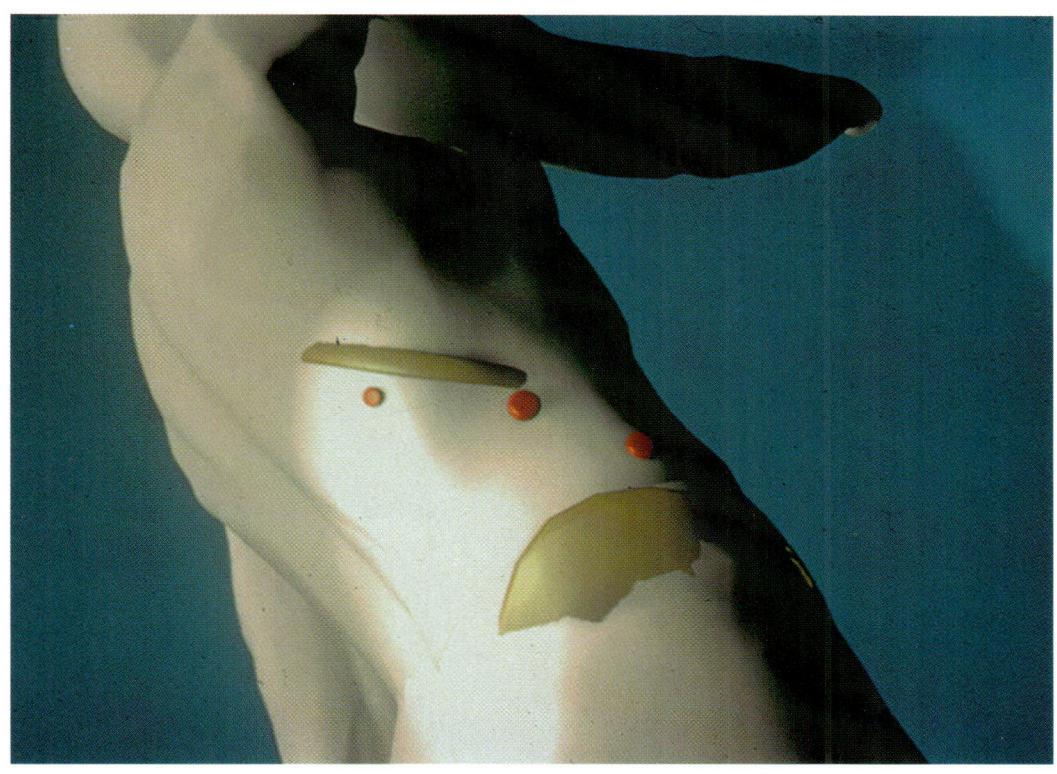

Fig. 18.1.1[1]. With the patient in full flank position, a 3-port approach is employed. The primary port is placed below the tip of the 12th rib. Two additional ports are introduced: one in the midaxillary line 3 cm superior to the iliac crest and another at the lateral border of the psoas muscle just below the 12th rib

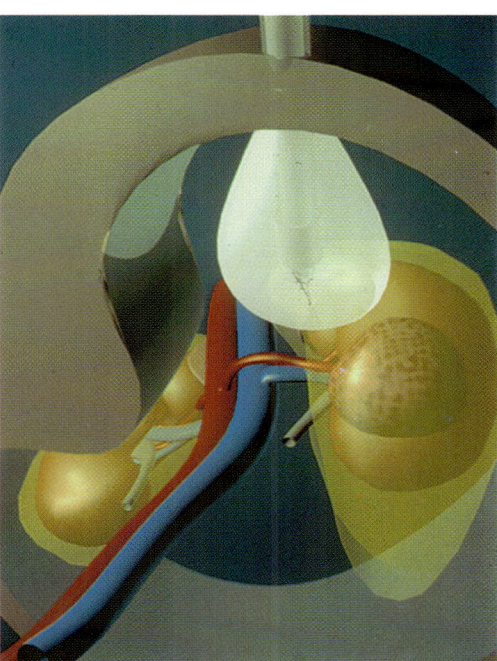

Fig. 18.1.2[1]. Following initial digital dissection, a balloon dissector is introduced in the retroperitoneal space

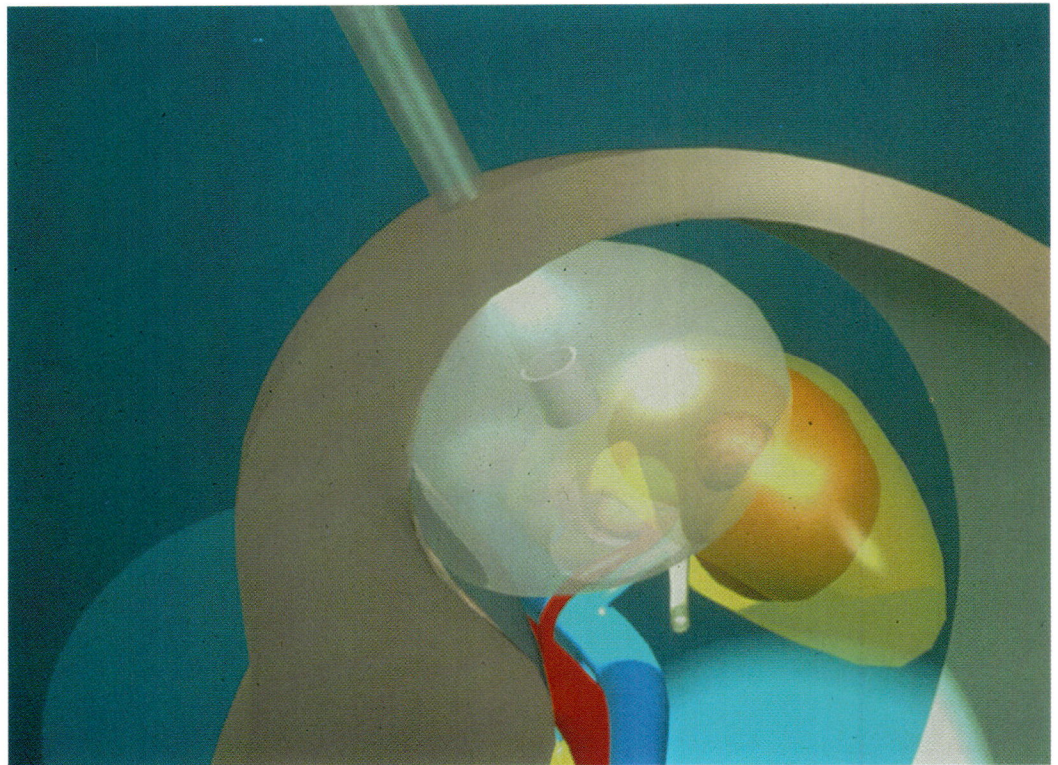

Fig. 18.1.3[1]. The balloon is distended with 800 cc of air and the inflation is maintained for 5–10 min to achieve hemostasis

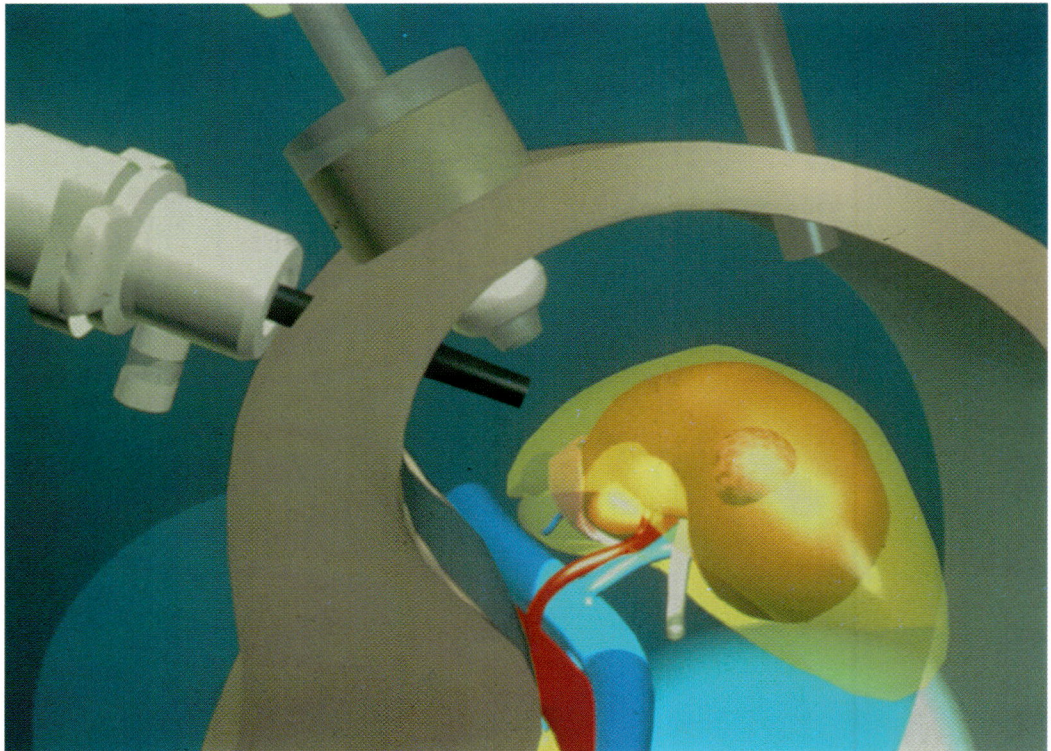

Fig. 18.1.4[1]. A 10 mm blunt-port with a retention balloon and a foam cuff is utilized as the primary port. In addition a 12 mm port is placed in the midaxillary line and a 5 mm port is introduced posteriorly

Section F   Clinical Aspects   **407**

**Chapter 18
Cryosurgical
Urology**

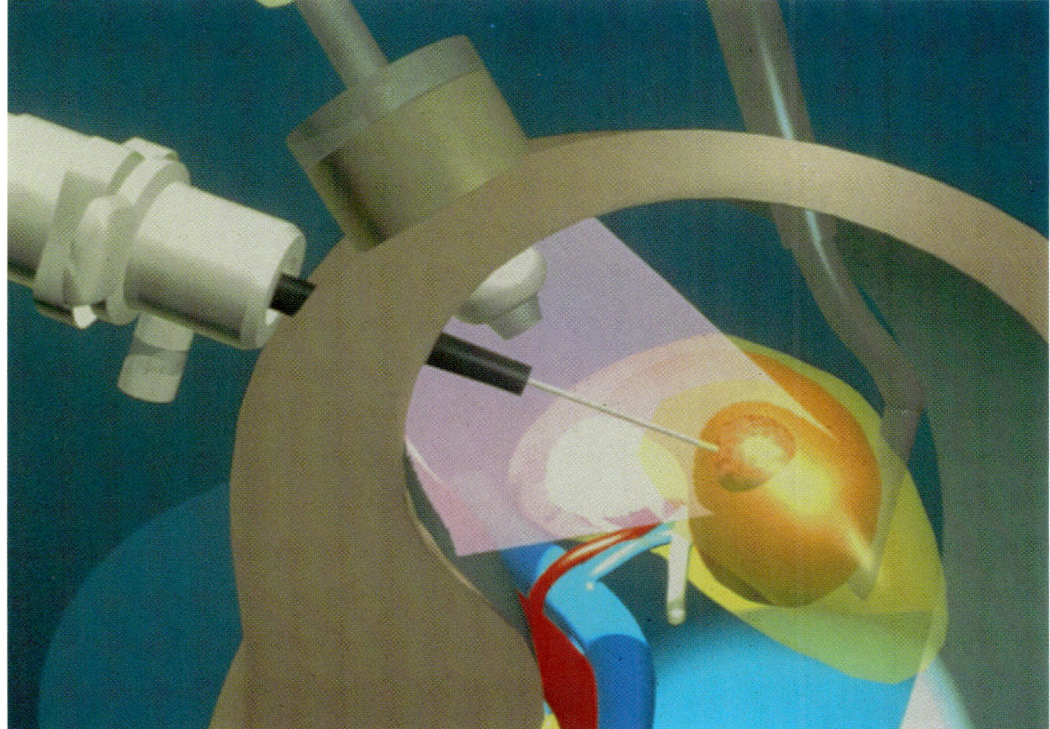

Fig. 18.1.5[1]. The mass is targeted utilizing intraoperative ultrasound, and a pre-cryoablation needle biopsy is obtained

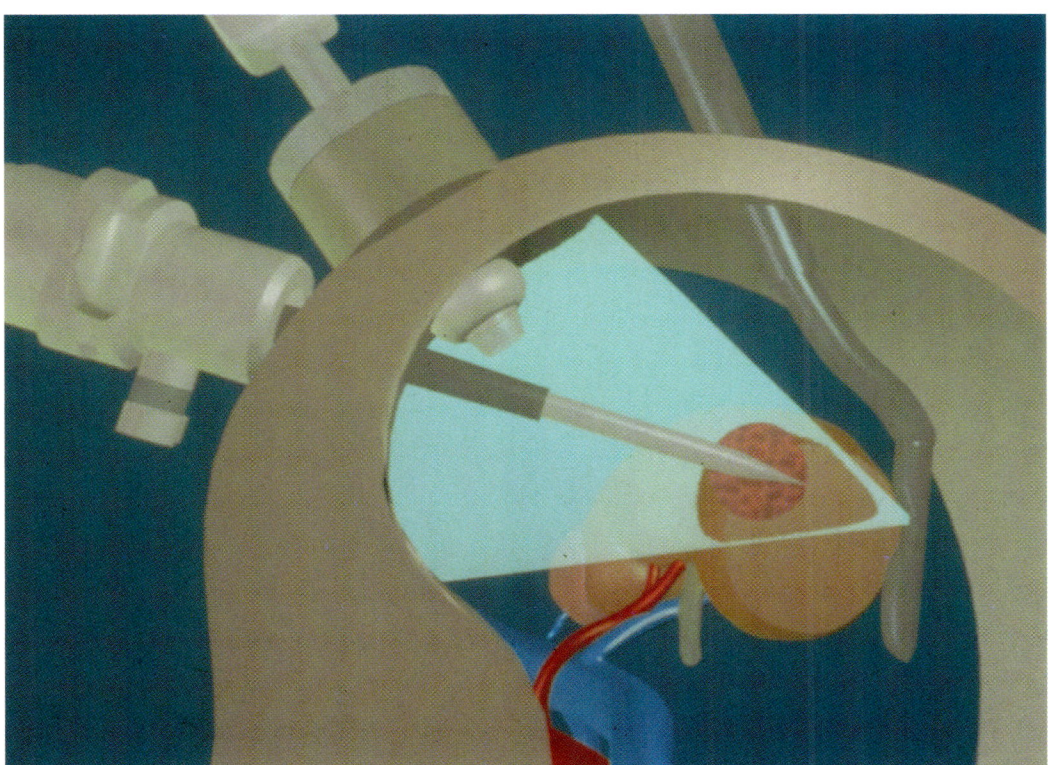

Fig. 18.1.6[1]. Under intraoperative ultrasound guidance the tip of the cryoprobe is positioned into the inner boundary of the tumor

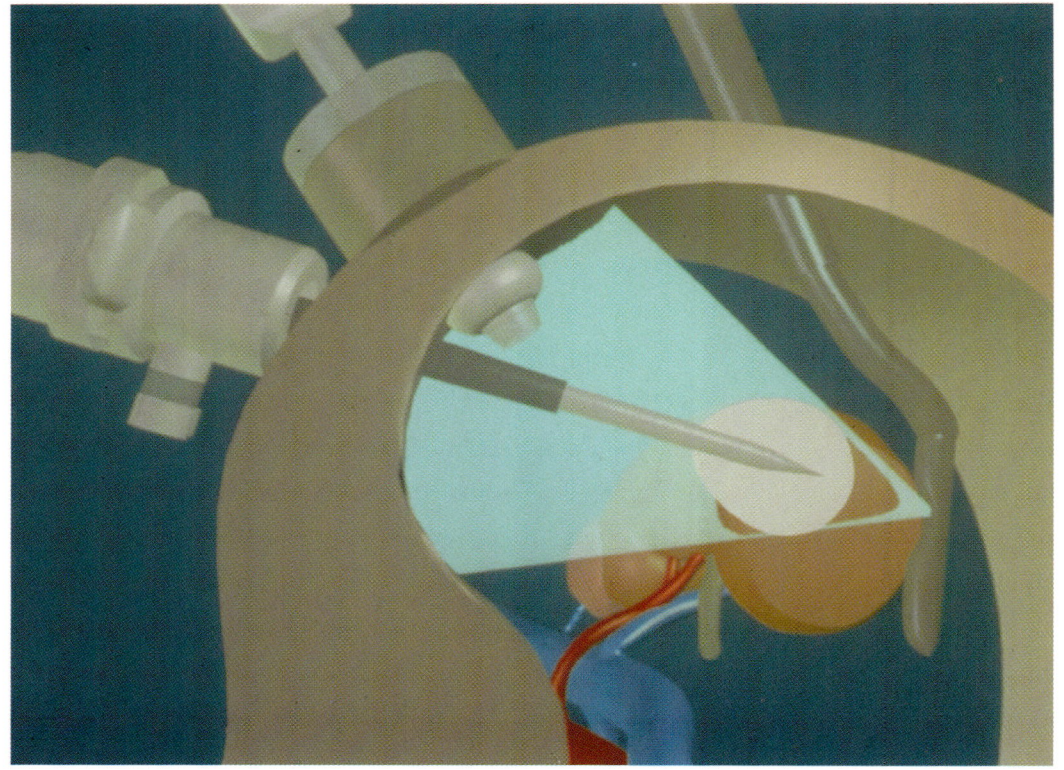

Fig. 18.1.7[1]. Cryoablation is initiated and a double freeze-thaw cycle is performed

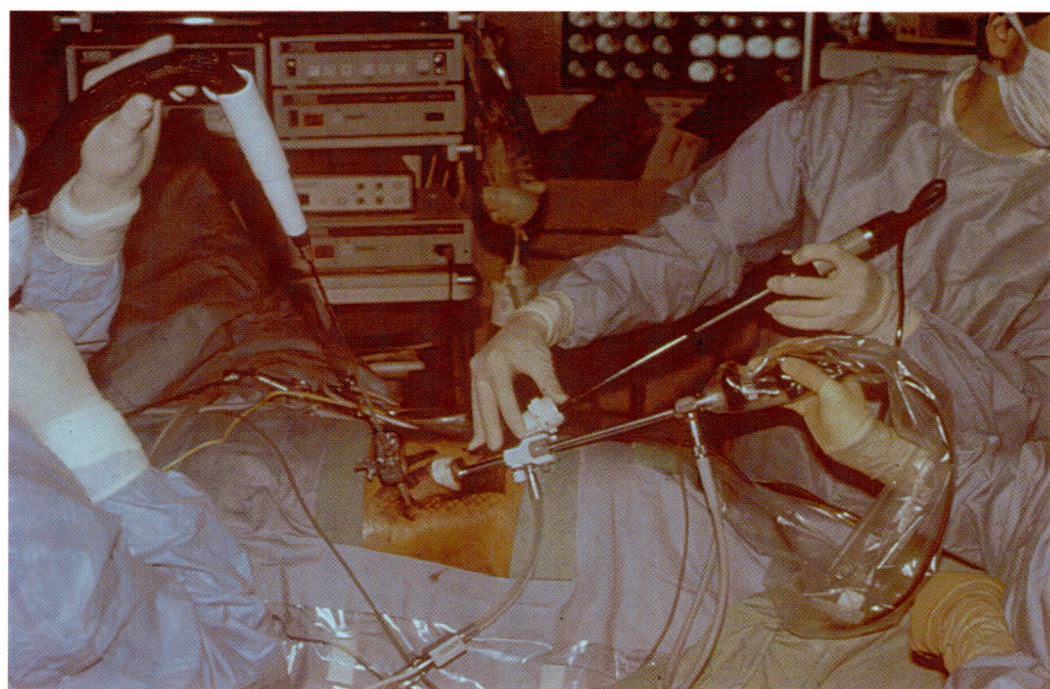

Fig. 18.1.8[1]. With the sonologist providing intraoperative real-time imaging of the tumor and the assistant providing laparoscopic visualization, the surgeon can accurately target the tumor with the cryoprobe

18.1.2 Equipment Utilized for Laparoscopic Renal Cryoablation

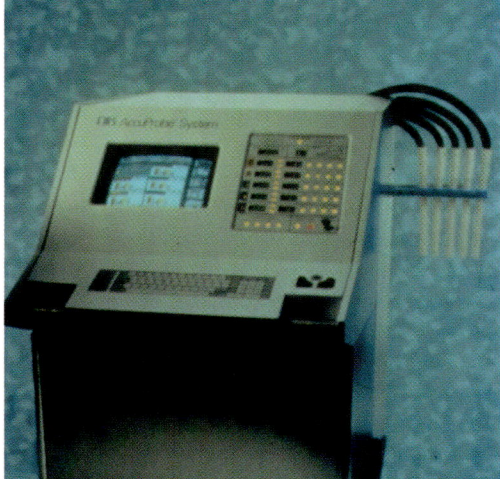

Fig. 18.1.9[1]. A liquid nitrogen based cryo-unit is used (Cryomedical Sciences, Rockville, MD)

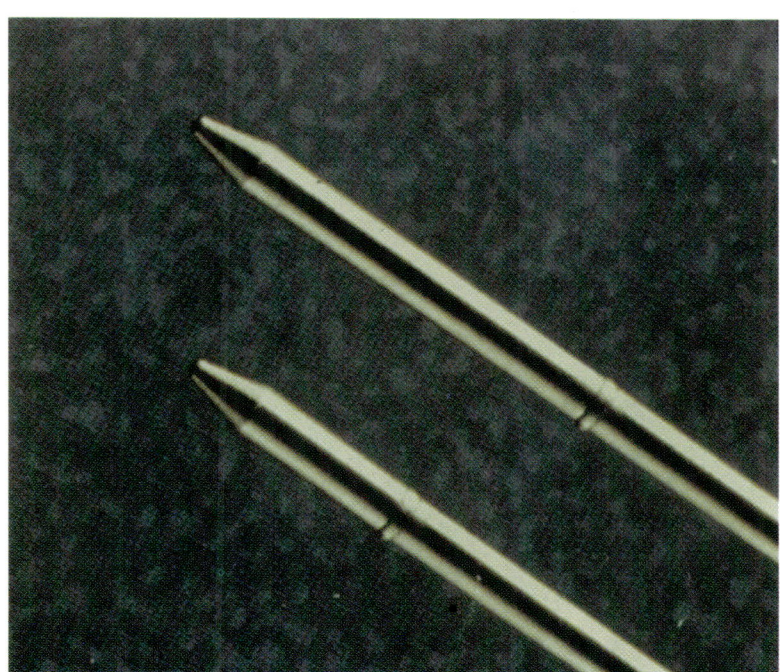

Fig. 18.1.10[1]. Cryoablation is performed utilizing insulated 4.8 mm diameter conical-tip cryoprobes

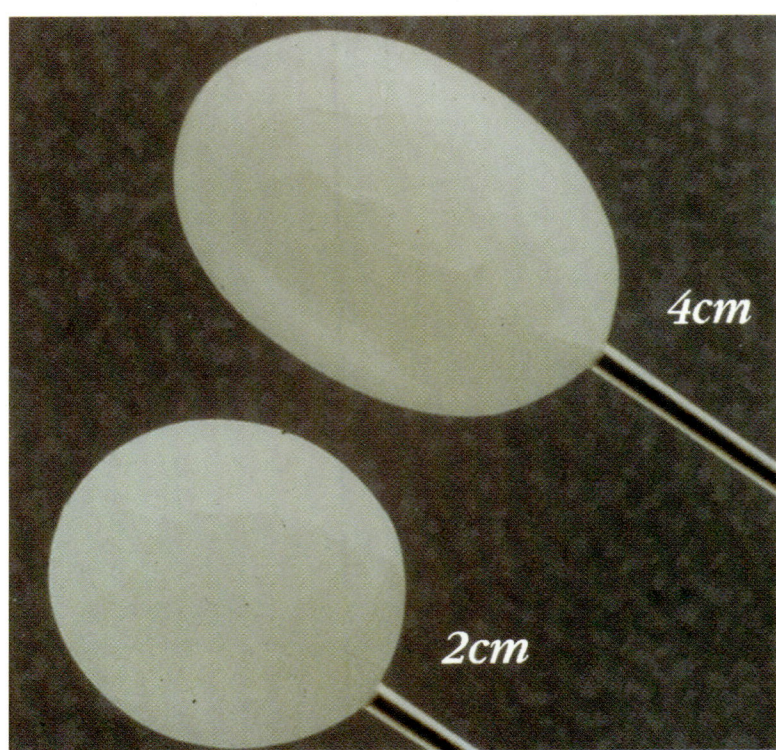

Fig. 18.1.11[1]. Utilizing these cryoprobes a freeze zone of either 2 cm or 4 cm is obtained

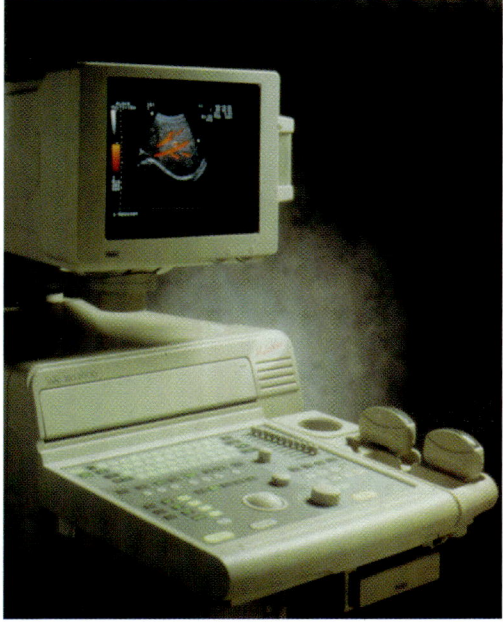

Fig. 18.1.12[1]. Real-time, color Doppler monitoring is performed with a B&K ultrasound machine (Panther 2002, Y-Ducer model 8555, Sadtoften 9, DK-2820, Gentoften, Denmark)

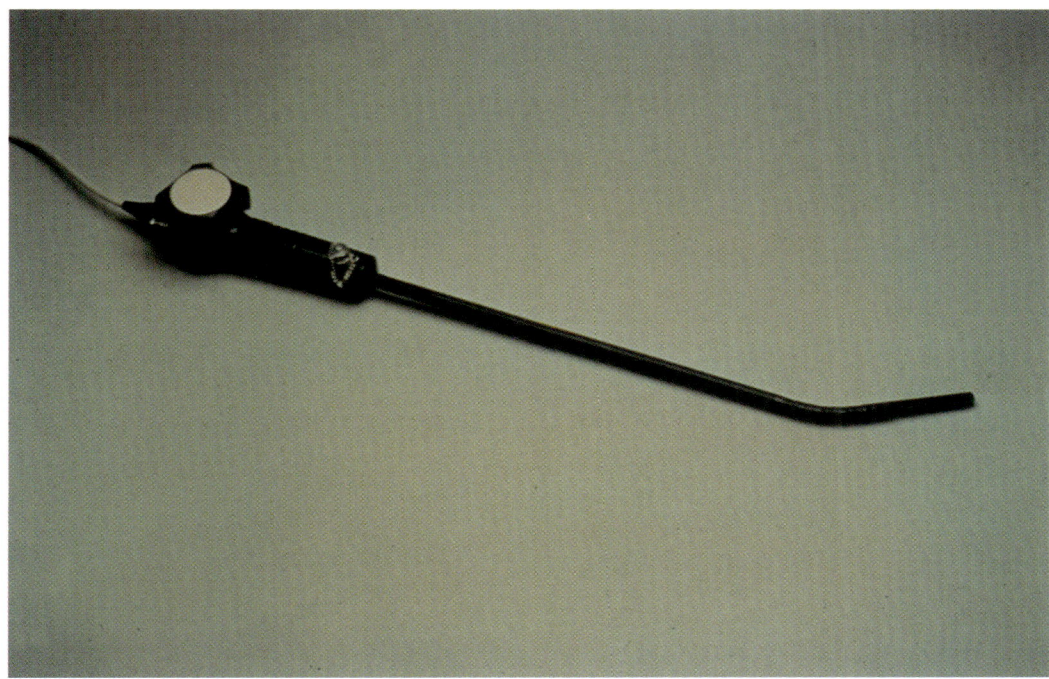

Fig. 18.1.13[1]. This endoscopic steerable ultrasound probe is 10 mm in diameter and can readily be inserted through a 12 mm port

18.1.3 Real-Time Intraoperative Ultrasound Images

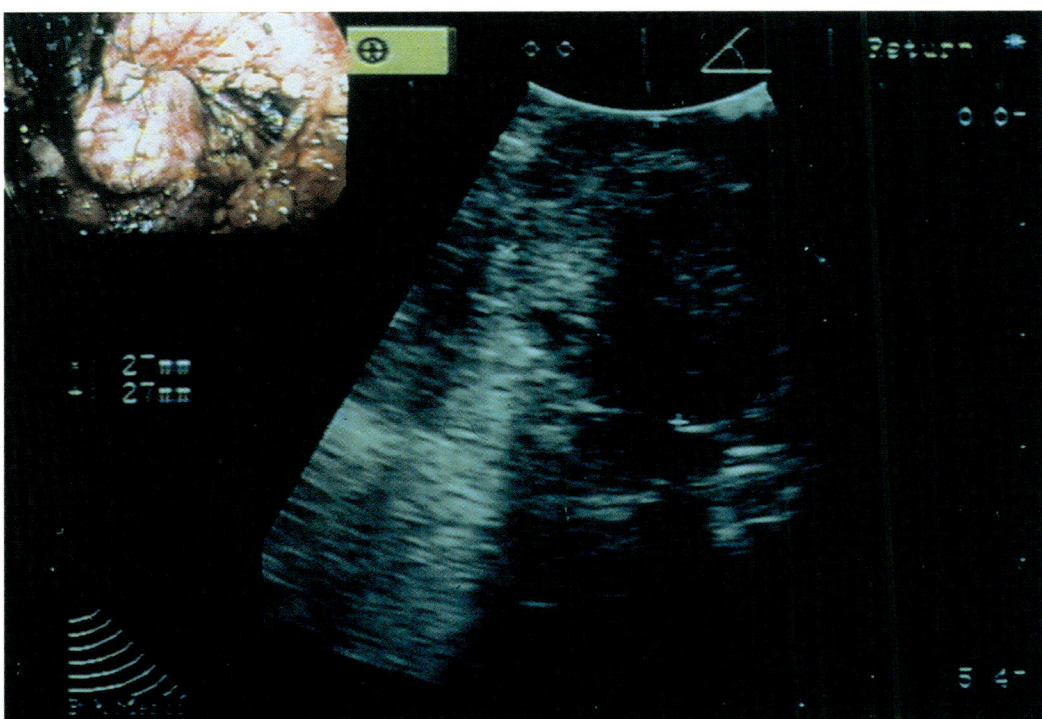

Fig. 18.1.14[1]. With the probe in direct contact with the renal surface, detailed ultrasound examination of the entire tumor is performed. Picture-in-picture display capability allows simultaneous visualization of the ultrasonographic and laparoscopic images

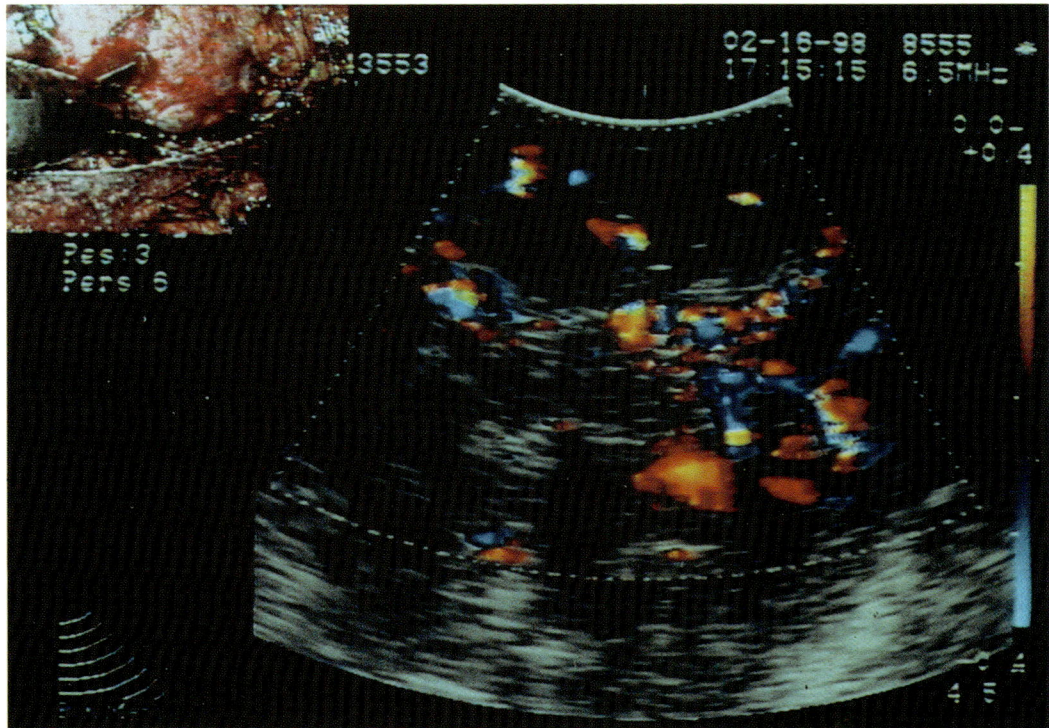

Fig. 18.1.15[1]. Intraoperative color Doppler images are employed to map the segmental renal vessels and to study the vascularity of the tumor

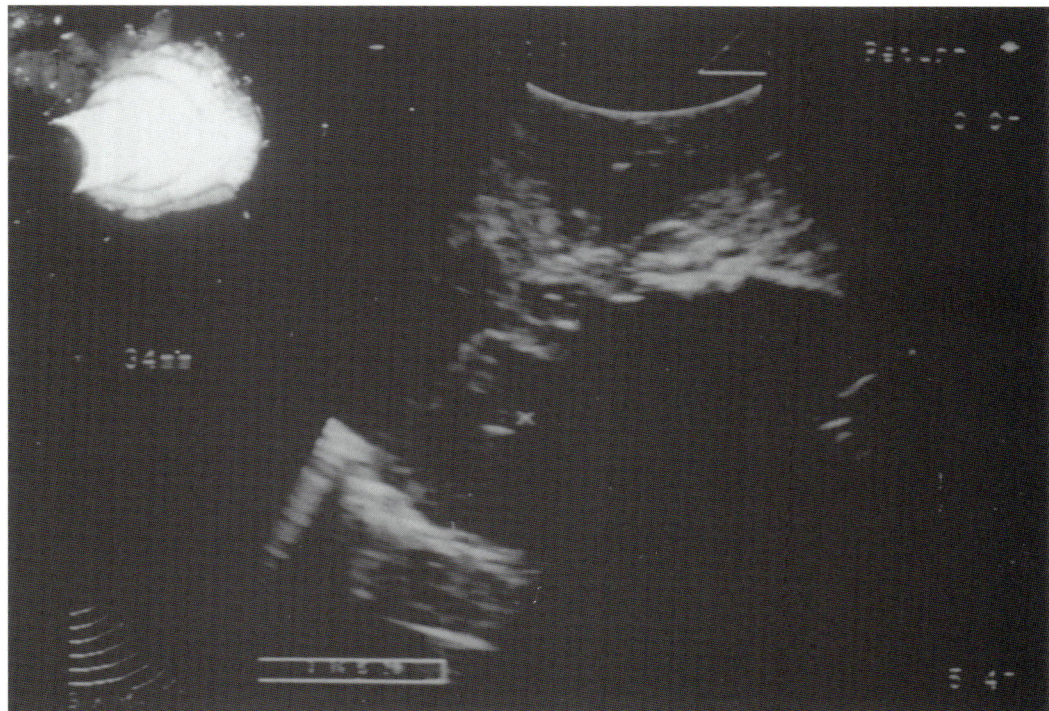

Fig. 18.1.16[1]. During renal cryoablation the advancing, hyperechoic, edge of the ice ball is monitored. It extends 1 cm beyond the tumor margin

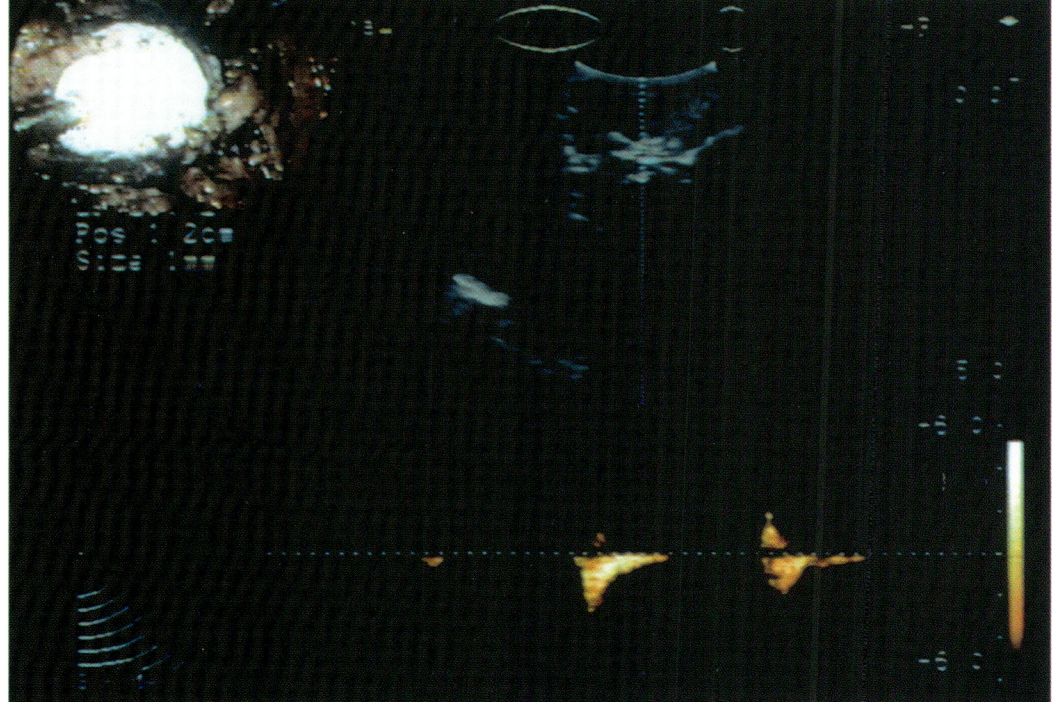

Fig. 18.1.17[1]. Obliteration of blood flow in the anechoic ice ball is confirmed by color Doppler imaging and spectral tracings

18.1.4 Laparoscopic Images

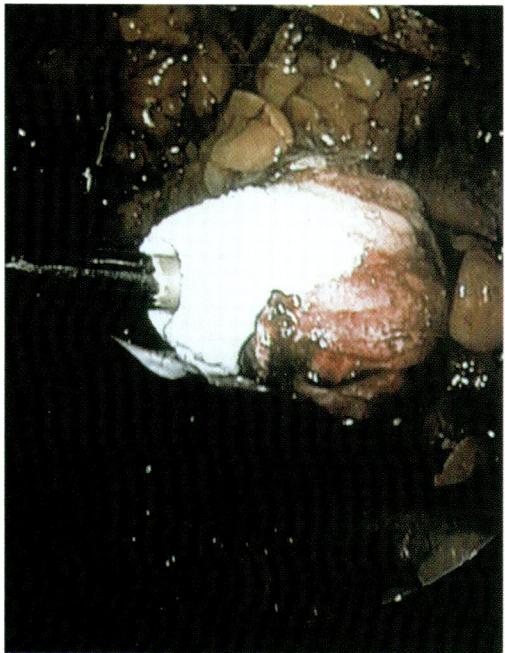

Fig. 18.1.18[1]. The external surface of the ice ball is seen to extend beyond the tumor margins circumferentially on laparoscopic visualization

Chapter 18
Cryosurgical Urology

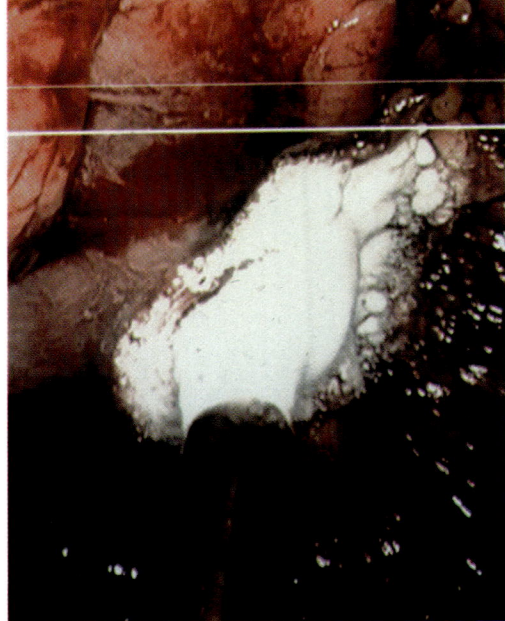

Fig. 18.1.19[1]. Extreme care is taken to ensure that the ice ball forming on the renal surface is exposed in its entirety and under clear laparoscopic visualization at all times in order to prevent cryoinjury to the peritoneum or the ureter

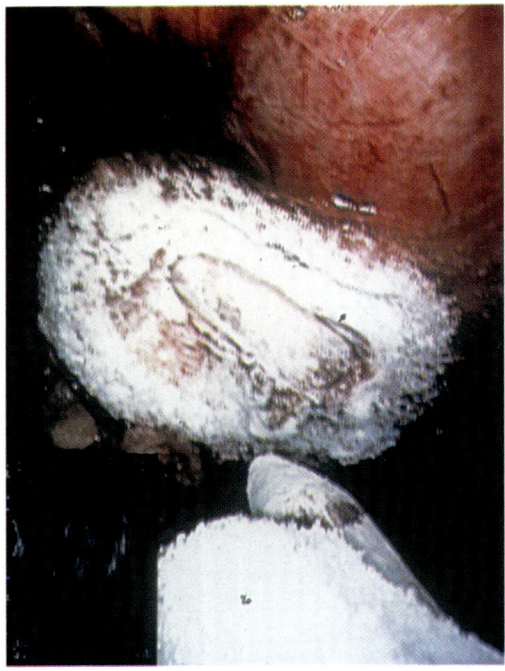

Fig. 18.1.20[1]. Upon final thawing, the probe is removed only after the ice ball begins to melt and "releases" the probe

Section F Clinical Aspects 415

Chapter 18
Cryosurgical
Urology

Fig. 18.1.21[1]. Post-cryoablation renal parenchymal hemorrhage is controlled with laparoscopic manual compression

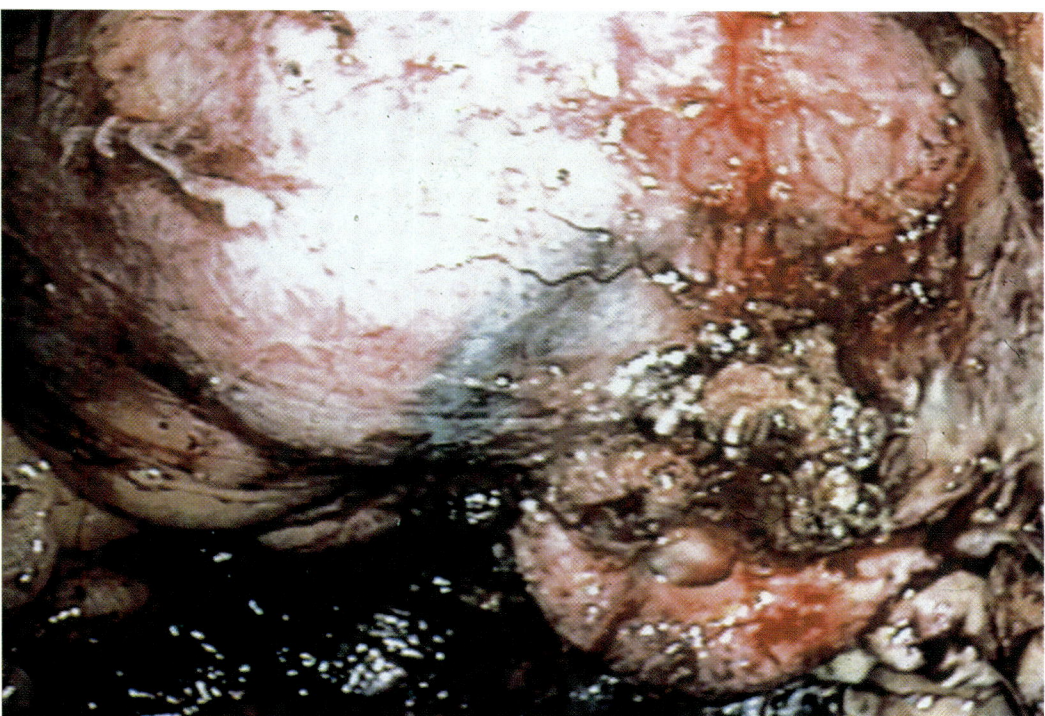

Fig. 18.1.22[1]. A purplish circular ring of demarcation is noted on the renal surface, signifying the hemorrhagic edge of the cryoablated area

18.1.5 CT/MRI Images

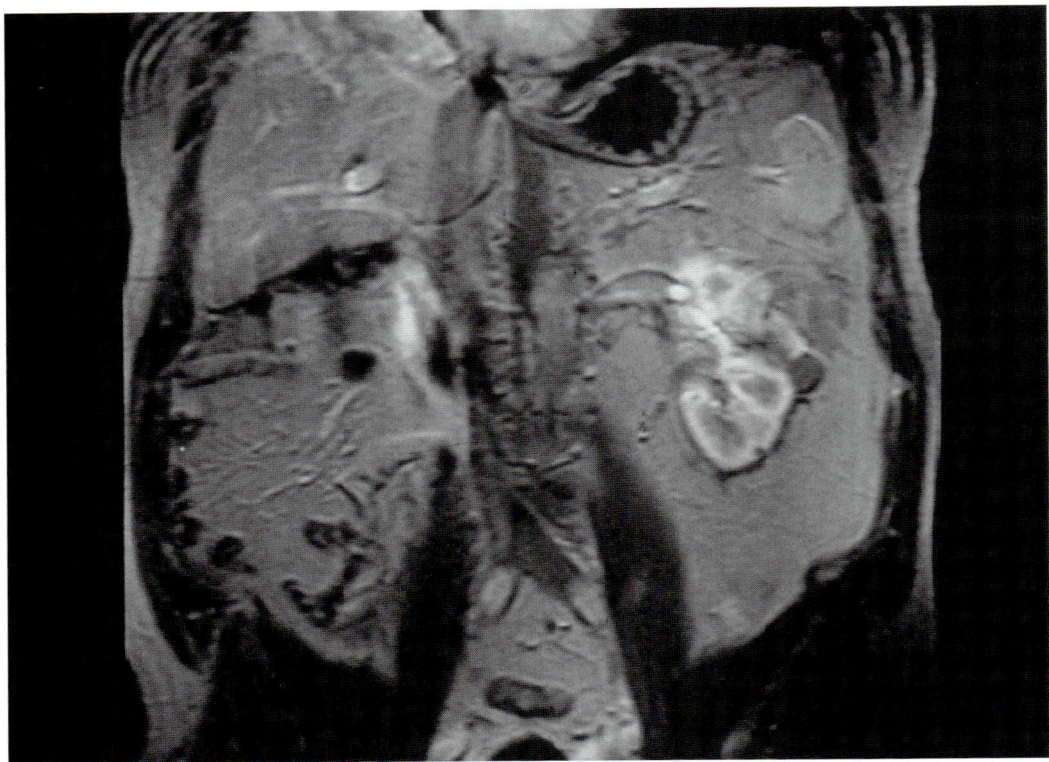

Fig. 18.1.23[1]. Preoperative gadolinium enhanced T-1 weighted MRI scan demonstrated a left mid polar, well-circumscribed, exophytic, renal mass

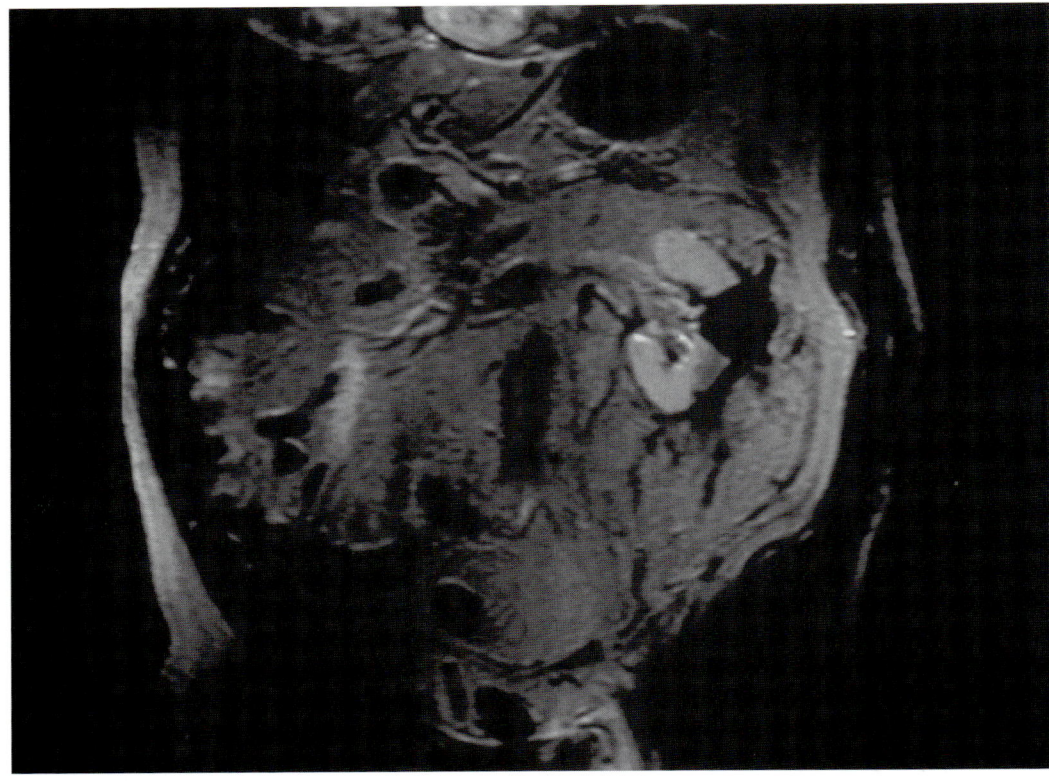

Fig. 18.1.24[1]. MRI scan on day 1 postoperatively demonstrating a crescentic cryolesion with signal void following gadolinium enhancement

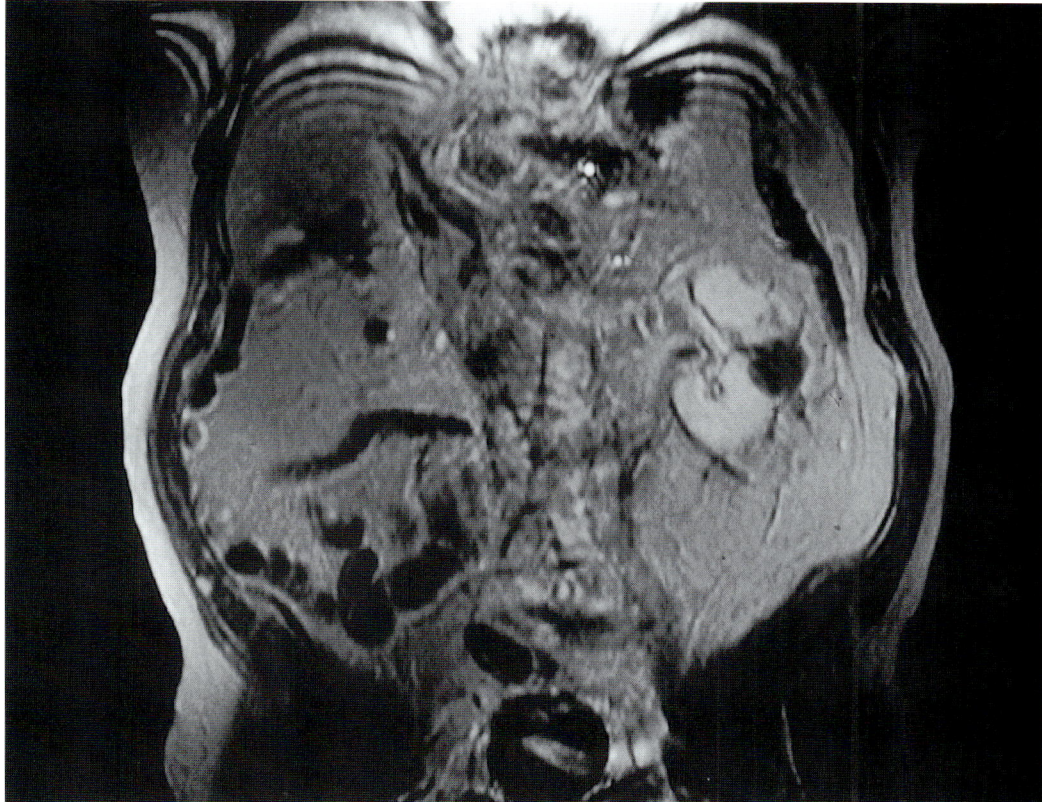

Fig. 18.1.25[1]. MRI scan at one month postoperatively demonstrates reduction in size of the lesion compared to the previous day-1 scan

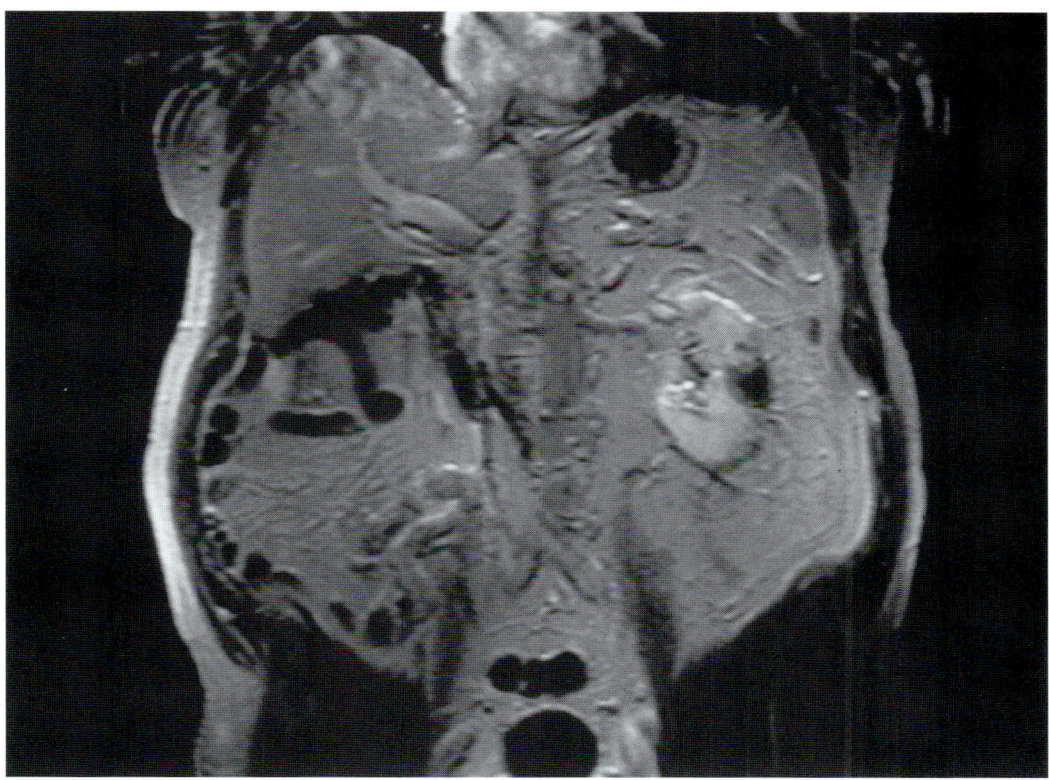

Fig. 18.1.26[1]. MRI scan at 3 months postoperatively shows further shrinkage of the cryolesion

18.1.6 Pre- and Post-Cryoablation Histology

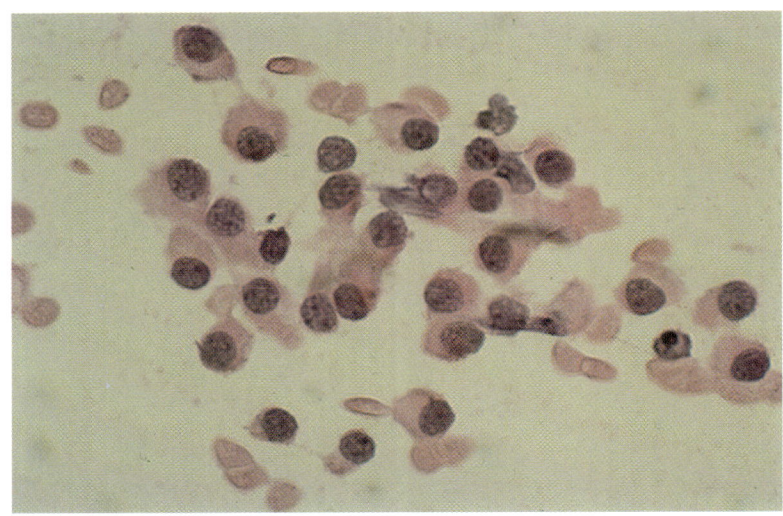

Fig. 18.1.27[1]. Pre-cryoablation needle biopsy confirming renal cell carcinoma

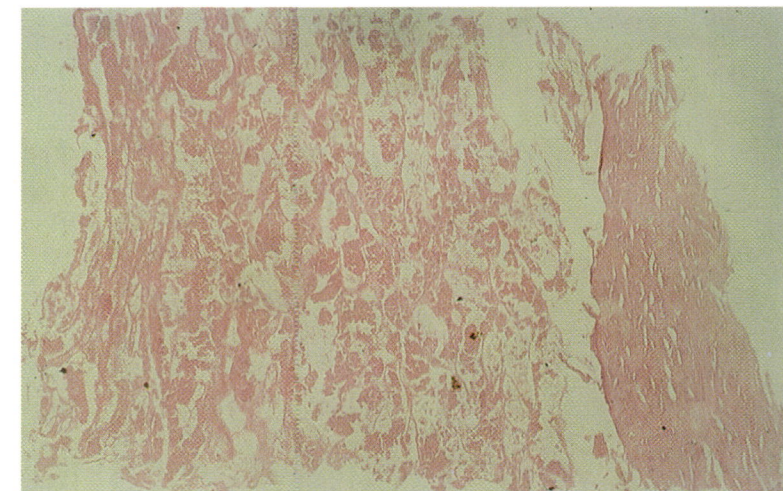

Fig. 18.1.28[1]. Needle biopsy at 6 months postoperatively demonstrating necrotic granulation tissue with fibrosis. There is no evidence of renal cell carcinoma

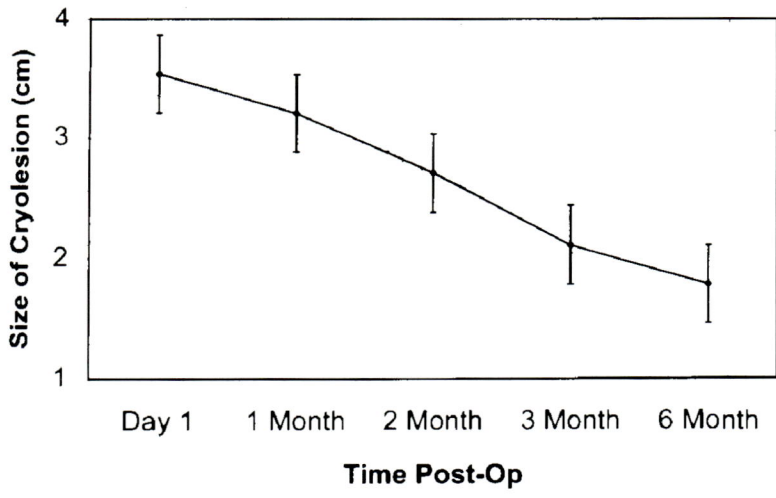

Fig. 18.1.29[1]. Graph depicting decrease in the size of cryolesion from the baseline size as seen on postoperative day 1

Orthopedic Cryosurgery

Martin M. Malawer[1], H.W. Bart Schreuder[2], James C. Wittig[1] and Jacob Bickels[1]

19.0 Introduction

The benefit of the use of cold for medical purposes has been known for a long time. The use of low temperatures, at first derived from snow and ice, was based on their anesthetizing properties and their slowing down of biological processes. Later, technical improvements made very low temperatures available which had the potential to destroy living tissue. Since then, low temperatures have found their use in virtual every specialty of medicine. But since 1968 only a few orthopedic surgeons dealing with skeletal tumors have adopted the cryosurgical technique. The clinical results and experimental data of cryosurgery with specific references to the skeletal system have been published in about 60 papers. Larger series of patients are, with only an occasional exception, not available, but are necessary for the benefits of the cryosurgical technique to be confirmed.

Cryosurgery is used as adjuvant treatment after resection (curettage) of active and aggressive benign and low-grade malignant, stage IA skeletal tumors. By spraying liquid nitrogen into the curetted lesion the surgical margin of resection is extended. Tumor cells left behind, which otherwise could be responsible for a recurrence of the tumor, are destroyed by this thermal injury. By this method the procedure can be considered to be marginal from the point of view of orthopedic oncologic principles. The advantage of this kind of treatment, as compared with local (en bloc) resection, is that as much as possible of the supportive function of bone is preserved and that reconstructive surgery can be limited.

A careful review of the literature reveals that cryosurgery is not as generally accepted in the treatment of diseases of the musculoskeletal system as it is in other categories of disease. It has been adopted only by a handful orthopedic surgeons. However, its use for bony pathology of the maxilla, mandible and facial bones is more commonly accepted and has resulted in a substantial body of basic research.

Since the early nineteen seventies, cryosurgery for orthopedic oncologic indications has been used in the University Hospital in Groningen and since 1991 in the University Hospital in Nijmegen, The Netherlands.

It seems that cryosurgery for orthopedic pathology is more generally practiced in Russia, considering the many (very) brief English abstracts appearing in Medline Express. Unfortunately the original articles are published in Russian journals, and are not easily available.

From the above-mentioned experimental data it is clear that cryosurgery is by far the most effective method of producing bone necrosis when compared to bone cement and phenol. It is therefore a valuable adjuvant, providing an extended surgical margin in almost every benign and low-grade malignant skeletal tumor. Its use as primary treatment without resection for carefully selected malignant tumors, e.g., chondroma, should still be considered experimental. Experience and improvements in technique have reduced the fracture rate to an acceptable level.

Chapter 19
Orthopedic Cryosurgery

The rate of other complications such as wound dehiscence and infection compare favorably to other treatments.

Although some experimental evidence suggests that articular cartilage is irreversibly damaged by cryosurgery, this has only been partially substantiated in clinical series.

The use of cryosurgery additional to an intralesional resection of the tumor is of value in order to diminish the risk for local recurrence.

In general orthopedic cryosurgery has summarized the theoretical, technical and practical requisites for the effective execution of a "state of the art" cryosurgical treatment as adjuvant to intralesional resection of benign and low-grade malignant bone tumors.

19.1 Bone Tumors

Chapter 19
Orthopedic Cryosurgery

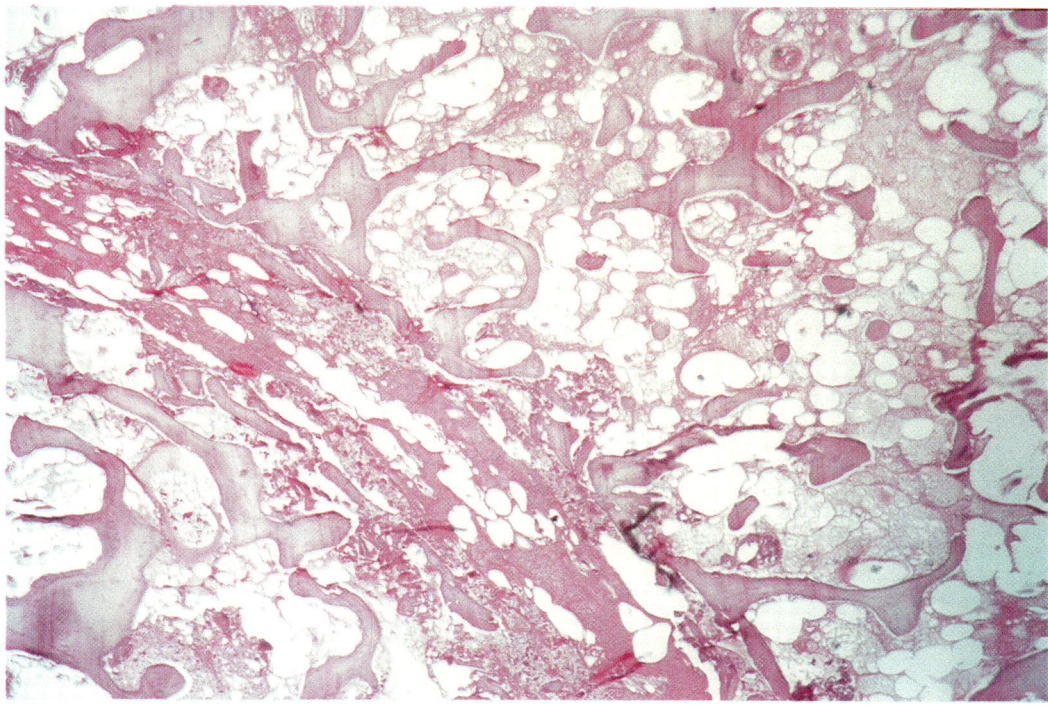

Fig. 19.1.1[1]. Effects of Cryosurgery on Bone: Photomicrographs of canine femora 3 weeks following cryosurgery. Cryosurgery induces extensive bone necrosis extending 10–12 mm around the bone cavity; however, it spares the articular cartilage. **A** Bone marrow demonstating widespread necrosis with necrotic trabeculae. **B** Subchondral region showing necrotic bone and bone marrow deep to viable articular cartilage

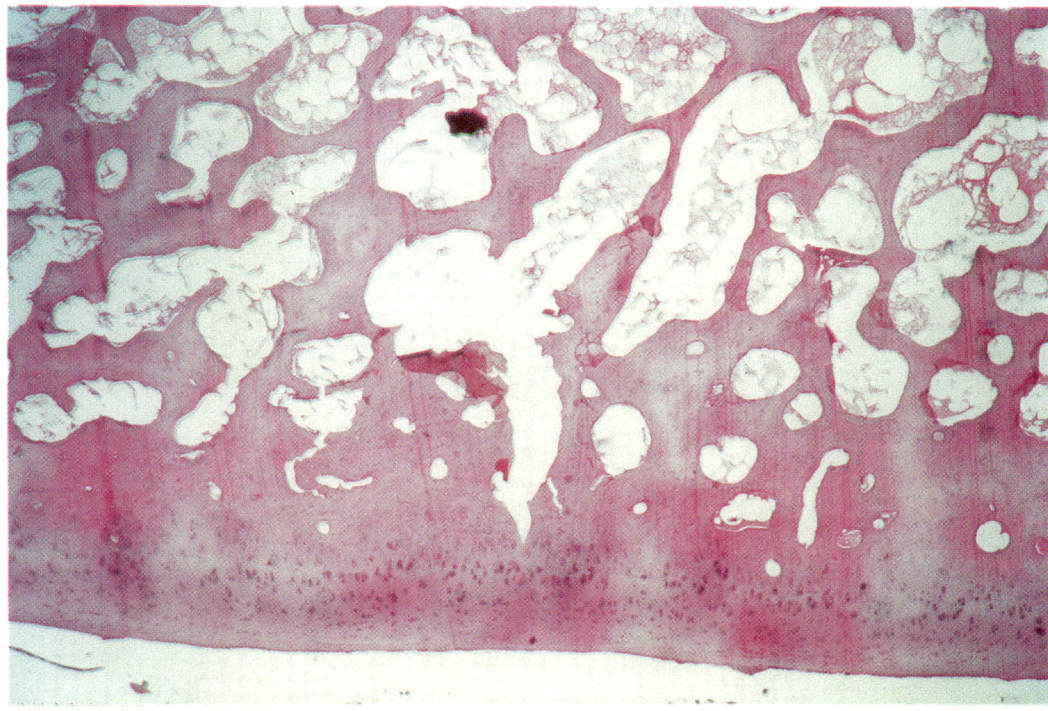

Chapter 19
Orthopedic Cryosurgery

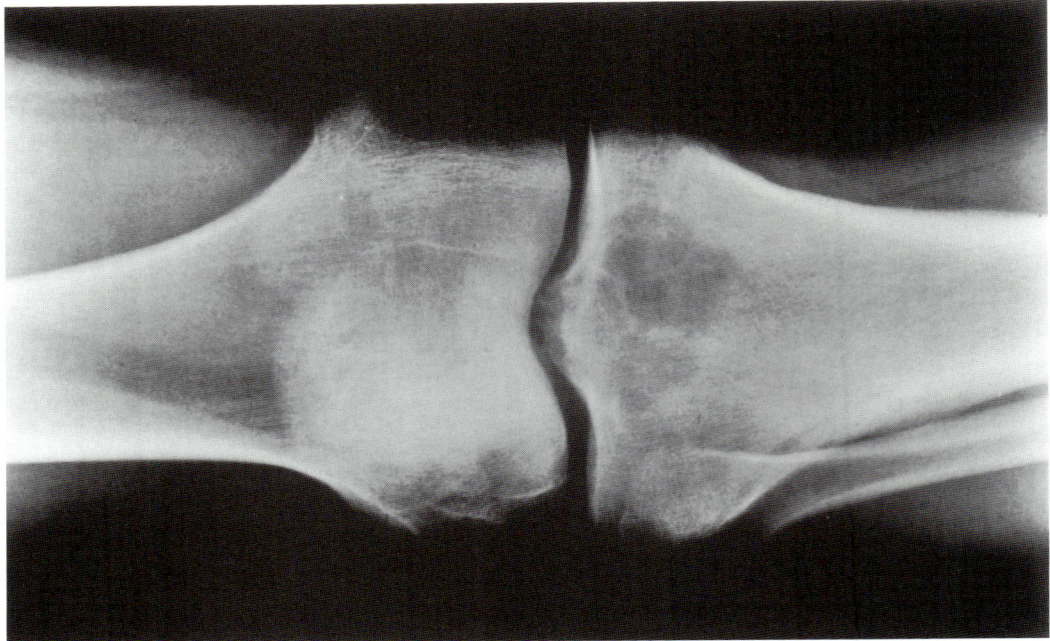

Fig. 19.1.2[1] A. Anteroposterior and lateral radiographs of a GCT of the proximal tibia

Fig. 19.1.2[1] (A–D). Radiographic Presentation of Giant Cell Tumor (GCT) of Bone: Cryosurgery has been used most extensively in the treatment of giant cell tumors. Giant cell tumors most commonly arise in the epiphysis of a skeletally mature distal femur or proximal tibia although any bone can be affected. It is purely lytic and surrounded by a variable rim of reactive sclerosis

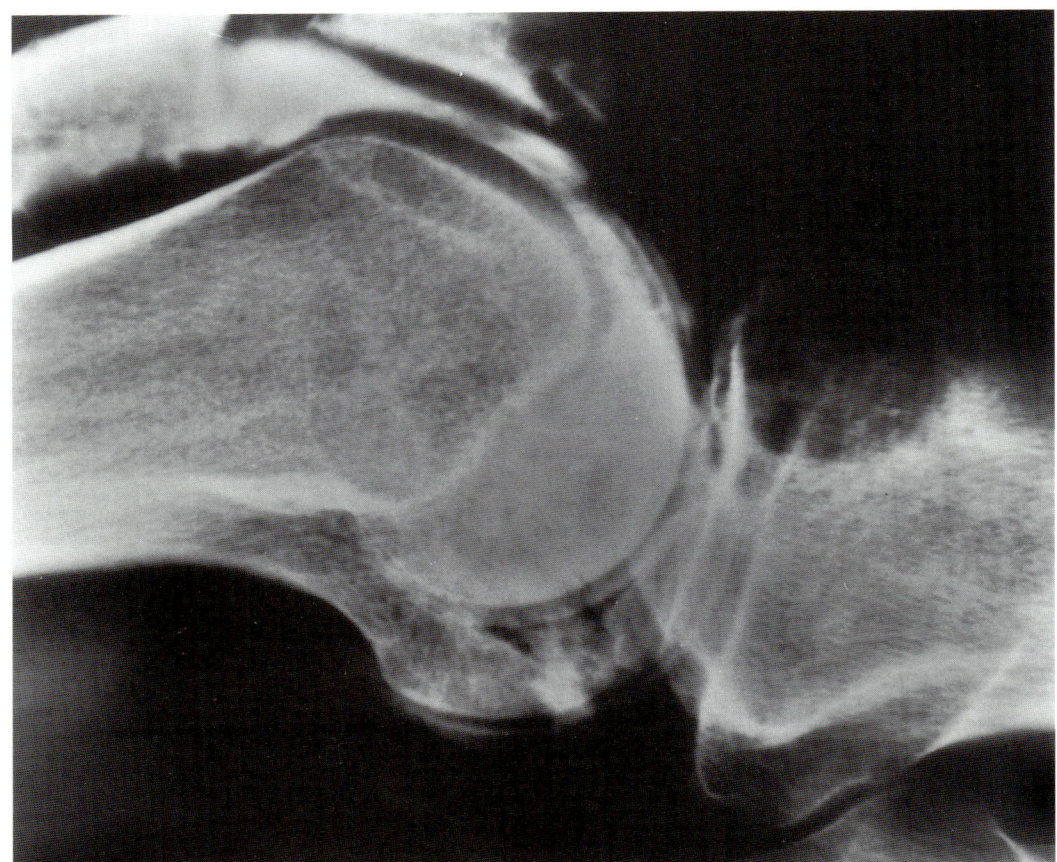

Fig. 19.1.2[1] B. Note the highly lytic nature on the lateral view

Section F Clinical Aspects 423

Chapter 19
Orthopedic
Cryosurgery

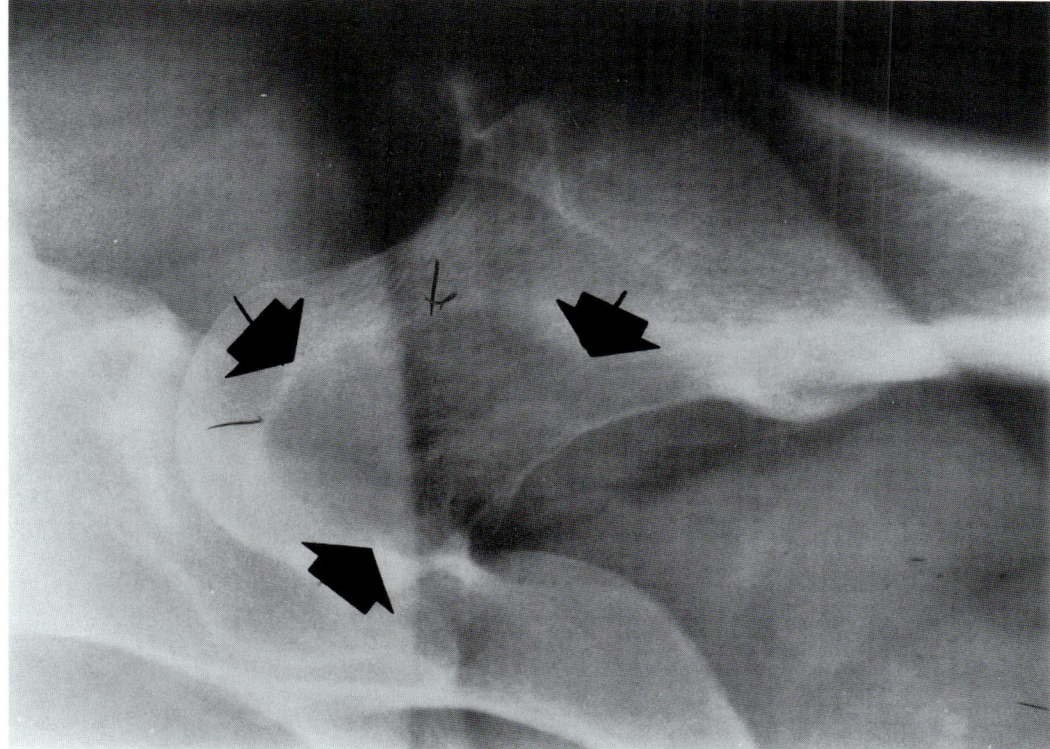

Fig. 19.1.2¹ C. Anteroposterior radiographs of a GCT in the proximal femur. Arrows demonstrate a surrounding rim of sclerosis. This finding is in contradistinction to the commonly viewed belief that GCTs characteristically lack a surrounding rim of sclerosis

Fig. 19.1.2¹ (A–D). Radiographic Presentation of giant cell tumor (GCT) of Bone: Cryosurgery has been used most extensively in the treatment of giant cell tumors. Giant cell tumors most commonly arise in the epiphysis of a skeletally mature distal femur or proximal tibia although any bone can be affected. It is purely lytic and surrounded by a variable rim of reactive sclerosis

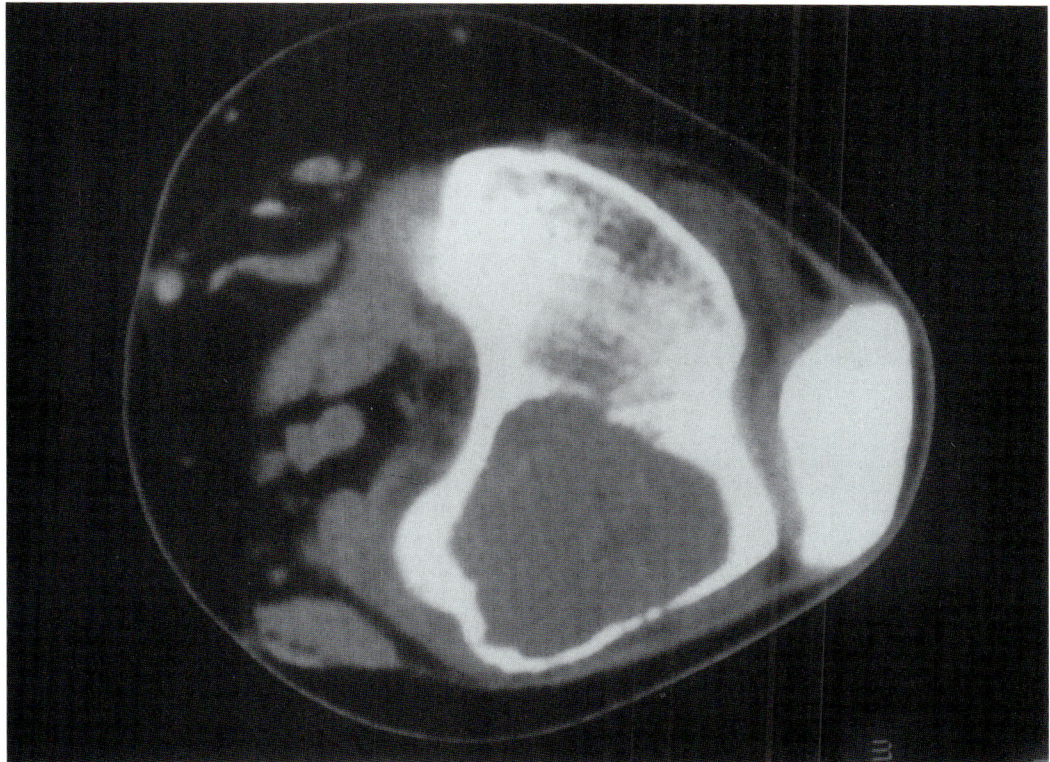

Fig. 19.1.2¹ D. CT scan demonstrating a highly lytic lesion in the distal femoral condyle which proved to be a GCT following biopsy

Anatomical Location	Recommended Surgical Approach	
Proximal femur	Watson-Jones approach	
Proximal humerus	Transdeltoid, anterior third approach	
Distal femur	Medial lesion:	Rectus femoris-vastus medialis interval, extracapsular approach
	Lateral lesion:	Rectus femoris-vastus lateralis interval, extracapsular approach
Proximal tibia	Medial lesion:	Direct, extracapsular incision over the medial border of the proximal tibia. After cryosurgery, the medial gastrocnemius muscle is mobilized anteriorly to cover the bone.
	Lateral lesion:	Direct, extracapsular incision over the lateral border of the proximal tibia. Lateral reflection of the lateral compartment and exposure of the lateral tibial metaphysis.

Fig. 19.1.3[1]. Recommended Surgical Approaches for Cryosurgery of Benign Aggressive and Low Grade Malignant Lesions Based on Anatomic Site of Origin (Bickels J, Rubert C, Meller I and Malawer M: Cryosurgery in the Treatment of Bone Tumors. Operative Techniques in Orthopaedics, 1999; 9(2): 79–83)

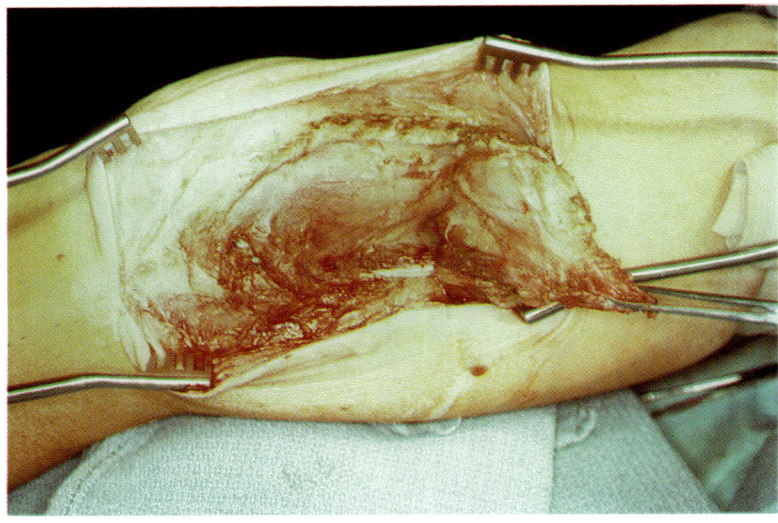

Fig. 19.1.4[1] A. Intraoperative photograph of surgical approach to a distal femoral GCT. Note the wide retraction of skin flaps, which is necessary to prevent thermal skin damage

Fig. 19.1.4[1] (A–F). An intralesional excision (resectional curettage) is performed for tumors amenable to cryosurgery. Wide skin flaps are raised to protect the skin from thermal damage. A wide, round, cortical window is made which encompasses the entire length of the tumor. Curettage is performed by hand first. This leaves an uneven surface with many craters and crevices which can serve as a reservoir for residual tumor cells. A high speed burr is then used to extend the hand curettage an additional 1–2 mm until a smooth surface is encounted (resectional curettage). Cryosurgery using liquid nitrogen is performed next

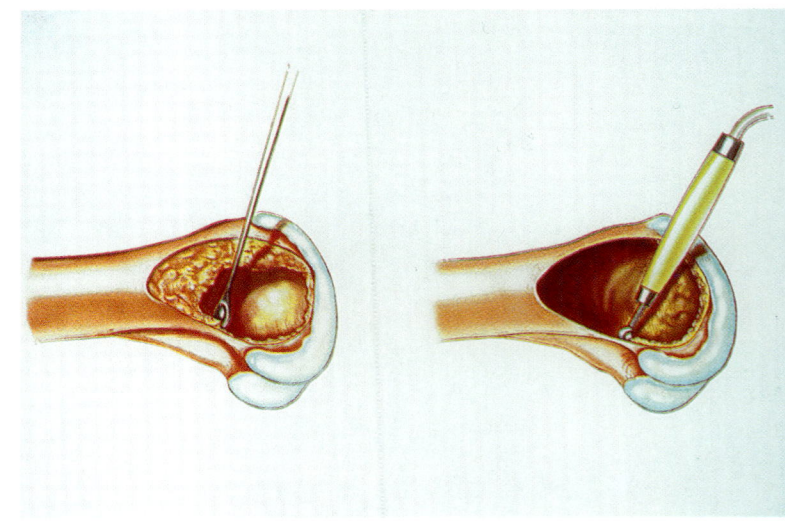

Fig. 19.1.4[1] B. Schematic demonstrating hand curettage followed by high speed burring of the tumor cavity. The cortical window is round and extends the entire length of the tumor cavity. The burr extends the hand curettage down to a smooth surface

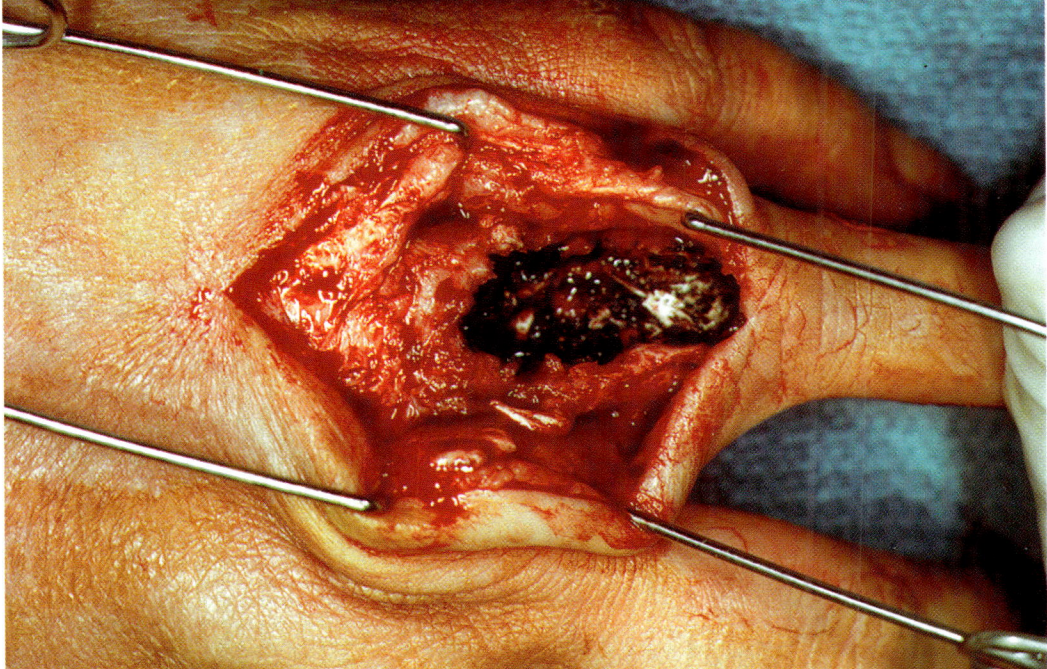

Fig. 19.1.4[1] C. Intraoperative photograph following hand curettage of a GCT arising in the proximal phalanx (intralesional excision). The walls of the tumor cavity are red, rough, irregular and composed of many craters which harbor tumor cells. This represents the reactive zone of the tumor. Hand curettage alone for the treatment of GCTs is associated with a 40–70% local recurrence rate

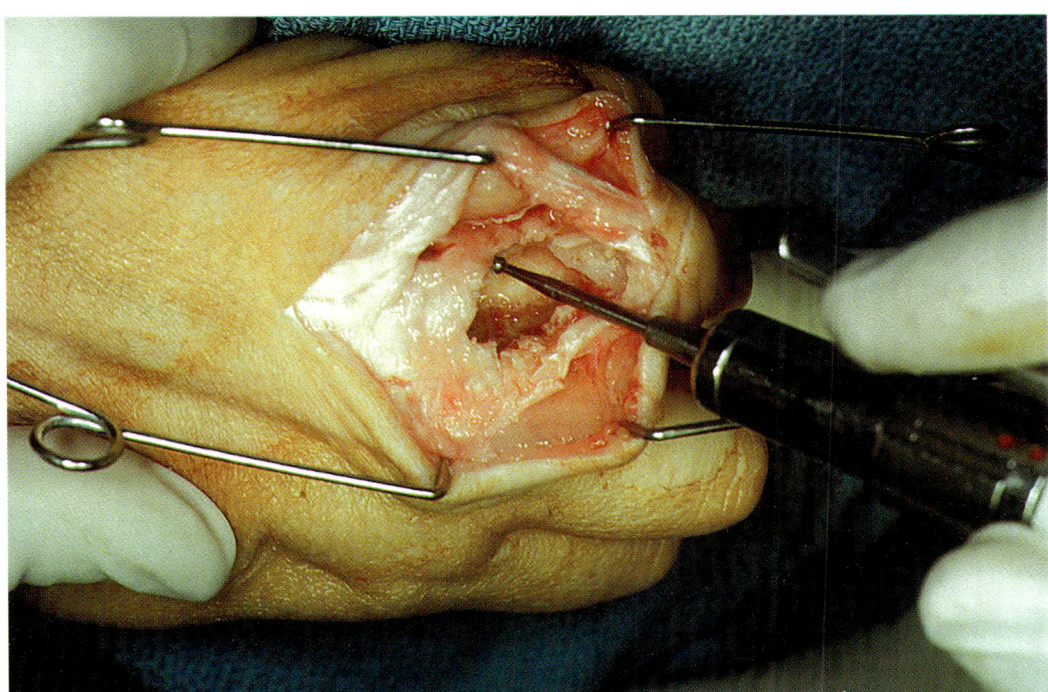

Fig. 19.1.4[1] D. Following hand curettage, a high speed burr is utilized to extend the resection an additional 1–2 mm. The wall of the cavity is smooth following resectional curettage. Resectional curettage without cryosurgery decreases the local recurrence rate to 15–20%. When performed in conjunction with cryosurgery the local recurrence rate drops to 2.3% for primary tumors

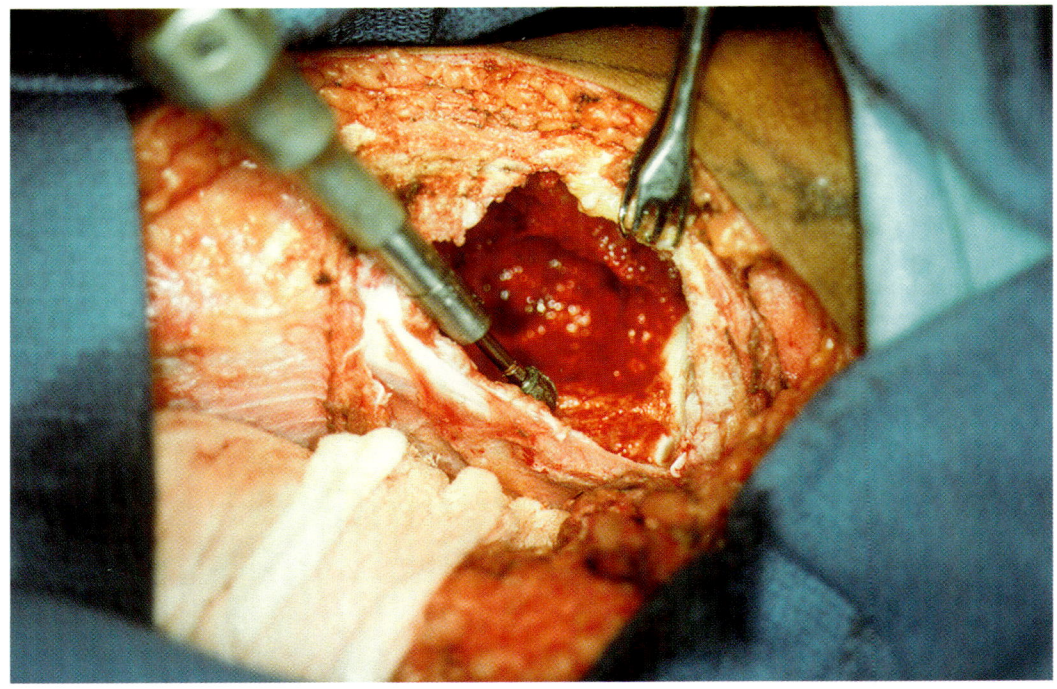

Fig. 19.1.4[1] E. Resectional curettage for GCT of the proximal tibia

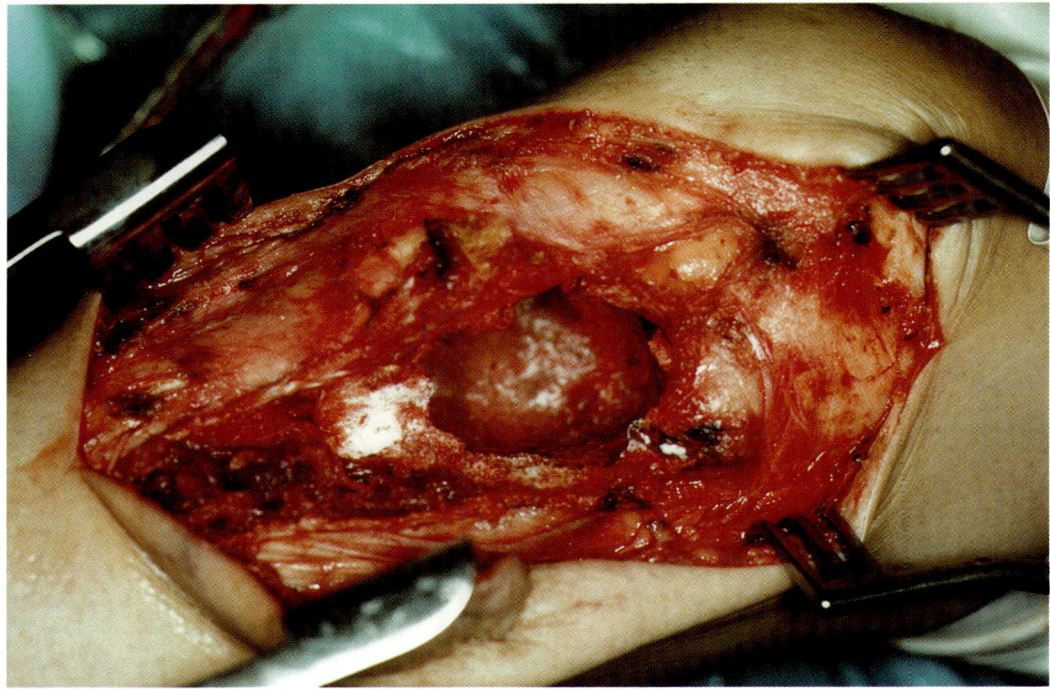

Fig. 19.1.4[1] F. Following high speed burr drilling the cavity walls are smooth. Cryosurgery of the tumor cavity can now be performed

Section F Clinical Aspects

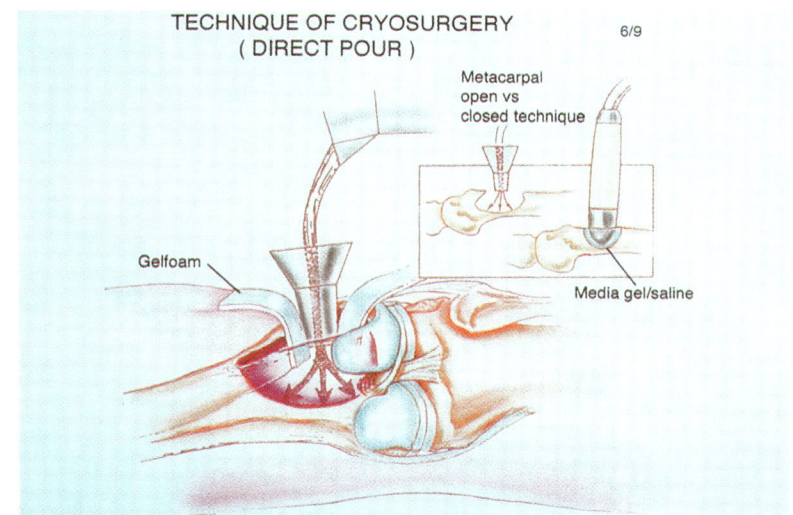

Fig. 19.1.5[1] A. Schematic demonstrating the open pour and closed techniques for freezing tumor cavities of various sizes

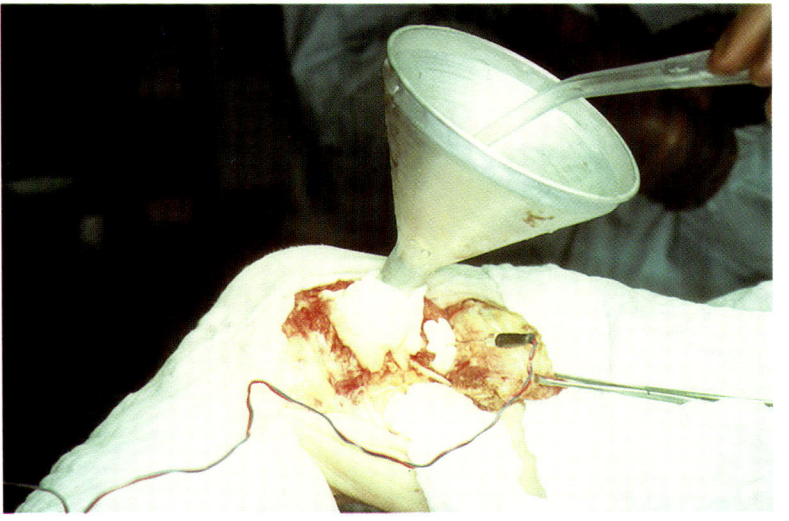

Fig. 19.1.5[1] B. Intraoperative photograph of cryosurgery for a distal femoral lesion. A stainless steel or aluminium funnel is placed into the tumor cavity and sealed with surrounding gel-foam. During cryosurgery, the gel-foam freezes and creates a seal around the funnel that prevents egress of liquid nitrogen from the tumor cavity into surrounding soft tissues and onto the skin. Liquid nitrogen should be permitted to freely evaporate and no attempt should be made to seal the mouth of the funnel as this may result in air embolism

Fig. 19.1.5[1] C. Following rapid freezing of the tumor cavity, a thermocouple is placed against the wall of the cavity to ensure the cavity wall temperature has dropped to $-20°C$. Additional liquid nitrogen is added if this goal has not been achieved

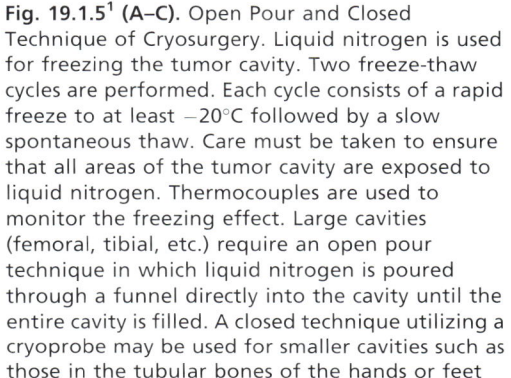

Fig. 19.1.5[1] (A–C). Open Pour and Closed Technique of Cryosurgery. Liquid nitrogen is used for freezing the tumor cavity. Two freeze-thaw cycles are performed. Each cycle consists of a rapid freeze to at least $-20°C$ followed by a slow spontaneous thaw. Care must be taken to ensure that all areas of the tumor cavity are exposed to liquid nitrogen. Thermocouples are used to monitor the freezing effect. Large cavities (femoral, tibial, etc.) require an open pour technique in which liquid nitrogen is poured through a funnel directly into the cavity until the entire cavity is filled. A closed technique utilizing a cryoprobe may be used for smaller cavities such as those in the tubular bones of the hands or feet

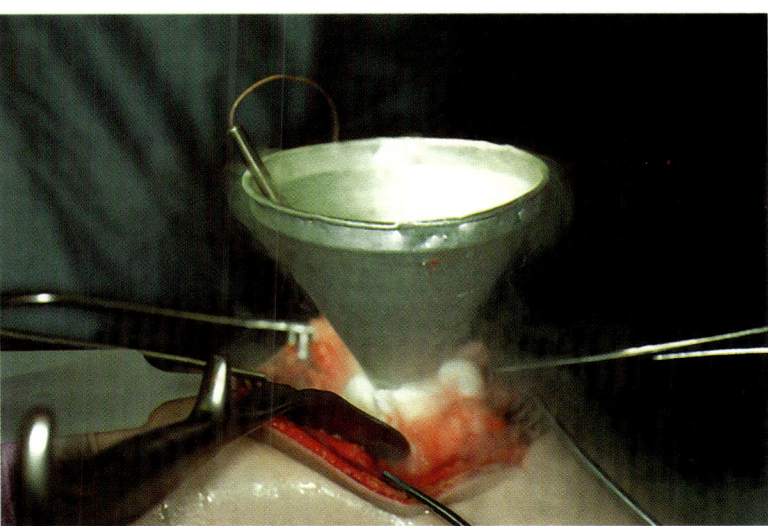

Chapter 19 Orthopedic Cryosurgery

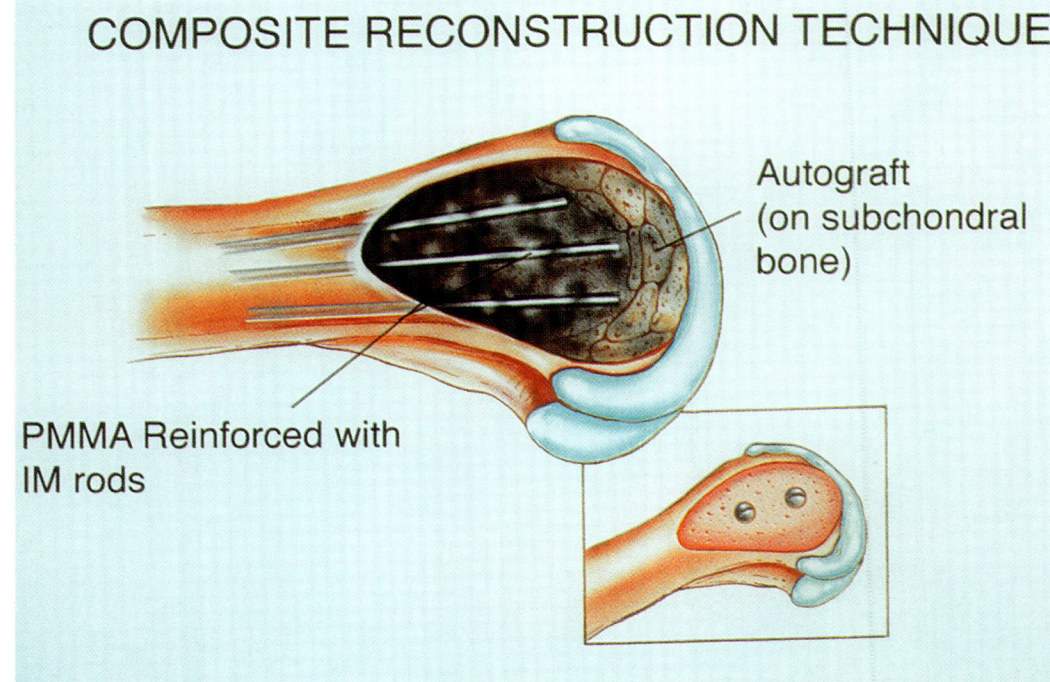

Fig. 19.1.6[1] A. Schematic demonstrating technique of composite fixation for a distal femoral lesion

Fig. 19.1.6[1] (A–D). Composite Reconstruction. Due to the typical epiphyseal presentation of GCTs, curettage commonly results in a large subchondral defect. Stable fixation of the tumor cavity must be obtained to prevent fracture and facilitate motion and early weight bearing. Composite reconstruction is typically performed. Autogenous corticocancellous iliac crest bone graft is placed against the subchondral surface. Rush rods or Ender's nails are placed retrograde through the tumor cavity into normal bone, bypassing the defect by at least a distance of 2 times the tumor cavity width. Cement (PMMA) is injected into the remaining cavity. An additional piece of corticocancellous graft containing two 22 mm screws is placed onto the surface of the defect, flush with surrounding cortex prior to the cement curing. In addition to providing immediate stable fixation, cement also provides a strong contrast medium, which allows early detection of local recurrence

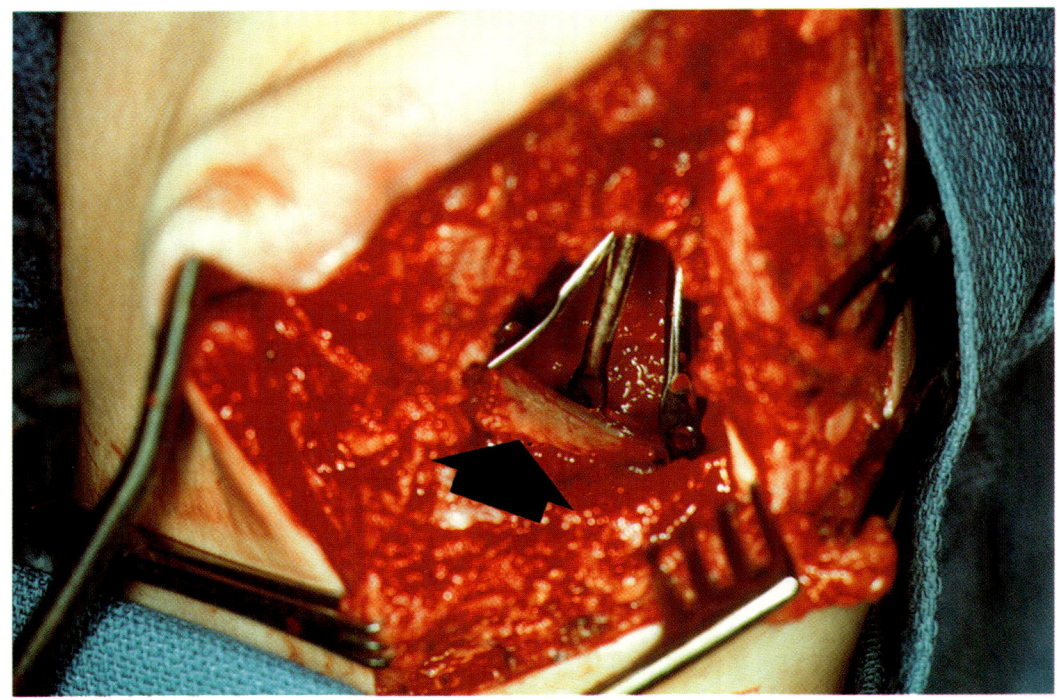

Fig. 19.1.6[1] B. Intraoperative photograph of composite reconstruction of the proximal tibia prior to cementation emphasizing subchondral placement of autograft (arrows) and positioning of Ender's nails for optimal structural support

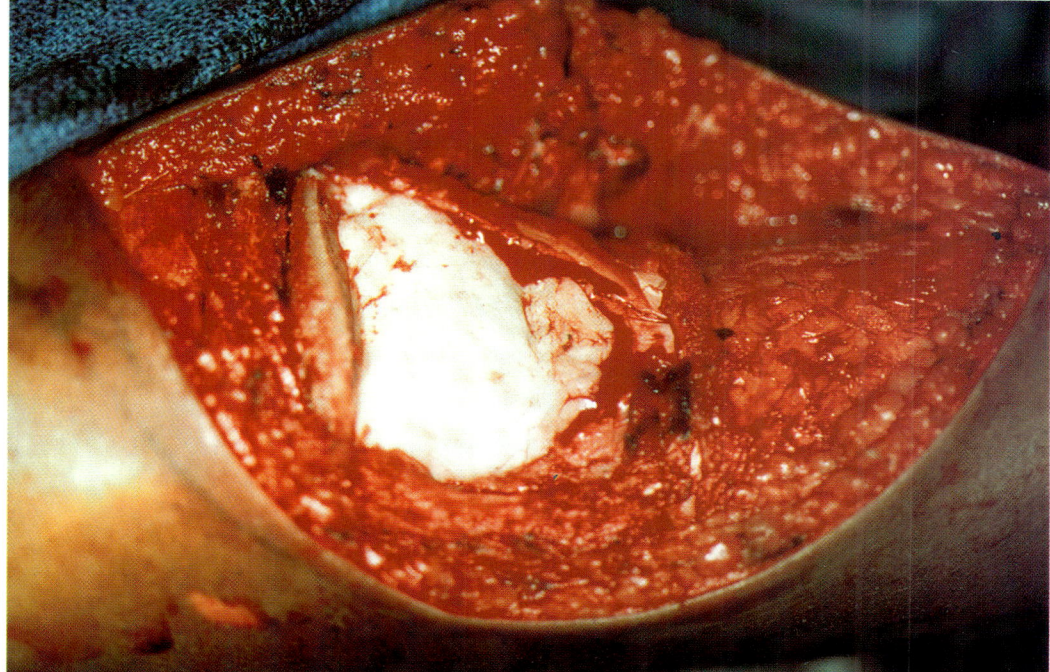

Fig. 19.1.6¹ C. Cementation follows subchondral bone grafting and placement of Ender's nails

Fig. 19.1.6¹ (A–D). Composite Reconstruction. Due to the typical epiphyseal presentation of GCTs, curettage commonly results in a large subchondral defect. Stable fixation of the tumor cavity must be obtained to prevent fracture and facilitate motion and early weight bearing. Composite reconstruction is typically performed. Autogenous corticocancellous iliac crest bone graft is placed against the subchondral surface. Rush rods or Ender's nails are placed retrograde through the tumor cavity into normal bone, bypassing the defect by at least a distance of 2 times the tumor cavity width. Cement (PMMA) is injected into the remaining cavity. An additional piece of corticocancellous graft containing two 22 mm screws is placed onto the surface of the defect, flush with surrounding cortex prior to the cement curing. In addition to providing immediate stable fixation, cement also provides a strong contrast medium, which allows early detection of local recurrence

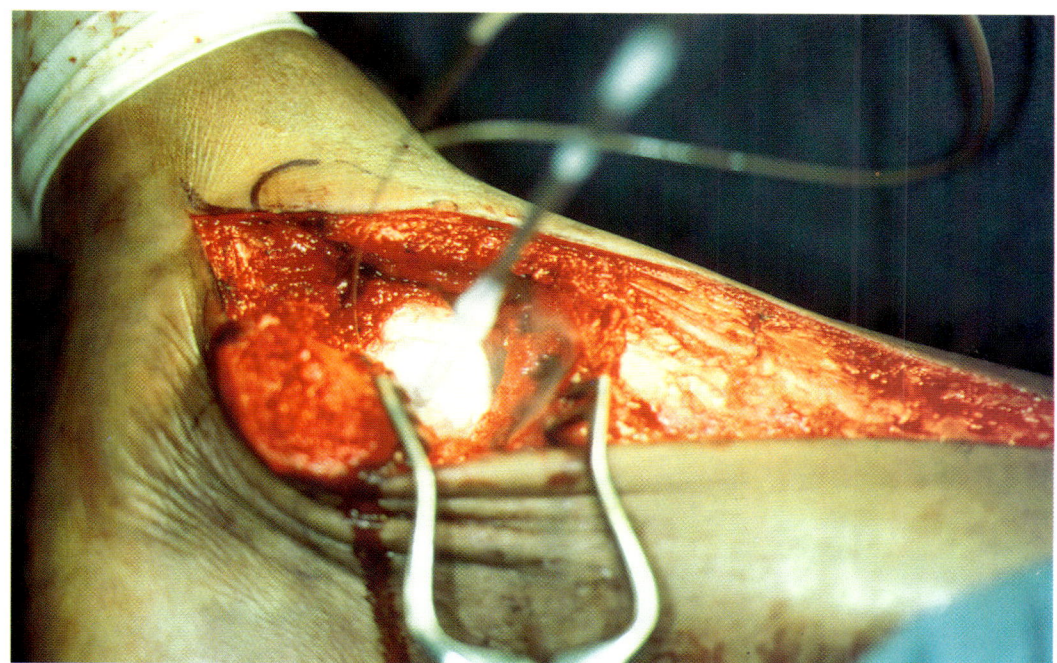

Fig. 19.1.6¹ D. Composite reconstruction of the talus following resectional curettage and cryosurgery for a GCT. Notice the wide exposure

Chapter 19
Orthopedic Cryosurgery

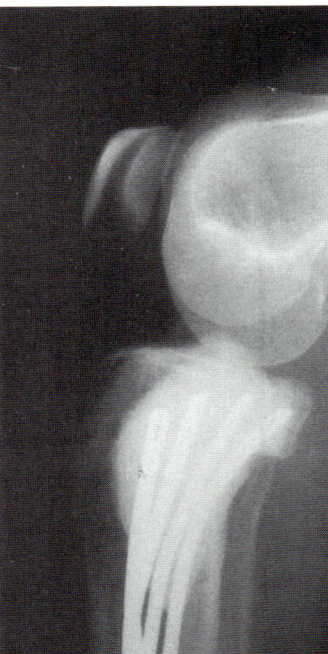

Fig. 19.1.7[1] A, B. Giant cell tumor of the proximal tibia treated with resectional curettage, cryosurgery and composite reconstruction

Fig. 19.1.7[1] (A–E). Postoperative Radiographs Following Curettage, Cryosurgery and Composite Reconstruction

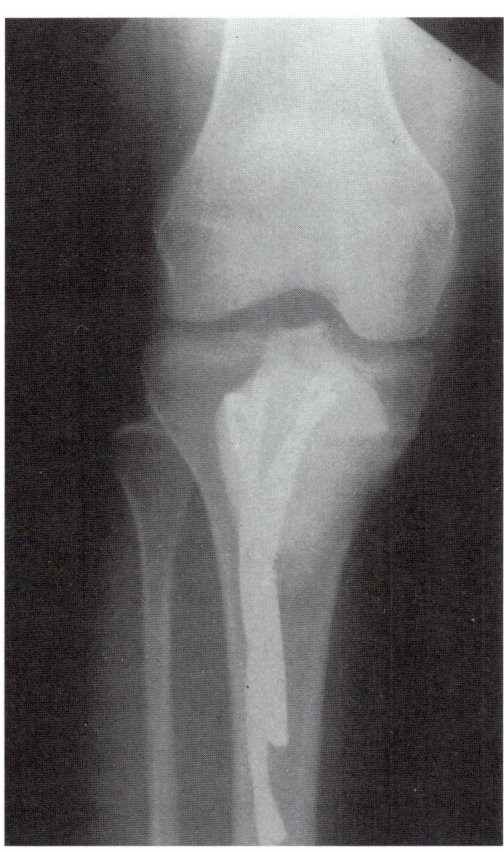

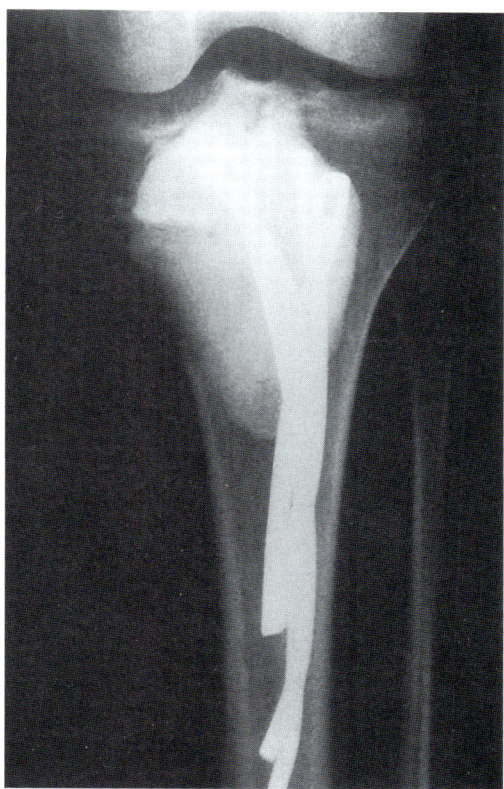

Fig. 19.1.7¹ C. Cementation permits immediate stable fixation and provides a strong contrast medium as demonstrated with this close-up view. This allows early detection and treatment of local recurrences

Fig. 19.1.7¹ (A–E). Postoperative Radiographs Following Curettage, Cryosurgery and Composite Reconstruction

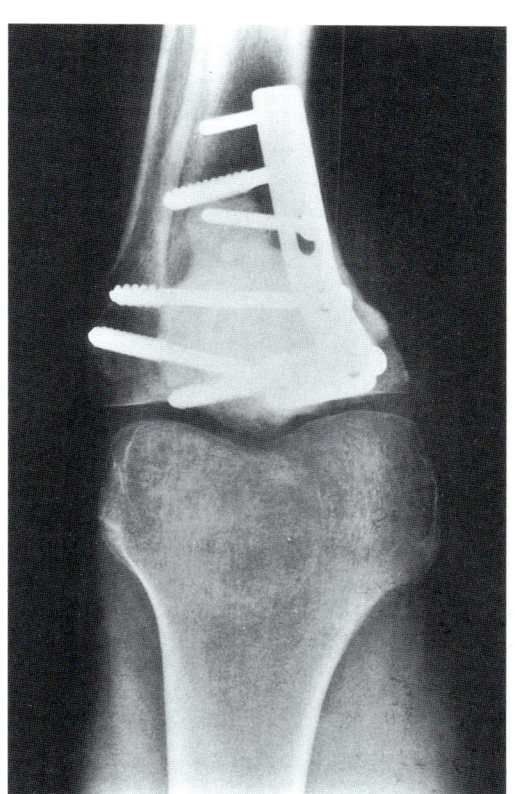

Fig. 19.1.7¹ D. Alternate method of composite fixation for proximal tibial tumors treated with cryosurgery

Chapter 19
Orthopedic Cryosurgery

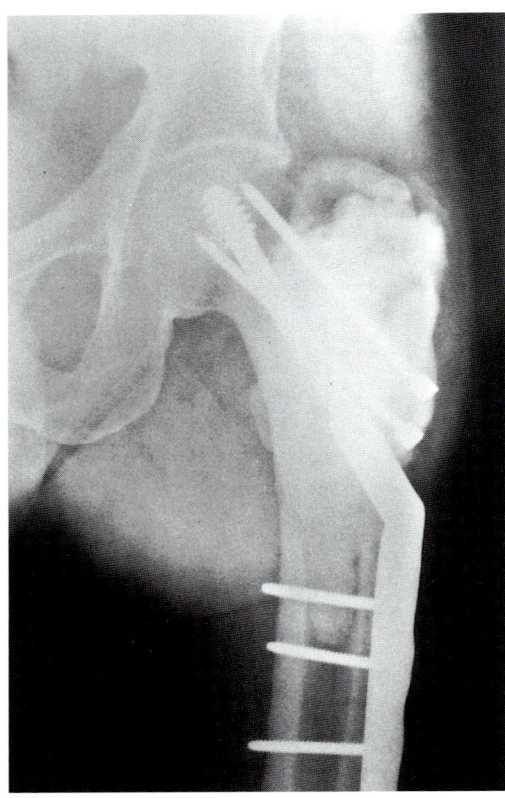

Fig. 19.1.7[1] E. Composite fixation following resectional curettage and cryosurgery of a proximal femoral GCT

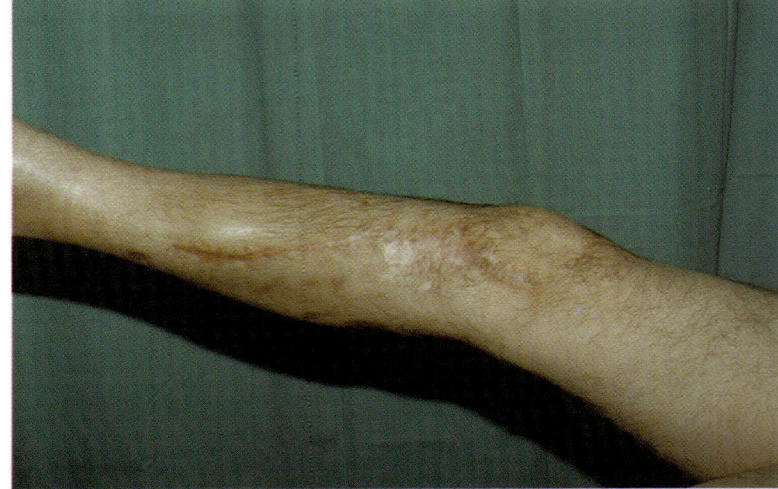

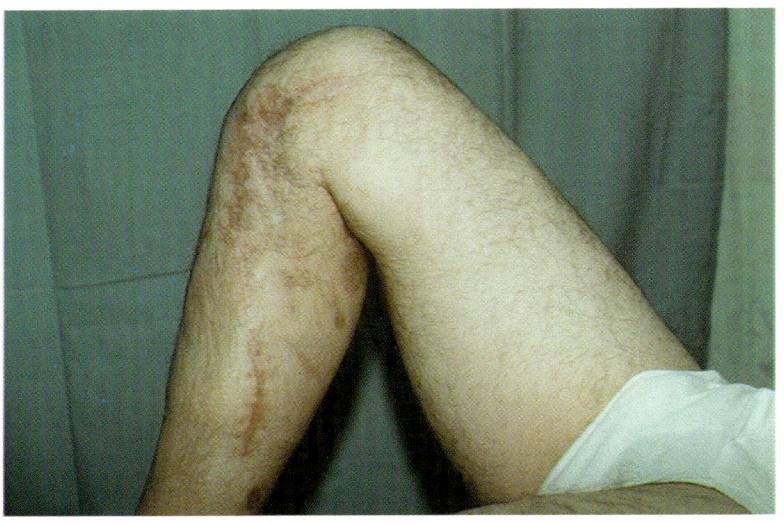

Fig. 19.1.8[1]. Postoperative function is virtually normal for all patients following cryosurgery since native bone and joint surface are preserved. Composite reconstruction achieves immediate stable fixation which obviates the need for postoperative immobilization and non-weight bearing ambulation. Early rehabilitation (range of motion and strengthening exercises) as well as early weight bearing is permitted, which facilitates prompt and complete functional recovery (A). Excellent range of motion three months after cryosurgery and composite fixation of a proximal tibial GCT (B)

Section F   Clinical Aspects

19.1.1 The Cryosurgical Principle for Bone Tumors[2]

Chapter 19
Orthopedic Cryosurgery

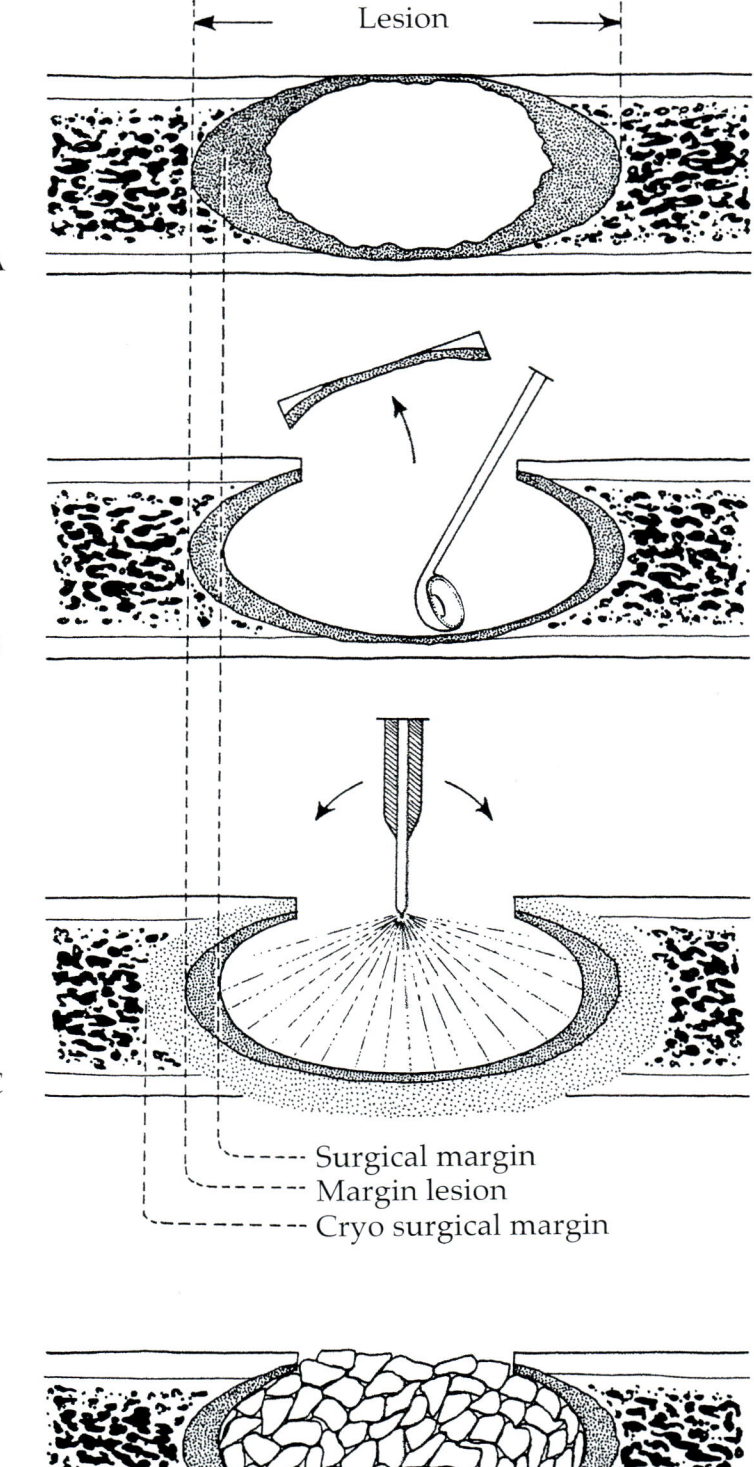

Fig. 19.1.9[2]. The bone tumor (**A**) is exposed via a sufficient oval window made in the cortex (**B**). Intralesional resection or curettage is done with curettes resulting in a surgical margin. Three cycles of cryosurgery are performed using a machine producing a liquid nitrogen spray. This spray is directed into the lesion in every direction, until the whole cavity is wetted and becomes frosted: the cryosurgical margin (**C**). The duration of each freeze is based on the temperature readings and visual observation. Intralesional temperatures of at least −50°C are pursued and necessary to induce tissue necrosis. Warming up until 20°C is done by spontaneous thawing. The defect remaining after curettage and cryosurgery is filled with autograft or allograft bone chips (**D**)

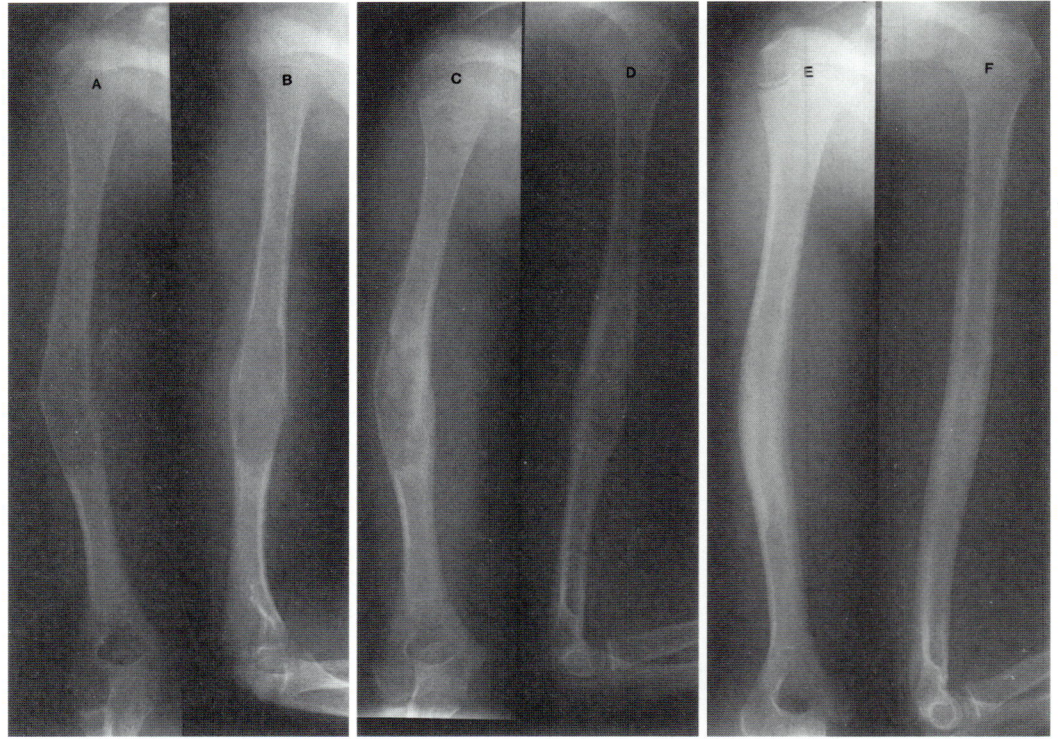

Fig. 19.1.10². Simple bone cyst of the humerus in an 11-year-old girl. Preoperative radiographs showing pathological fracture (**A, B**). Postoperative radiographs at 2 months after curettage, cryosurgery and bone grafting (**C, D**), and at 13 months demonstrating complete consolidation of the grafted site and humeral remodelling (**E, F**)

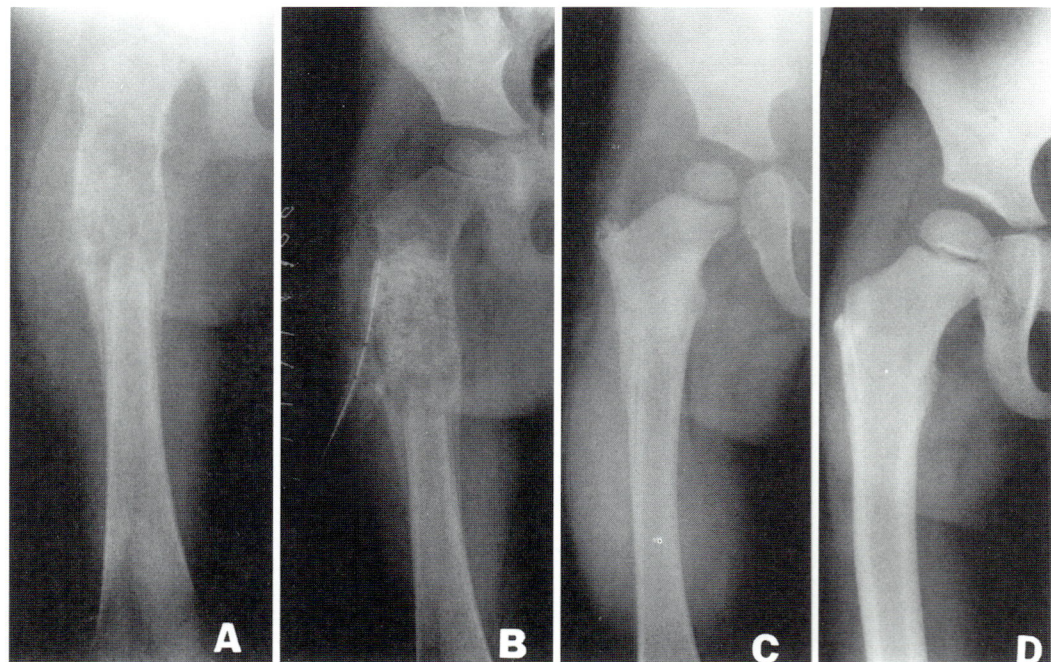

Fig. 19.1.11². Antero-posterior radiographs of right femur of a 6-year-old boy. Osteolytic lesion due to eosinophilic granuloma of bone (histiocytosis X) with pending pathologic fracture (**A**). After curettage, cryosurgery and homologous bone graft (**B**). Follow-up at 6 (**C**) and 33 (**D**) months. A complete normalization of the proximal femur has occurred

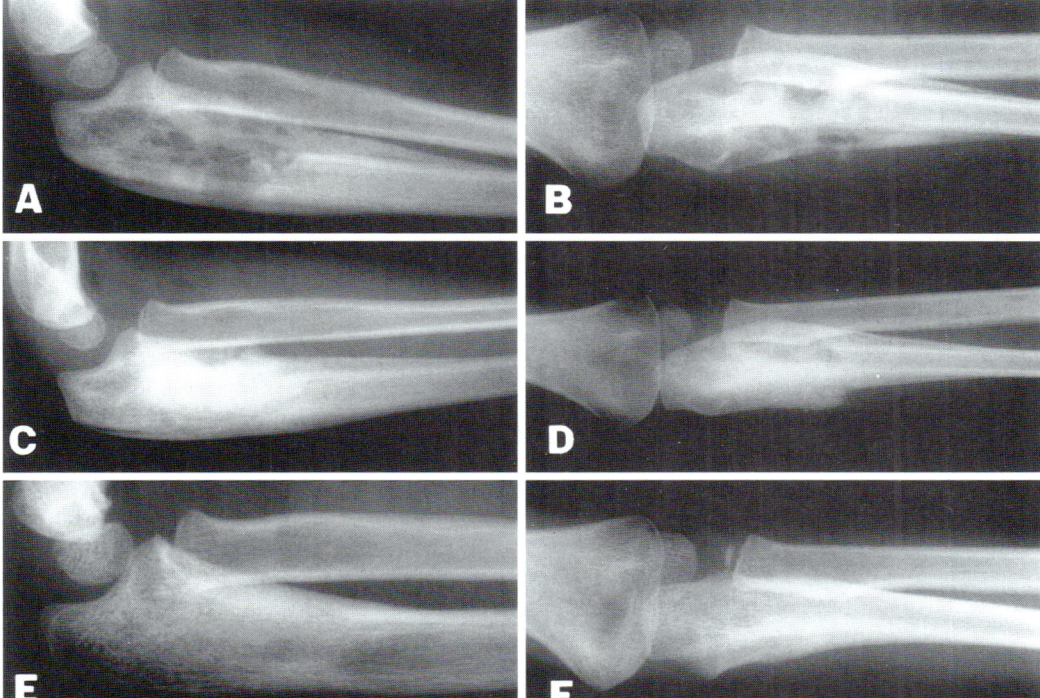

Fig. 19.1.12². Antero-posterior and lateral radiographs of left elbow of a 3.5-year-old boy. Eosinophilic granuloma of bone (histiocytosis X) lesion close to joint (**A, B**). Follow-up at 7 months after curettage, cryosurgery and homologous bone graft (**C, D**) and at 15 months, normalization of the intramedullar space (**E, F**)

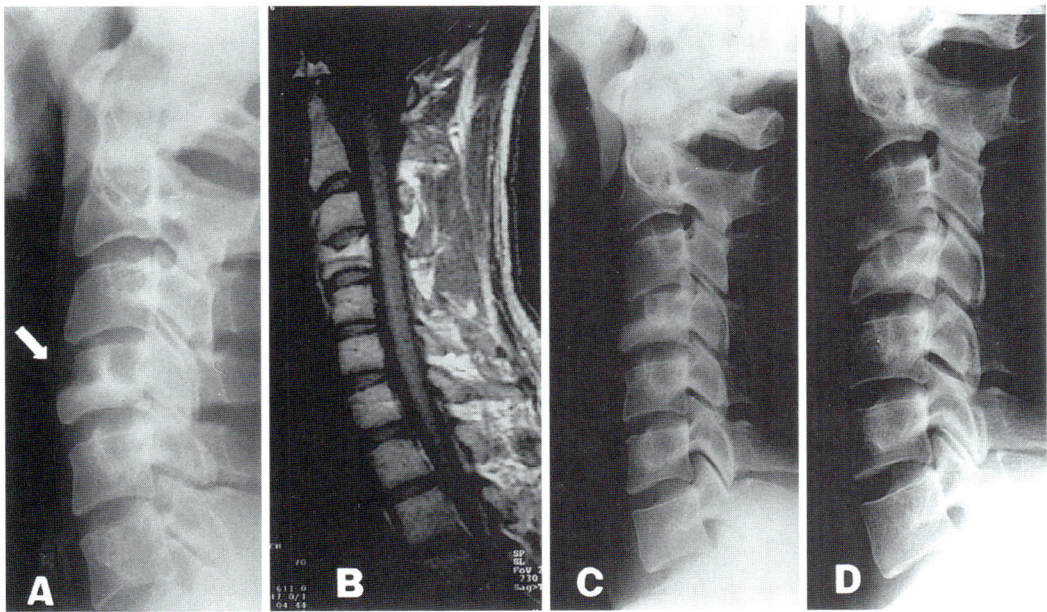

Fig. 19.1.13². Lateral radiograph of cervical spine of a 23-year-old man. **A**: lytic lesion of body C4 due to eosinophilic granuloma of bone (histiocytosis X). T1 weighed magnetic resonance image, partial collapse of vertebral body (**B**). Follow-up at 4 months after curettage, cryosurgery and autologous strut bone graft (**C**) and at 10 months (**D**)

Chapter 19
Orthopedic Cryosurgery

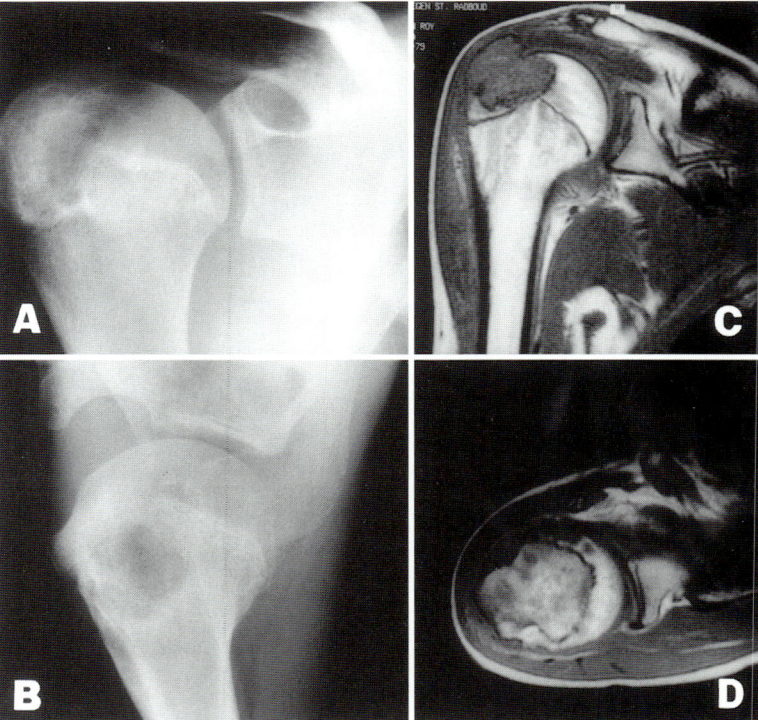

Fig. 19.1.14[2]. Routine radiographs of chondroblastoma located in proximal epiphysis of humerus of a 18-year-old man (**A, B**). The lesion was painful, because of pathologic, minimally displaced fracture of tuberculum majus. T1 weighted MRI studies, the extent of the lesion is accurately depicted (**C** coronal, **D** transversal)

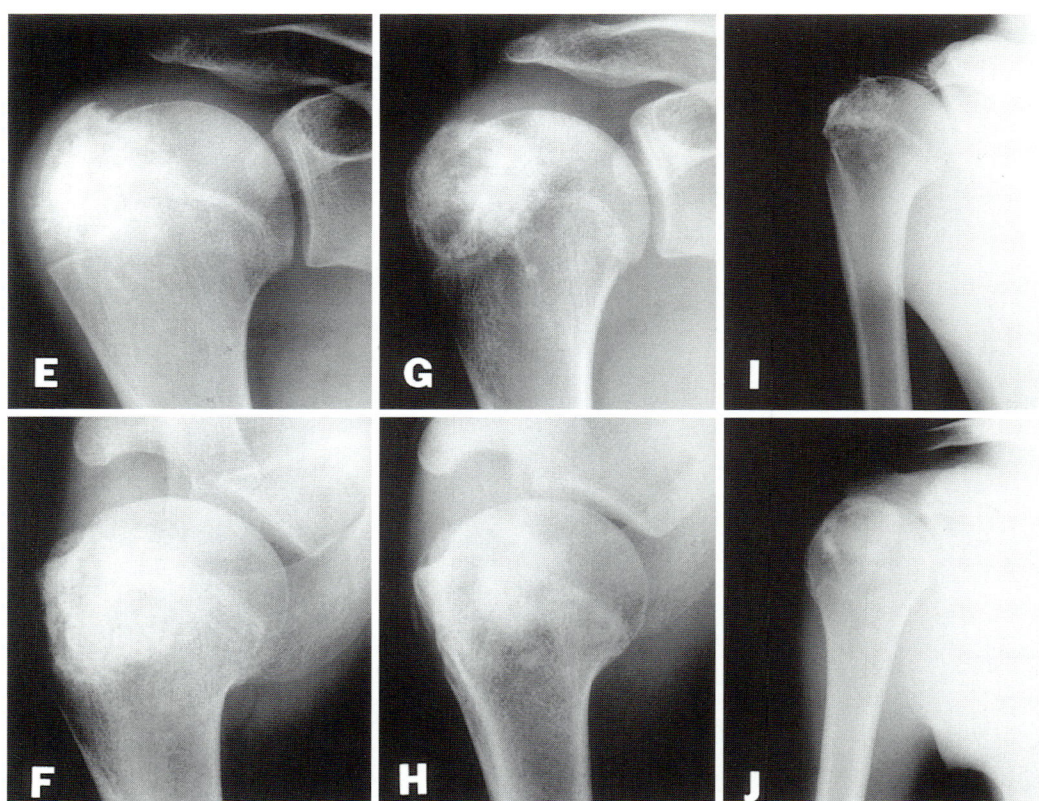

Fig. 19.1.15[2]. 3 (**E, F**), eight (**G, H**) and 30 months after curettage, cryosurgery and homologous bone grafting. Progressive incorporation and remodeling of the graft, resulting in nearly normal bone structure at latest follow-up. No evidence of recurrence. Normal, pain free function (**I, J**)

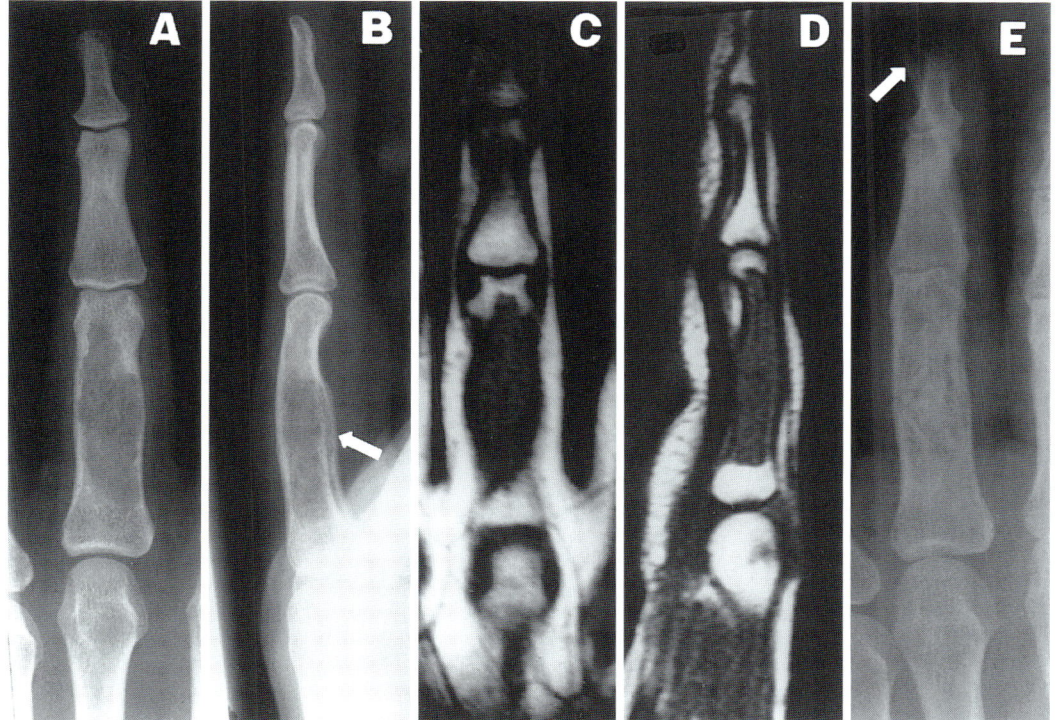

Fig. 19.1.16². Radiographs of painful enchondroma (**A, B**) located in first phalanx of digit 3 of a 30-year-old woman. Periosteal reaction (arrow). T1 weighted MRI: coronal (**C**) and sagittal (**D**). Postoperative view after curettage, cryosurgery and autologous bone graft, wound drain *in situ* (arrow) (**E**)

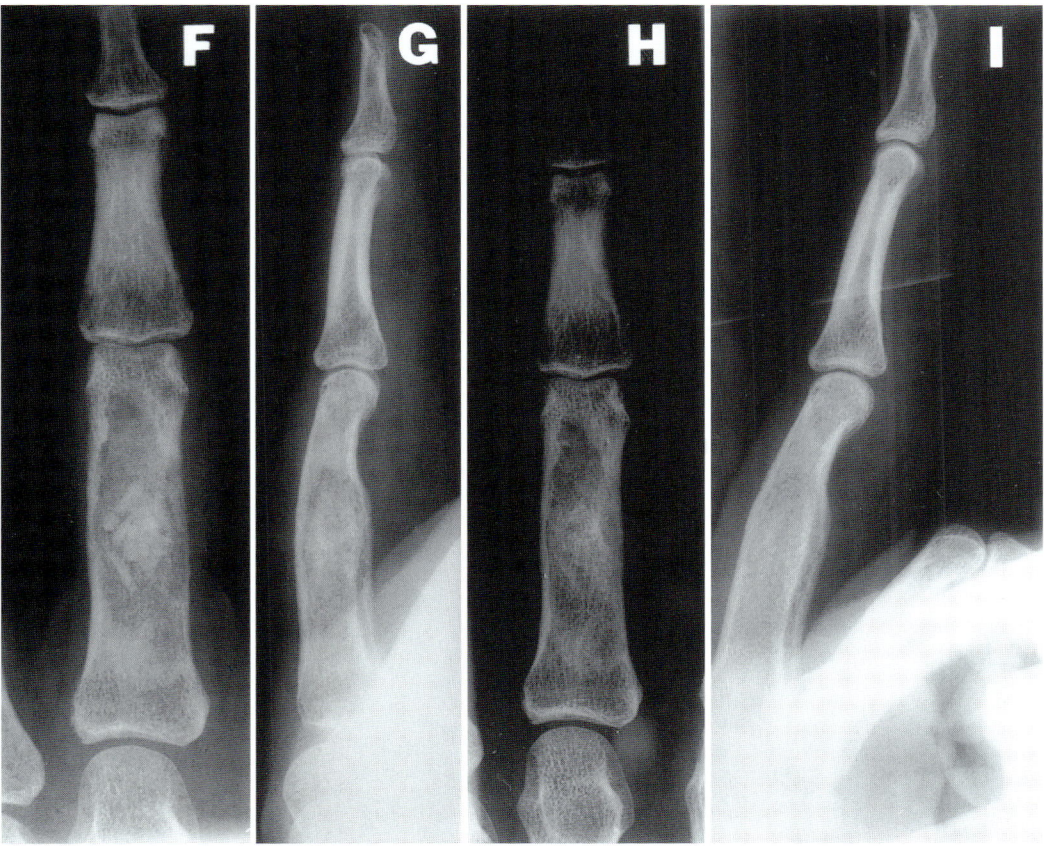

Fig. 19.1.17². 7 weeks (**F, G**) and 12 months (**H, I**) postoperatively, progressive incorporation of bone graft, normal function

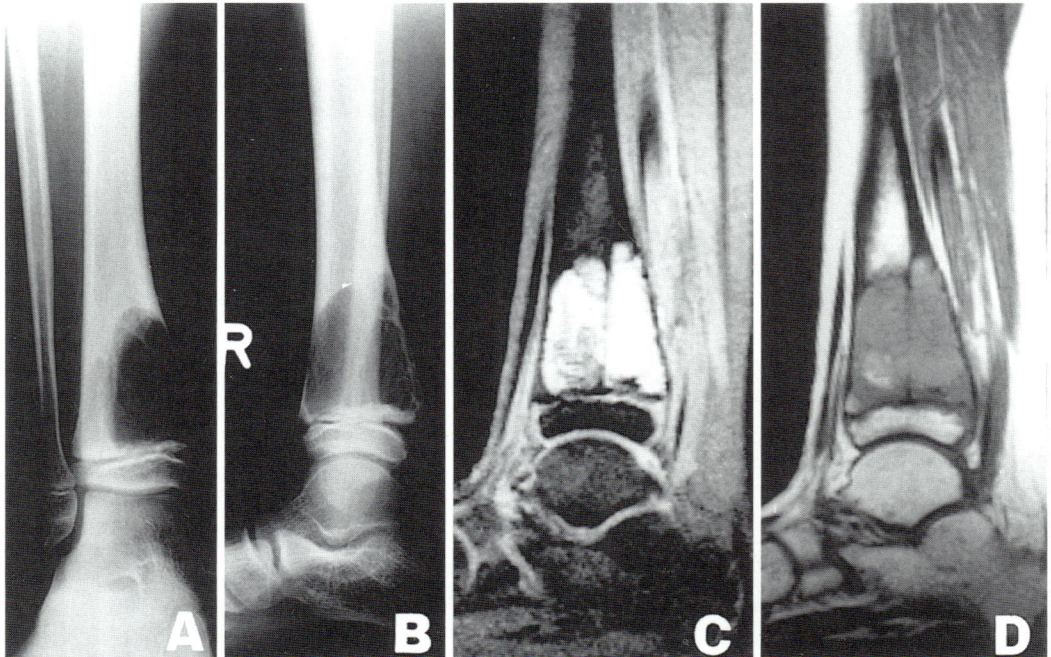

Fig. 19.1.18². Routine radiographs of an 11-year-old boy with aneurysmal bone cyst in the distal tibia, extending very close to the growthplate (**A, B**). Magnetic resonance imaging, T2 (**C**) and T1 (**D**), showing erosion of cortex and a fairly homogenous intensity of the contents of the cyst consistent with fluid. The cyst seems not to have damaged the epiphysis

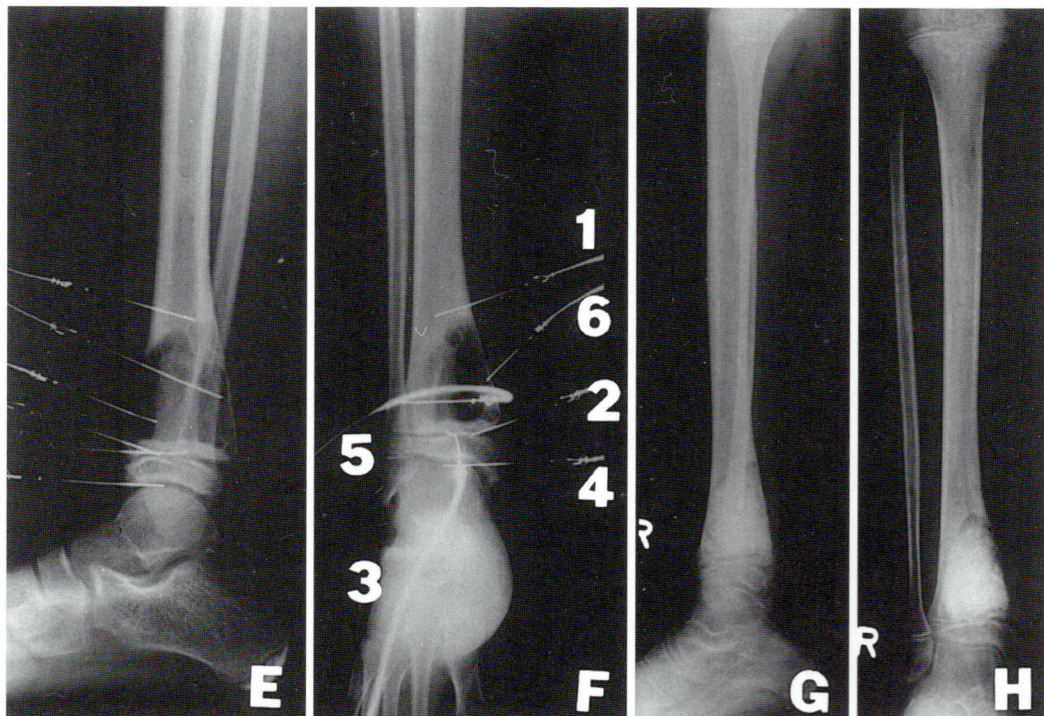

Fig. 19.1.19². Intraoperative radiographs showing location of the temperature couples. Number 2 and 3 are situated in the growth plate, number 4 is intra-articular (**E, F**). An intralesional temperature couple was added later. After curettage and cryosurgery the cyst is filled a homologous graft (**G, H**)

Section F   Clinical Aspects

Chapter 19
Orthopedic
Cryosurgery

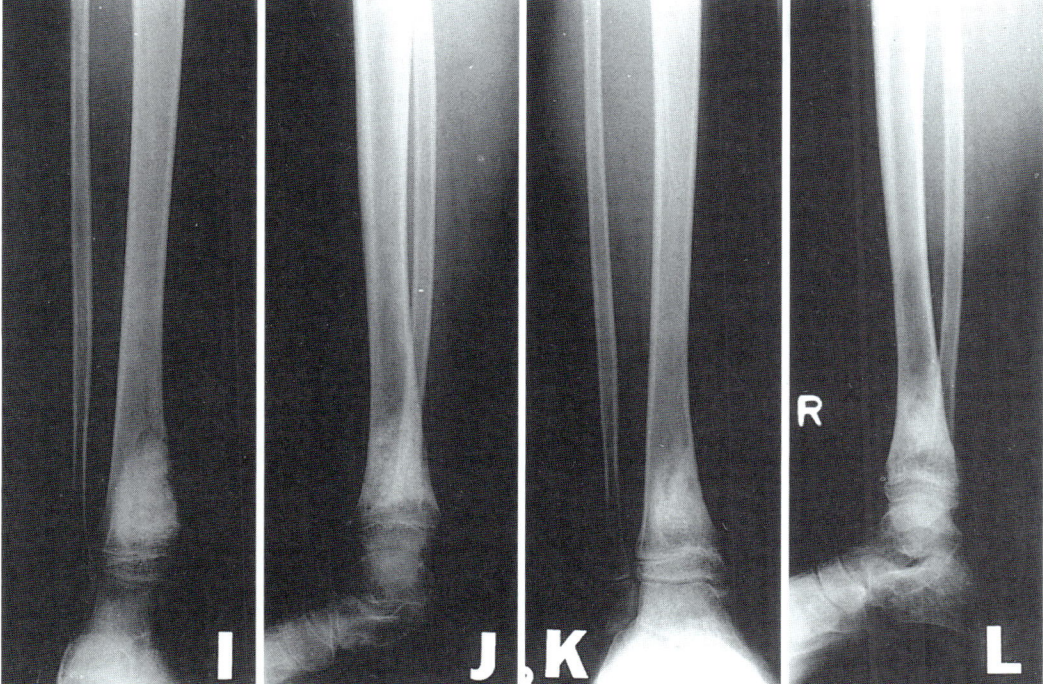

Fig. 19.1.20[2]. Routine radiographs at 9 (**I, J**) and 16 (**K, L**) months postoperatively: no evidence of recurrence

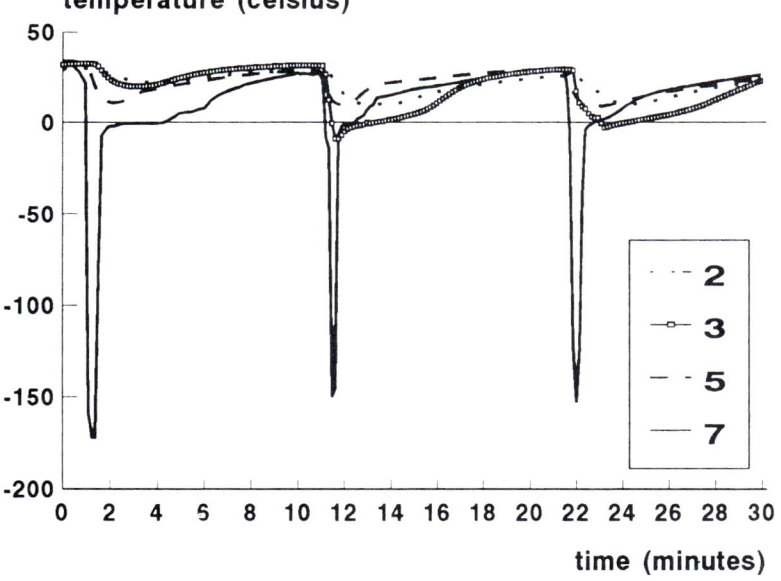

Fig. 19.1.21[2]. Temperature recordings of patient in Fig. 19.1.19 numbers correspond with those in Fig. 19.1.19 E and F. The recording number 3, next to number 2 of the epiphysis, shows sub-zero levels during the second and third freeze cycle, which may damage the epiphysis. The temperatures measured by the thermocouples 1, 4 and 6 were at all times above 25°C. For reasons of clarity of the graph they are not shown

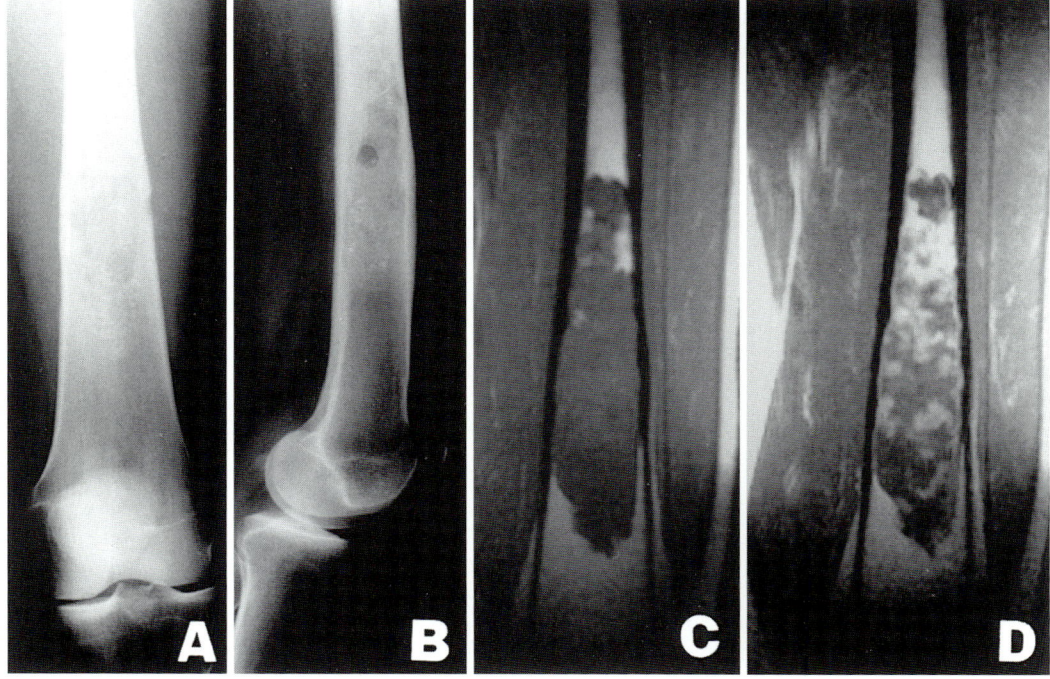

Fig. 19.1.22². Postbiopsy routine radiographs of a 29-year-old female with chondrosarcoma, grade 1 of diaphysis of the femur (**A, B**). Magnetic resonance imaging, T1 (**C**) and T2 (**D**) weighted showing erosion of cortex and an inhomogeneous signal intensity consistent with enchondroma or low-grade chondrosarcoma

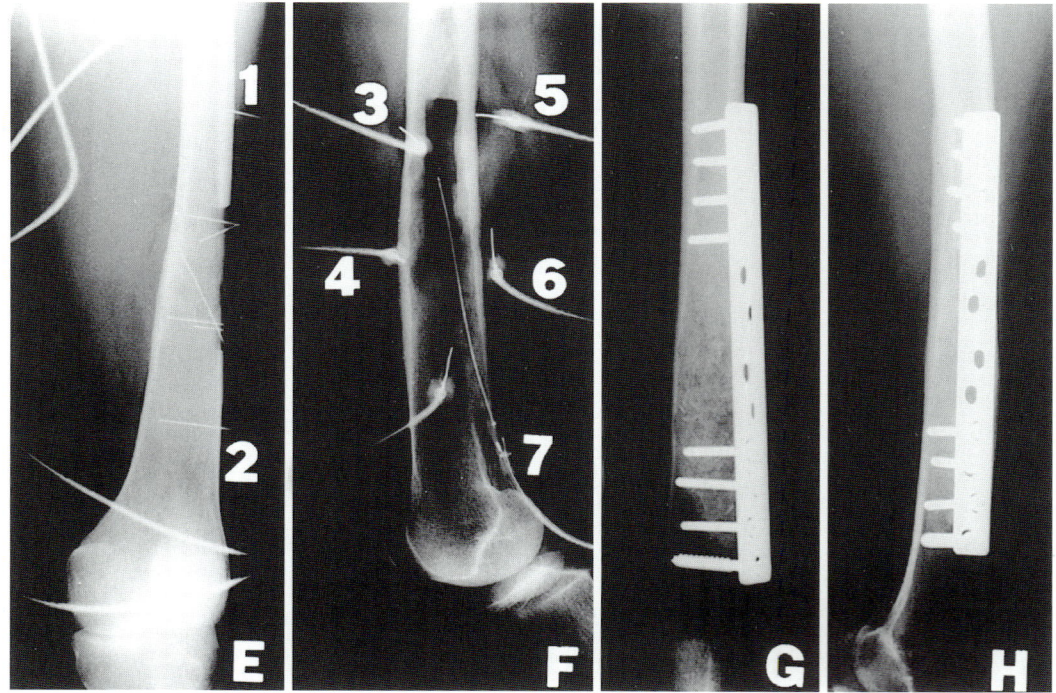

Fig. 19.1.23². Intraoperative radiographs of patient in Fig. 19.1.22 showing localization of the temperature couples (**E, F**). Number 7 is situated in the curetted lesion. Numbers correspond with those in Fig. 19.1.24. After curettage and cryosurgery the cyst is filled with a homologous bone graft. To prevent postoperative fracture a prophylactic osteosynthesis was added (**G, H**)

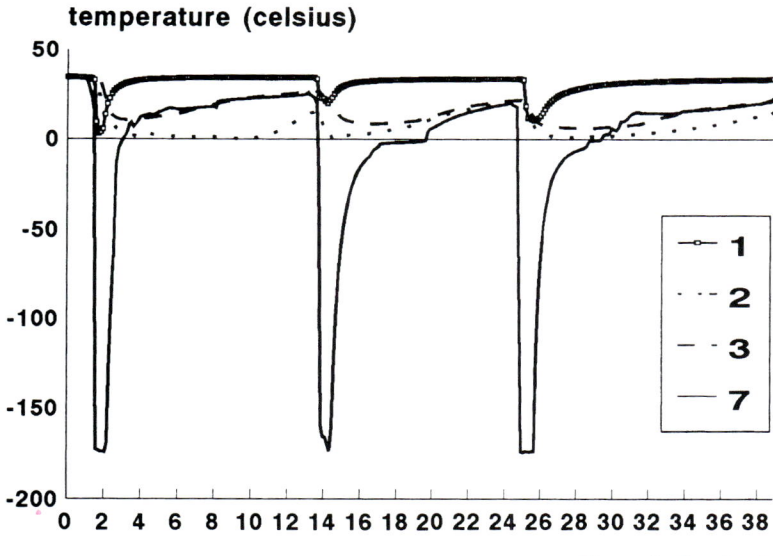

Fig. 19.1.24[2]. Temperature recordings of patient in Fig. 18.22; numbers correspond with those in Fig. 18.23 E and F. The temperatures measured by the thermocouples 4,5 and 6 were at all times above 10°C. For reasons of clarity of the graph they are not shown

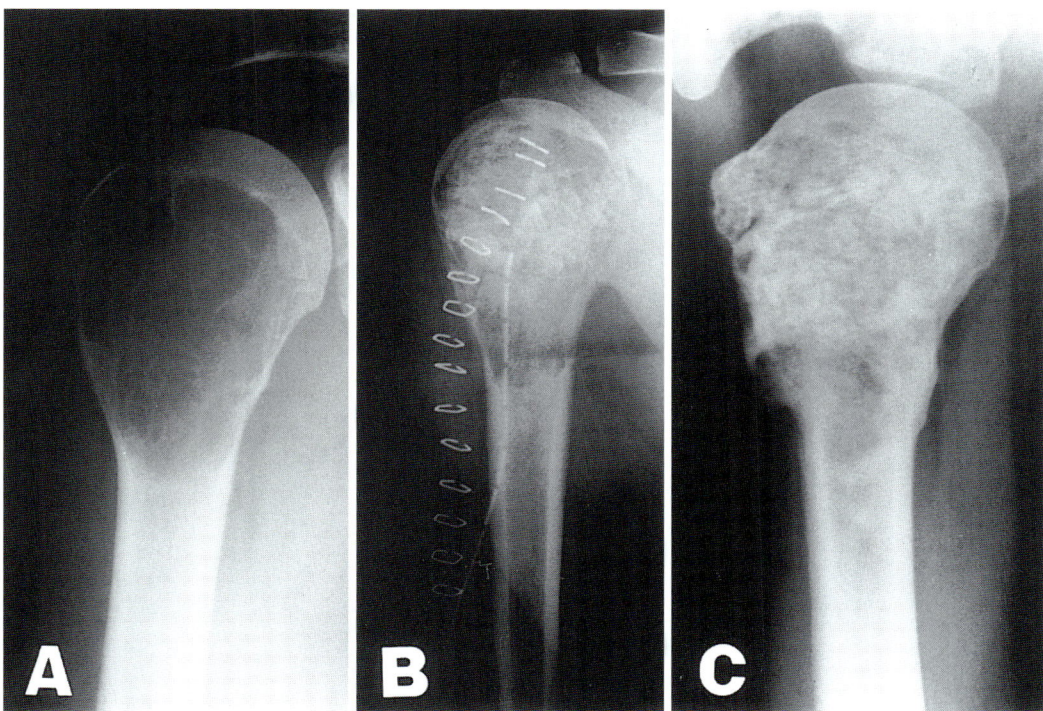

Fig. 19.1.25[2]. Giant cell tumor in the proximal part of the humerus in a 24-year-old woman: only a thin layer of bone supporting the articular surface is preserved (**A**). Status after curettage, cryosurgery and homologous bone grafting (**B**) and at 3 months after the operation (**C**)

Chapter 19
Orthopedic
Cryosurgery

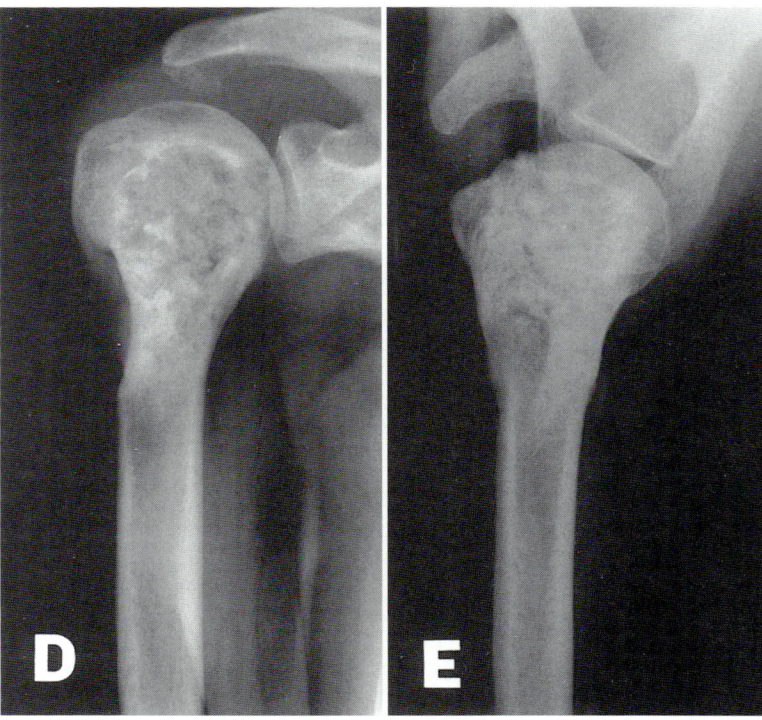

Fig. 19.1.26[2]. One year postoperatively; no signs of arthrosis, excellent range of motion

Fig. 19.1.27[2]. 22 months after the operation: AP (F) and lateral view (G): some arthrosis of the glenohumeral joint

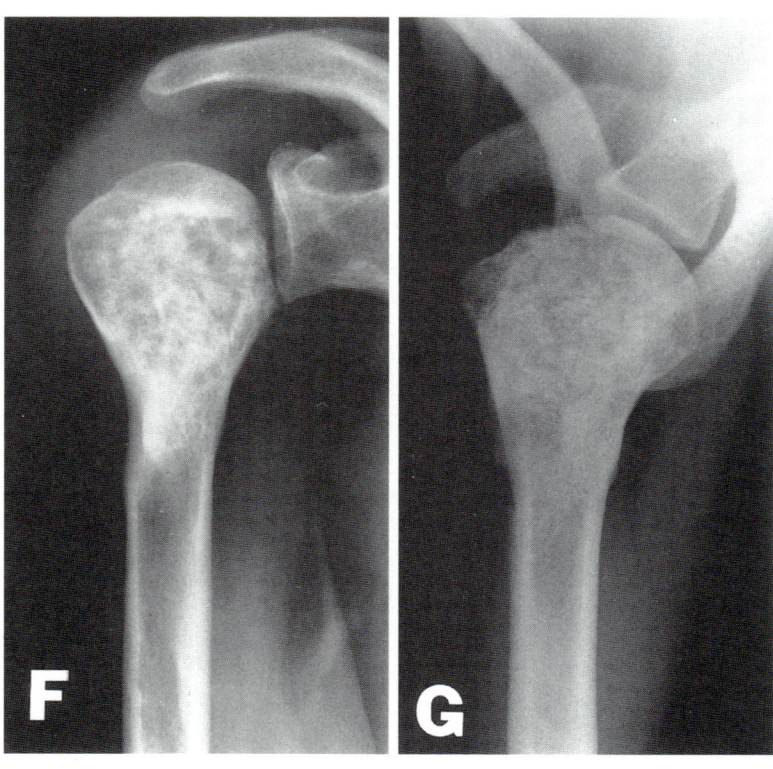

Section F   Clinical Aspects   443

Chapter 19
Orthopedic
Cryosurgery

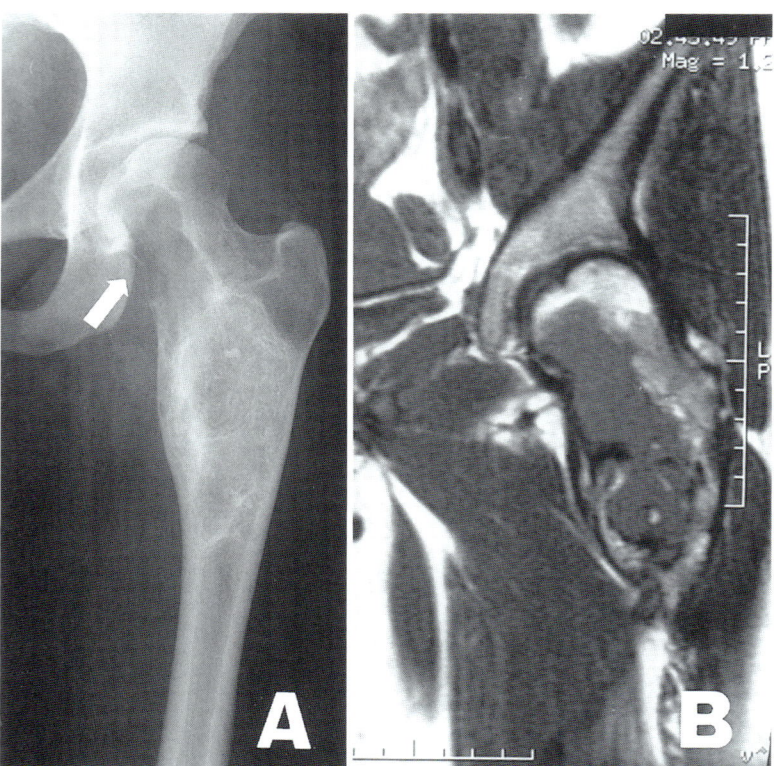

Fig. 19.1.28². A, B. Fibrous dysplasia of the left femur in a 23-year-old woman: pending pathological fracture of the collum femoris, see arrow (A). On MRI the extent of the lesion is accurately depicted (B)

Fig. 19.1.29². C, D. Status quo 4 months after curettage, cryosurgery and a combination of homologous fibula strut graft and homologous morselised allograft (C), 12 months postoperatively: incorporation of bone graft and restoration of the medial part of the collum femoris (D)

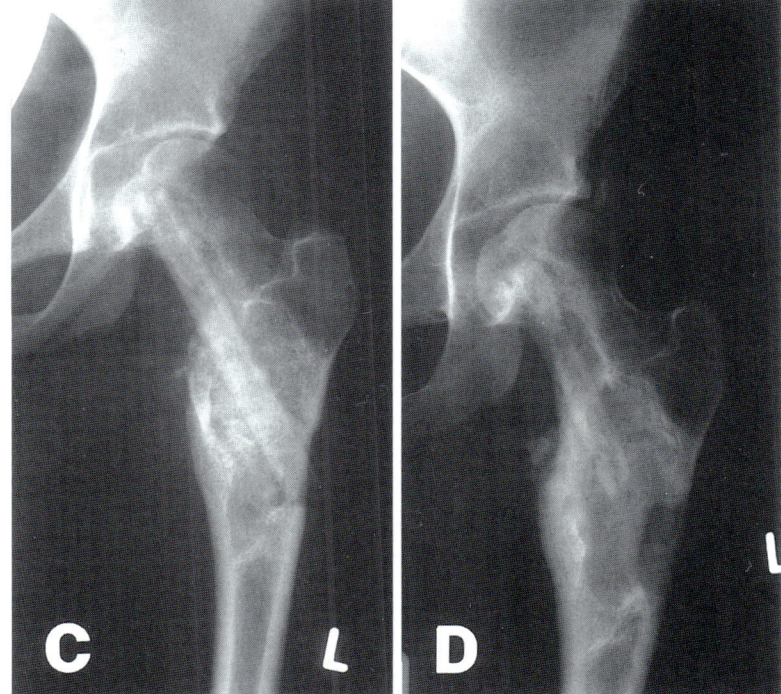

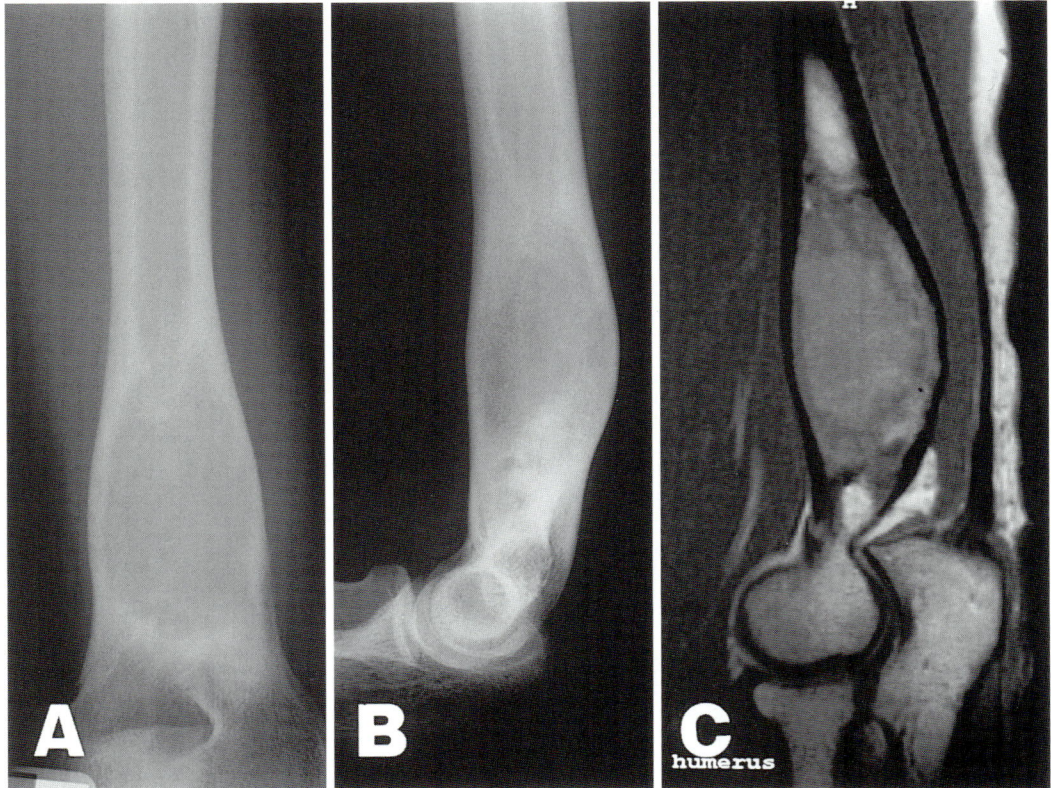

Fig. 19.1.30². 21-year-old woman with fibrous dysplasia in the distal part of the left humerus; routine radiographs (**A, B**) and MRI, T1 weighted (**C**)

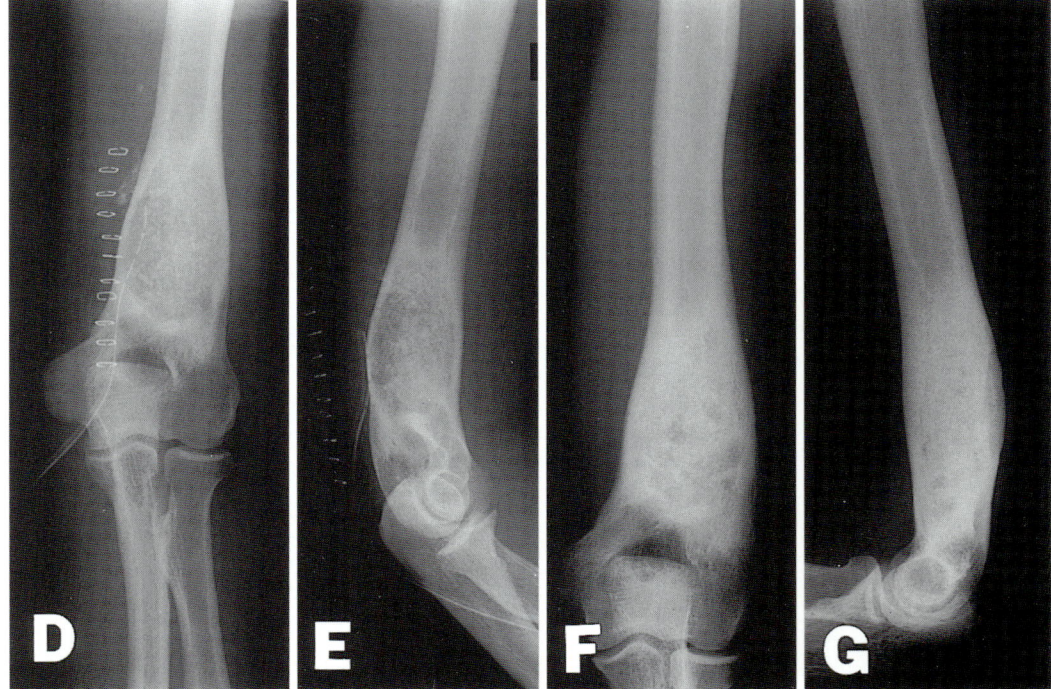

Fig. 19.1.31². Antero-posterior and lateral views postoperatively (**D, E**) and at 13 months (**F, G**): no recurrence and clinically asymptomatic, normal range of motion

Chapter 20

Cosmetic Cryosurgery

Nikolai N. Korpan[1] with contributions by Yoshiaki Hosaka[2]

20.0 Introduction

Hypertrophic scars and keloids are uncommon complications of superficial wounds but are not uncommon in full-thickness wounds, particularly in certain locations.

We prefer the cryogenic method for nondestructive treatment, such as that for scars or skin peeling. But cryosurgery is also a method of therapy that uses freezing to achieve destruction of tissue. It is medically indicated for the treatment of various benign, premalignant, and malignant lesions.

Eradication of simple cutaneous lesions by freezing was first attempted at the turn of the century. Liquid air was applied with a cotton swab or solidified carbon dioxide was placed on the lesion, but destruction was limited. When liquid nitrogen became available, it was initially applied with a cotton swab, but in the 1960's new techniques and equipment were developed that permitted deeper destruction. Thus malignant as well as benign lesions became amenable to cryosurgical treatment.

Cryosurgery is used alone, in combination with intralesional steroid injection, or combined with surgery to treat keloids and hypertrophic scars.

The standard cryosurgical procedure is carried out for the treatment of such scars. As a rule the freeze time ranges between 10 and 30 seconds, but large keloids require a longer freeze time. A single or double freeze-thaw cycle is performed, and more than one treatment session is usually needed. Complete flattening can be achieved. This procedure is repeated as often as necessary.

We use a different, simple cryotechnique for the treatment of hypertrophic scars and keloids – i.e., cryosurgical shaving. With shaving cryosurgery, the final scar is much smaller than the primary scar. The cryosurgical procedure is not difficult and the cryosurgical shaving of scars has excellent clinical and cosmetic results. Furthermore, incidence of complications after the cryosurgery is low. Shaving cryosurgery is therefore a safe and effective technique for treating hypertrophic scars and keloids.

Other techniques, such as laser therapy, have theoretical advantages but have been of little practical help.

In Japan nevus Ota is estimated to affect approximately 0.4% of the dermatology out-patient population and 2.6% of plastic surgery out-patients. The ratio of male to female patients is reported to be approximately 1:3.

During the past 15 years, from 1977 to 1991, Yoshiaki Hosaka with other collegues treated a total of 164 Japanese patients with nevus Ota using Cryo-Mini (Nagai Manufacturing Company, Ltd, Tokyo, Japan), a portable gun-type liquid nitrogen cryogenic instrument with a removable disk-shaped copper probe. The authors found this method to be not only simple and effective, but also advantageous and beneficial in the treatment of the extensive and deep-situated type of nevus Ota.

Application time of the cryogenic probe to the lesion is determined by taking into consideration the age and sex of the patient and depth of dermal melanocytes, and thickness of the skin to be treated. It is important to keep the application time of the liquid nitrogen, which is applied at the extremely low temperature −196°C, as short as possible, to hold the instrument lightly, and to place as little pressure as possible on the lesion. Since children have thinner skin than adults, the application time for a child is reduced to about two-thirds of the time for an adult. In the treatment of extensive cases with uncertain depths of dermal melanocytes, trial tests should be routinely done on a marginal area of the lesion before treatment and ascertain whether the selected application time is appropriate. Usually, one application is administered to each lesion site during a session, this being sufficient to obtain good results in most cases of a superficially situated nevus Ota. In severe and extensive cases with deeply situated dermal pigmentation, however, repeated applications of liquid nitrogen in combination with dermabrasion are usually required, and patients may receive two applications to the same site during a session. In such cases, the second application time is shorter than the first. As a rule, dermabrasion is employed lightly immediately after cryosurgery at the first session and is repeated in later sessions, if necessary.

Compared with carbon dioxide snow cryosurgery, liquid nitrogen cryosurgery has the following advantages in plastic surgery: (1) it is easier to manipulate and control; (2) the number of treatments can be reduced from one-third to one-quarter of those necessary with the carbon dioxide snow cryotherapy technique; (3) cosmetic appearance after cryosurgery is better; and (4) there is less scar formation and fewer depigmentation problems after cryosurgery.

However, the pigmented lesions in the palpebral area are the most difficult to treat even using this technique. Due to the fact that the palpebral skin is thin and excessive treatment easily leads to necrosis of the skin with a tendency toward scarring, it is risky to abrade this area. To avoid the potential hazard of injuring the eyelids, the authors now employ the Q-switched ruby laser in combination with liquid nitrogen cryosurgery for the treatment of nevus Ota in this region. The clinical experience of the author (Yoshiaki Hosaka) indicates that this laser therapy seems to result in excellent clearance with less edema formation and less postoperative pain than when liquid nitrogen is applied in such cases.

Clinical care after cryosurgery in which liquid nitrogen is used is basically the same as with carbon dioxide snow therapy. When cryosurgery is over, the treated area is kept cold with gauze soaked in physiological saline, in combination with an ointment containing steroids and antibiotics, and covered by silicone-coated gauze or sterilized bactericidal dressing. Then the entire area undergoing treatment is covered with regular gauze. The following day, small blisters develop, but are left untouched, and only the outermost gauze is changed. The bulla dries in 7 to 10 days and the crusts that develop fall off spontaneously. About 2 weeks after cryosurgery, the patients are allowed to wash their faces. For at least 3 months, the patients are advised not to expose the treated area to solar radiation, covering it with gauze and protecting it with sunscreen preparations and/or appropriate cosmetics.

The following figures show the liquid nitrogen instrument and some of the clinical pictures before and after the cryosurgery.

Section F Clinical Aspects

20.1 Hypertrophic Scars (postoperative, posttraumatic)

Chapter 20
Cosmetic Cryosurgery

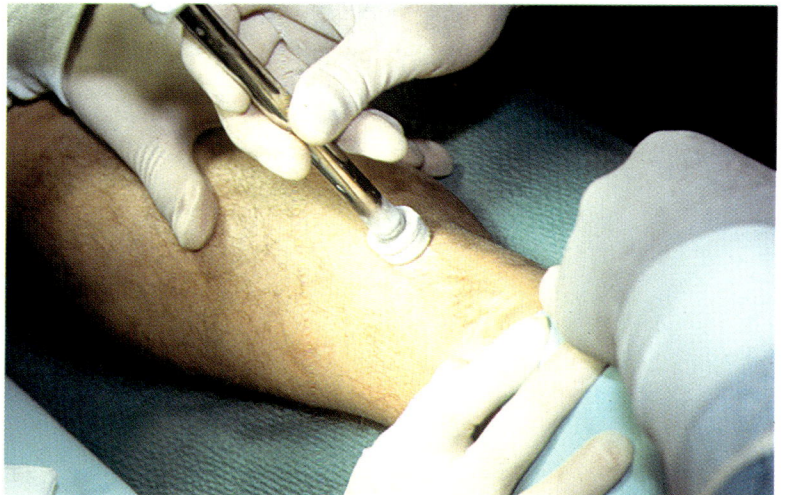

A

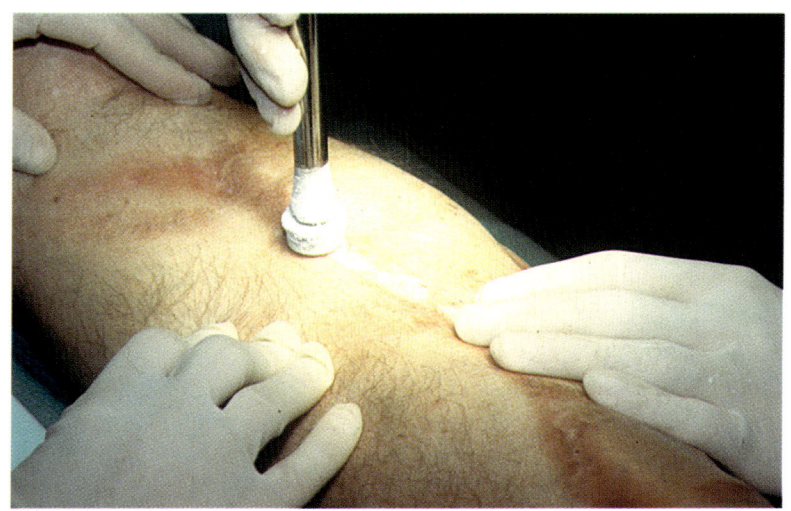

B

Fig. 20.1.1[1]. Posttraumatic, postoperative hypertrophic scars on the leg of a 27-year-old man. A cryoshaving is performed by means of a disc cryoprobe with a diameter of 20 mm at a temperature of −80°C without local anesthesia

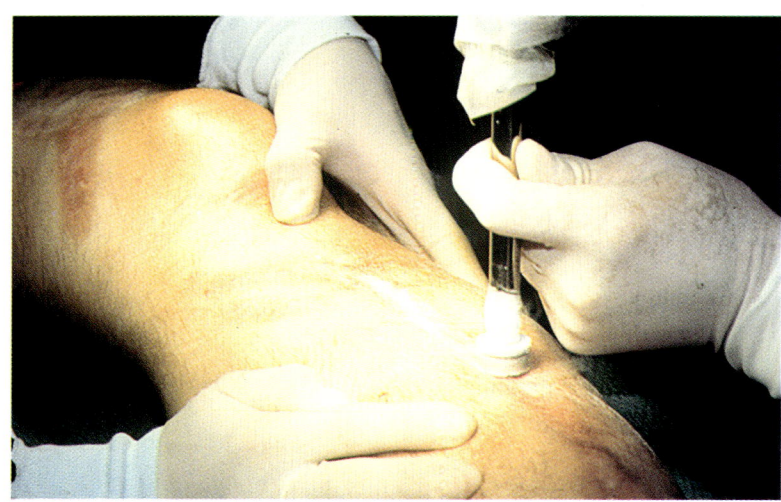

C

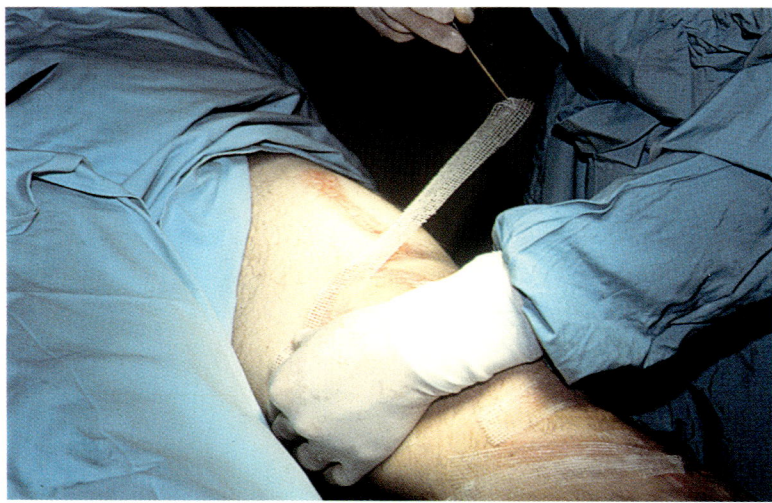

A

B

Fig. 20.1.2¹. Immediately after the cryoshaving, a simple wound dressing is applied for the first postoperative days. As a contact layer between the surface of the dressing and the wound a layer of "Jelonet" ointment is applied

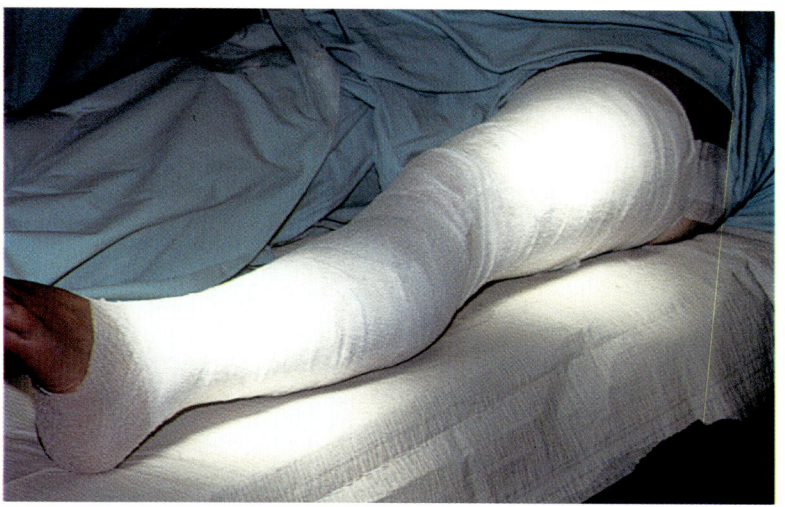

C

Section F   Clinical Aspects   449

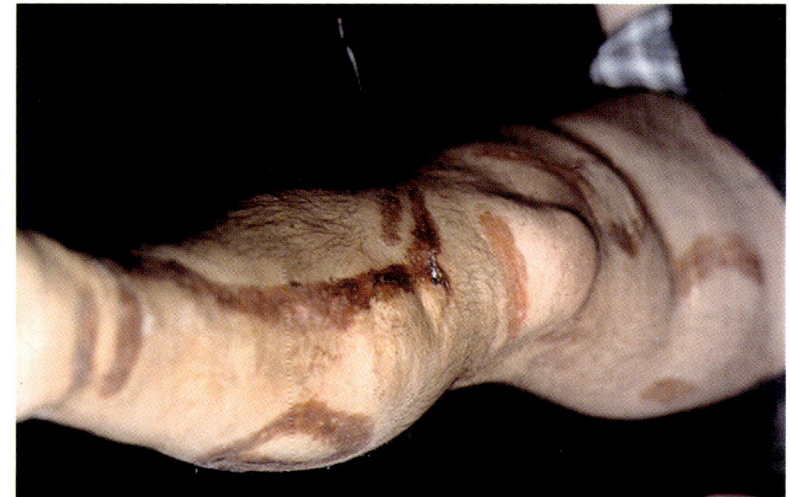

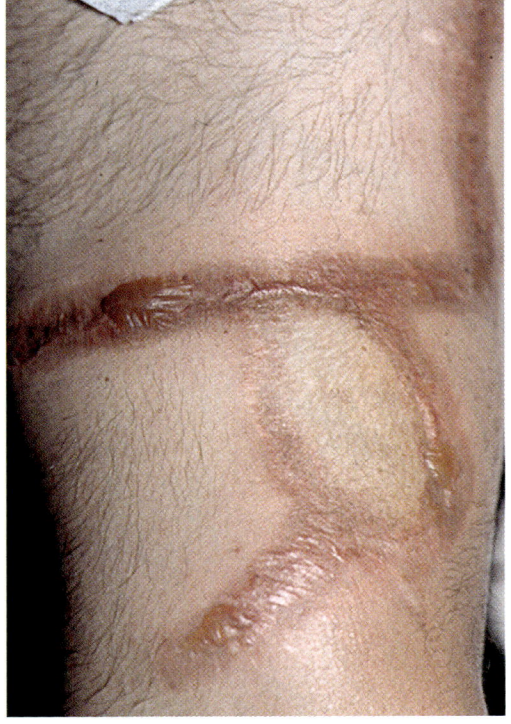

Fig. 20.1.3[1] **A–C.** Postoperative view. The first day after cryoshaving. No pain

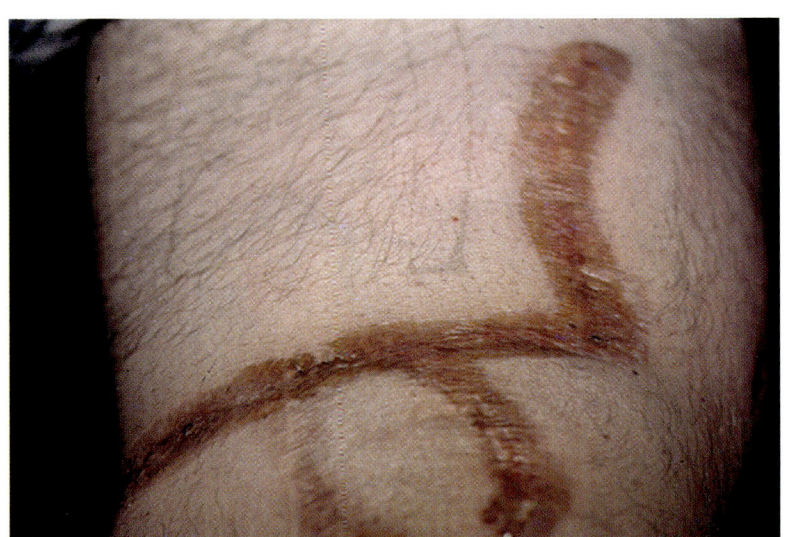

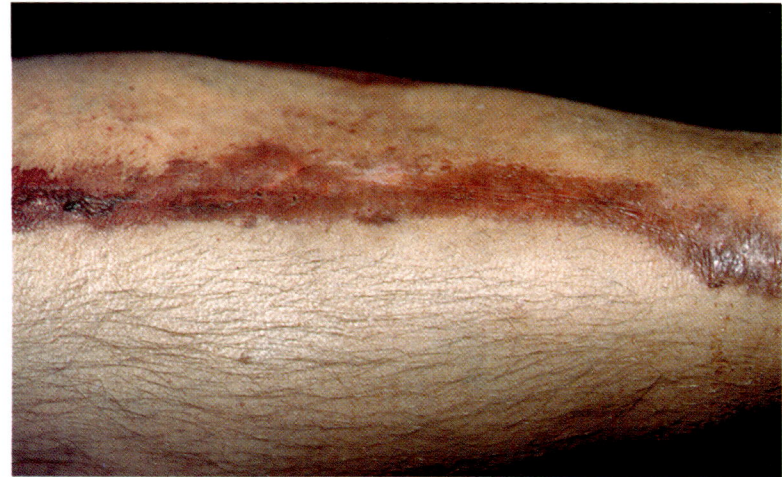

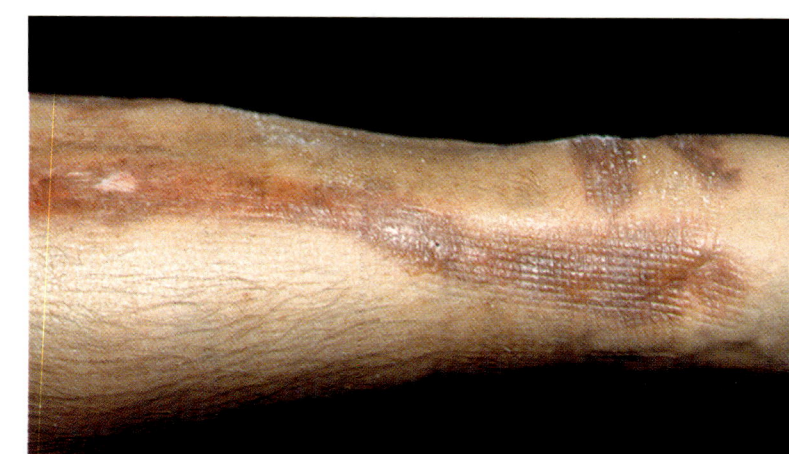

Fig. 20.1.4[1] **A–C.** Postoperative view. The same area seven days after cryoshaving. No pain

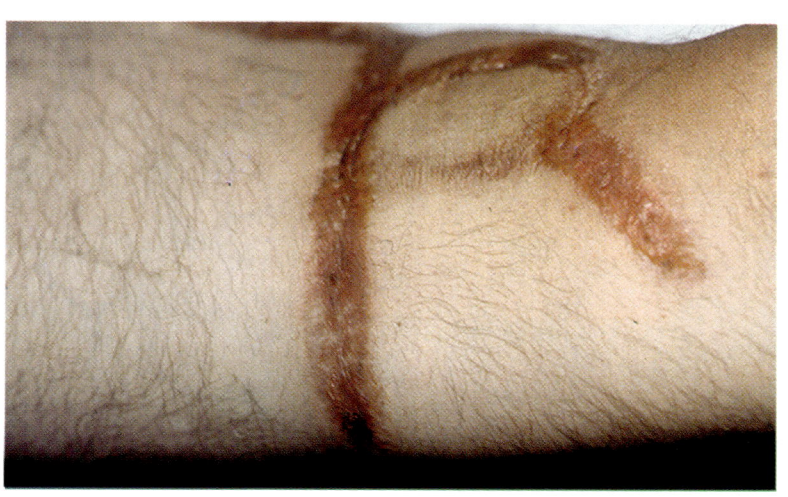

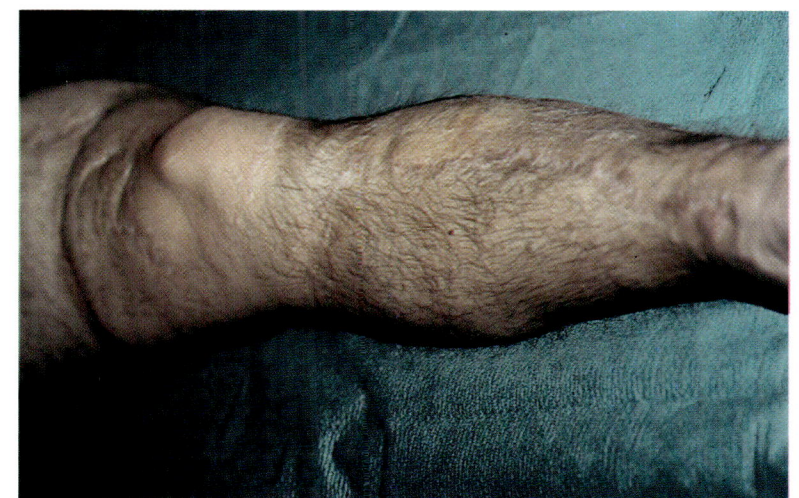

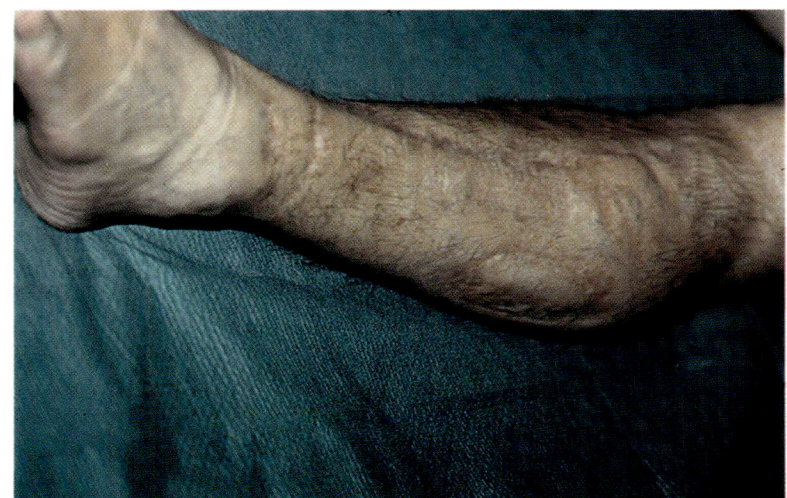

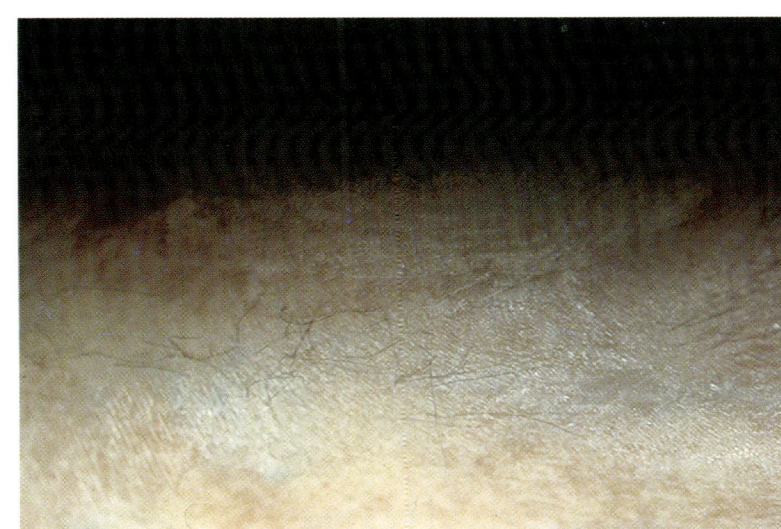

Fig. 20.1.5¹ A–F. Excellent cosmetic and curative results 3 months after cryoshaving. The patient is free of complaints after a 4-year observation period

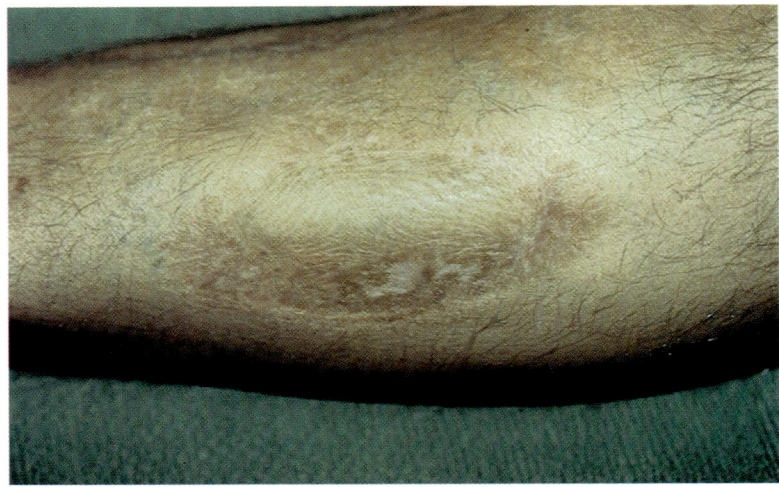

D

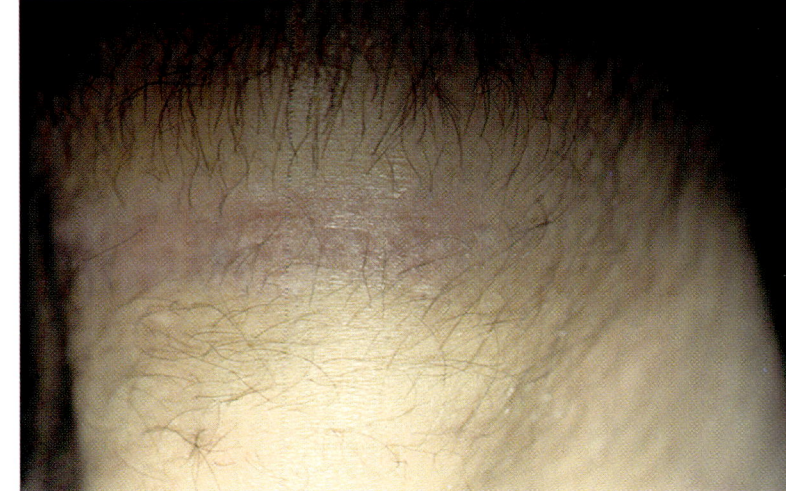

E

Fig. 20.1.5¹ A–F. Excellent cosmetic and curative results 3 months after cryoshaving. The patient is free of complaints after a 4-year observation period

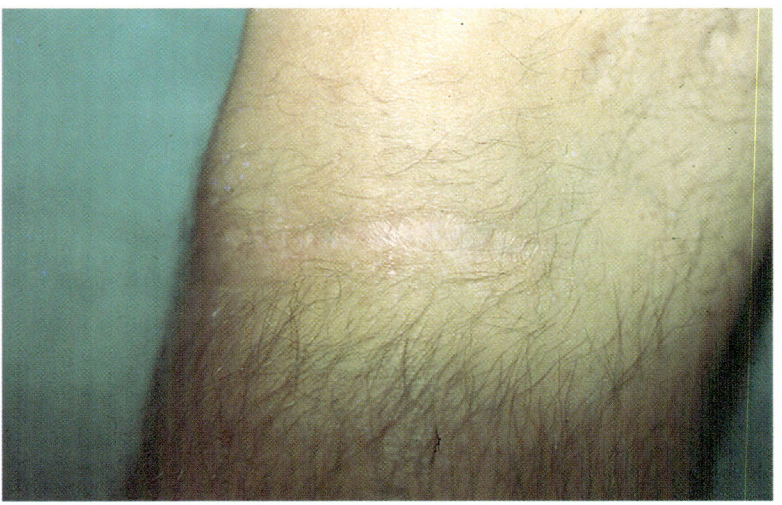

F

Section F   Clinical Aspects

20.2 Skin Lesions

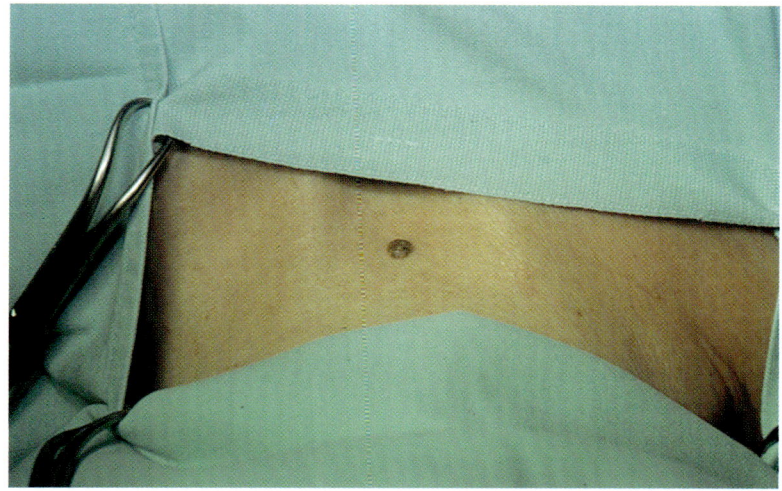

Fig. 20.2.1[1]. A 46-year-old woman with pigmented skin lesion on the neck

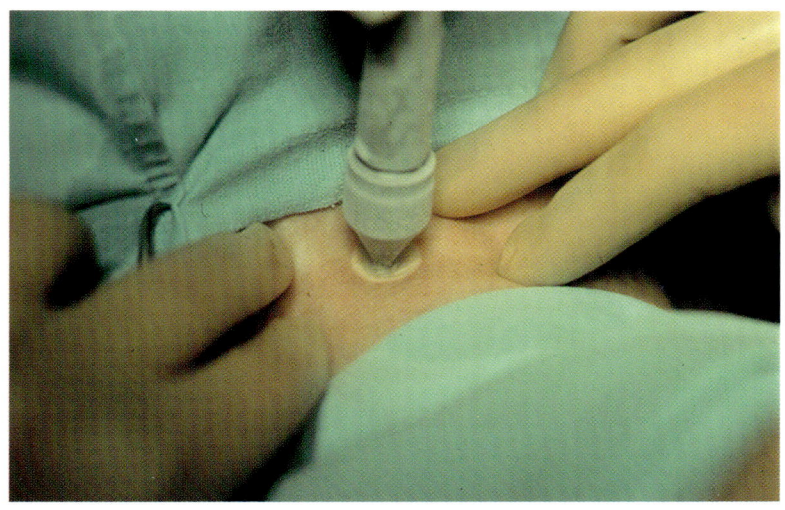

Fig. 20.2.2[1] **A, B.** A simple cryosurgical session by with a 5 mm disc cryoprobe which is placed on the skin lesion at a temperature of −180°C. No exposure time

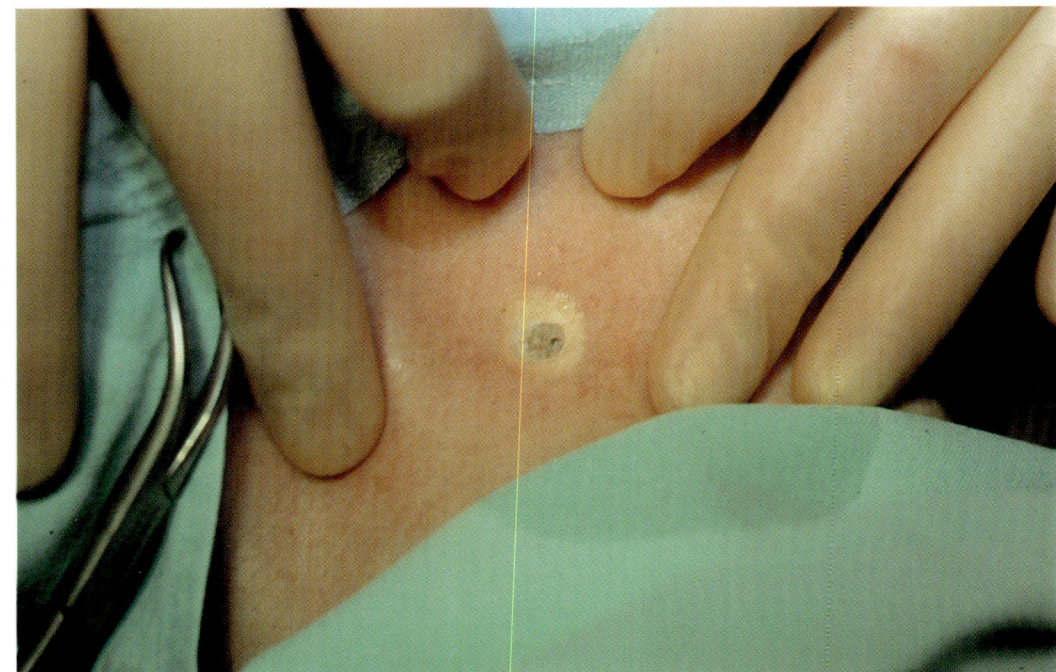

Fig. 20.2.3[1] A, B. Post-cryosurgical view of the same patient. The skin lesion immediately after the cryosurgical session

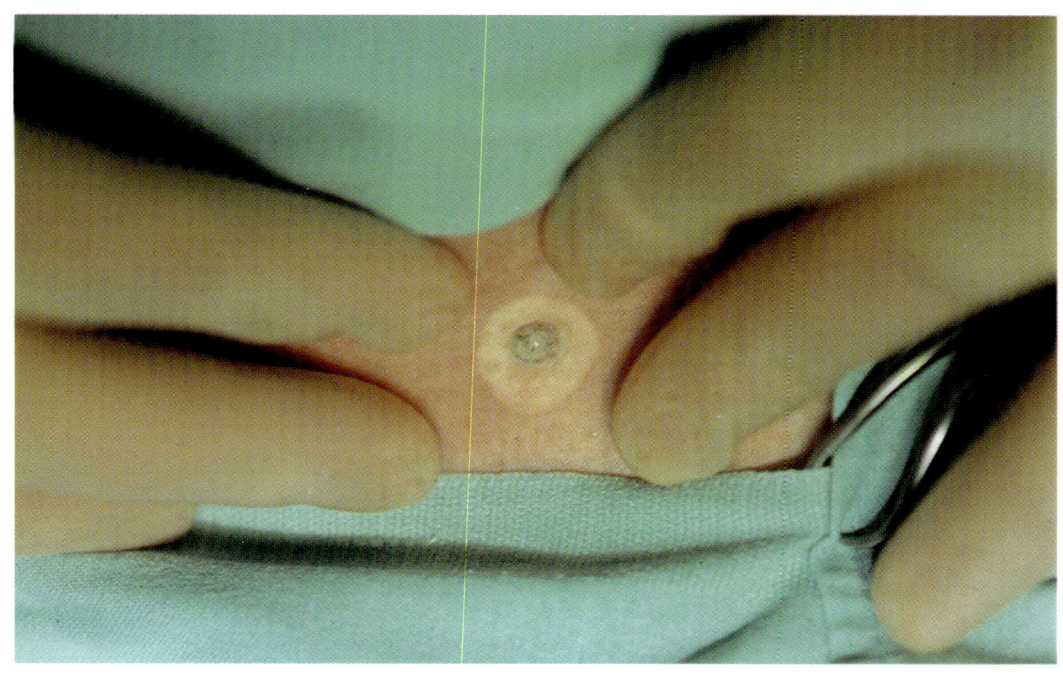

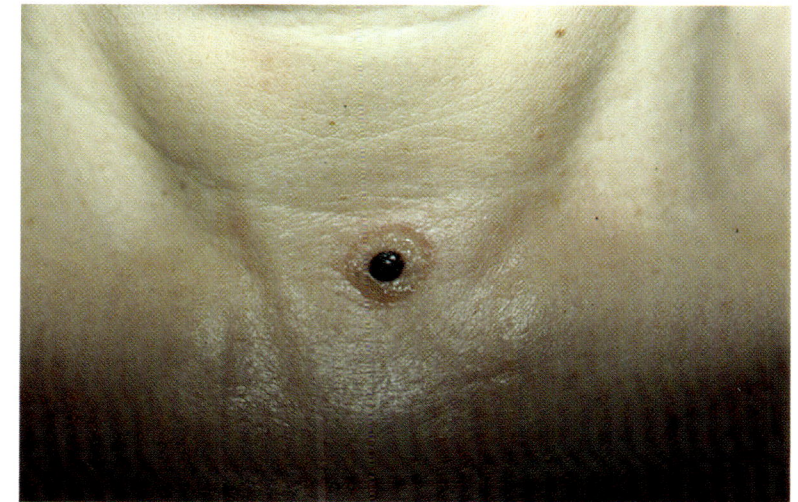

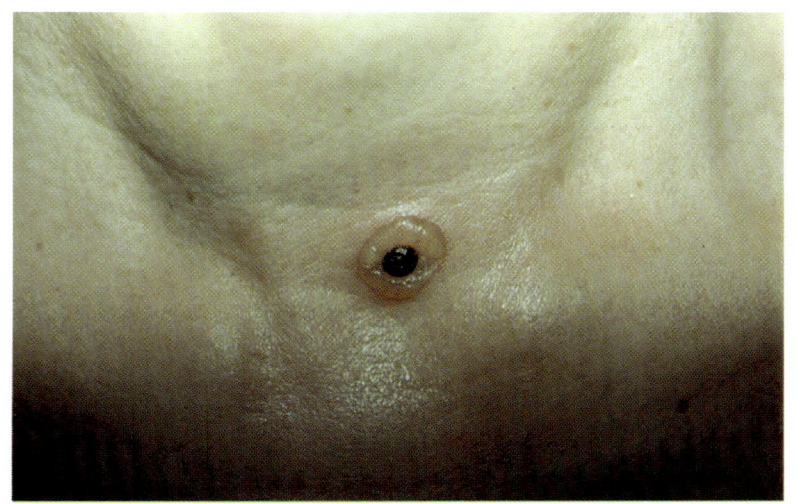

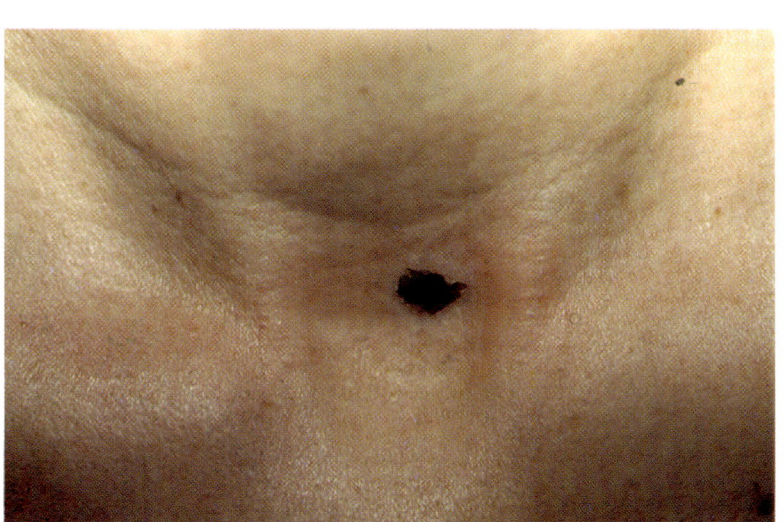

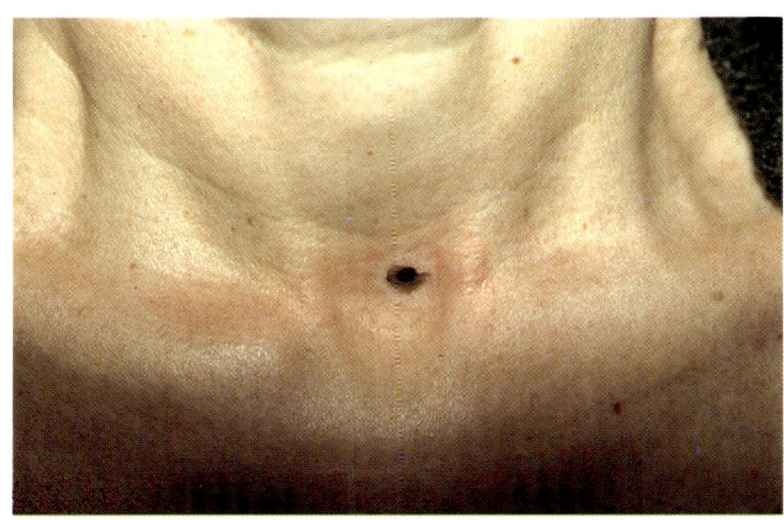

Fig. 20.2.4¹. Post-cryosurgical view: The skin lesion 1 day (**A, B**) and 7 days (**C, D**) after the cryosurgical session

Chapter 20
Cosmetic Cryosurgery

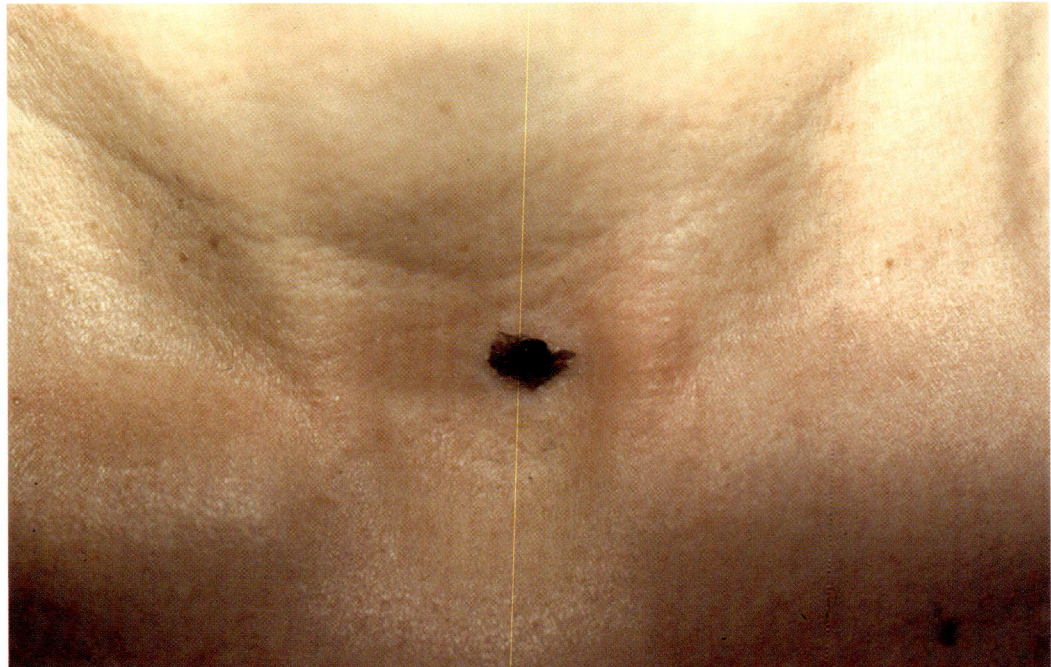

Fig. 20.2.5[1] A, B. Wound healing. 2 weeks after cryosurgical treatment showing that the crust has fallen off

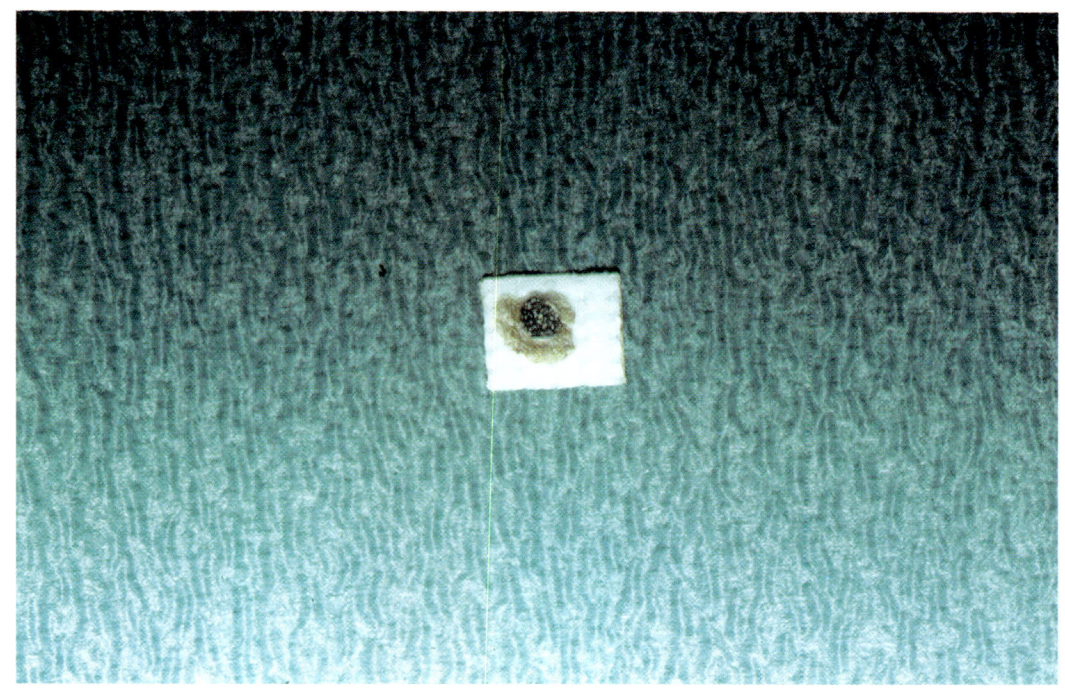

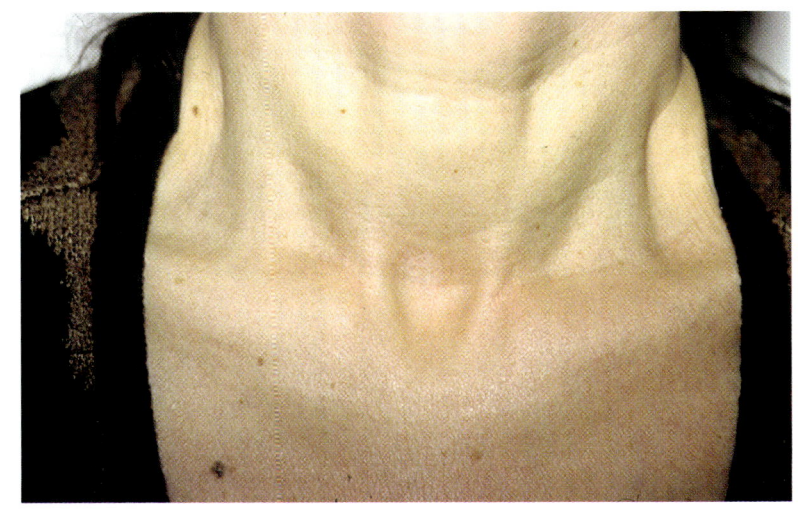

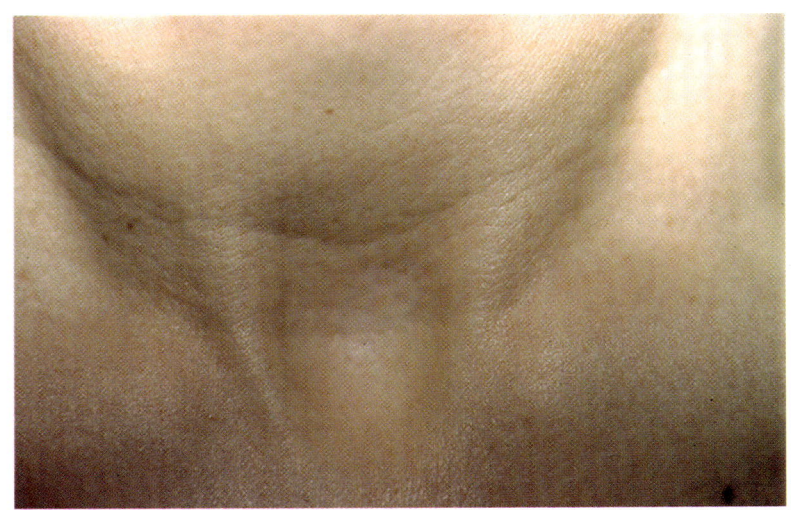

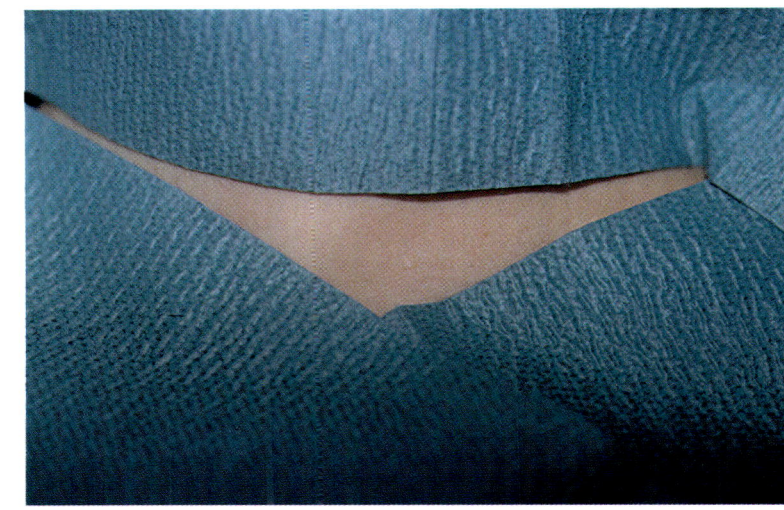

Fig. 20.2.6¹. Excellent cosmetic and curative result 6 weeks (**A, B**) and 12 weeks (**C**) after the cryosurgical treatment

20.3 Nevus Ota

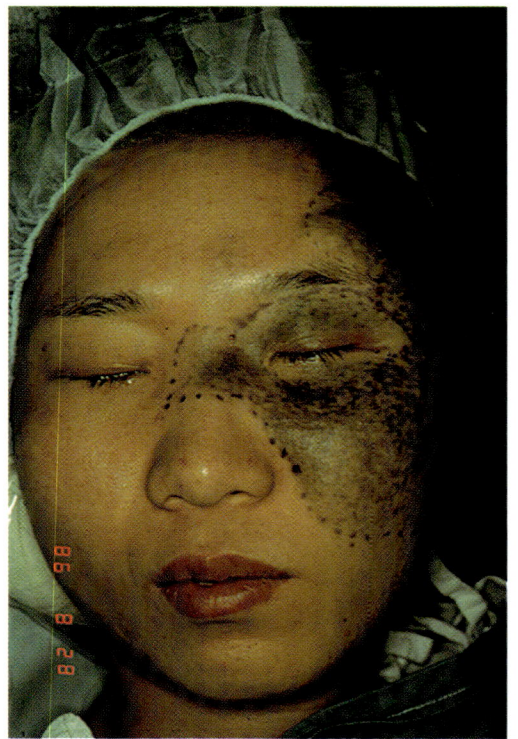

Fig. 20.3.1[2]. A 25-year-old woman with nevus Ota. Preoperative frontal view. The intensive pigmentation spread over the eyelid, forehead and cheek regions

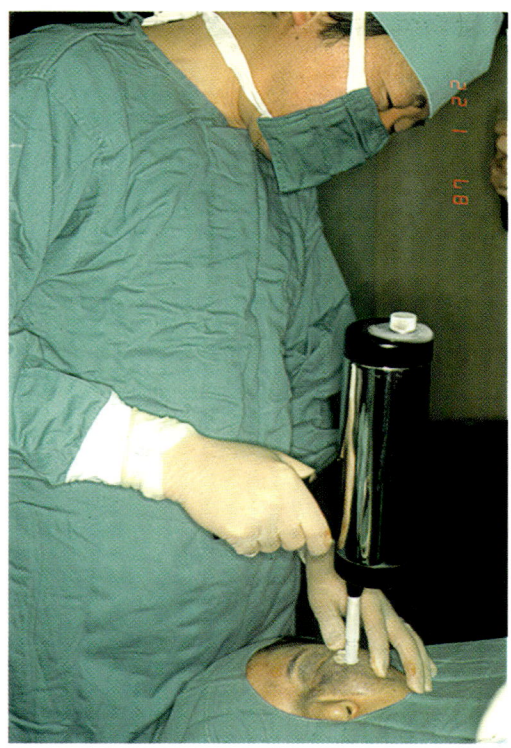

Fig. 20.3.2[2]. Cryosurgery using CRYO-MINI

Section F   Clinical Aspects   459

Chapter 20
Cosmetic
Cryosurgery

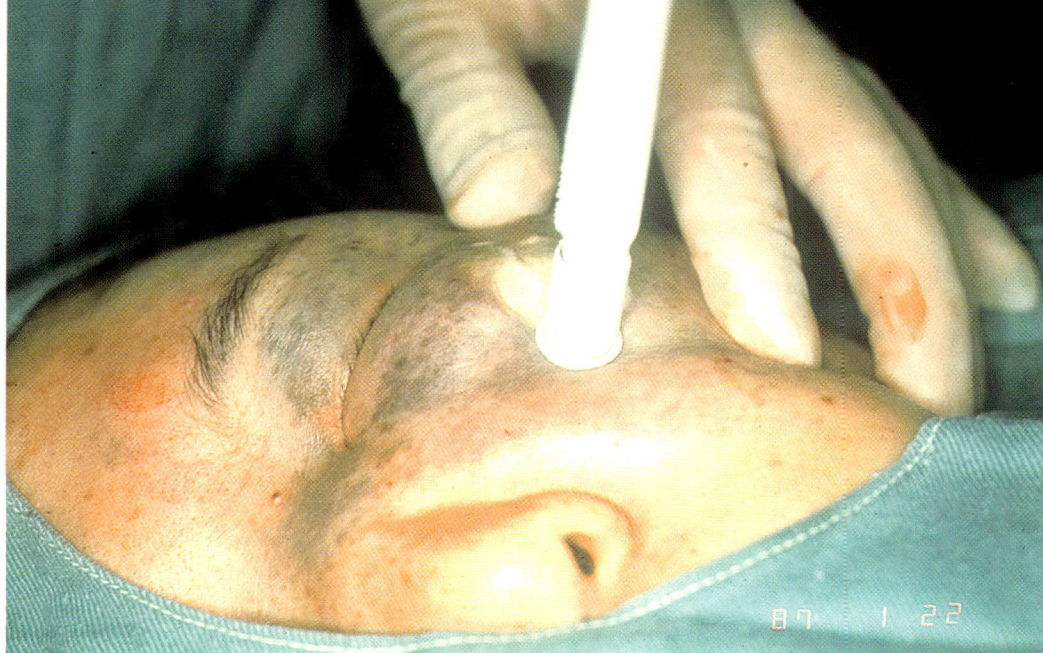

Fig. 20.3.3[2]. A highly magnified view of the tip area is shown. The cryoprobe is applied to affected skin with only the pressure necessary to hold the instrument. The contacted skin is frozen

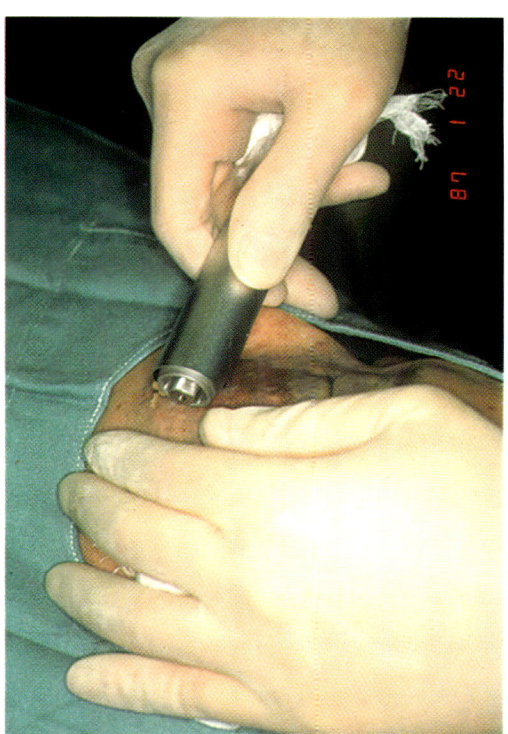

Fig. 20.3.4[2]. Dermabrasion is employed lightly immediately after cryosurgery at the first session and is repeated in later sessions, if necessary

Chapter 20
Cosmetic
Cryosurgery

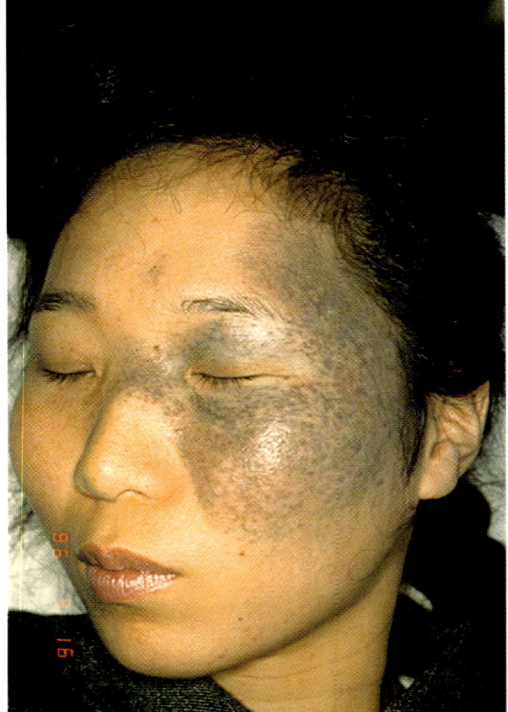

Fig. 20.3.5[2]. Postoperative lateral view.
1 month after the first cryosurgical session

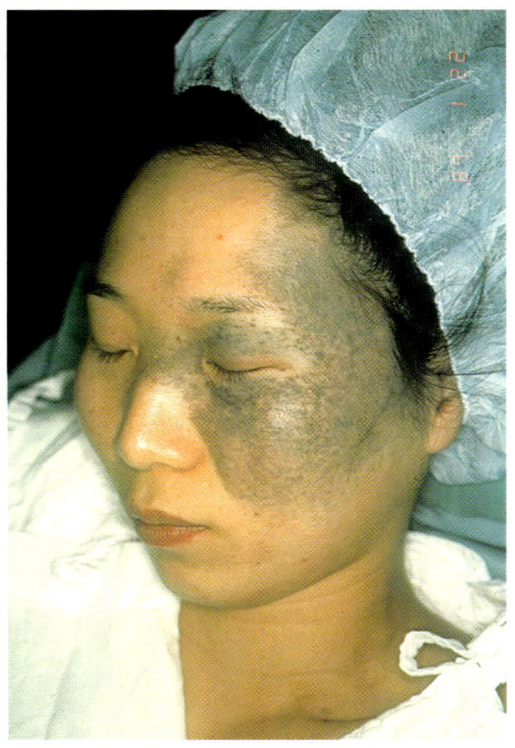

Fig. 20.3.6[2]. Postoperative lateral view.
5 months after the first cryosurgical session

Section F   Clinical Aspects   461

Chapter 20
Cosmetic
Cryosurgery

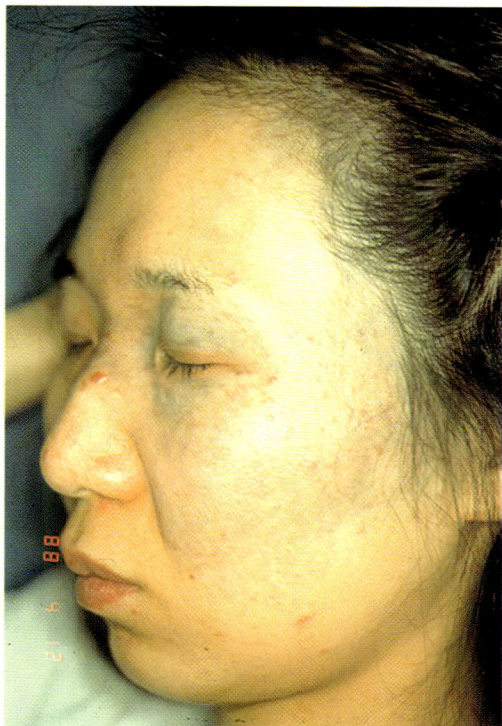

Fig. 20.3.7². Postoperative lateral view. 3 months after the fourth cryosurgical session

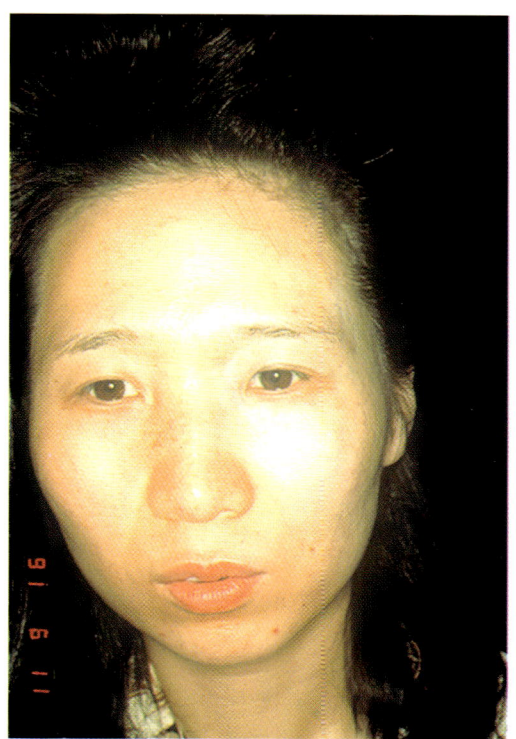

Fig. 20.3.8². Postoperative frontal view. 3 years and 5 months after the fourth cryosurgical session

Chapter 20
Cosmetic
Cryosurgery

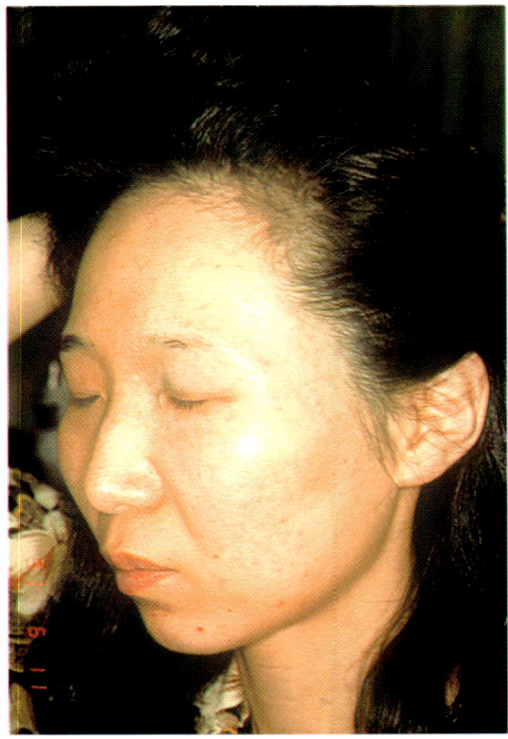

Fig. 20.3.9². Postoperative lateral view. 3 years and 5 months after the fourth cryosurgical session

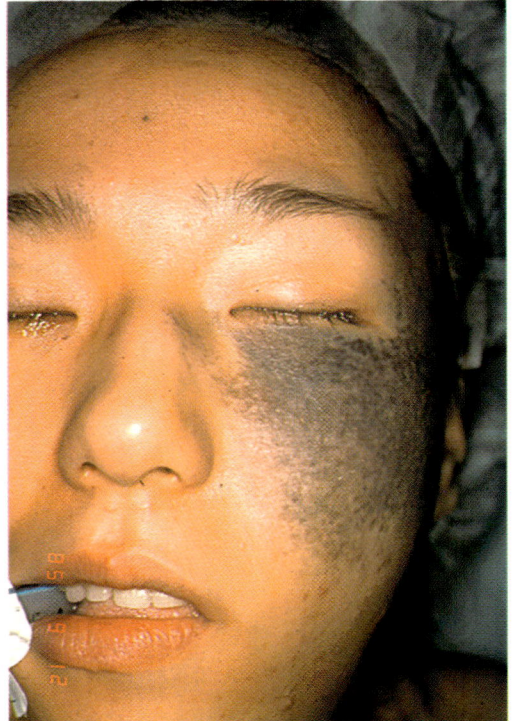

Fig. 20.3.10². A 21-year-old woman patient with nevus Ota. Preoperative frontal view. Intensive pigmentation spread over the zygomatic region

Section F Clinical Aspects 463

Chapter 20
Cosmetic
Cryosurgery

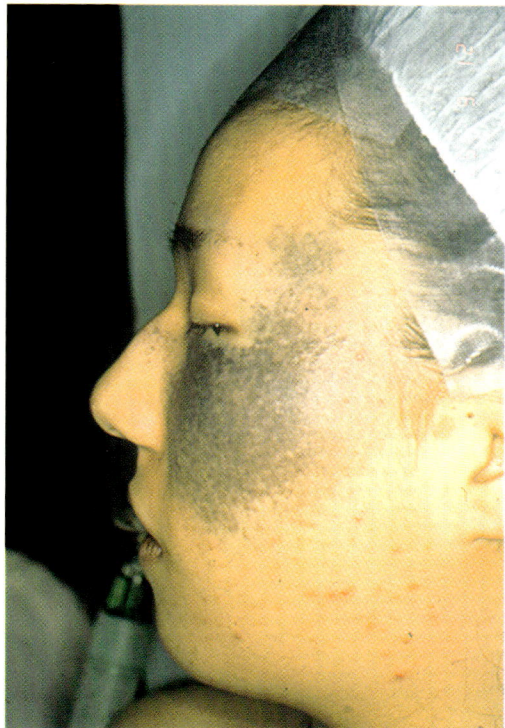

Fig. 20.3.11². Preoperative lateral view

Fig. 20.3.12². Postoperative lateral view. 6 months after the first cryosurgical session

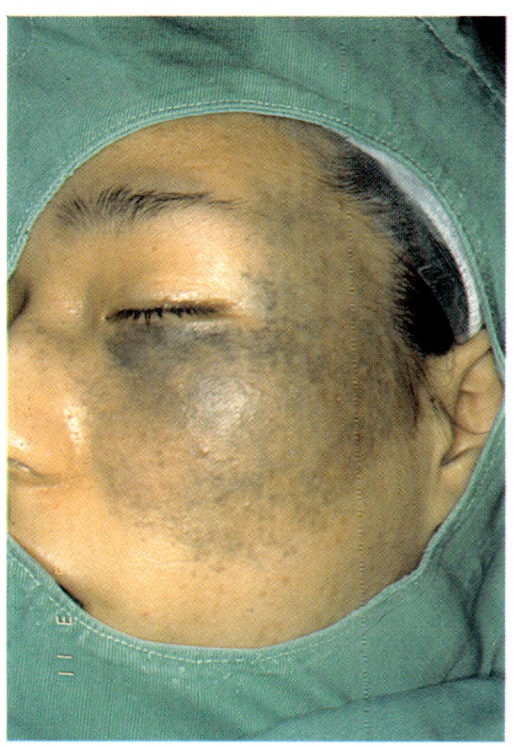

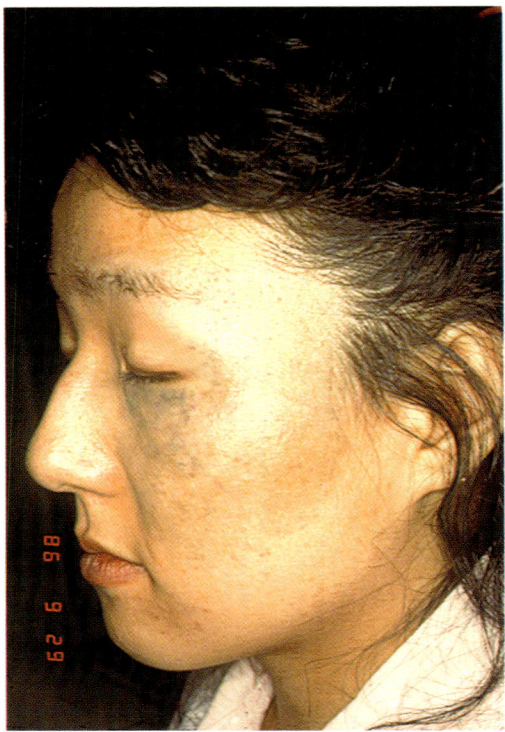

Fig. 20.3.13². Postoperative lateral view. 6 months after the second cryosurgical session

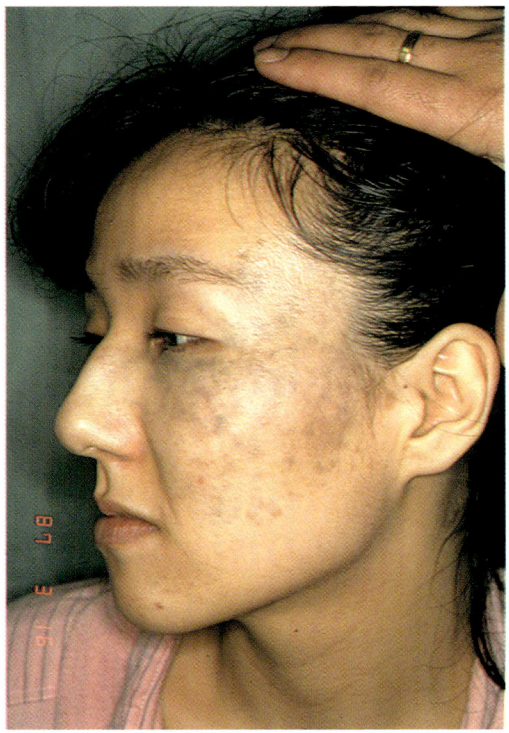

Fig. 20.3.14². Postoperative lateral view. 6 months after the third cryosurgical session

Section F   Clinical Aspects   465

Chapter 20
Cosmetic
Cryosurgery

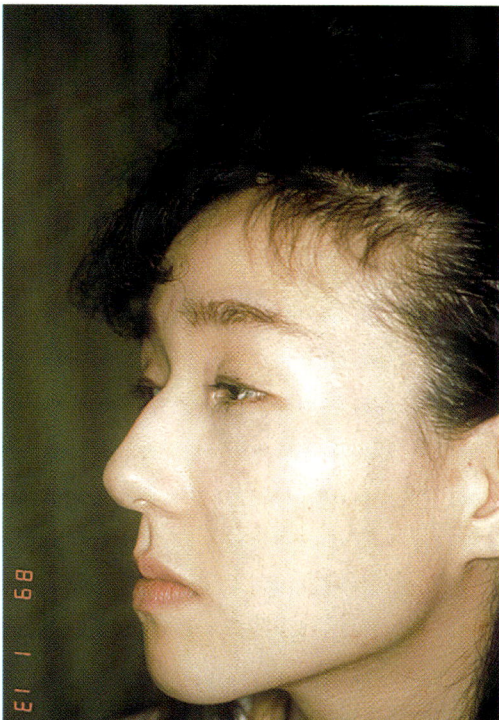

Fig. 20.3.15². Postoperative lateral view. 1 year and 10 months after the fourth cryosurgical session

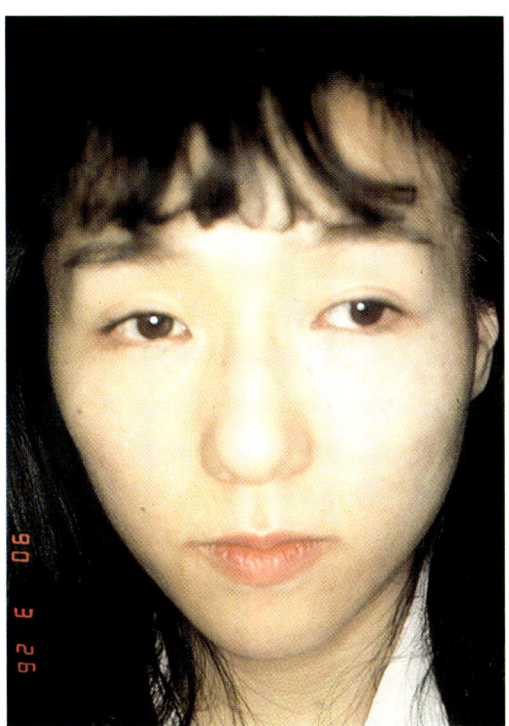

Fig. 20.3.16². Postoperative frontal view. 3 years after the fourth cryosurgical session

Chapter 20
Cosmetic
Cryosurgery

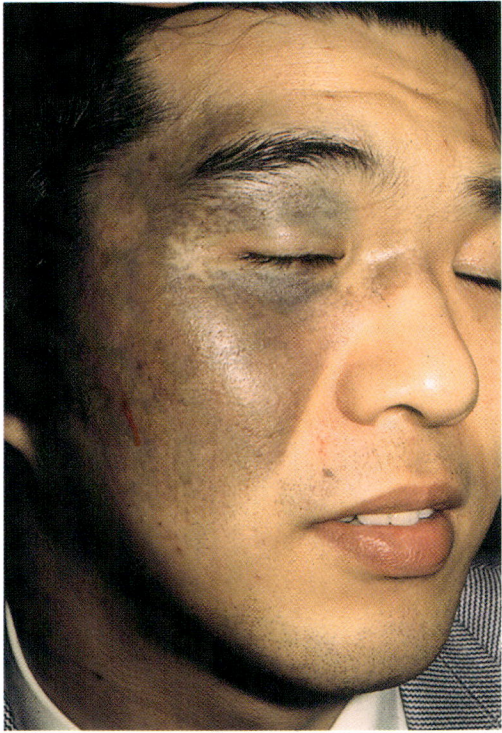

Fig. 20.3.17[2]. A 26-year-old man with nevus Ota. The distribution of pigmentation was the same as in the first patient

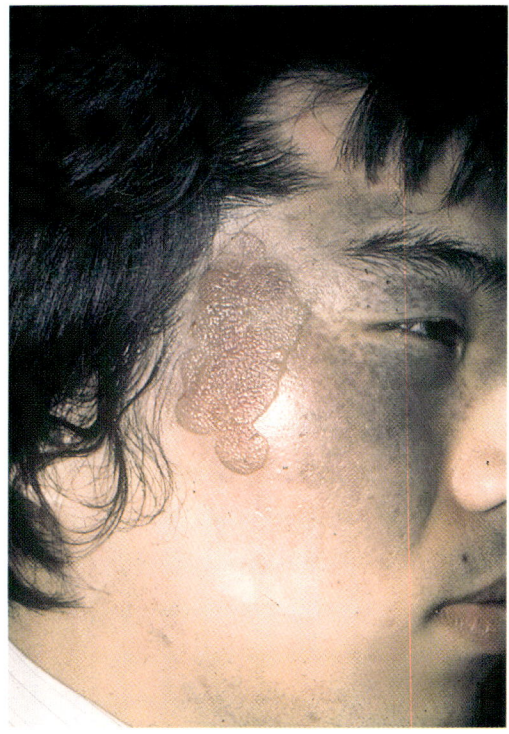

Fig. 20.3.18[2]. Lateral view showing the bulla formed after trial applications of the cryoprobe

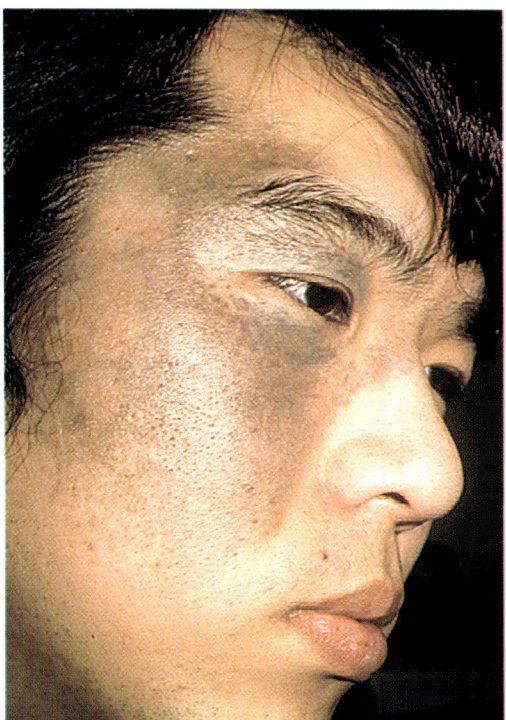

Fig. 20.3.19². Postoperative lateral view. 3 months after the trial application

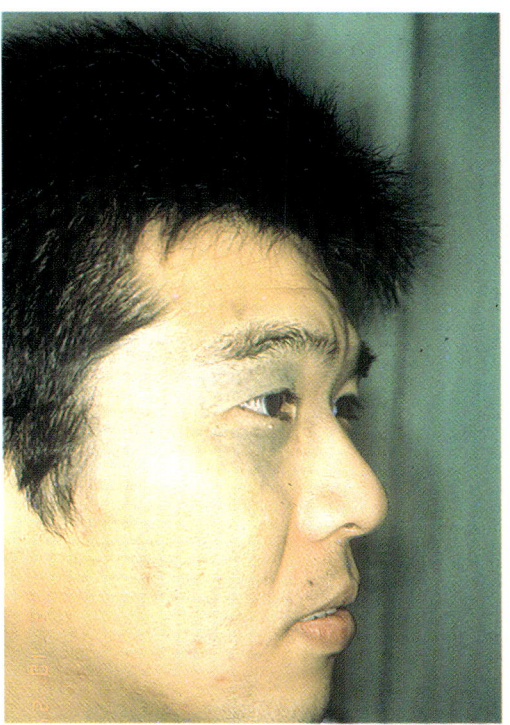

Fig. 20.3.20². Postoperative lateral view. 2 years and 5 months after the second cryosurgical session

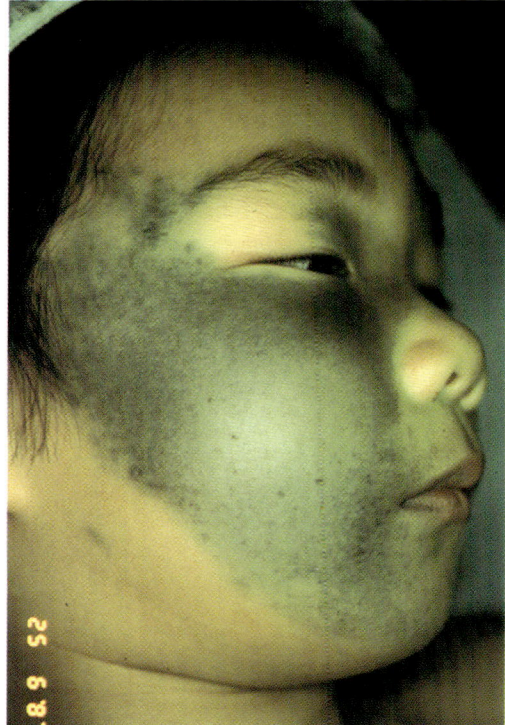

Fig. 20.3.21[2]. A 6-year-old boy with nevus Ota. This is a special case in which slate-bluish pigmentation extended from the zygomatic region to the cheek and maxillary region. Preoperative lateral view

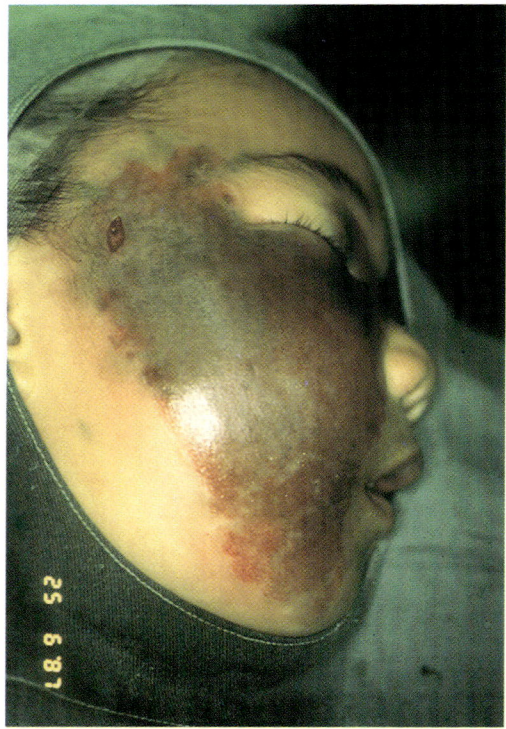

Fig. 20.3.22[2]. Postoperative lateral view after dermabrasion in the first cryosurgical session

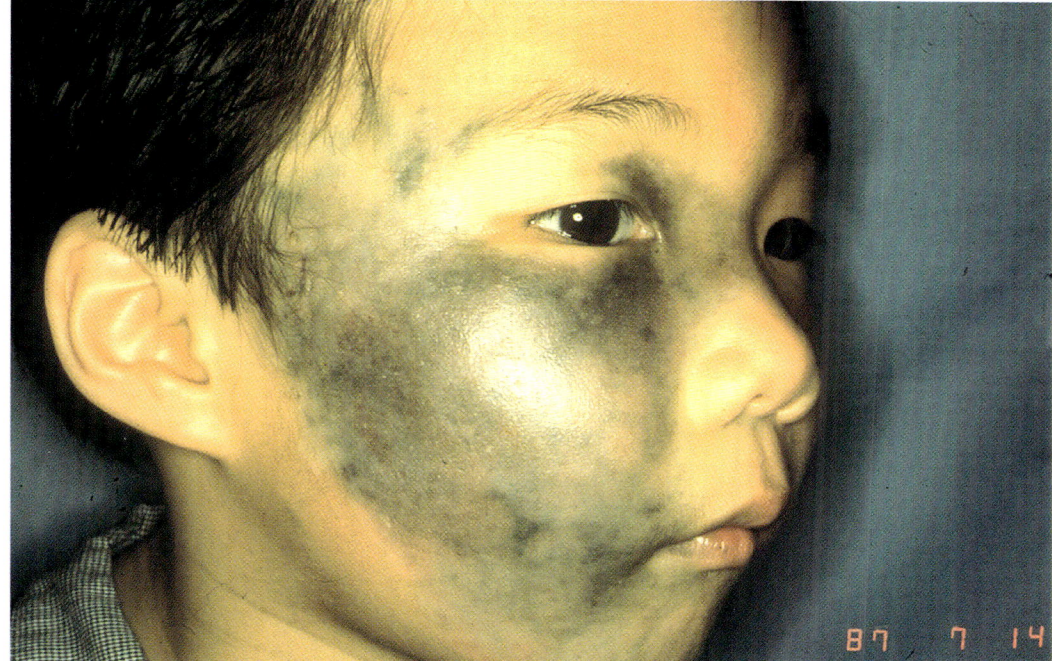

Fig. 20.3.23². Postoperative lateral view. 3 weeks after the first cryosurgical session

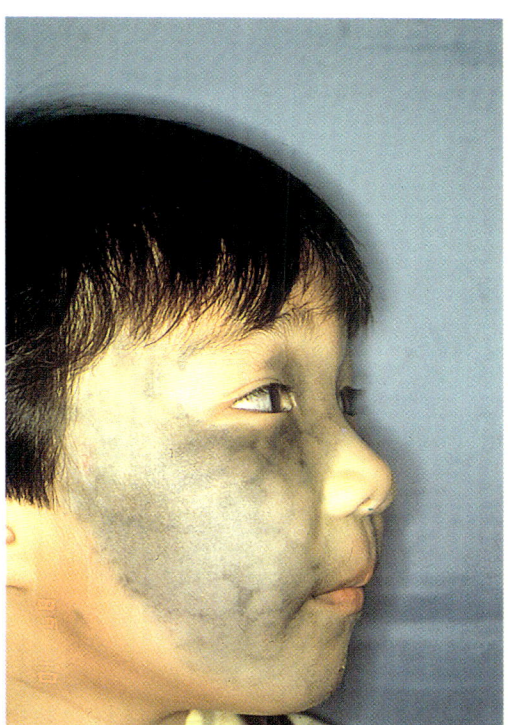

Fig. 20.3.24². Postoperative lateral view. 3 months after the first cryosurgical session

Chapter 20
Cosmetic
Cryosurgery

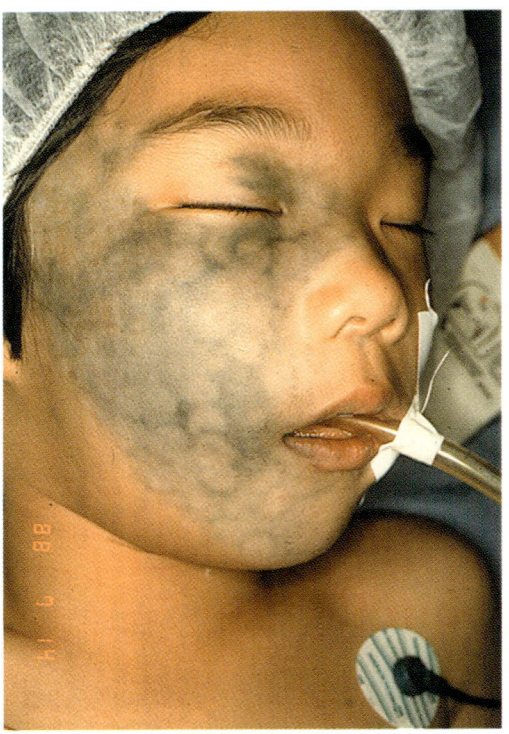

Fig. 20.3.25[2]. Postoperative lateral view.
7 months after the third cryosurgical session

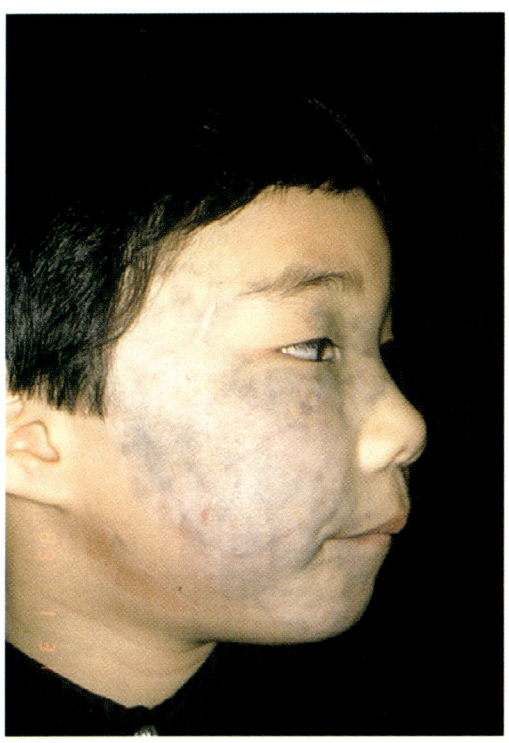

Fig. 20.3.26[2]. Postoperative lateral view.
2 months after the fourth cryosurgical session

Chapter 20
Cosmetic Cryosurgery

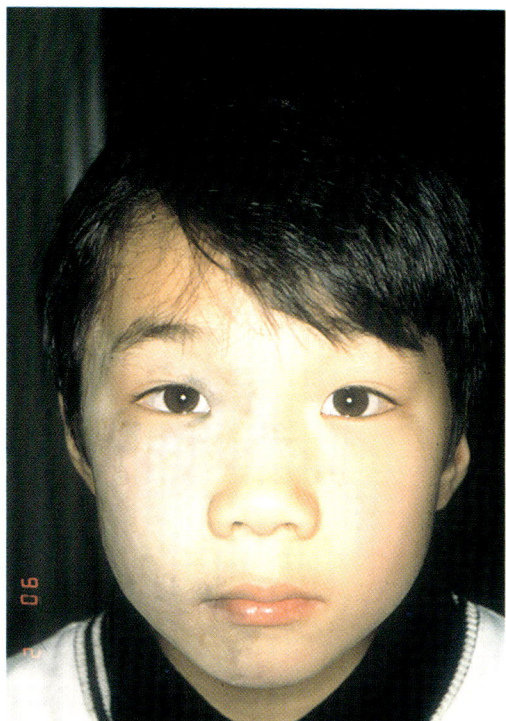

Fig. 20.3.27[2]. Postoperative frontal view. 9 months after the fifth cryosurgical session

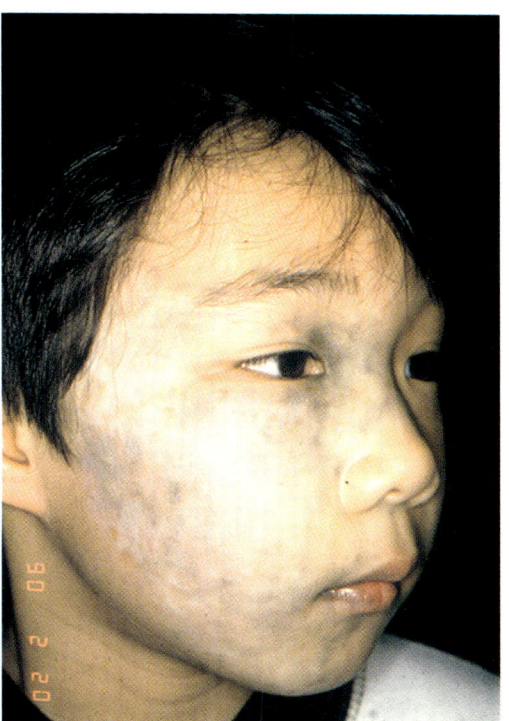

Fig. 20.3.28[2]. Postoperative lateral view. 9 months after the fifth cryosurgical session

Chapter 20
Cosmetic
Cryosurgery

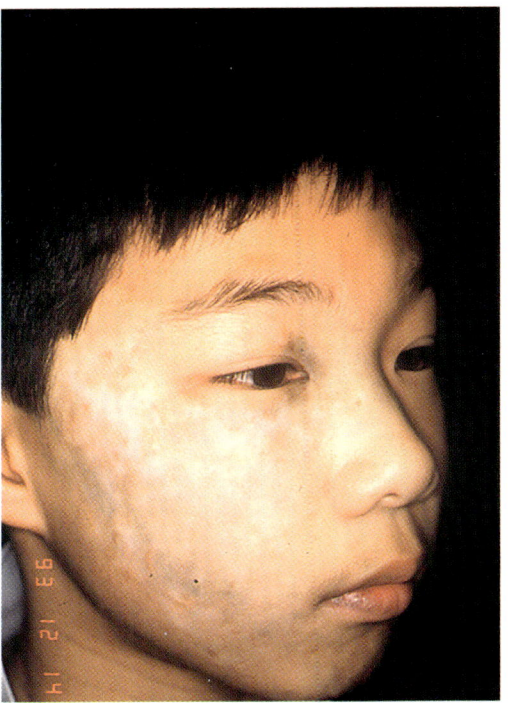

Fig. 20.3.29². Postoperative lateral view. 4 years and 7 months after the fifth cryosurgical session

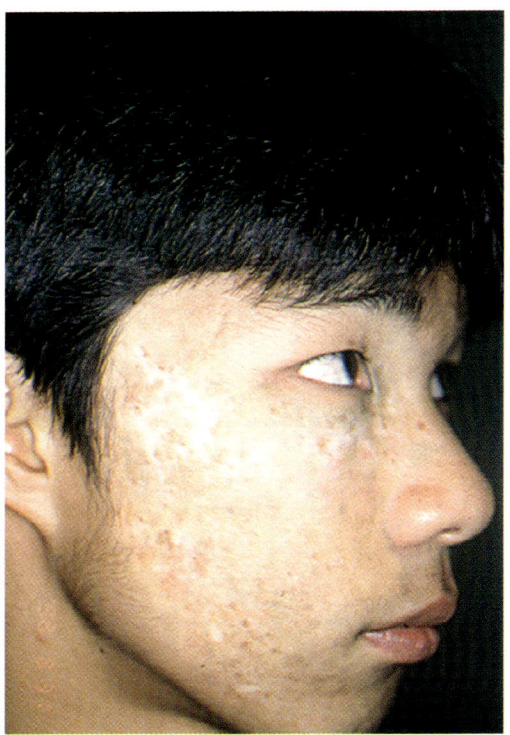

Fig. 20.3.30². Postoperative lateral view. 9 years and 3 months after the fifth cryosurgical session

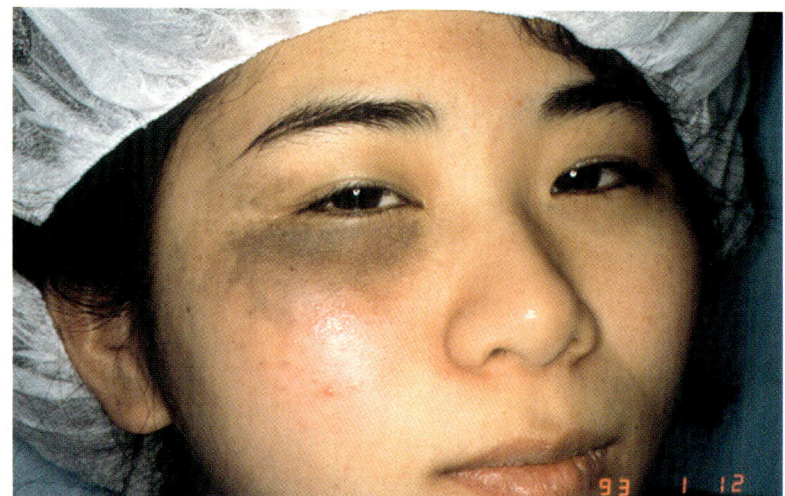

Fig. 20.3.31[2]. A 23-year-old woman with nevus Ota. Postoperative frontal view. After the first cryosurgical session

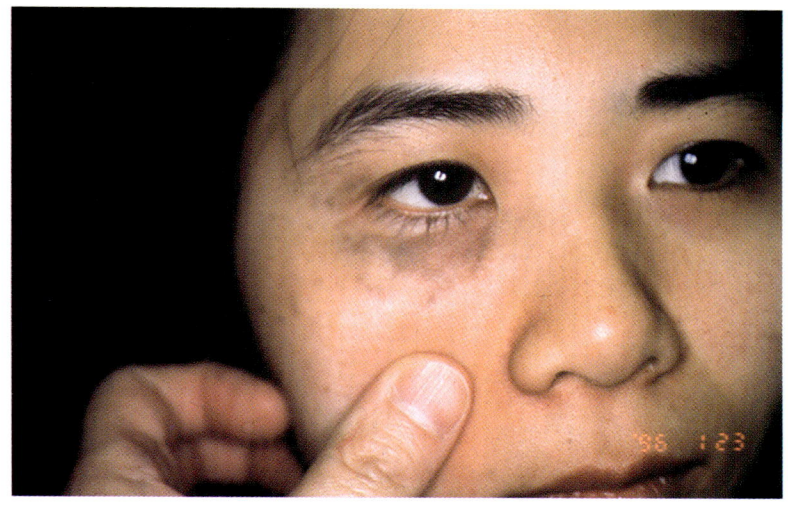

Fig. 20.3.32[2]. Postoperative frontal view. After the second cryosurgical session

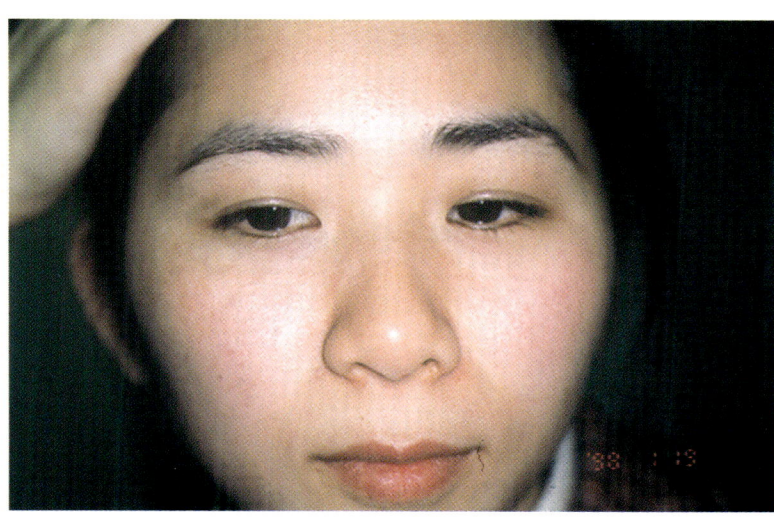

Fig. 20.3.33[2]. Postoperative frontal view. 6 months after Q-switched ruby laser irradiation (3 times)

Chapter 21

Cryosurgical Otorhynolaryngology

Nikolai N. Korpan[1] with contributions by Marco Scala[2]

21.1 Benign Neoplasms

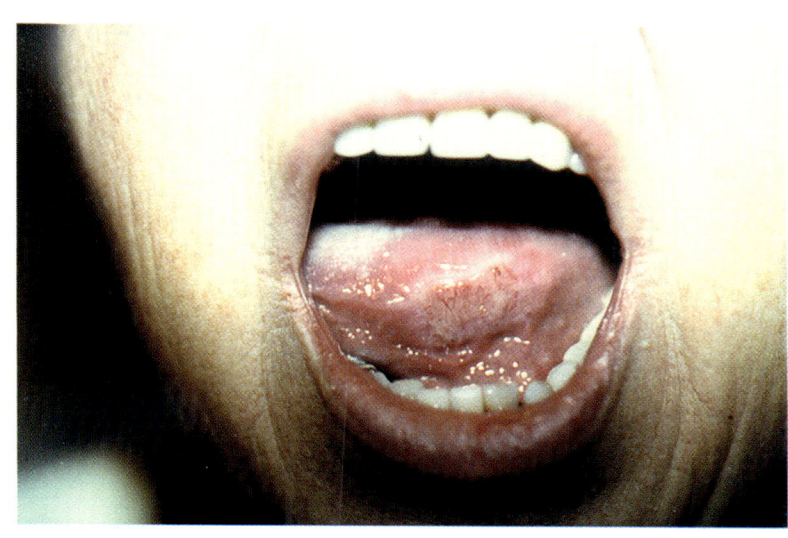

Fig. 21.1.1[1] (*right*). Preoperative view of the leukoplakia on the left side of the tongue in a 63-year-old woman

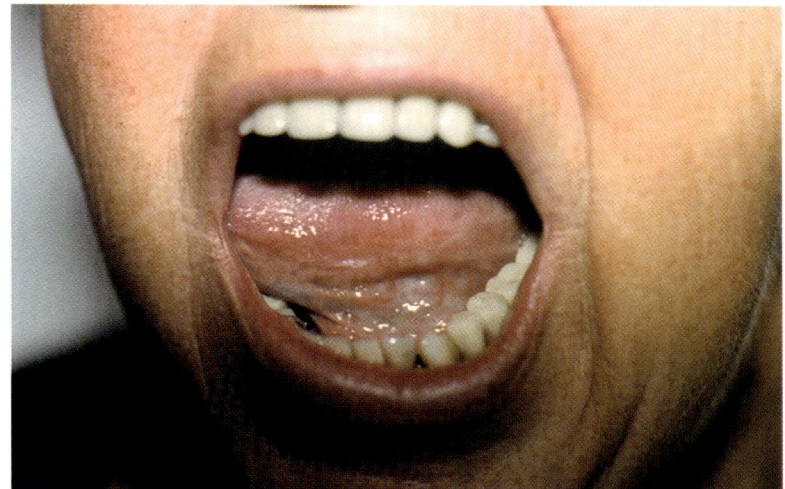

Fig. 21.1.2[1] (*left*). 1 month after a cryosurgical operation on the tongue with complete response to treatment

Fig. 21.1.3[1]. Excellent result 5 years after cryosurgical treatment (**A**, **B**). The patient is disease-free

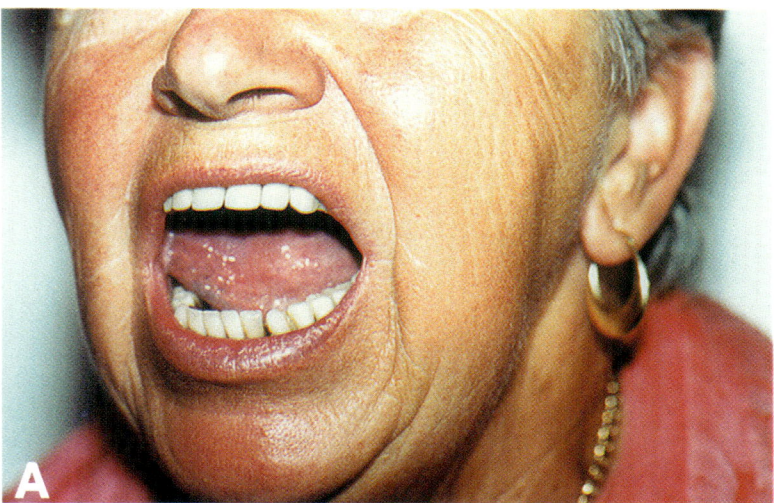
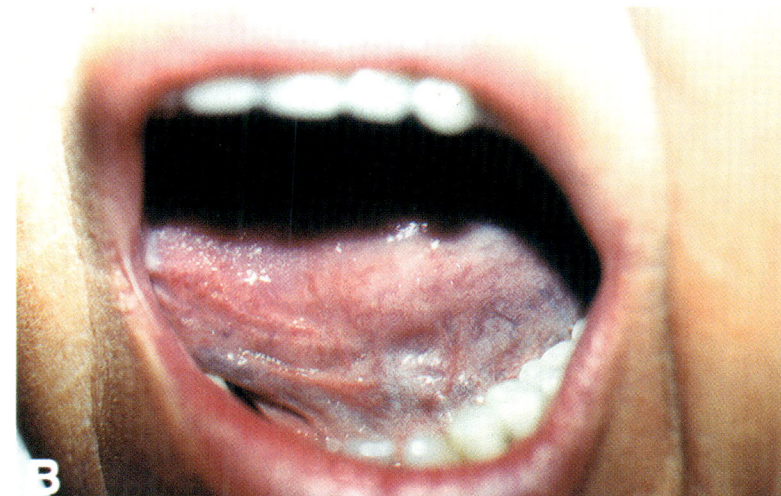

Chapter 21
Cryosurgical Otorhynolaryngology

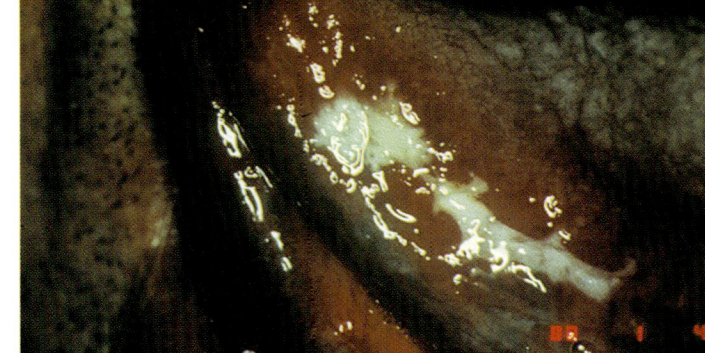

Fig. 21.1.4². Leukoplakia of left side of the tongue

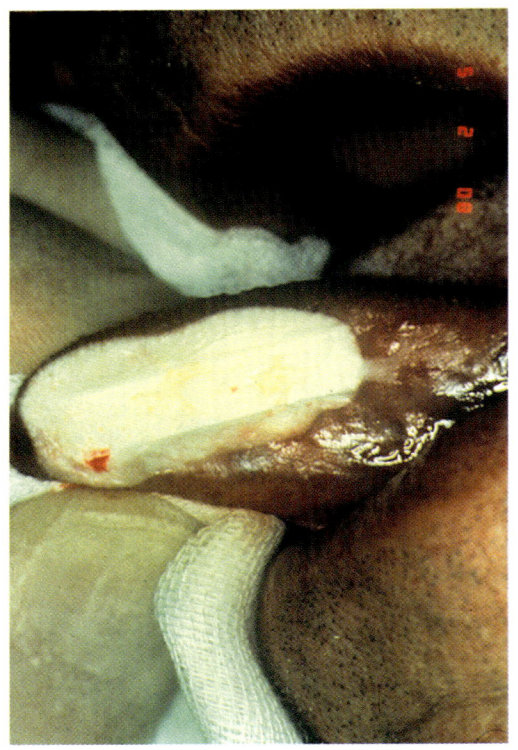

Fig. 21.1.5². Ice ball immediately after cryosurgical treatment

Section F   Clinical Aspects   477

Chapter 21
Cryosurgical
Otorhyno-
laryngology

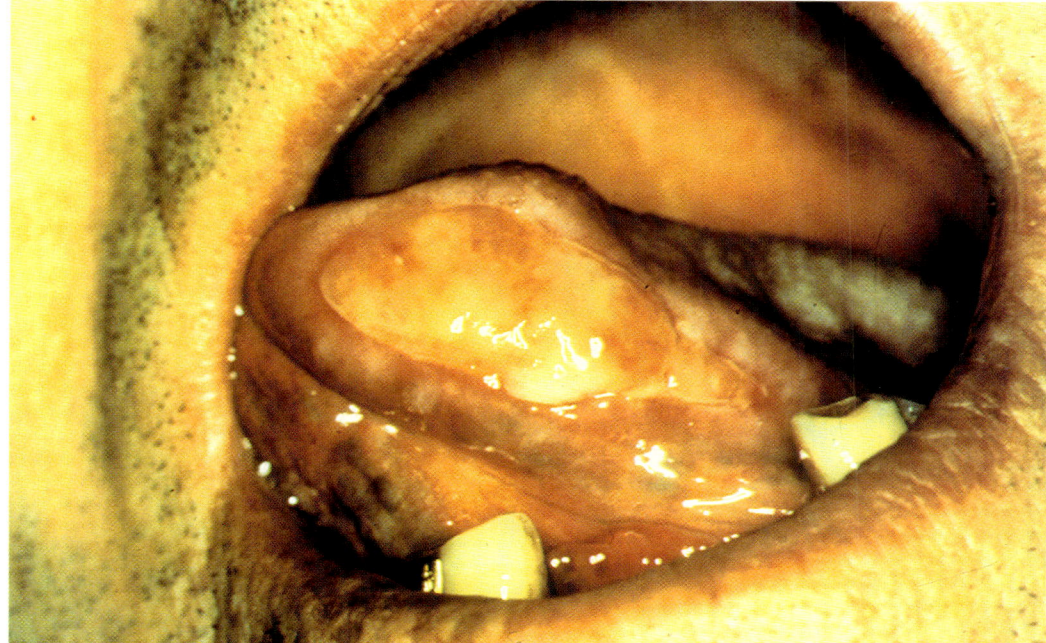

Fig. 21.1.6². A patient seven days after cryosurgical treatment

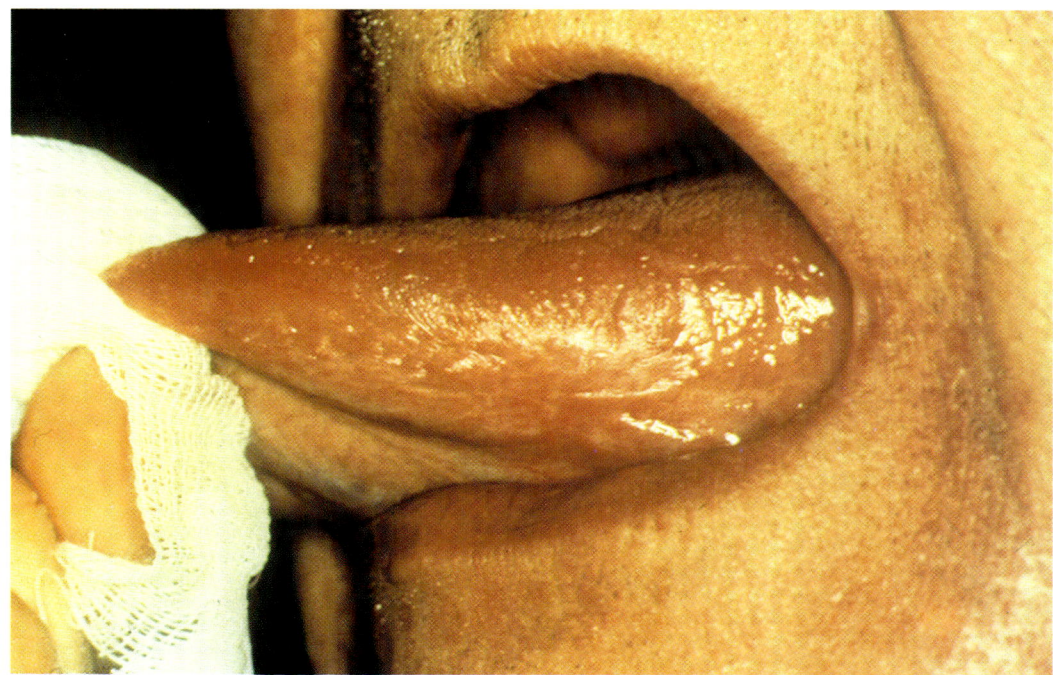

Fig. 21.1.7². One month after treatment; complete response to cryosurgery

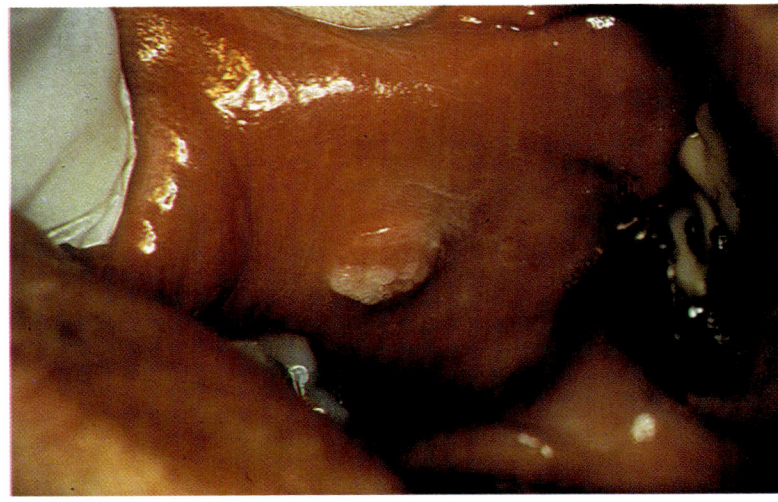

Fig. 21.1.8². Verrucous leukoplakia of the right cheek

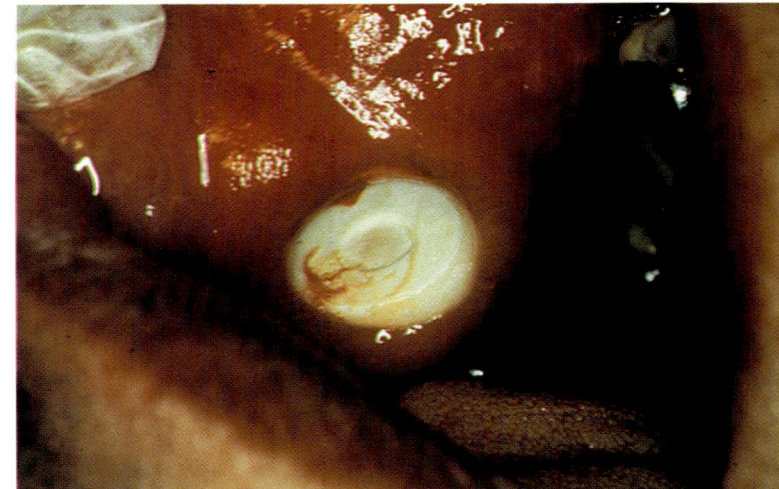

Fig. 21.1.9². Ice ball after cryosurgical treatment

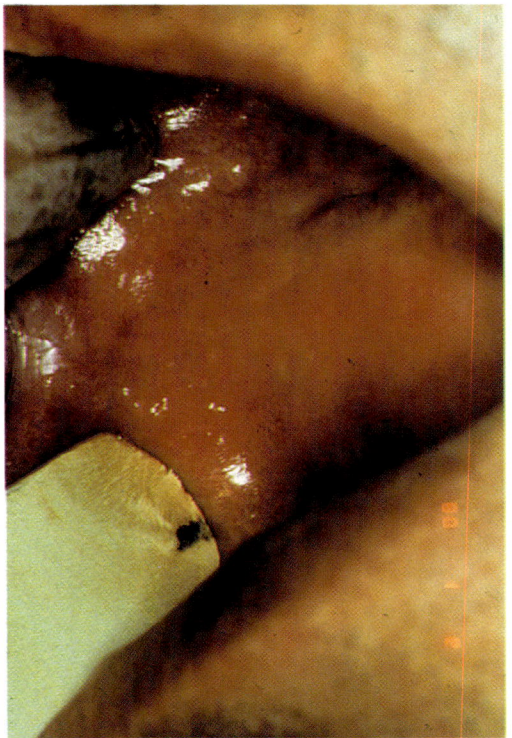

Fig. 21.1.10². Restitutio ad integrum one month after cryosurgical treatment

Chapter 21
Cryosurgical Otorhynolaryngology

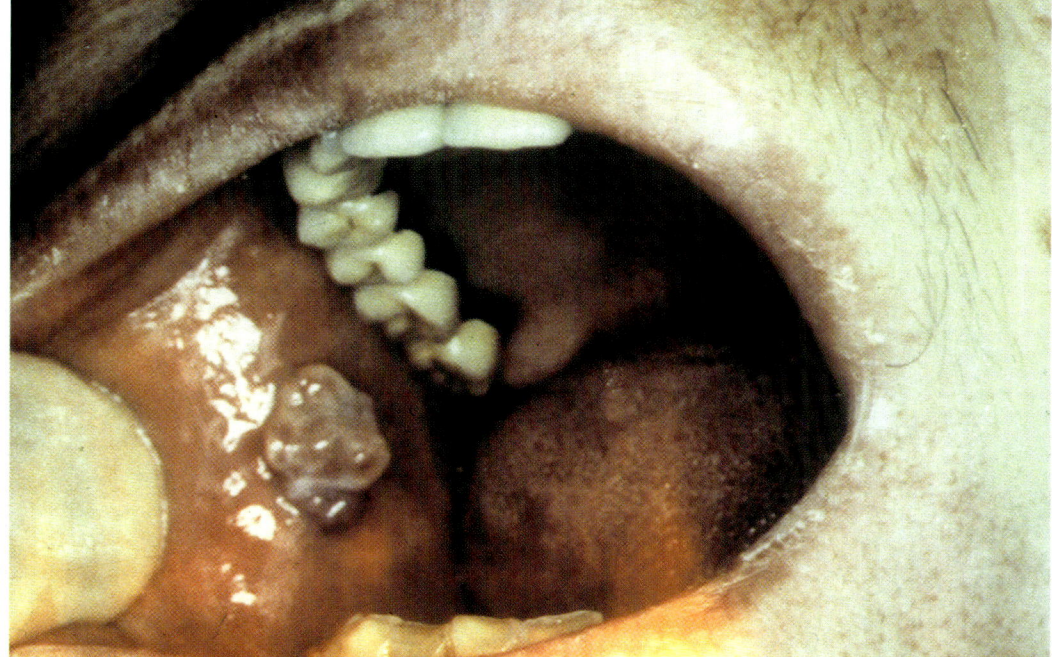

Fig. 21.1.11[2]. Leukoplakia of the right cheek

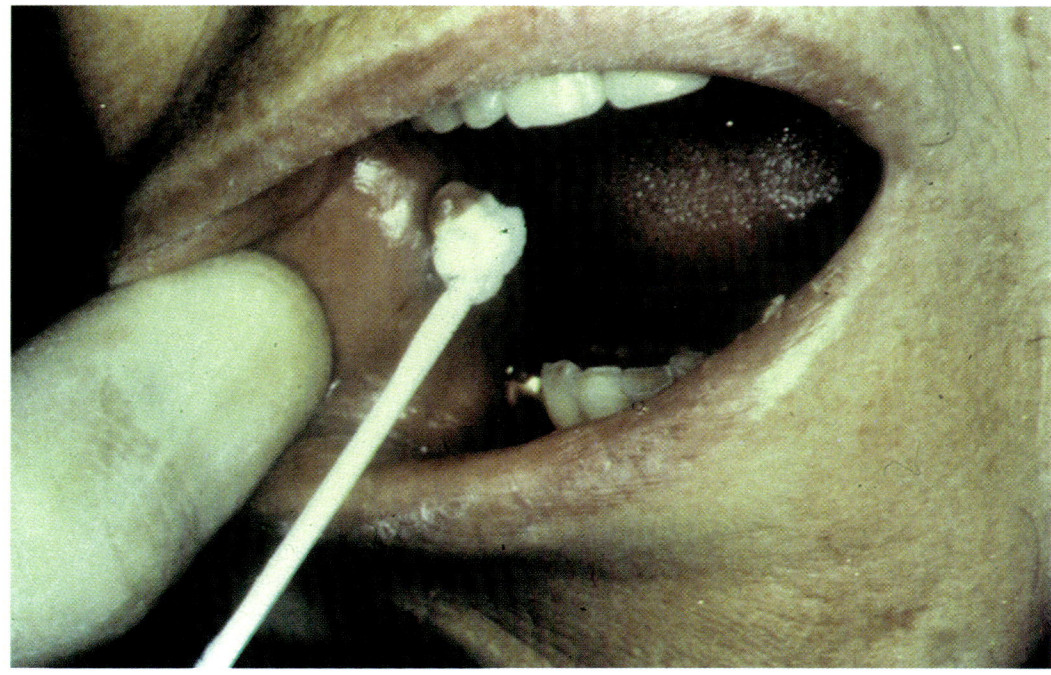

Fig. 21.1.12[2]. The same patient after toluidine blue coloring

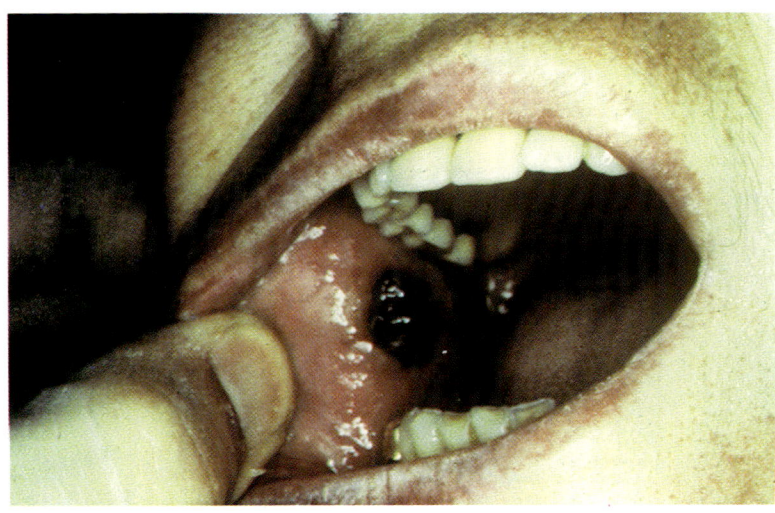

Fig. 21.1.13². Ice ball covers entire lesion

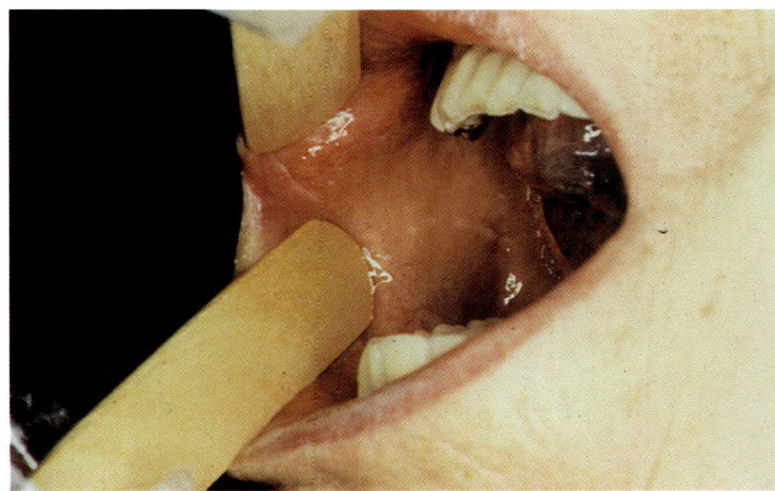

Fig. 21.1.14². The lesion seven days after cryosurgical treatment

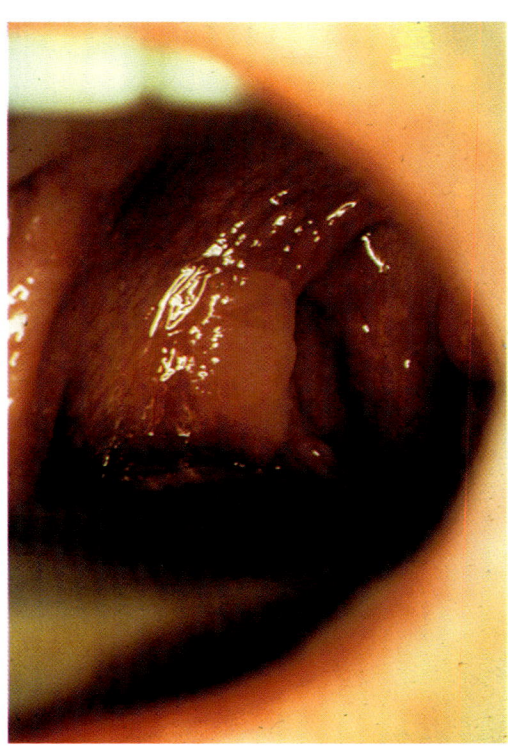

Fig. 21.1.15². Same patient six months after cryosurgery

Section F Clinical Aspects 481

Chapter 21
Cryosurgical
Otorhyno-
laryngology

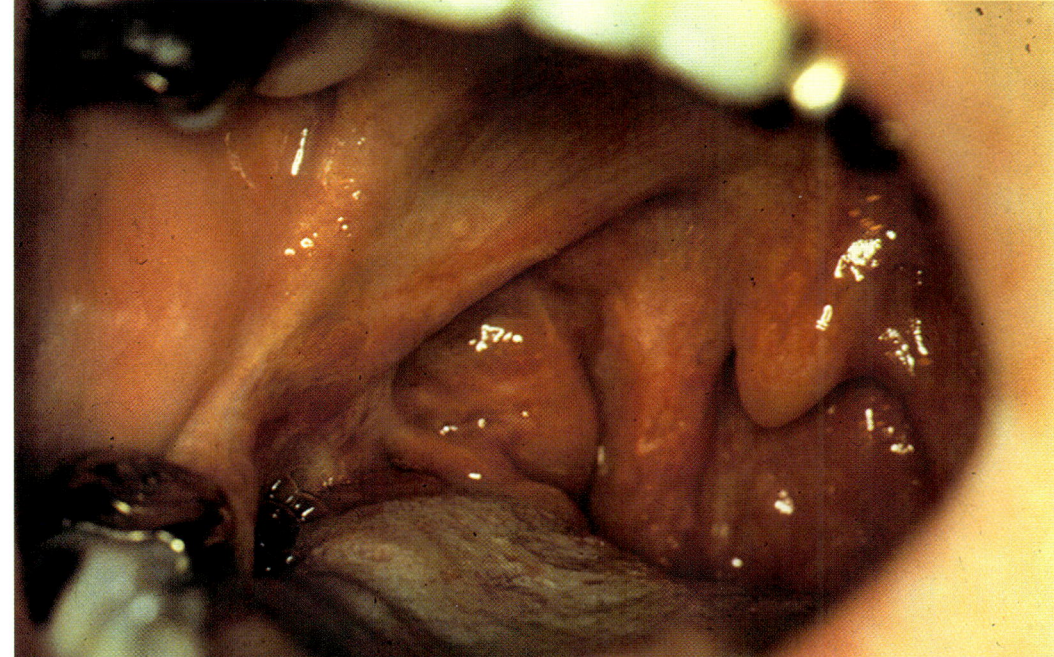

Fig. 21.1.16². Hemangiopericytoma of the right cheek

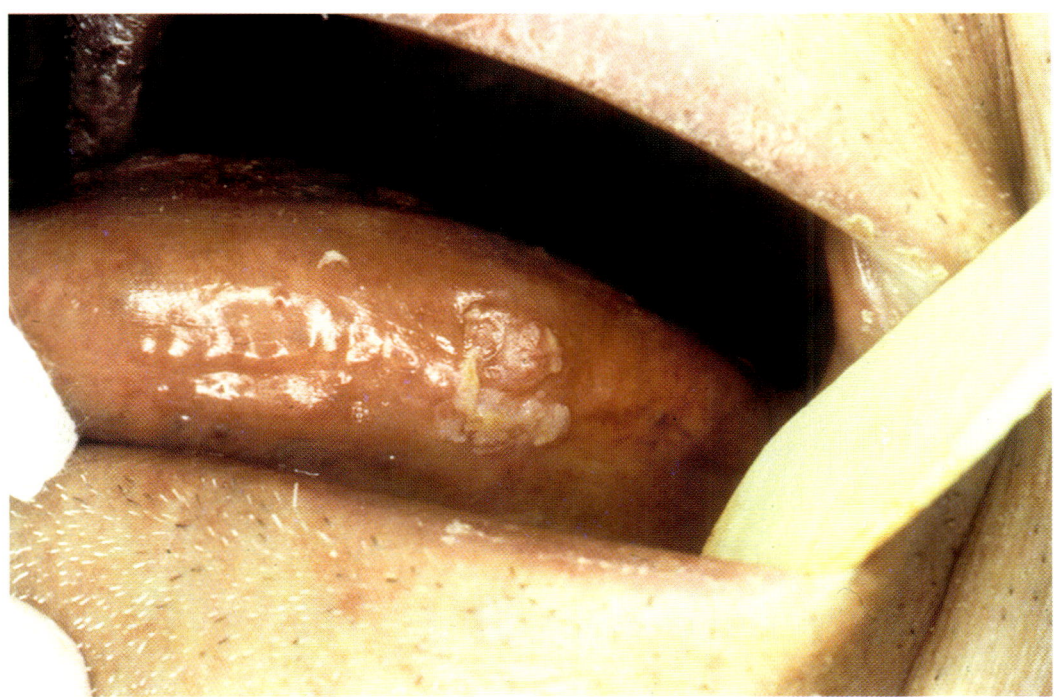

Fig. 21.1.17². Lesion during cryosurgical treatment

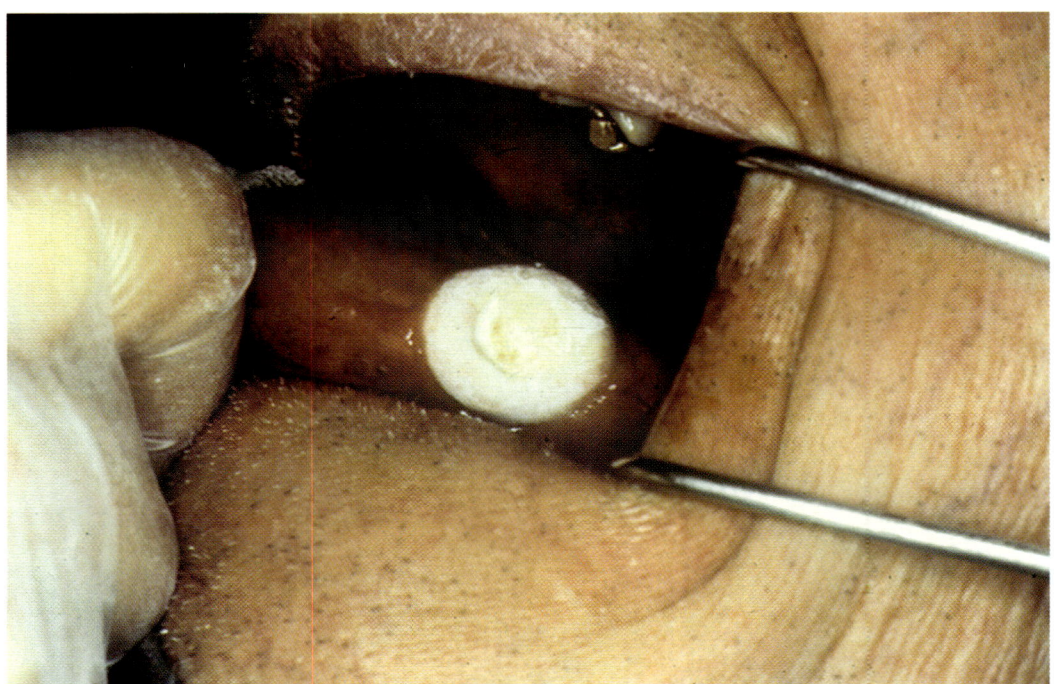

Fig. 21.1.18². Necrosis five days after treatment

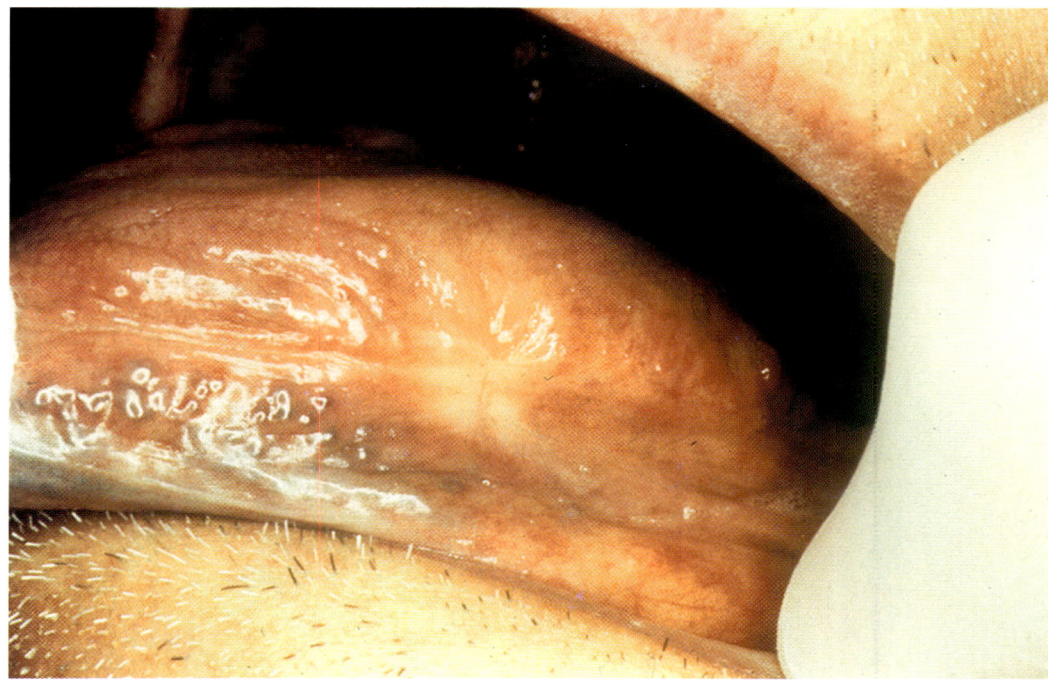

Fig. 21.1.19². Complete response 1 month after cryosurgical treatment

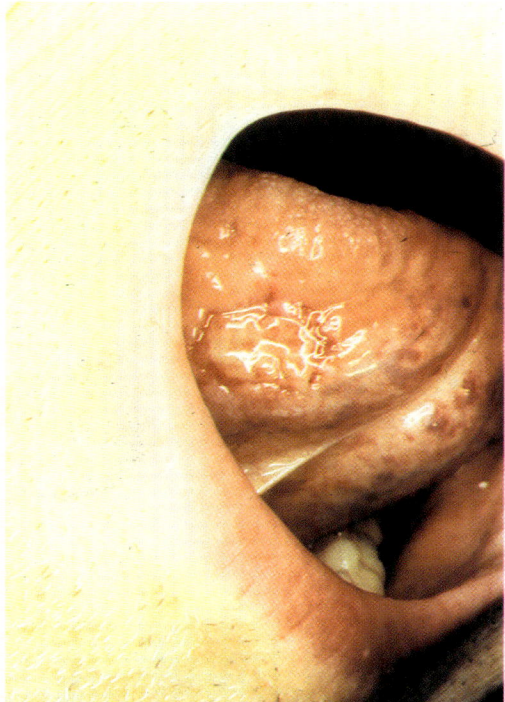

Fig. 21.1.20². Serious dysplasia of the anterior faucial pilar of the tonsillar fossa

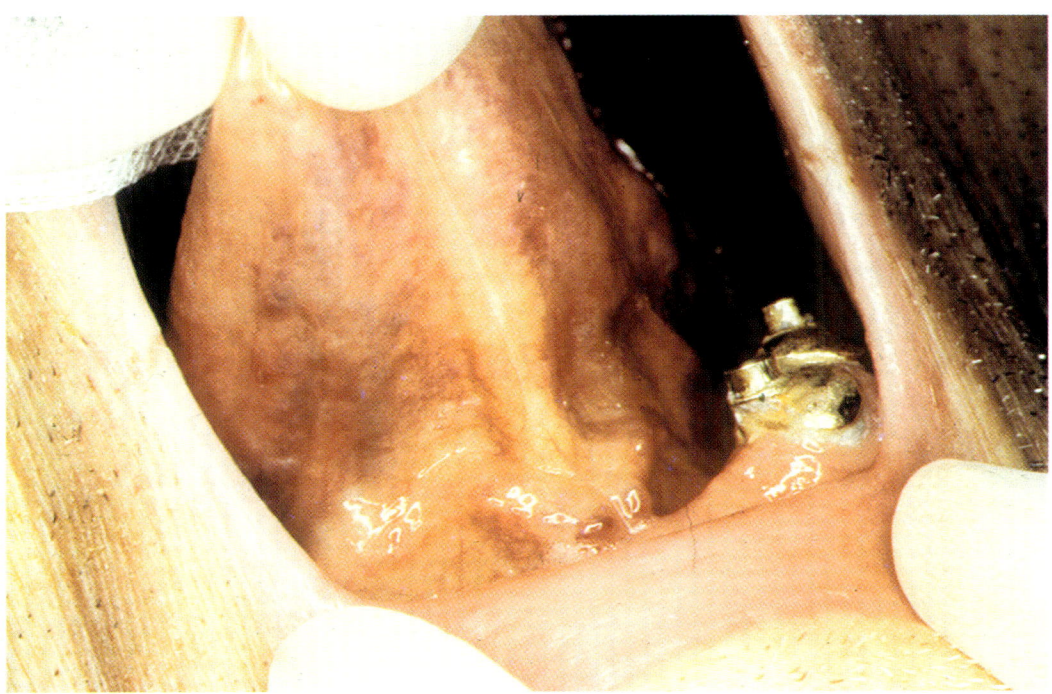

Fig. 21.1.21². Lesion twenty days after cryosurgical treatment

21.2 Malignant Tumors

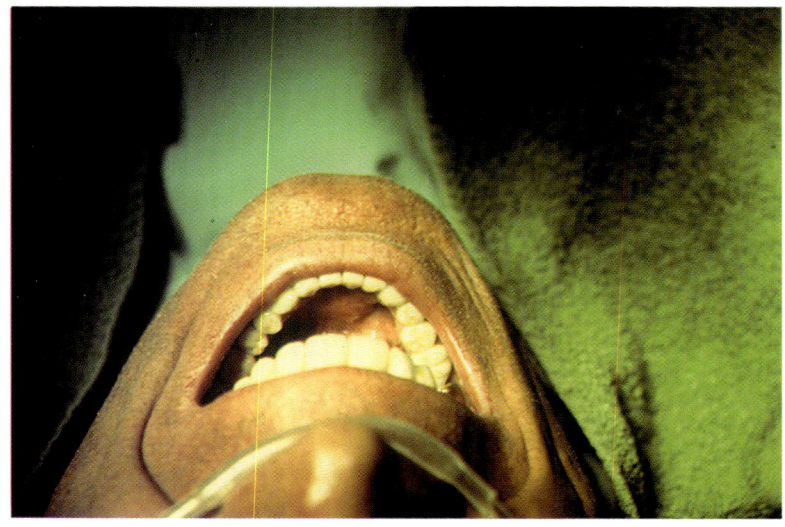

Fig. 21.2.1[1]. Recurrence of the carcinoma of the floor of the mouth of a 71-year-old man. Preoperative view

Fig. 21.2.2[1]. Cryosurgical treatment using a disc cryoprobe 20 mm in diameter which is placed on the tumor mass of the floor of the mouth at a temperature of −180°C for 3 min. A single freeze-thaw cycle is used for the complete destruction of the tumor mass

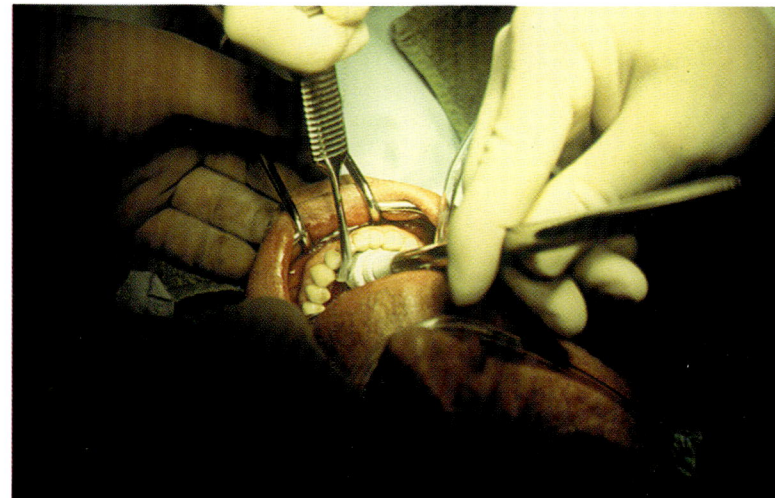

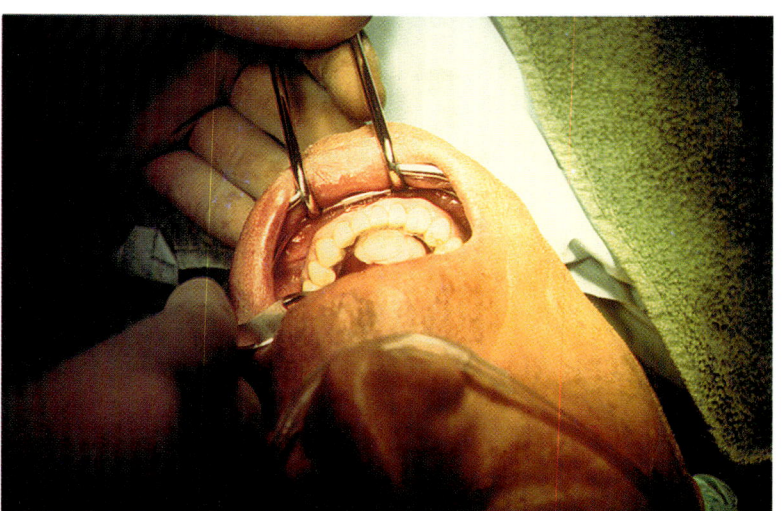

Fig. 21.2.3[1]. Post-cryosurgical appearance of the malignant lesion of the floor of the mouth immediately after the cryosurgical session. After cryosurgery, no local recurrence after a 2-year observation period

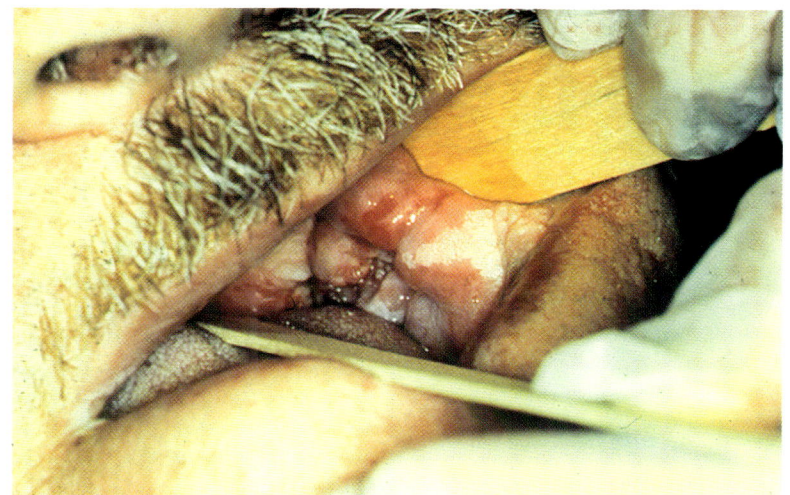

Fig. 21.2.4². Squamous cell carcinoma of the left side of the tongue $T_1N_0M_0$

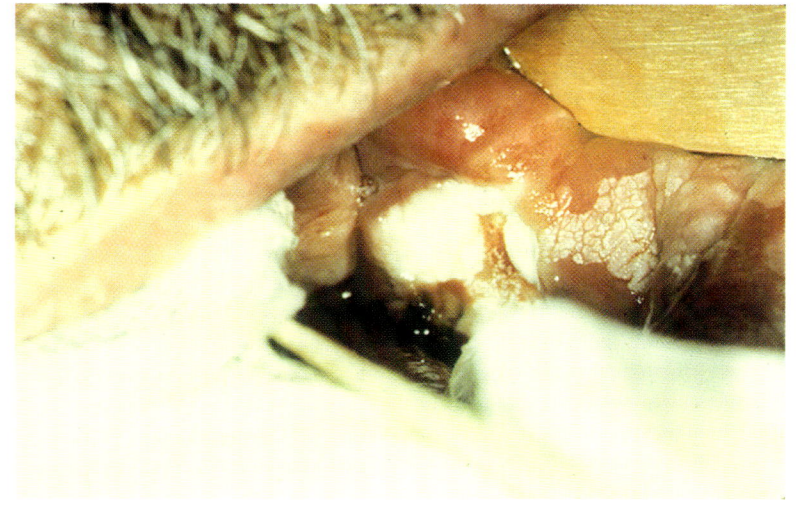

Fig. 21.2.5². The ice ball covers the entire lesion

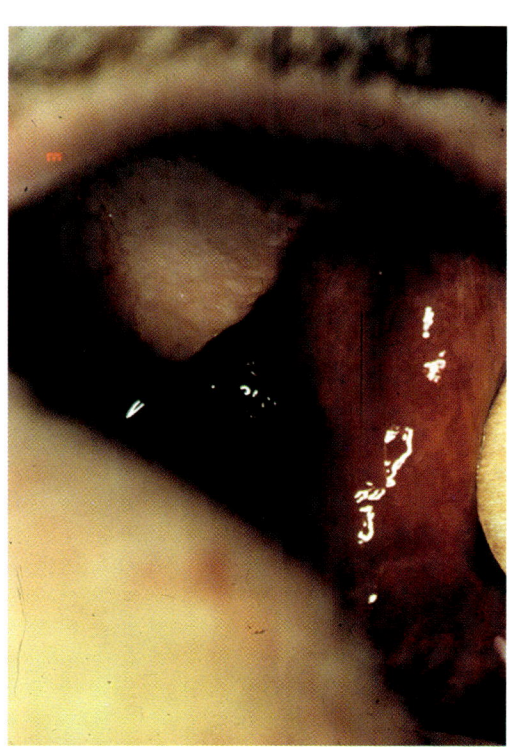

Fig. 21.2.6². Recovery two months after cryosurgery

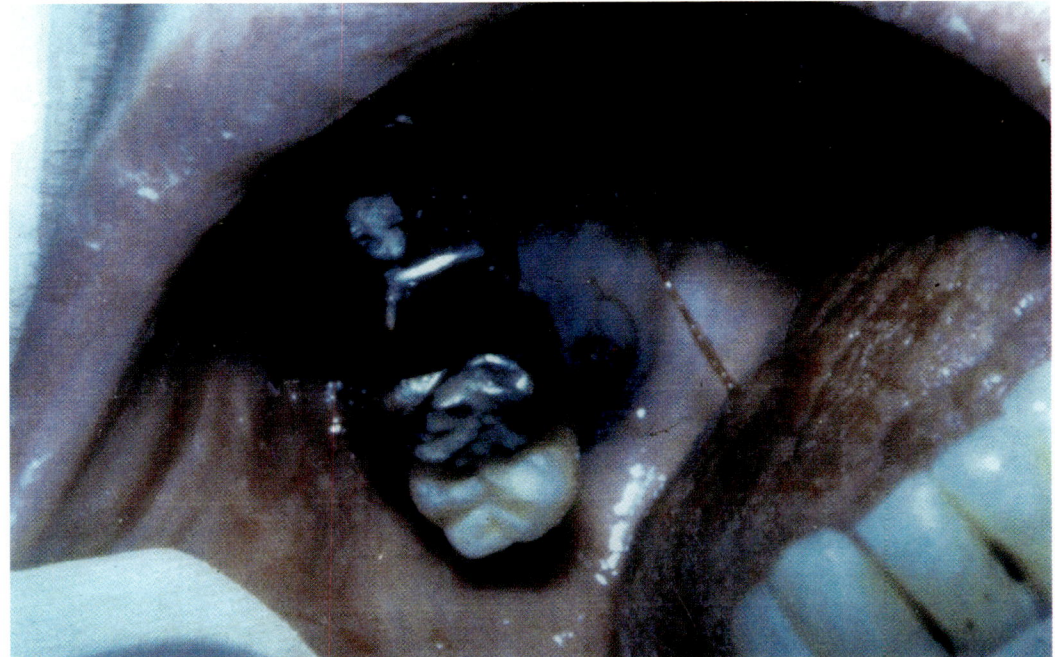

Fig. 21.2.7². Squamous cell carcinoma on the ventral surface of the tongue

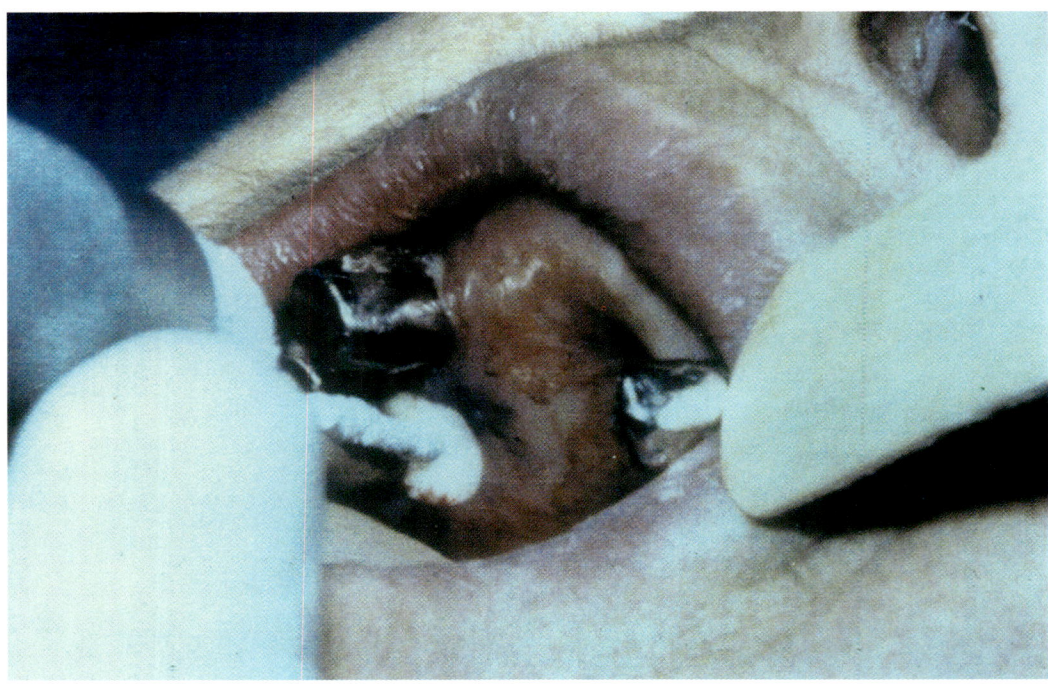

Fig. 21.2.8². Restitutio ad integrum one month after cryosurgical treatment

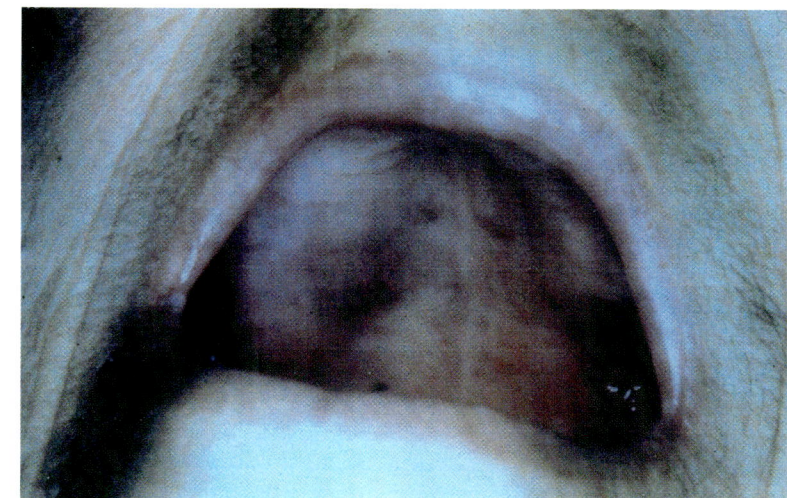

Fig. 21.2.9². Squamous cell carcinoma of the left side of the cheek with anterior leukoplakia

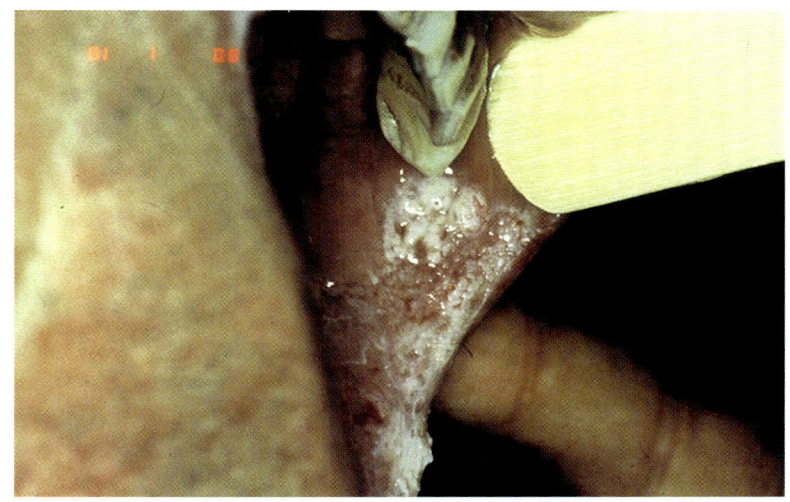

Fig. 21.2.10². Single cryosurgical session, same patient as below

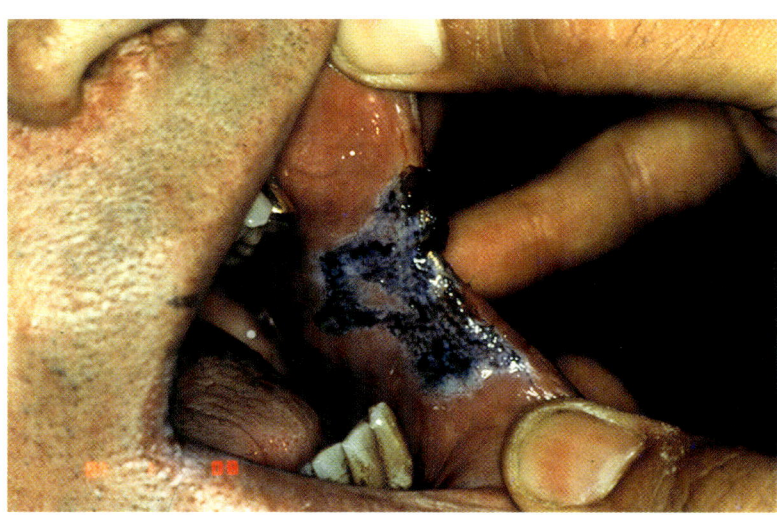

Fig. 21.2.11². The same patient three months after treatment: lesion disappeared and there was restitutio ad integrum of the tissue

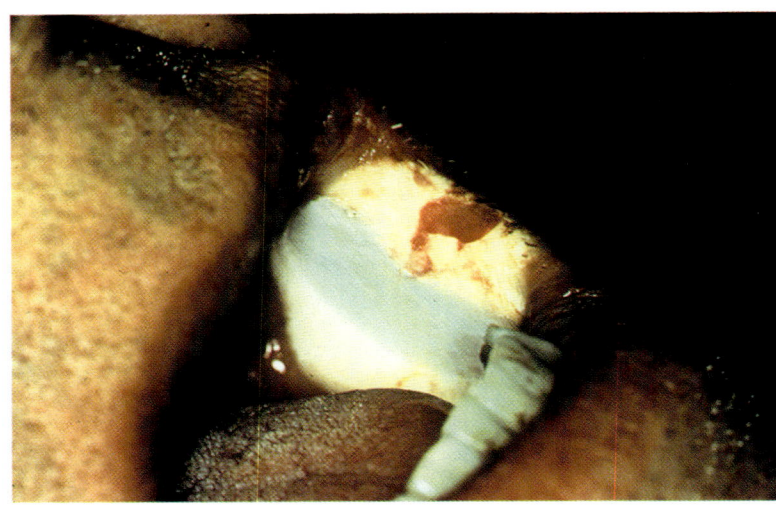

Fig. 21.2.12². Malignant mucous melanoma of the right hard palate and the bucco-alveolar sulci

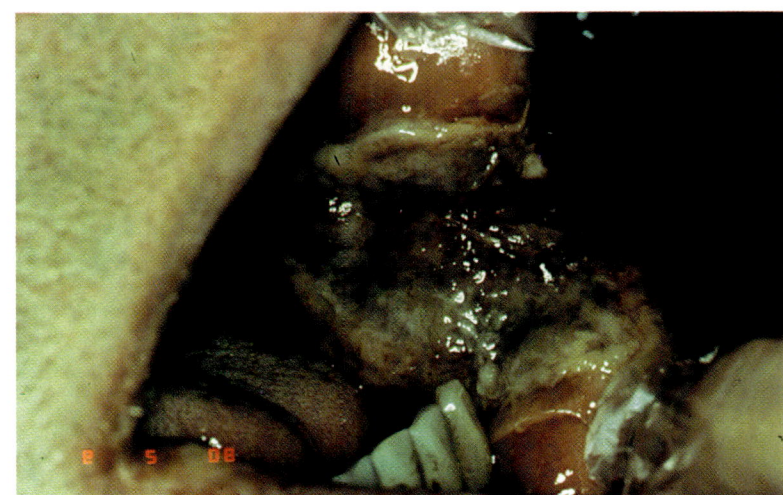

Fig. 21.2.13². The cryoprobe is inserted into the lesion

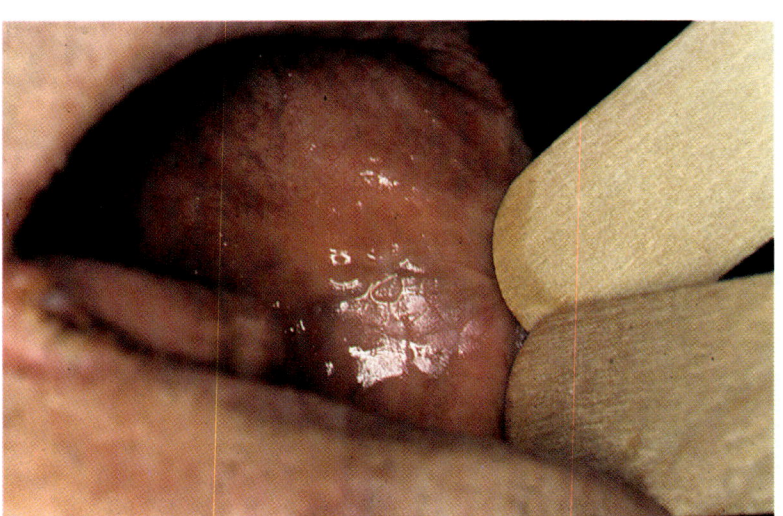

Fig. 21.2.14². The same case two months after cryosurgery (teeth fell out following treatment)

Cryophlebology

Patrick J.M. Le Pivert[1] and Laszlo Vizsy[2]

22.0 Introduction

The operating technique for treating primary varicosity has recently undergone a change. Subcutaneous cryosurgical methods are being used today, the use of an angiological cryoprobe being a fairly modern practice.

By using cryovaricectomy or cryo-stripping we can remove the dilated venous branches by making a 3–4 mm-wide incision in the skin and thus preserve the insufficient main vein.

The authors underline the importance of performing exact varicectomy. The basic operating technique includes crossectomy in the inquinal bend, stripping of insufficient saphenous vein and local removal of dilated collateral veins. This method has become standard medical practice in the author's surgical department since the spring of 1993.

The principal thing is to remove the main and collateral venous branches by means of an angiocryoprobe. After placing the freezing probe into the cavity of the saphenous vein and operating the pedal of the appliance, the surgeon can freeze it and then pull it out. The smaller branches can be pulled out through the 3–4 mm incision in the skin, and it is not necessary to place the probe into the cavity, as the branches freeze on the cryoprobe. The ruptured branches will coagulate as a result of the freezing effect and hematoma will be reduced.

Summarizing the experience the author acquired through performing 416 cryo-stripping operations over the past 4 years, it is evident that the cryovaricectomy (cryo-stripping) is an effective technique suitable for performing minimally invasive surgery; furthermore, the operation is less time-consuming, the esthetic-cosmetic results are the very best, the hospital stay is far shorter, the postoperative complications and the complaints of patients are by far fewer compared to conventional surgical techniques.

Chapter 22 Cryophlebology

22.1 Cryo-Stripping

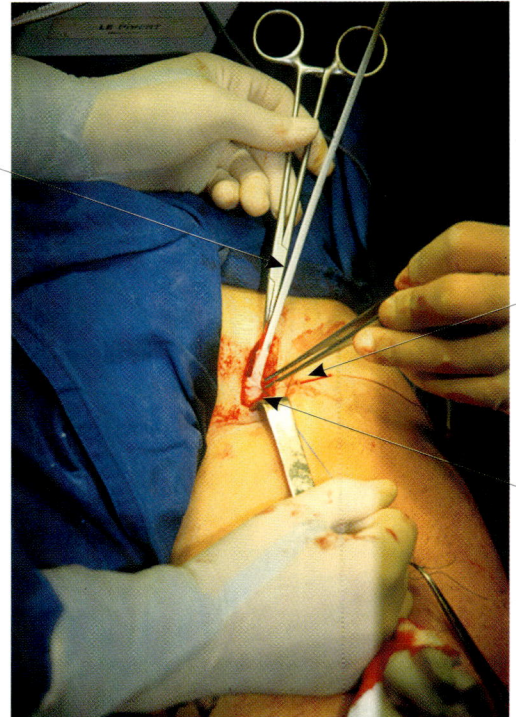

Cryoprobe catheterizing SM trunk at the SF junction

Fig. 22.1[1]. Vein cryo-obliteration. Part 1

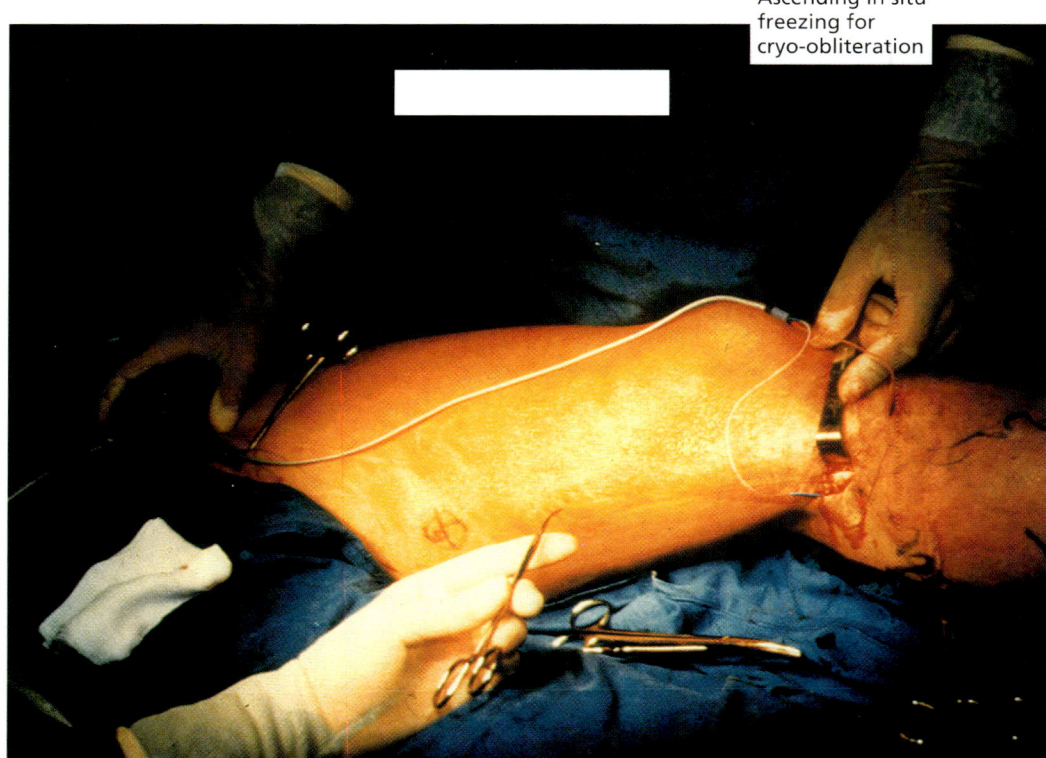

Ascending in situ freezing for cryo-obliteration

Fig. 22.2[1]. Vein cryo-obliteration. Part 2

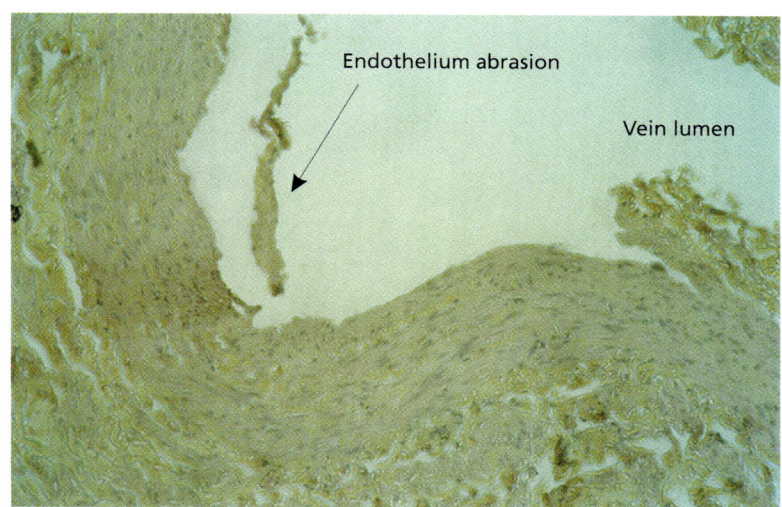

Fig. 22.3[1]. Histology: 6 to 36 hours after cryo-obliteration

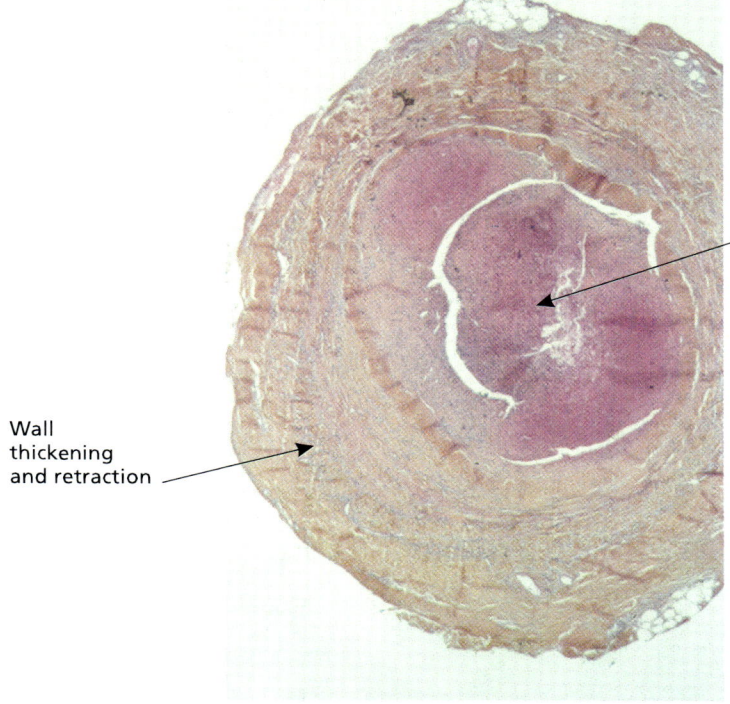

Fig. 22.4[1]. Histology: 80 days after cryosurgical treatment

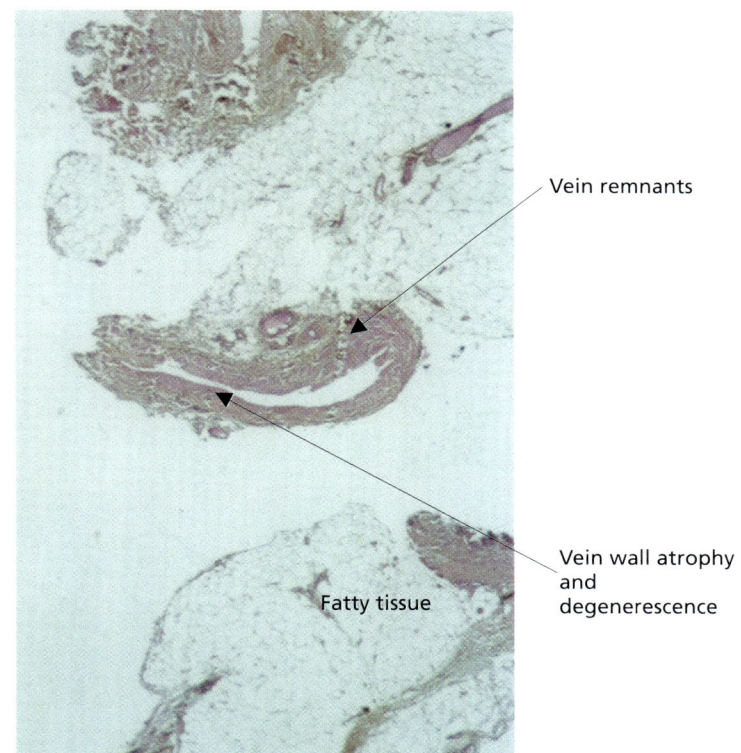

Fig. 22.5[1]. Histology: 8 months after cryosurgical treatment

Chapter 22
Cryophlebology

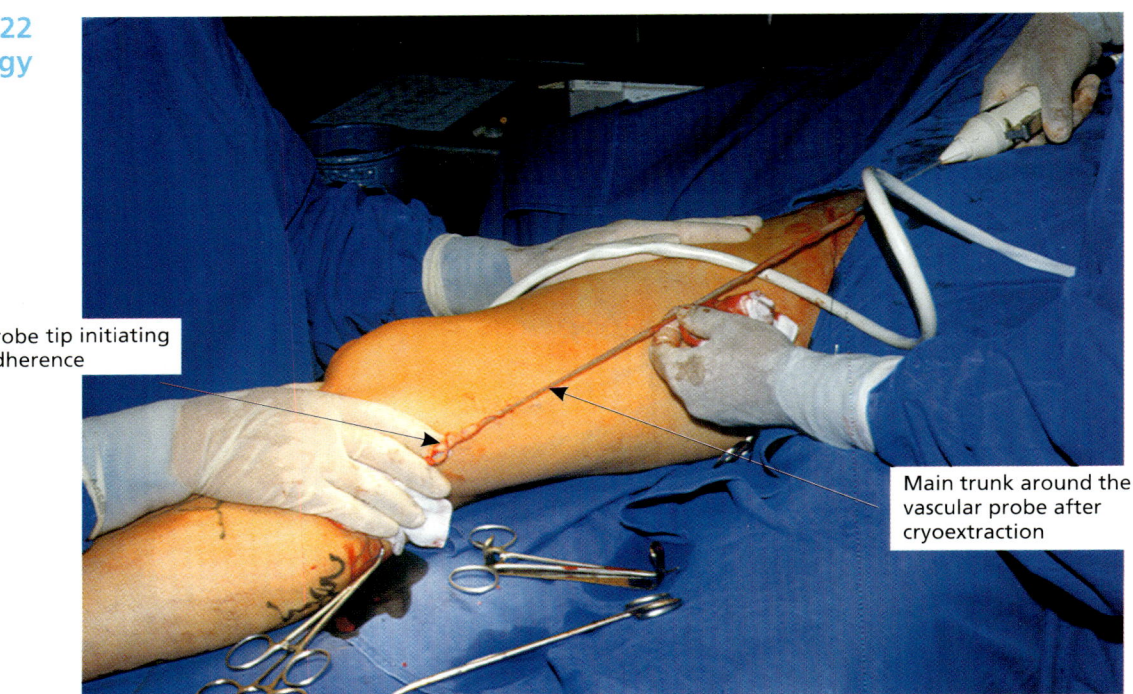

Fig. 22.6[1]. Vein cryo-stripping: saphena magna

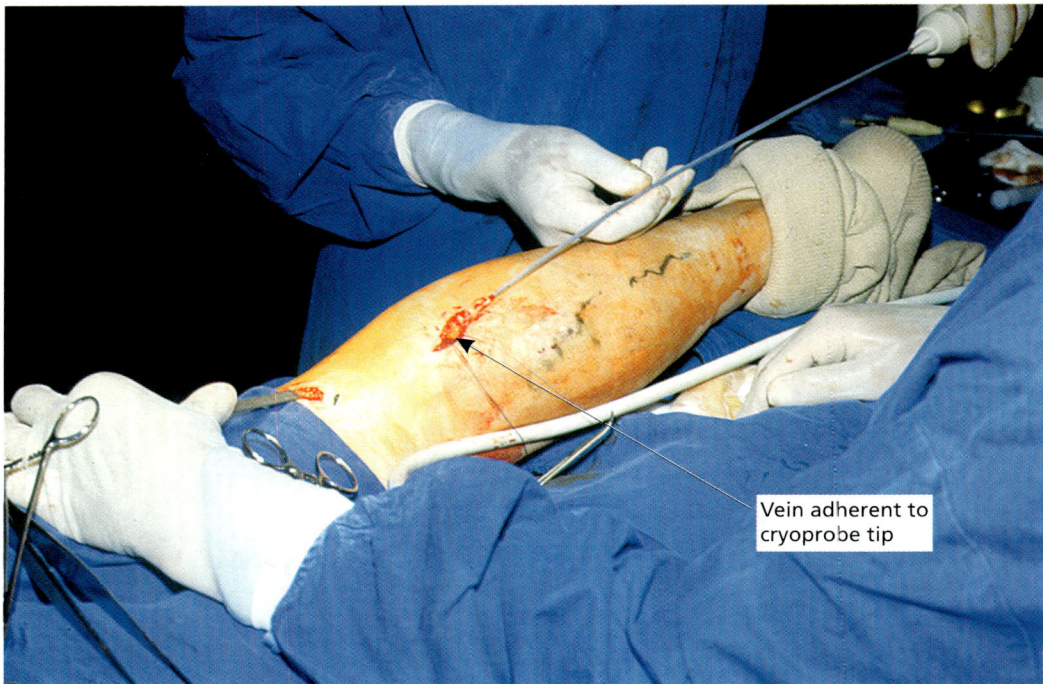

Fig. 22.7[1]. Vein cryo-stripping: saphena parva

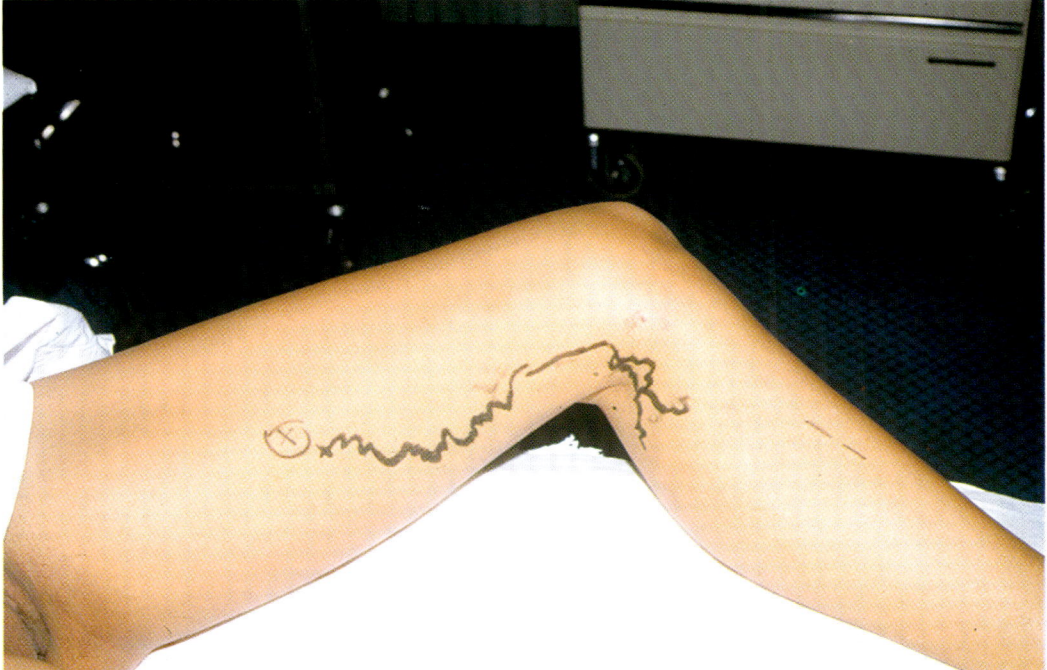

Fig. 22.8[1]. Vein cryosurgery (1): cryo-stripping+cryo-obliteration

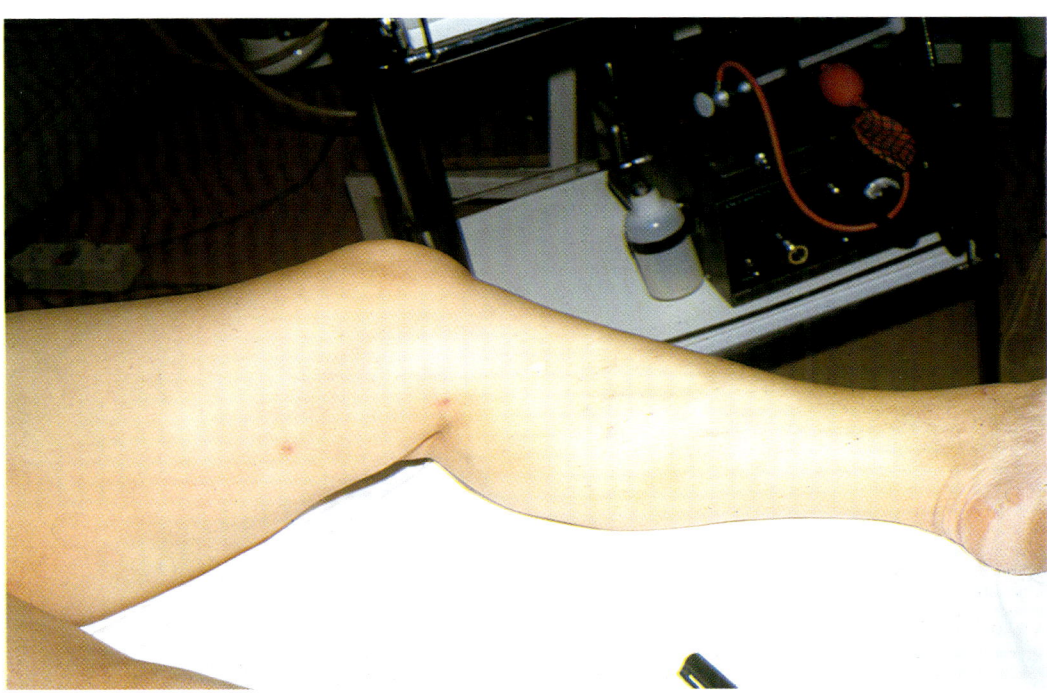

Fig. 22.9[1]. Vein cryosurgery (1): result

Chapter 22
Cryophlebology

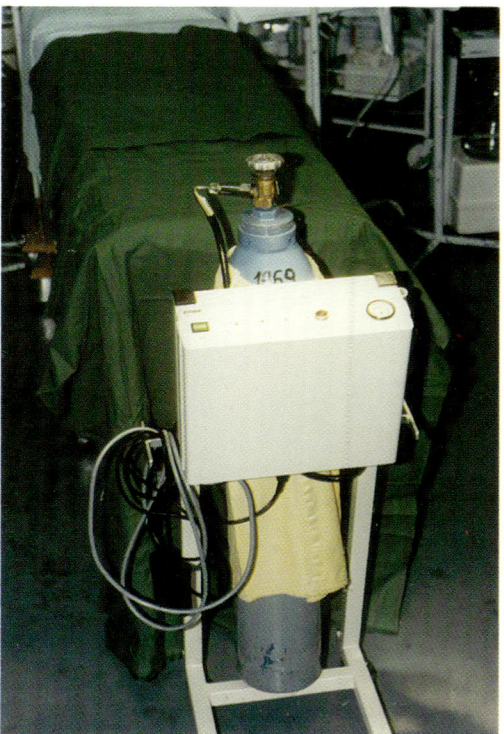

Fig. 22.10[2]. The cryosurgical device

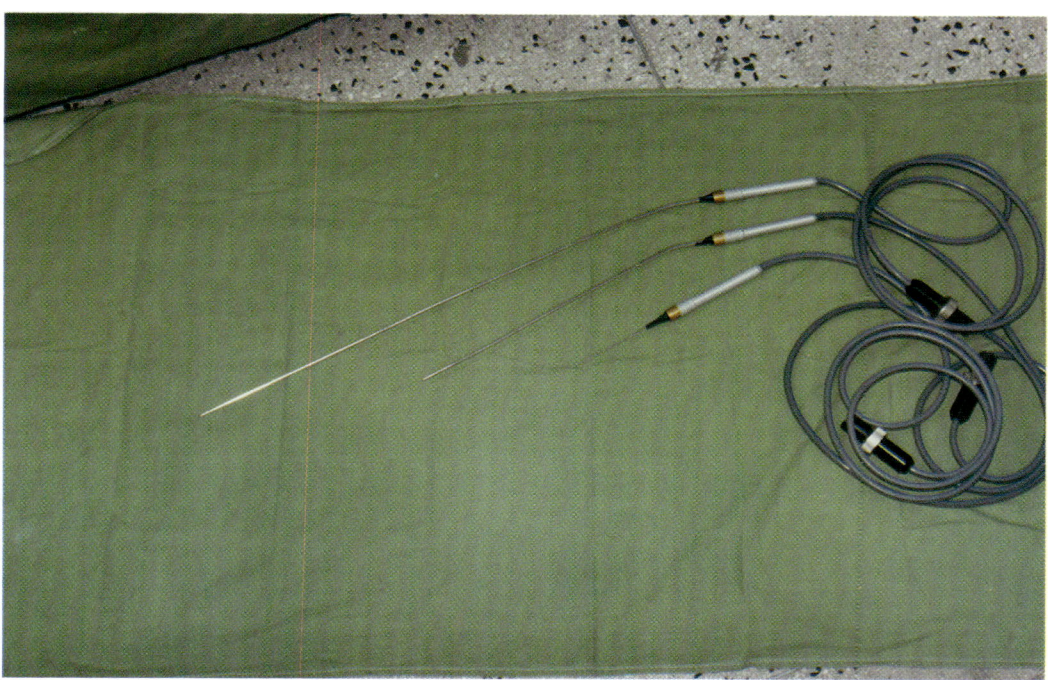

Fig. 22.11[2]. The cryoangioprobes for cryovaricectomy (cryo-stripping)

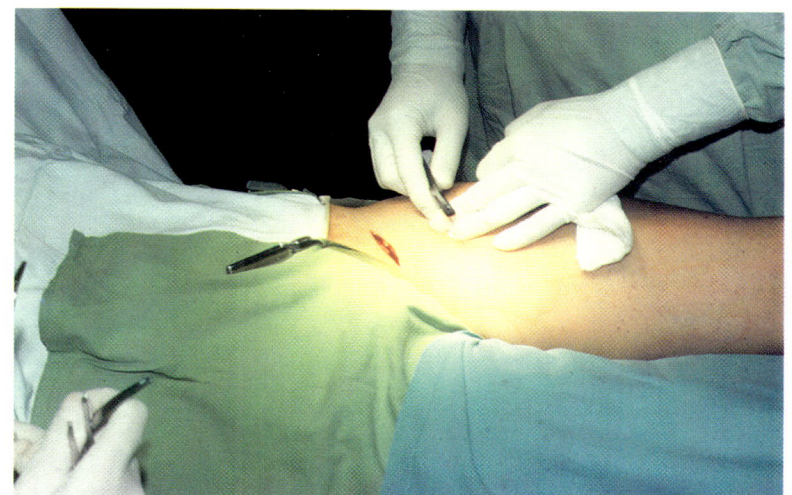

Fig. 22.12². The crossectomy

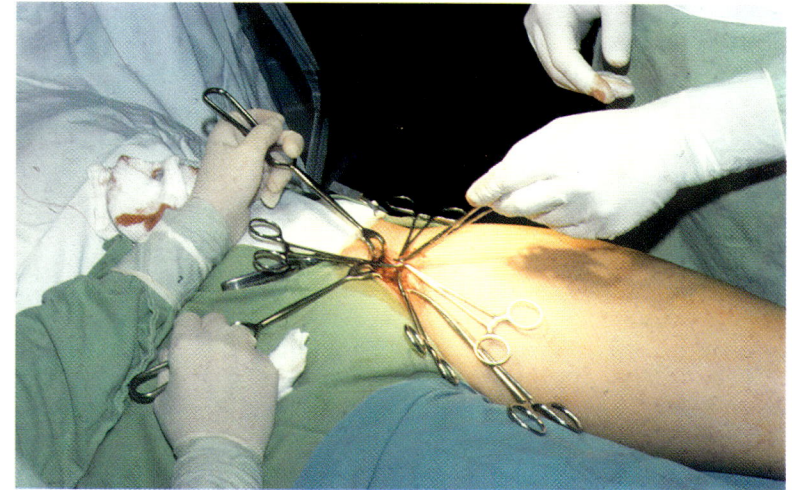

A

B

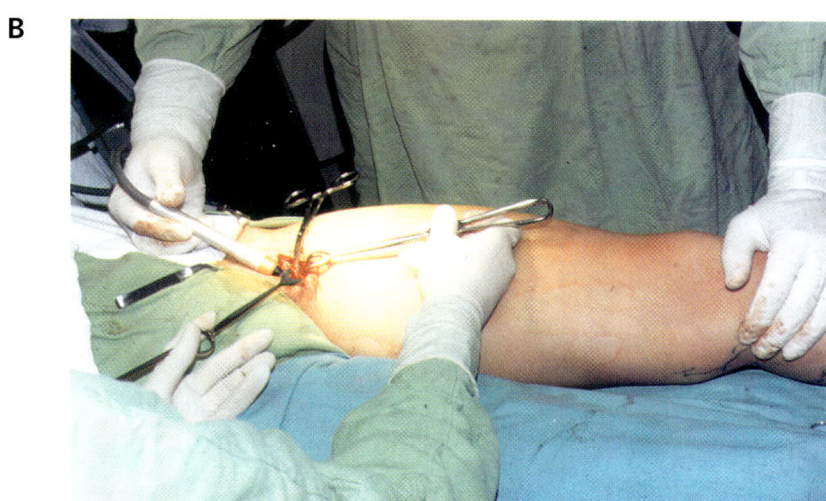

Fig. 22.13². Proximal femoral cryo-stripping

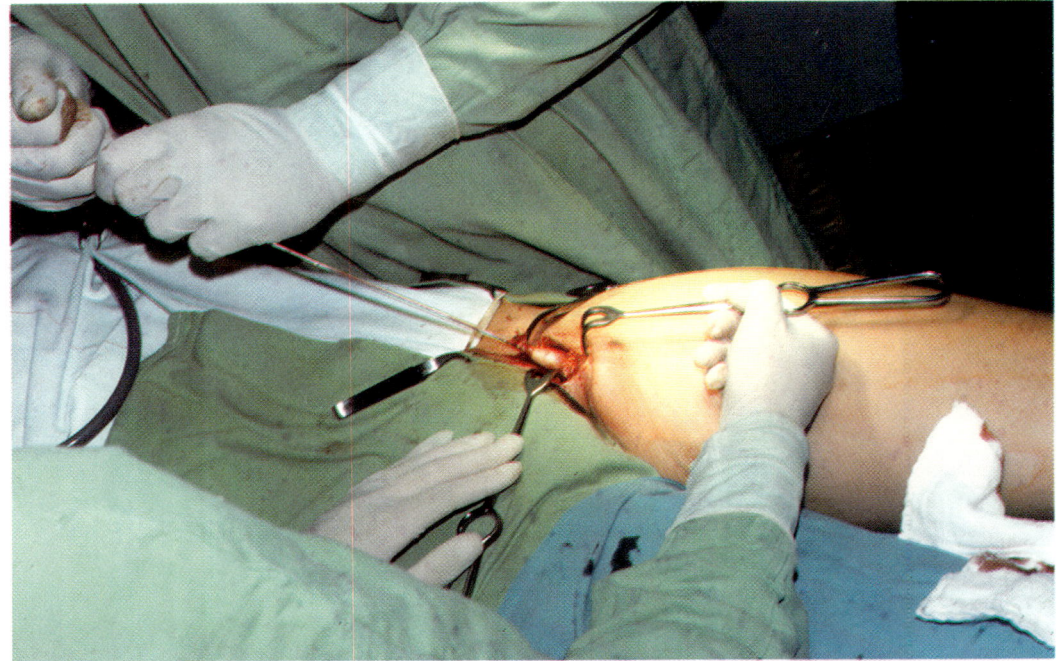

Fig. 22.14[2]. A, B. The removed insufficient part of the long saphenous vein

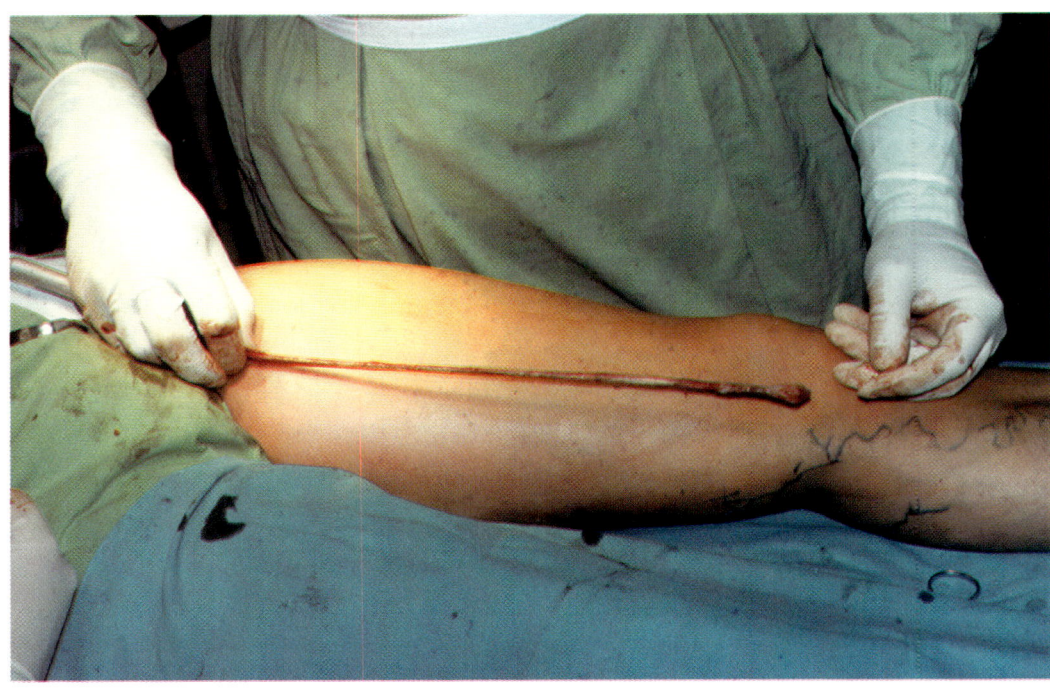

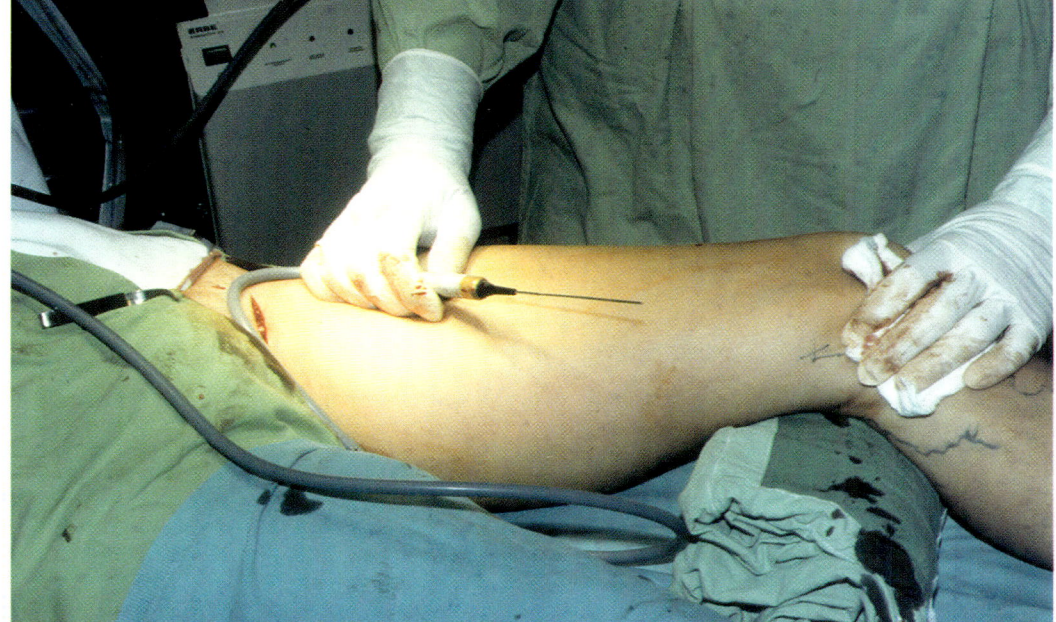

Fig. 22.15². A, B. The local (collateral) cryovaricectomies

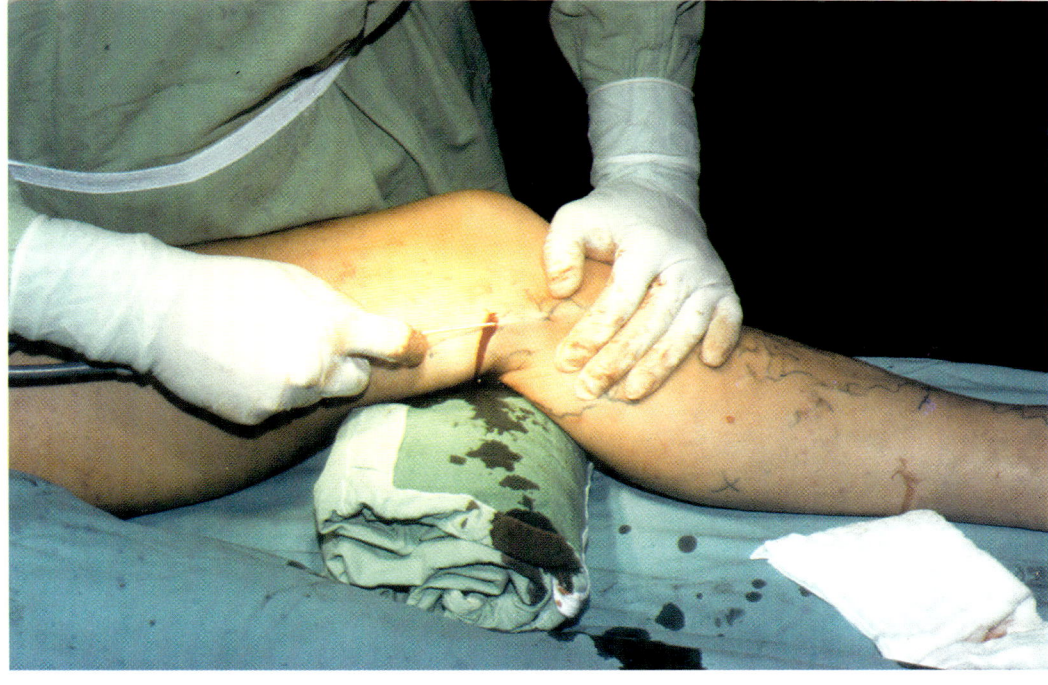

Chapter 22
Cryophlebology

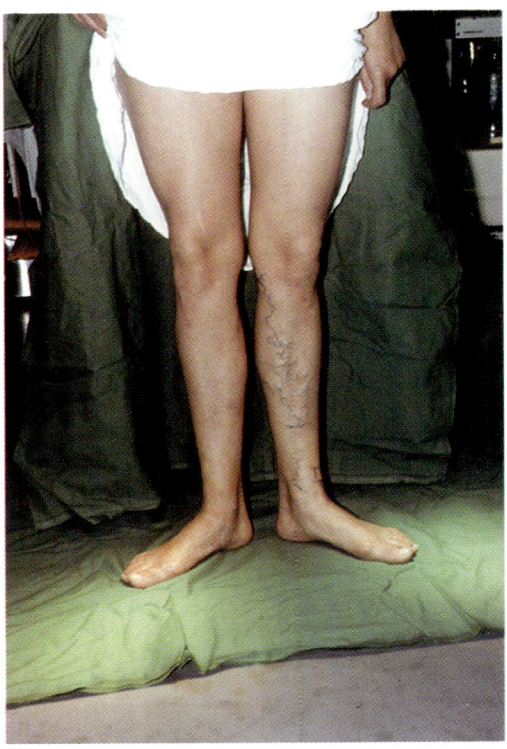

Fig. 22.16[2]. The lower extremity preoperatively

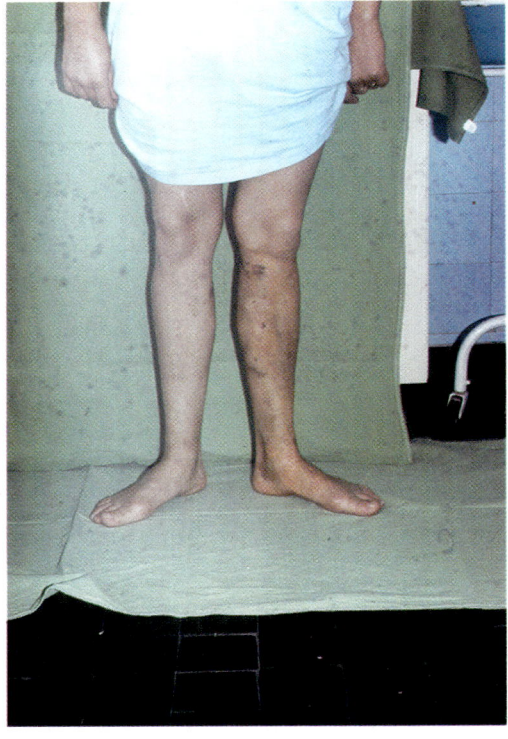

Fig. 22.17[2]. The same extremity 2 days after the cryo-stripping

Chapter 23

Cryosurgical Gynecology

Jose Carlos d'Almeida Gonçalves

23.1 Advanced Cancer of the External Genital Organs

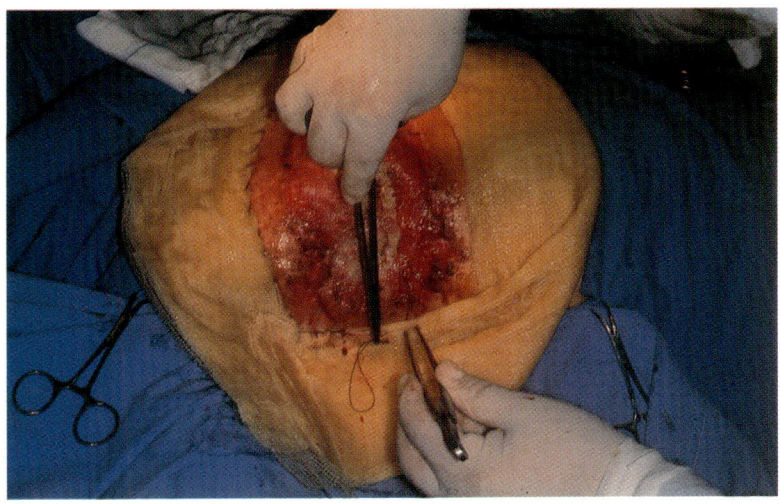

Fig. 23.1.1. The flexible plaques are stitched on the rim of the contour of the area to be frozen, a vulva with an advanced and inoperable cancer

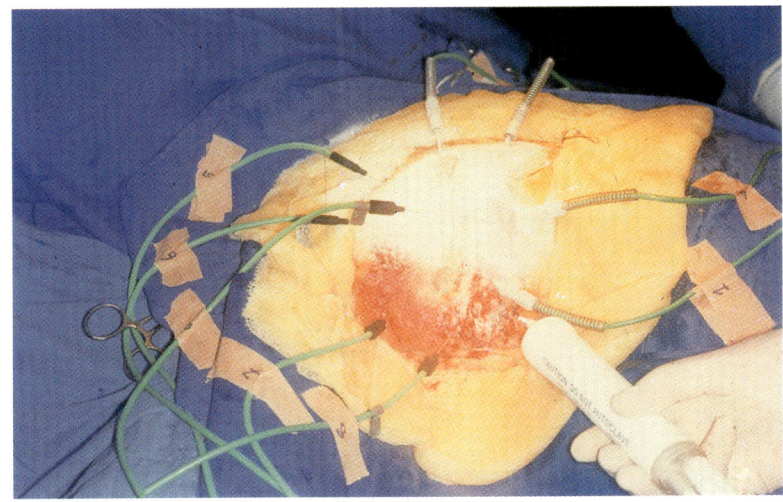

Fig. 23.1.2. In order to freeze the tumor, one point is chosen, and the spray is persistently applied until a temperature of between −50°C and −80°C is obtained at the tip of the thermocouple inserted 2–3 cm into the cancer. The contour of the 'ice ball' is then slowly and progressively widened to cover the whole vulvar region

Chapter 23
Cryosurgical Gynecology

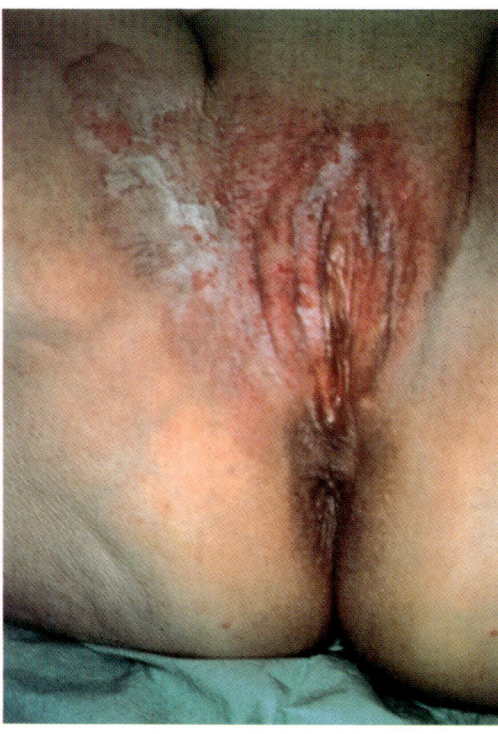

Fig. 23.1.3. A large and thick example of Paget's disease of the vulva, inoperable by conventional surgery

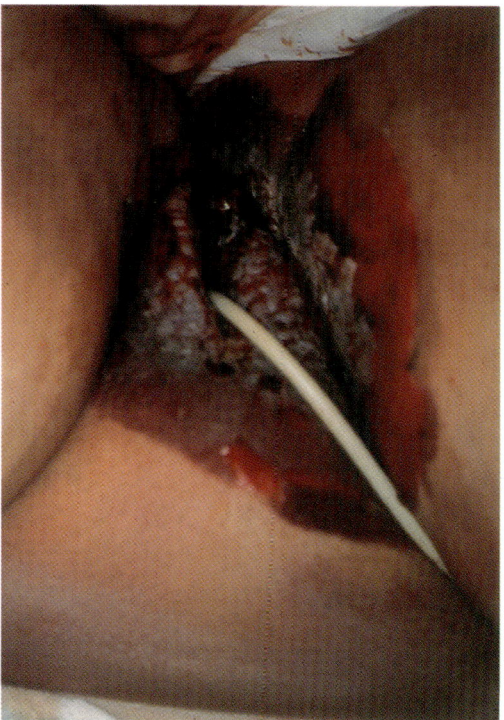

Fig. 23.1.4. Twenty-four hours after cryosurgery. The method of stitching the folded gauze dressings around the target permits an accurate and predictable limit of the freezing (even when the tumor is asymmetric, as in this case) and application of the spray for as long necessary to obtain cancericidal temperatures inside the cancer. The necrosed tissue was easily removed three weeks later, without pain. A clean ulceration resulted that healed by second intention

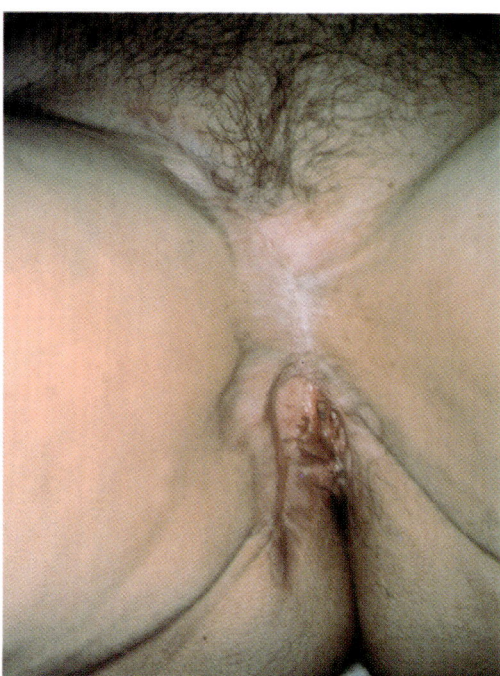

Fig. 23.1.5. This photo was taken three months after cryovulvectomy. No pain or discomfort persisted. The patient remained under observation for 6 years without recurrence

Chapter 24

Cardiovascular Cryosurgery

Vincent Dor[1] and Jean-Marc Frapier[2]

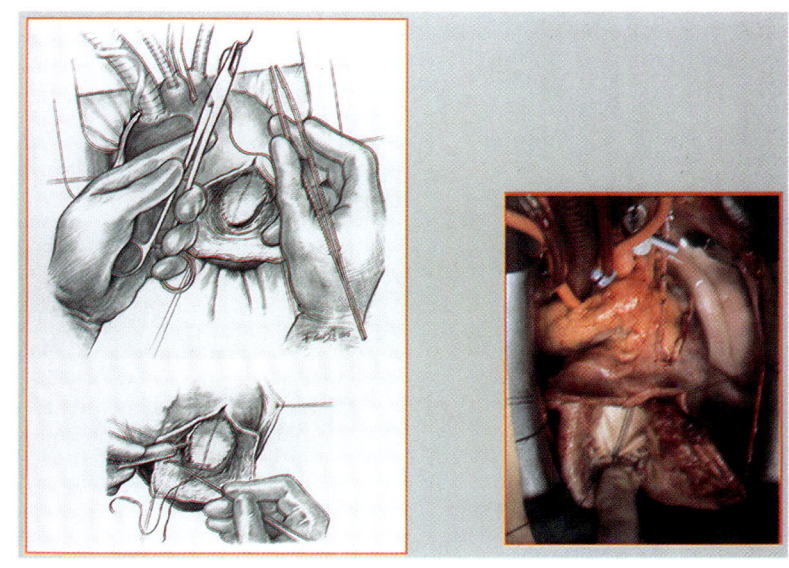

Fig. 24.1[1]. Comparative picture of cryosurgery in a patient who had a left ventricular aneurysm. A schematic explaining how the probe is placed, and the borderline between the fibrous tissue and the normal myocardium

Fig. 24.2[1]. Same ventricle by patch with operative view and schematic

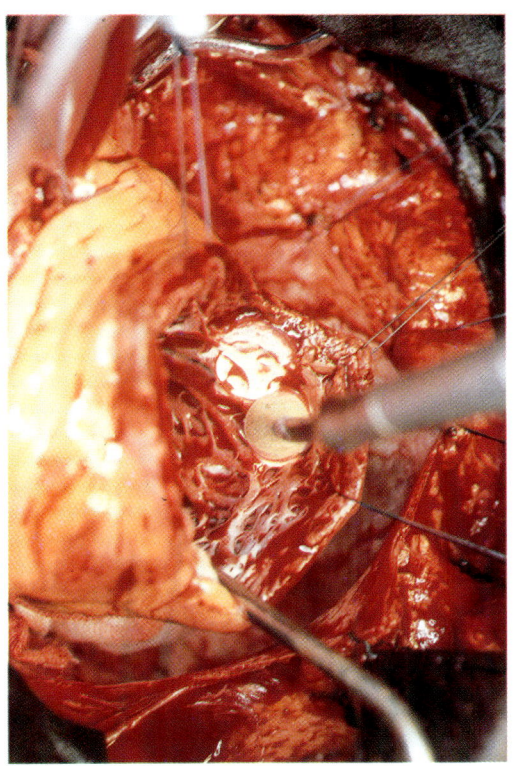

Fig. 24.3[2]. After left ventriculotomy through the center of the scar, extensive encircling cryosurgery is performed in a clockwise manner. Points of cryolesion (1.5 cm diameter probe) are applied along the border zone and are edge-to-edge or overlapping

Cryomassage

Irina R. Khramova

25.0 Introduction

Cryomassage denotes repeated short applications of superficial cold on healthy body tissue with a cryo-instrument to accelerate the process of stimulation and biological regeneration in the case of an anemic or hyperemic skin surface.

A cryoinstrument driven by liquid nitrogen is used for the cryomassage. The cryoinstrument consists of a special lightweight bottle. The special cryoprobes are cylindrically formed. Cryoprobes varying in size with a diameter ranging from 5 to 30 mm can be used so that different parts of the body can be effectively massaged. A temperature ranging from $-40°C$ to $-50°C$ is applied. The cryomassage cycle lasts for 1 to 3 min. A complete treatment includes 3 to 6 cycles, once a month.

Cryomassage is especially indicated in the case of dry or 'aged and withered skin'. Why so? Because no injury to lipid- and protein-containing complexes and no vascular stasis in the skin occurs in the course of this effective cryosurgical treatment.

The effectiveness of cryomassage is enhanced when the skin is cleansed beforehand.

Metabolic processes and microcirculation are improved in the course of this cryogenic procedure, regenerating the patient's anemic or hyperemic skin surface. As a general rule, a stimulation and biological regeneration process can be observed in the skin.

Under the microscope, a regenerated new skin layer – epidermis – consisting of 10 to 20 layers of cells is observed. In the regenerated epithelium one can make out the basal, spinous and corneal skin layers. These histological changes resulting from the cryomassage therapy could form the basis for the treatment of baldness. Future studies will provide clinical results in this regard.

Chapter 25 Cryomassage

25.1 Technique

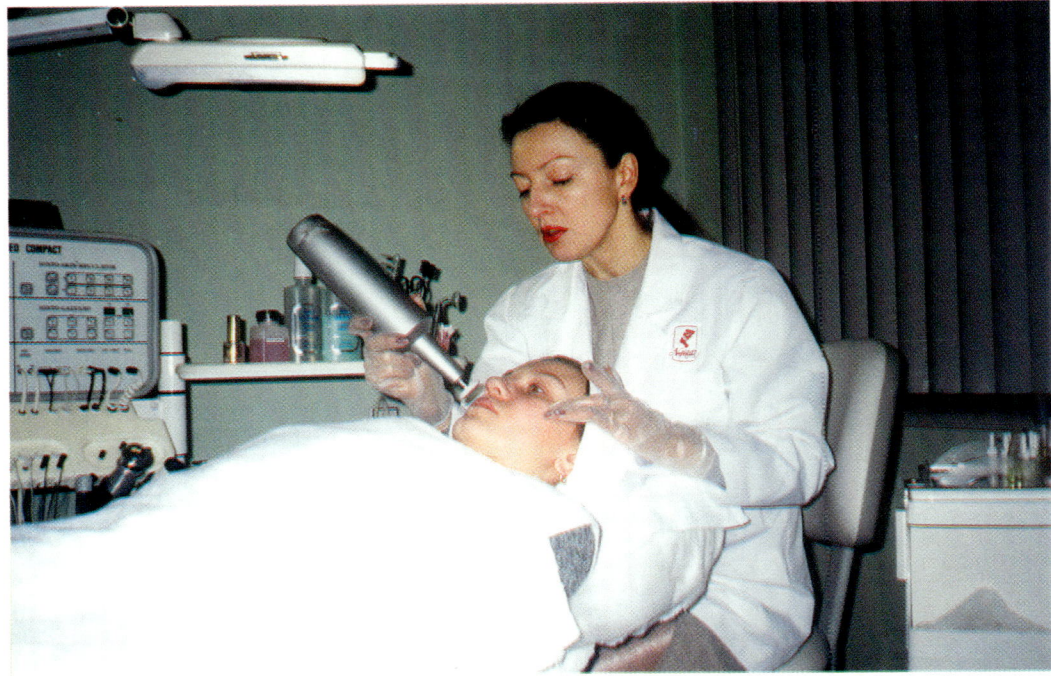

Fig. 25.1.1. Cryomassage using a special cryoprobe on a patient with dry skin to achieve good cosmetic results

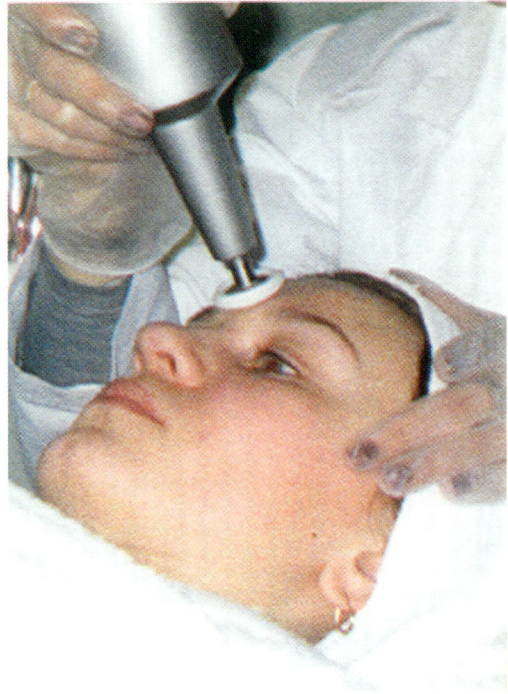

Fig. 25.1.2. A special cryogenic unit with liquid nitrogen, equipped with a cryoprobe the temperature of which is lowered to −50°C, is used for cryomassage in cosmetic medicine

Section G

Tumor Anemia

Chapter 26

Causes of Anemia in Cancer Patients

Nedjeljka BALDASS

26.1 Introduction

Anemia frequently is associated with cancer or its treatment. Anemia may manifest itself in symptoms that include fatigue, shortness of breath, chest pain, weakness, loss of appetite, and headache. Even mild to moderate anemia may cause fatigue at rest, and may deleteriously affect a cancer patient's ability to perform normal daily activities. Along with functional impairment, anemic cancer patients may suffer a decline in their sense of well-being. The quality-of-life domains of exercise tolerance, work capability, social interaction, and leisure enjoyment may each be affected by anemia symptoms.[1] Left untreated, anemia in cancer patients may become severe, necessitating red blood cell (RBC) transfusion.

Otherwise inexplicable anemias associated with malignancies and certain chronic inflammatory conditions have been generically termed *anemia of chronic disease*, or ACD. Although anemia may result from blood loss from mucosal surfaces, cachexia and poor nutrition, tumor infiltration of the bone marrow, or hemolysis,[2] anemia in cancer patients is frequently characterized as hypoproliferative ACD.[3] ACD is usually attributed to a deficit in bone marrow production of the erythroid progenitor cells.[4] Pincus et al. demonstrated that the ACD associated with rheumatoid arthritis responds favorably to hormone supplementation with recombinant human erythropoietin,[5] suggesting that hormonal regulation may influence the development and course of anemia in bone marrow disease (see Fig. 26.1).

26.2 Origin and Characteristics of ACD

Patients with ACD typically have a blunted erythropoietin response; that is, their endogenous serum erythropoietin levels, while higher than normal, are low for their degree of anemia.[6,7] In contrast to iron-deficiency anemia, ACD is associated with a decrease in RBC survival as well as a decrease in RBC production related to disturbed iron metabolism. The bone marrow's iron stores are increased,[8] but its ability

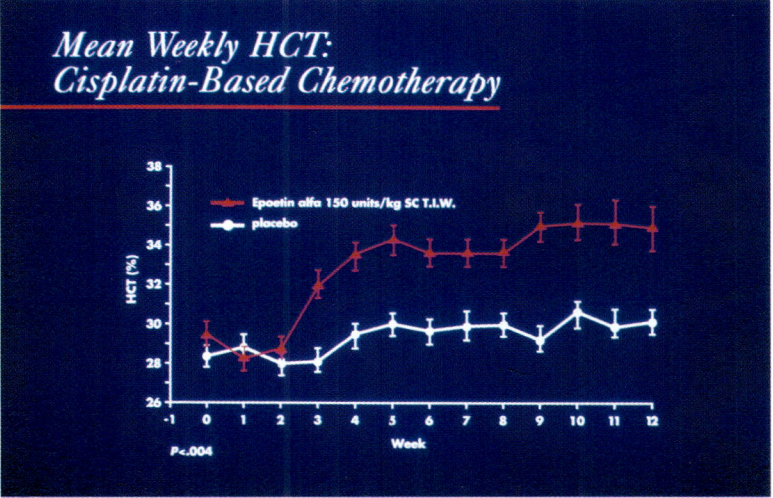

Fig. 26.1

to transport and utilize iron is impaired,[9] resulting in a reticuloendothelial blockade, subsequent hypoproliferation of precursor cells, and diminished hemoglobin (Hb) production.

26.3 The Erythropoietin Feedback Loop

RBC level is regulated by the erythropoietin hormonal feedback loop. Erythropoietin, released primarily by the kidneys in response to hypoxia, sends a highly specific signal prompting committed erythroid progenitor cells in the bone marrow to produce RBCs.[10]

RBCs proliferate and differentiate during their first 4 days and mature in another 3 days. Thus a delay of approximately one week may occur between the erythropoietin signalling event and the release of RBCs into the circulation, where they typically survive for about 120 days. The demise of RBCs results from a loss of cell membrane pliability that renders them easily damaged.[11] Maintenance of a proper RBC level is a function of the rates of erythropoiesis and RBC destruction. When the RBC level and subsequent tissue oxygenation are adequate, erythropoietin release is down-regulated (see Fig. 26.2).

26.4 Symptoms of Anemia

The primary physiologic consequence of anemia is reduced oxygen-carrying capacity of the blood,[12] which produces a variety of symptoms. Fatigue is common even with mild (grade 1) anemia,[13] and may be expressed as both physical weakness and mental lethargy. Due to respiratory compensation for the reduced oxygen flow, patients with mild to moderate (grades 1 und 2) anemia may have difficulty breathing after exercise; those with more severe (grades 3 and 4) anemia may have breathing difficulties at rest.[13,14]

On exertion, anemic patients experience greater than normal increases in cardiac output, resulting in reduced exercise capacity; with severe anemia, resting cardiac output may increase as well.[12] Heartbeat irregularities may occur after exercise or, in patients with severe anemia, at rest.[13] Anemic patients with preexisting arteriosclerosis may suffer angina pectoris, myocardial infarction, and transient ischemic attacks.[14] In severe cases of anemia, the increased circulatory load can even lead to cardiac failure.[13,15]

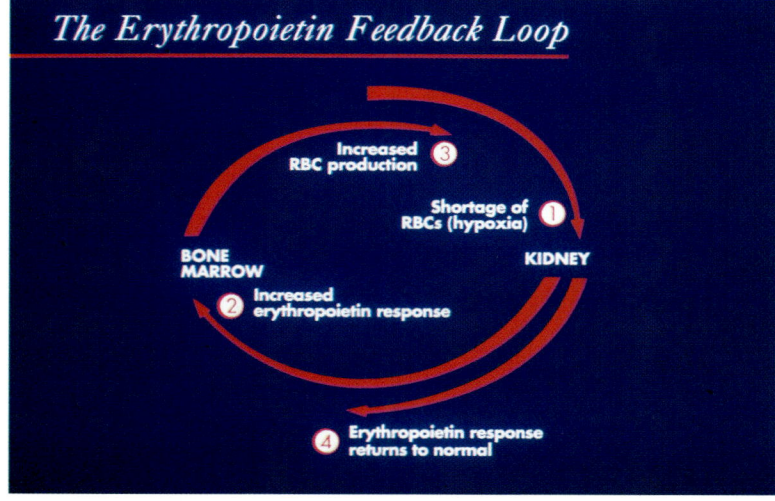

Fig. 26.2.

26.5 Risk Factors for Anemia in Cancer Patients

An understanding of the risk factors for anemia in cancer patients would allow early therapeutic intervention in patients at risk.

Several factors may be related to increased risk of anemia in cancer patients. Tumor type, particularly hematologic vs solid, may be a risk factor for anemia. Among patients with solid tumors, lung cancer patients are particularly prone to anemia and, because of their compromised respiratory capacity, tolerate it poorly.[16] Replacement of healthy bone marrow with tumor mass, a common occurrence in hematologic cancers, might also increase the risk of anemia.

The type and intensity of chemotherapy may influence the development of anemia; cisplatin-based therapy in particular is associated with significant renal toxicity.[17] In addition, a low baseline Hb level or a significant drop in Hb level after the first cycle of chemotherapy might also be predictive of anemia.

26.6 Anemia Associated with Platinum-Based Chemotherapy

Chemotherapy can cause hypoproliferative anemia by suppressing either kidney or bone marrow function. For example, cisplatin may cause significant renal injury by damaging both proximal and distal tubules.[17]

Two comparative studies carried out by the National Cancer Institute of Canada (NCIC) and Southwestern Oncology Group (SWOG) investigated platinum-based chemotherapy regimens using cisplatin or carboplatin for the treatment of ovarian cancer.[18] As the table shows, significant anemia necessitating transfusion developed in patients receiving either drug. While 8% to 24% of patients developed anemia of grade 3 or greater (with an Hb level less than 8 g/dl), it is important to note that approximately 90% of patients in both studies developed anemia of at least grade 1 (with an Hb level less than 11 g/dl). Although less nephrotoxic than cisplatin,[18] carboplatin still induced substantial anemia and the need for transfusion.

26.7 Frequency of Anemia with Nonplatinum Chemotherapeutic Agents

High incidences of anemia also are observed with a number of widely used nonplatinum agents.

Paclitaxel and docetaxel, frequently used to treat breast and ovarian cancers, were associated with anemia in 78% and 90% of patients, respectively, in single-agent trials.[19,20] Anemia was also seen in 65% of patients receiving gemcitabine as single-agent therapy for pancreatic cancer.[21] Many patients with ovarian or colorectal cancer may receive topotecan or irinotecan; trials with both agents revealed substantial incidences of anemia.[22,23] With topotecan, nearly all patients developed anemia, and the incidence of anemia of grade 3 or greater was 40%.

26.8 Hb Level as a Risk Factor for Anemia— Skillings' Study

Skillings et al. carried out a retrospective study in 381 cancer patients receiving chemotherapy to determine the frequency of transfusion for anemia and to examine possible risk factors.[16]

They found a correlation of transfusion frequency with Hb level prior to chemotherapy. An inverse relationship was seen between baseline Hb level and frequency of transfusion, with a higher risk for patients who are anemic prior to chemotherapy.

26.9 Hb Levels as a Risk for Anemia— Abels' Study

Abels and his colleagues[24] looked at Hb level at baseline and after the first cycle of chemotherapy in patients with small-cell lung cancer on mainly platinum-based regimens. They found that risk of transfusion increased with lower baseline Hb levels irrespective of changes in Hb level occurring after the first cycle of chemotherapy. Likewise, greater declines in Hb level after the first cycle were associated with increased risk of transfusion regardles of baseline Hb level.

Both the Skillings and Abels studies show that Hb level can be predictive of anemia in cancer patients receiving chemotherapy. Particular risk is associated with either a low initial Hb level or a significant drop in Hb level after the first chemotherapy cycle.

26.10 Management of Anemia

Iron deficiency and ACD often occur together in patients with cancer. Correction of iron or vitamin deficiency, improvement of catabolic states, and prevention and treatment of infection all accelerate recovery from anemia.

Transfusion, while providing only short-term benefits, is an option for patients with moderate to severe anemia, but the physician must consider the benefits and risks of blood transfusion in each clinical situation.

Therapy with Epoetin alfa has been found to be effective in treating anemia resulting from impaired production of endogenous serum erythropoietin or impaired erythropoietic response in cancer patients receiving chemotherapy.[3]

26.11 Patient Candidate for Epoetin Alpha Therapy

Epoetin alfa is indicated for use in anemic cancer patients with non-myeloid malignancies receiving concomitant chemotherapy. However, not all patients are appropriate candidates for Epoetin alfa therapy. Patients with grossly elevated endogenous serum erythropoietin levels may fail to respond to Epoetin alfa therapy, and Epoetin alfa is not recommended for patients with baseline levels higher than 200 mU/mL. Before starting therapy with Epoetin alfa, a patient's iron status should be assessed by measuring transferrin saturation and serum ferritin levels. To support Epoetin alfa-stimulated erythropoiesis, these values should be at least 20% and 100 ng/ml, respectively. In addition, anemia resulting from hemolysis, occult blood loss, folic acid or vitamin B_{12} deficiencies, infection, or bone marrow infiltration should be ruled out prior to initiating Epoetin alfa therapy. The recommended initial dose of Epoetin alfa for anemic patients receiving chemotherapy for nonmyeloid malignancies is 150 units/kg subcutaneously (SC) three times weekly (T.I.W.), or approximately 10.000 units for a 70-kg patient.

26.12 Titration

If response to Epoetin alfa therapy is not satisfactory in terms of reducing transfusion requirements or increasing Hb level after 4 weeks of therapy, the dose may be increased to a maximum of 300 units/kg T.I.W., or approximately 20.000 units for a 70-kg patient.[25] Patients who do not respond to this increased dose are unlikely to respond to higher doses. If Hb level exceeds 13 g/dl, Epoetin alfa should be withheld until Hb level falls to $\leq$12 g/dl. The dose of Epoetin alfa should be reduced by 25% when treatment is resumed and then titrated to maintain desired Hb level. If Hb level rises by more than 1.3 g/dl in any 2-week period, the Epoetin alfa dose should be reduced based on the physician's clinical judgement.

Since absolute or functional iron deficiency may develop during Epoetin alfa therapy, transferrin saturation and serum ferritin levels should be monitored. Virtually all patients receiving Epoetin alfa will eventually need iron supplementation to maintain response.

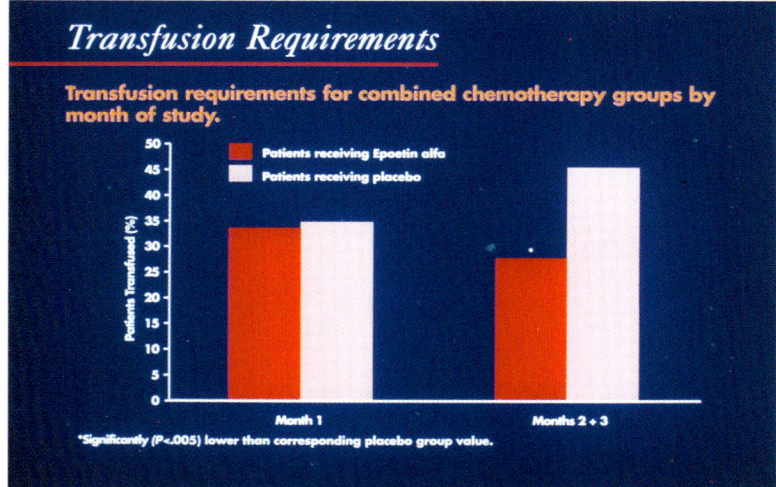

Fig. 26.3.

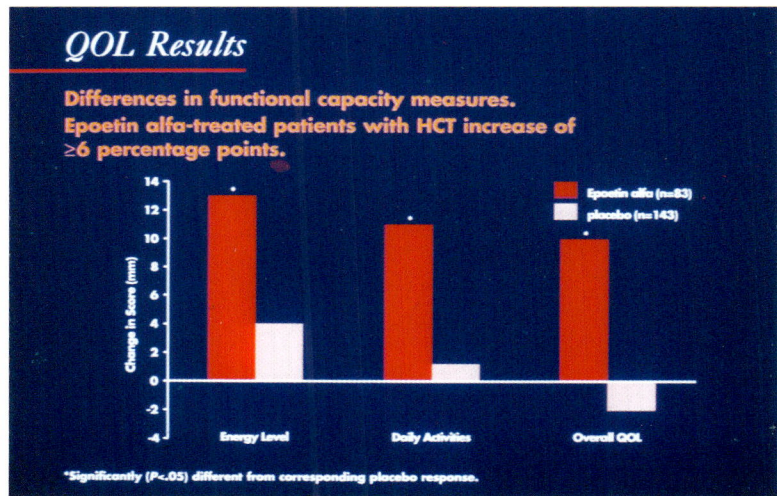

Fig. 26.4.

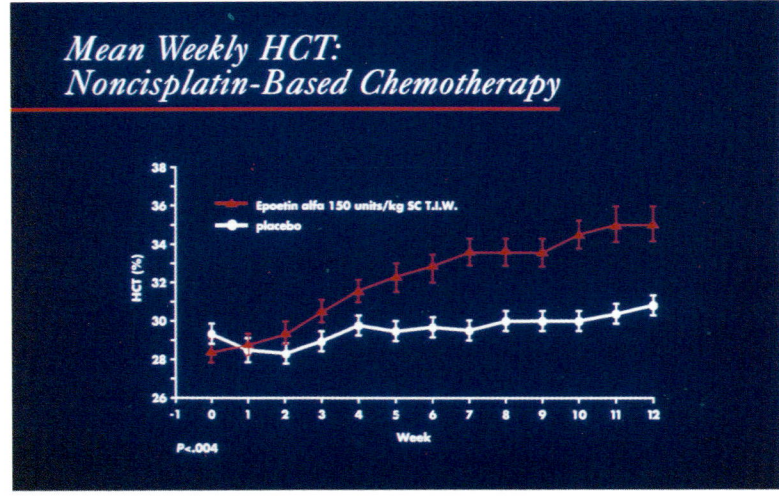

Fig. 26.5.

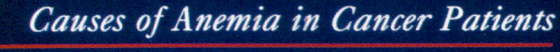

Fig. 26.6.

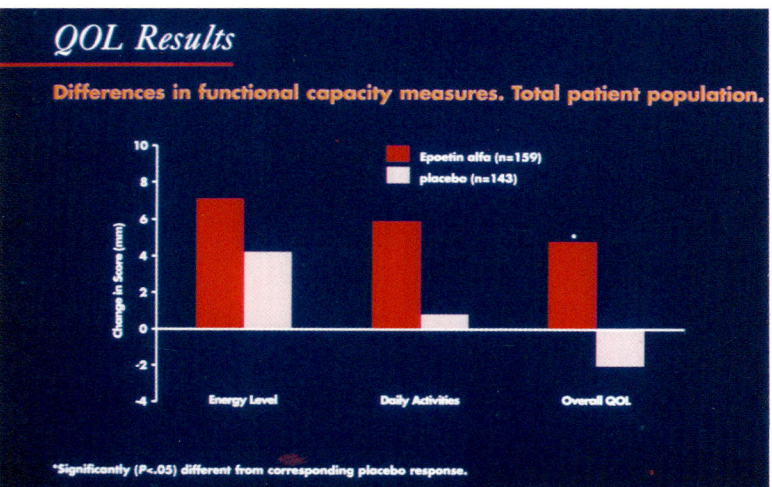

Fig. 26.7.

References

1. Yellen et al. J Symptom Pain Manage 1997; (13): 2
2. Spivak JL. Sem Oncol 1994; 21 (suppl 3): 3s–8s
3. Abels et al. In: Murphy, Blood Cell Growth Factors: Their Present and Future Use in Hematology and Oncology. Dayton, Ohio: Alpha Med Press 1991; 121–141
4. Krantz SB. Am J Med Sci 1994; 307: 353–359
5. Pincus et al. Am J Med 1990; 89:161–168
6. Doweiko et al. Oncology 1991; 5: 31–44
7. Miller et al. N Engl J Med 1990; 322: 1689–1692
8. Schilling RF. Ann Int Med 1991; 115: 572–573
9. DeRienzo et al. Tex Med 1990; 86: 80–83
10. Krantz SB. Blood 1991; 77: 414–434
11. Brunn HF. In: Harrison's Principles of Internal Medicine, 13th ed. New York, 1994; 1717–1721
12. Varat et al. Am Heart J 1972; 83: 415–426
13. Bunn et al. Harrisons's Principles of Internal Medicine, 13th ed. New York, 1994; 313–317
14. Jain et al. Med Clin North Am 1992; 76: 727–744
15. Graettinger et al. Ann Int Med 1963; 58: 617–626
16. Skillings et al. Am J Clin Oncol 1993; 16: 22–25
17. Patterson et al. Sem Oncol 1992; 19: 521–528
18. Paraplatin prescribing information. Medical Economics 1997; 713–717
19. Taxol prescribing information. Medical Economics Co 1997; 723–727
20. Taxotere prescribing information. Medical Economics Co 1997; 2204–2207
21. Gemzar prescribing information. Medical Economics Co 1997; 1482–1485
22. Hycamtin prescribing information. Medical Economics Co 1997; 2665–2667
23. Camptosar prescribing information. Medical Economics Co 1997; 2060–2064
24. Abels et al. Risk of transfusion in small cell lung cancer patients receiving chemotherapy. Blood 1994; 84: 664A, Abstract 2642
25. Glaspy et al. J Clin Oncol 1997; 15 (3): 1218–1234

Subject Index

A
Ablation, 12
Acid, salicilic, 178
Adenocarcinoma, 315, 339, 341, 383, 390
  -ductal, 353, 390
  -medullo-tubular, 378, 385
  -rectum, 11, 242, 315
Adenoma, tubulo-villous, 337
Adenomatous polyp, 336
Advance, 403
  -cryosurgical technology, 21, 105, 137
Advanced
  -cancer, 10
  -cancer of the external genital organs, 499
  -pancreatic cancer, 296
  -primary anal canal tumors, 320
Advantage, 11
Alveococcal cavern, 284, 287
Anal region epidermoid cancer, 320
Aneurysmal bone cyst, 438
Angiocryoprobe, 489
Animal, 12, 105, 116, 137, 144, 351
  -experiment, 137, 144
  -pancreas, 144, 145
Anorectal carcinoma, 319
  -tumor, 320, 336
Anoscope, 325
Application, 3–5, 7–11, 13, 22, 78, 85, 86, 95, 105, 137, 165, 289, 343, 445, 446
  -cold, 5
  -local, 3
  -temperature, 4, 5, 12, 81, 167, 446
  -time, 446
  -trial, 466, 467
Approach
  -nonoperative, 319
  -surgical , 424
Areas, well-demarkated, 3
Aspect
  -clinical, 163
  -dorsal, 219–222
  -theoretical, 15
  -volar, 219–221

Atrophy, focal of rectal mucosa, 338

B
Biopsy, intraoperative, 285
Biopsy punch, 222, 225
Bleeding, 159, 278, 316, 319, 341, 376, 378, 383, 392, 399
Bone
  -cavity, 421
  -cement, 419
  -chips alograft, 433
  -contour of the orbit, 210
  -cyst of humerus, 434
  -facial, 419
  -giant cell tumors, 422, 423
  -graft, 434, 435, 437, 440, 443
  -graft iliac crest, 428, 429
  -grafting, 434, 436, 441
  -grafting, subchondral, 429
  -marrow, 421, 507–510
  -necrosis, 419, 421
  -normal, 428, 429
  -producing, 11
  -structura normal, 436
  -tubular, 427
  -tumors, 420, 421, 433
Bronchoscopes, fibreoptic, 303
Bronchoscopy, fibreoptic, 306

C
Cancer
  -anal canal, 320
  -anaplastic, 390
  -basosquamous, 225
  -breast, 13, 97, 343, 353, 354, 357, 365, 371–376, 391–396
  -cell, 8
  -colorectal, 96, 274, 509
  -diagnosis, 343
  -external, 212
  -extremity, inoperable, 213
  -inflammatory, 387
  -inoperable, 10, 499
  -invasive, 320
  -larynx, 317
  -liver, unresectable, 235
  -Paget, 389
  -penis, advance, 217
  -rectal, 12, 94, 319, 320, 340
  -research, 343

-survival, 404
-temperature inside, 500
Carbon dioxide, 3, 4, 9, 10, 12, 165, 445, 446
Carcinoma
  -breast, 12, 355
  -bronchus, 310, 311
  -ductal, 376
  -erysipelatous, 387
  -medulary, anaplastic, 380
  -metastatic of the liver, 95
  -trachea, 310
Cell
  -basal and squamous, 320
  -carcinoma basal (BCC), 12, 186, 188, 196, 199–201, 206, 207, 209, 218, 223, 224, 230, 231
  -carcinoma, basal ill-defined, 222, 226, 227
  -carcinoma, squamous, 202–204, 215, 217, 220, 304, 306, 485–487
  -destruction, 131, 134, 158
  -epithelial of glands, 352
  -lines, 105 11, 89, 92, 435
  -red blood, 351, 353, 507
  -tumor giant (GCT) of bone, 422, 423, 430, 441
Chemotherapy, 258, 261, 263, 392, 509, 510, 513
  -anticancer, 389
  -resistance, 343, 391
Chloride
  -2,3,5-triphenyltetrazolium (TTC), 351
  -iron solution, 225
Chondroblastoma, 436
Chondroma, 419
Chondrosarcoma, 440
Cold, 3–5, 7–9, 85, 95, 98, 419, 446
Cold
  -cautery, 4
  -clamp, 4
  -extreme, 3–5, 95
  -injury, 5, 7, 8
  -packs, 3
  -sensitiveness, 4
  -substances, 4
  -surgery, 3
  -therapy, 3
  -urticaria, 5
Condyloma, 166
Condylomata, 166, 319
  -acumulata, 319
Corpora cavernosa, 217
Cosmetic, 451, 452, 457, 446

  -appearance, 446
  -difficulties, 211
  -medicine, 504
  -results, 165, 167, 197, 371, 398, 401, 445, 489, 504
Crossectomy, 489, 495
Crymo, 5
Crymotherapy, 5
Cryo, 4, 5
Cryoablated area, 415
Cryoablation, 4, 11, 12, 137, 235, 404, 408, 409, 415, 418
Cryoalgesia, 4
Cryoanalgesia, 4, 12
Cryoanesthesia, 4
Cryobiology, 5, 144
Cryocautery, 4
Cryoclamp, 3
Cryodestruction, 4, 73, 77, 78, 81, 82, 95, 108, 137, 166, 289, 290, 294, 295
Cryoechinococcotomy, 278
Cryoesthesia, 4
Cryoextirpation, 4, 95
  -liver, 268, 271
Cryoextraction, 4
Cryoextractor, 4
Cryogen, 5, 9, 10, 75, 165
Cryogenic, 5, 8, 9, 21, 22, 73, 75, 77, 78, 108, 117–119, 123, 144, 171, 189
  -applicator, 319
  -clamp, 3, 102
  -effect, 167
  -lesion, 137
  -method, 445
  -probe, 324, 325, 445
  -procedure, 503
  -surgery, 11, 167
  -technique, 10, 105, 137
  -unit, 73
Cryoglobulin, 5
Cryoglobulinemia, 5
Cryohypophysectomy, 5
Cryoimmunology, 5
Cryoinfluence, 22, 235
Cryoinjured region, 352, 353
Cryoinjury, 403, 414
Cryoinstrument, 3, 4, 17, 21, 78, 81, 330, 331, 333, 503
Cryolesion, 10, 13, 86, 265, 267, 403, 416–418, 501
Cryolumpectomy, 5, 12
Cryolymphadenectomy, 5
Cryomassage, 4, 503, 504

Cryomastectomy, 5, 343, 391, 392
Cryometer, 4
Cryonecrosis, 107, 129–136, 140, 142, 146–148, 158–162, 253, 360, 374
Cryopolypectomy, 338
Cryopreservation, 5
Cryoprobe, 3, 4, 11, 17, 21, 23–54, 56–70, 85, 95, 101, 102, 109, 140, 141, 143, 146, 167, 169, 170, 172, 175, 189, 235, 254, 289, 290, 299, 303, 340, 344, 345, 359, 367, 377, 394, 400, 403, 407–409, 427, 447, 453, 459, 466, 484, 488, 489, 504
 -cylindrical, 18
 -disc-shapes, 4, 21, 96, 97
 -PR-6, 377
 -SK-51865-1, 381
 -technique, 166, 169, 170
Cryoresection, 3, 295
 -hepatic, 102
 -liver, 278, 284
Cryoscalpel, 3, 278, 279, 284
Cryoscopy, 4
Cryoshaving, 4, 447–452
Cryostripping, 5, 489, 490, 492–495, 498
Cryosurgery, 1, 3, 5, 7–13, 15, 17–19, 21, 22, 73, 77–79, 81, 82, 85, 95, 98, 102, 105, 107–109, 111, 114, 116, 137–140, 144–146, 149, 150, 165–167, 169, 170, 178–180, 182, 183, 198–205, 210, 212–215, 217, 235, 278, 284, 287, 289, 290, 292, 303, 304, 310–314, 316, 319–322, 328–331, 333–335, 346, 374, 375, 379, 380, 383–385, 388, 390, 398, 401, 403, 419–427, 429–438, 440, 441, 443, 445, 446, 458, 459, 477, 480, 484, 485, 488, 500, 501
 -abdominal, 235, 289
 -breast, 343–345, 396, 399
 -breast cancer, 343, 359–372, 395, 396
 -cardiovascular, 501
 -contact, 166
 -curative, 319
 -endoscopic, 315, 319
 -fructional, 12, 206, 211
 -hepatic, 4, 12, 105, 106, 235–237, 241, 256, 257, 261, 263–268, 278
 -local, 3
 -orthopaedic, 419, 420
 -preoperative, 340
 -pulmonary, 303

 -rectal cancer, 319, 339
 -shaving, 165, 445
 -snow, 446
 -tracheobronchial, 303
 -vein, 493
Cryosurgical
 -application, 86–88, 107–109, 140, 145, 291, 293, 375
 -approach, 341
 -equipment, 11, 12, 22, 71, 73, 81, 105, 166, 171, 247, 248, 278
 -exposure, 87, 116, 122–128, 137, 144, 152
 -instrument, 4, 9, 73, 76, 78, 81, 171, 248, 273, 290
 -knife, 4
 -literature, 105
 -liver resection, 284
 -management, 165
 -margin, 433
 -measure, 284
 -method, 7, 73, 82, 105, 166, 320, 489
 -necrosis, 142
 -operation, 95, 194, 268, 278, 284, 290, 316, 362, 377, 475
 -otorhynolaryngology, 475
 -palliation, 319
 -principle, 433
 -procedure, 4, 78, 81, 95–98, 102, 165, 166, 206, 243–246, 445
 -removal, 3, 4
 -response, 21, 137
 -segment, 5
 -session, 5, 21, 109, 117–121, 129, 141, 142, 146, 157, 169, 170, 172, 176–179, 185, 218, 255, 269–271, 282–284, 286–288, 300, 303, 332, 333, 336, 337, 339, 340, 362–372, 374, 394–398, 400, 453–455, 460–465, 467–473, 484, 487
 -system, 10, 73–76, 78, 81, 110, 277
 -technique, 21, 22, 78, 81, 83, 85, 95, 137, 144, 190, 206, 250, 284, 289, 419
 -technology, advanced, 21, 73, 81
 -treatment, 11, 13, 85, 169, 170, 173–177, 181, 184, 195–197, 206, 207, 316, 317, 401, 445, 456, 457, 475–478, 480–484, 486, 491, 503
 -unit, 21, 73, 76, 77, 81, 82, 102, 110, 139, 171, 277, 330, 331, 333, 359
 -urology, 403

-zone, 87, 93, 96, 97, 189, 190, 254, 266, 269, 271, 361, 367, 394
Cryotechnological Research Institute "Pulse", 110
Cryotechnology, 11
Cryothalamectomy, 5
Cryothalamotomy, 5
Cryotherapy, 3, 5, 12, 13, 305, 446
Cryotolerant, 5
Cryotreatment, 323
Cryovaricectomy, 5, 489, 494
Cryovulvectomy, 500
Cryozone, 21–70, 88–91, 95, 108–110, 112, 113, 120–122, 126–128, 140, 141, 146–148, 156, 169, 170, 189, 191, 192, 253–255, 268, 269, 271, 277, 300, 333, 360, 362
Cure, 7, 8, 320
  -clinical, 198, 200, 206, 215
  -rate, 95, 165, 166, 343
Curettage, 222, 226, 227, 419, 424, 428–431, 433–438, 440, 441, 443
  -cryosurgery, 12, 219–221, 226, 227
  -meticulous, 219–221, 223–225
Cystectomy, 278

D

Damage
  -breast lobules, 353
  -epiphysis, 438, 439
  -ischemic, 351
  -mechanism, 22
  -skin, 108
Demarcation
  -line, 21, 91, 93, 95, 108, 137, 146, 253, 360, 361, 365, 394
  -ring, 415
Dermabrasion, 446, 459, 468
Dermatofibroma, 166
Diathermy, bipolar, 319
Disease
  -Bowen's, 219–221
  -Crohn's, 319
  -hemorrhoidal, 321, 332–334
  -musculoskeletal system, 419
  -Paget's, 320, 500
  -pancreatic, 137
  -recurrence, 355, 393
  -sexually transmitted, 319
  -tissue, 4, 7, 95, 375, 403
  -unresectable, 235
Dissector balloon, 405
Doppler monitoring, 410
Doppler-ultrasound images, 343, 344

Dysplasia
  -anterior faucial pilar, 483
  -fibrous, 443, 444
Dyspnoea, 303

E

Echinococcectomy, 278
Echinococcal cystic disease, 278, 280–283
  fibrous capsule, 282
Echinococcosis, 278, 280, 281
Electrocautery, 316
Electrocoagulation, 13, 319
Emphysema, 315
Enchondroma, 437, 440
Ender's nails, 428, 429
Endothelium, 150, 151, 156
Epidermal
  -tumor, 315
  -graft, 375
Epidermis, 503
Epiphysis, 422, 423, 436, 439
Equipment, 9, 165, 235, 273, 404, 409, 445
Experiment, 13, 105, 114, 137, 291
  -animal, 351
  -*in vitro* and *in vivo*, 22, 105, 235
Experimental
  -aspects, 103
  -based discussion, 21, 105, 137,
  -basis, 138
  -data, 419
  -evidence, 420
  -freezing, 138
  -interest, 303
  -observations, 105
  -research, 289
  -studies, 22, 81, 105
  -work, 404
Experimental and clinical
  -cryosurgical research, 137
  -experience, 167
  -investigation, 284
  -knowledge, 343
Exposure, wide, 429

F

Filiform verrucae, 181
Fistula, 403
Formaldehyde, 351
Freeze
  -cycle, 112, 113, 277, 439
  -depth, 10
  -lesion, 11
  -surgery, 3
  -time, 165, 166, 445
  -zone, 226, 227, 410

Freeze-thaw cycle, 21, 82, 86, 88–91, 93–95, 98, 102, 107–111, 129–136, 140, 141, 145, 151, 154, 158–162, 165, 166, 169, 170, 189, 191, 192, 206, 219–227, 230, 231, 249, 251–253, 255, 257, 271, 299, 301, 303, 333, 359, 367, 403, 408, 427, 445, 484
Freezing, 3–5, 8–12, 21–70, 75, 95, 102, 105, 112, 113, 116, 137, 144, 149, 150, 165, 166, 169, 170, 206, 209, 212, 218–222, 225–227, 235, 303, 316, 343–350, 373, 386, 391, 427, 445, 489, 500
 -agent, 166
 -contact, 377, 381
 -effect, 427, 489
 -fibroma, 177
 -granuloma, 317
 -liver tumor, 105
 -liver, 105
 -penetration, 377
 -point, 3, 5
 -procedure, 82
 -rapid, 403, 427
 -sites, 377
 -spray, 386
 -technique, 8, 235
 -temperature, 5, 9, 77
 -tip, 377
 -tissue, 3, 4, 17
 -tumor, 427

G Gadolinium, 404, 416
Germination, 284
Granulation
 -secondary, 403
 -tissue, 303
Granuloma, 317
 -bone, Eosinophylic, 434, 435
Growing ice ball, 18

H Haemostatic effect, 268, 303, 341, 377, 403
Halo
 -freeze, 222
 -thaw time, 219–222
Hand
 -curettage, 424, 425
 -function, 214
Hemangioma, 166, 174, 182, 184
Hemangiopericytoma, 481
Hemoptysis, 303, 316
Hemorrhoids, 94, 319, 321, 322
Hemorrhage, 341, 403

Histiocytosis X, 434, 435
Histologic
 -appearances, 303, 307, 308, 315
 -data, 404
 -section of pig liver, 114
Histological
 -changes, 503
 -confirmation, 305
Histology, 418, 491
Histopathological
 -examination, 339
 -findings, 222, 225
Hyperchromasia, 352
Hyperechoic, 412
 -rim, 143
Hypothermia, 3
 -artificialis, 3
 -localis, 3
 -regionalis, 3

Ice, 3, 8, 146, 192, 257, 301, 419 **I**
 -ball, 4, 17, 21, 108, 109, 112, 113, 140, 146, 166, 230, 231, 249, 257, 301, 326, 327, 336, 340, 343–350, 386, 403, 412–414, 476, 478, 480, 485, 499
 -crater, 21, 109, 141, 146, 255, 269, 271, 300, 333
 -margin, 21, 109, 141, 145, 146, 255, 269, 271, 300, 333
Imaging
 -breast cryosurgery, 344
 -cryodestruction, 18
 -Doppler, 413
 -intraoperative real-time, 408
 -magnetic resonance (MRI), 239, 240, 404
Infiltrating
 -lesion, 303
 -tumor, 380
Infiltration vessel, 235
Injury
 -eyelid, 446
 -tissue, ischemically, 351
Ink
 -contour, 207
 -India, 114
Investigation, 21
 -clinical, 77, 105
 -experimental, 13

Keloid, 165, 445 **K**
Keratolytic agents, 178
Kidney, 11, 241, 403, 508, 509

L

Lagophthalmus, 206
Laparoscopic cryosurgery, 74, 95, 114, 115, 274, 403
  -era, 105
  -hepatic cryosurgery, 105, 114
  -images, 411, 413
  -liver cryosurgery, 4, 101, 273, 275, 277
  -manual compression, 415
  -manual, controllable, 403
  -renal cryoablation, 403–405, 409
  -technique, 405
  -trocar, 115
  -ultrasound, 114
  -visualisation, 408, 413, 414
Laparoscopy, 4, 101, 403
Laparotomy, 106, 107, 138, 139, 242
Laser, 78, 303
  -ablation, 235
  -treatment endoscopic, 316
  -therapy, 445, 446
Lateral
  -spread of freeze, 166
  -tangential contact, 303
Layer
  -bone, 441
  -cell, 503
  -hyperkeratotic, 178
  -muscular, 340
Leiomyoma, 307
Lesion, 3, 10, 11, 114, 165, 166, 168, 172, 173, 175, 178, 187–190, 206, 230–233, 303, 387, 399, 400, 417, 433, 435, 436, 443, 445, 446, 453–455, 480, 481, 483, 485, 488
  -benign, 165, 166, 445
  -bronchial, 303
  -curetted, 419, 440
  -cutaneous, 168–170
  -cutaneous eradication, 165, 445
  -femoral, 427, 428
  -laparoscopic freeze, 114
  -liver in, 274
  -lytic, 423, 435
  -margin, 320
  -multiple, 165
  -noninvasive, 320
  -osteolytic, 434
  -pigmented, 166, 172, 446
  -polipoid, 303
  -skin malignant, 193
  -suspicion, 167
  -target, 114
  -thawing, 166

Leukoplakia
  -cheek, 478, 479, 487
  -tongue, 475, 476
Liver
  -alveococcosis, 284–288
  -areas, "dangerous", 286
  -bleeding, 278
  -blood circulation, 278
  -carcinoma, metastatic, 95
  -cryodestruction, 4
  -cryoextirpation, 4
  -cryosurgery, 95–98, 102, 105, 235, 242, 249, 251–255, 258, 269, 270
  -cryosurgical resection, 102, 286
  -echinococcal cystic disease, 278
  -freezing, 105
  -healthy, 108, 137, 144, 253, 254
  -malignancy, 105
  -metastasis, 87, 95–98, 101, 236, 247, 265, 269, 271, 277
  -parasitic disease, 278
  -resection, 98, 278, 284
  -tissue, 105, 111, 116–129, 132, 136, 265
  -tumors, 4, 95, 98, 101, 102, 105, 137, 144, 235, 284
  -ultrasonography, intraoperative advantage, 235
Long-Term Follow-up Post-Cryosurgery, 352
Lymphadenectomy, 217

M

Malignancy
  -hepatic, 105
  -melanoma, 166
Malignant
  -condition, 403
  -lesion, 165, 167, 424, 445, 484
  -tumor, 10, 11, 21, 22, 85, 95, 186, 289, 303, 319, 484
  -tumor bone, 13
  -tumor liver, 11
  -tumor skeletal, 419
Malodorous, 378
Mass, 336, 392, 407
  -hilar right, 315
  -necrotic, 289
Mechanism, tissue destruction, 105
Medium, contrast, 428, 429, 431
Melanocyte, 445, 446
Melanoma, 88–90, 166, 205
Metastasis, 5, 12, 89, 90, 92, 96–98, 102, 105, 205, 214–217, 235–240, 242–246, 251, 252, 258, 261, 263,

268–271, 274, 276, 284, 303, 304, 319, 343, 398
 -adenocarcinoma, 315
 -dissemination, 403
 -endobronchial, 315
 -hepatic, 261
 -renal cell carcinoma, 403
Method, open cone-spray, 222
Minimal invasive liver cryosurgery, 4
Model
 -pig, 115
 -sheep breast, 344–350, 352
 -theoretical, 17
 -Y-Ducer, 410
Monitoring, 111, 212, 249, 302, 403
 -electrical, 18
 -intraoperative, 142, 301
Morbidity, 8, 98, 105, 319
Morphology, 105
Morphological study, 157
Mucous
 -discharge, 319
 -melanoma malignant, 488
Myocardium, 501

N

Necrosis
 -biological, 167
 -cold, 3
 -fibrous capsule, 283
 -focal superficial, 336
 -ischemic, 353
 -skin, 446
 -tumor, 315
Necrotomy, 377, 379, 382, 385, 390
Neoplasm benign, 475
Nephrectomy, 403
Nevus
 -congenital giant, 166
 -dysplastic, 166
 -ota, 445, 446, 458, 462, 466, 468, 473
Nitrogen liquid, 3, 4, 10, 11, 13, 73, 77, 102, 110, 116, 144, 149, 150, 165, 166, 171, 209, 219–221, 223, 224, 235, 303, 324, 373, 419, 424, 427, 445, 446
 -based cryo-unit, 409
 -based universal system, 139
 -cryogenic instrument, 445
 -cryogenic unit, 504
 -cryosurgery, 12, 446
 -cryosurgery device, 324
 -driven cryoinstrument, 503
 -driven device, 377
 -instrument, 446
 -spray, 177, 433
Nodular tumor, 225
Nodule, hemorrhoidal, 326

Obstruction, 319
 -bronchial, 303
 -tracheal, 303
Option
 -therapeutic, 105
 -treatment, 7, 144
Organ, 3, 10, 82, 167
 -specificity, 5
 -structure, pathological, 4
Oxidation-reduction indicator, 351
Oxide nitrous, 18, 165, 303, 324

Palliation, 12, 303, 319, 320
Palliative
 -cryosurgery, 12, 319
 -liver resection, 284
 -treatment, 303
Palpebral
 -area, 446
 -region, 207
 -skin, 446
Pancreas, 11, 12, 86, 137–142, 144–150, 156, 157, 161, 289–292, 295–299, 301, 302
 -animal freezing, 137
 -cryosurgery, 12, 137, 142–144, 289, 299–302
 -operating area, 138
 -ultrasound intraoperative, 142
Pancreatic
 -cancer advanced, 12, 509
 -malignancy, 137
 -neoplasm, 137
 -parenchyma, 137, 144
 -tissue, 137, 157, 159–161
 -tumor, 137
Pancreatitis, 289–293
Papilloma, 316
Papillomatosis tracheal, 316
Papule, 206
Parenchyma
 -breast, 343
 -healthy, 98
 -normal, 114
Parenchymal
 -hemorrhage, 403
 -organs, 10, 22, 105, 137
Pathohistological, 137
Penis glans, 217

O

P

Perianal
- skin carcinoma, 320
- warts, 319

Phenomenon, 137, 144, 269–272
- Raynaud's, 5

Photocoagulation infrared, 319
Photomicrograph, 114, 421
Pile, 319
Polypoid tumor, 336, 337
Post-cryoablation images, 404
Post-cryosurgery, 351–353
Post-cryosurgical view, 110, 141, 148, 255, 267, 269, 271, 300, 333, 397, 398, 454, 455
Post-thaw hemorrhage, 403
Pre-cryoablation, 407, 418
Pregnancy, 165
Pregnant sheep breast model, 352
Primary
- breast cancer, advanced, 91
- cancer, 390
- hepatocellular carcinoma, 235
- port, 405, 406
- resection abdomino-perineal, 320
- scar, 445
- treatment, 419
- tumor, 425
- tumor liver, 105
- varicosity, 489

Q Quality of life, 85, 95, 289, 319, 392
Q-switched ruby laser, 446, 473

R Rate
- complications, 420
- cooling, 167
- fructure, 420
- low resectability, 235
- recurrence, 425

Remnant, 337, 375, 377, 379
Renal
- cancer, 404
- cell carcinoma, 403, 418
- cryolesion, 404
- cryosurgery, 403
- mass, 403, 416
- parenchymal hemorrhage, 415
- surface, 411, 414, 415
- tumors, 13, 403
- vessels, 412

Resection
- conventional, 235
- intralesional, 420, 433
- quadrant, 5
- surgical, 289, 337
- tumor, avascular, 289

Resectional curettage, 424–426, 429, 430, 432
Respiratory
- distress, 304
- distress, acute, 303
- function, 303
- mitochondrial enzymes, 351

Restitutio ad integrum, 328, 478, 486, 487
Retroperitoneal
- renal cryoablation, 405
- space, 405

S Saline
- medium, 18
- physiological, 446

Scalp, 218
Scar, 165, 186, 212, 214, 388, 445
- hypertrophic, 165, 445, 447
- tissue, 202, 203

Sclerotherapy, 319
Sensorial incontinence, 323
Shaving cryosurgery, 165, 445
Sinus pilonidal, 215
Skeletal
- tumor, 419
- system, 419

Skin
- aged and withered, 503
- children, 446
- cryosurgery, 165
- damage, 424
- dry, 504
- flaps, 424
- frozen, 459
- grafting, 320
- layer, 11, 503
- malignant tumors, 165, 167, 190
- metastases, 88, 355, 397, 398
- normal, 232, 233, 377, 386
- peeling, 445
- surface, 4, 503
- thickness, 445
- tumors, benign, 165
- tumors, epidermal benign, 166
- vascular stasis, 503

Slough, 306, 308, 309, 403
- area, 304

Sore, 322, 328
Sphincter preservation, 320
Stridor, 317
Surgery conventional, 85, 165, 167, 215, 500

System
  -biological, 5, 105
  -calyceal, 403
  -fluid, 105

T Technology, 71
Teflon, 115
Temperature
  -application, 21, 144
  -body, 3
  -cavity wall, 427
  -cold, 3, 7
  -constant, 21, 23–70, 95
  -couple, 438, 440
  -intralesional, 433
  -local, 3
  -low, 3–5, 7, 8, 11, 13, 16, 81, 82, 105, 144, 235, 419
  -minimal, 17, 165
  -monitoring, 383
  -monitoring, subcutaneous, 388
  -recording, 13, 439, 441
  -sub-zero, 3, 8, 22, 81, 95, 105, 137, 165, 278, 284
Thaw, 21, 109, 303, 403, 427
  -time, 166, 219–222
Thawing, 4, 11, 21, 77, 81, 86, 98, 101, 110, 120, 121, 124, 127, 128, 137, 141, 144, 148, 156, 277, 351, 377, 391, 414, 433
  -gradual, 403
Thermal
  -damage, 424
  -injury, 419
Thermocouple, 15, 209, 212, 217, 391, 427, 439, 441, 499
Thermometer, 4, 8
Thermography, 12
Thomson Joule effect, 303
Tissue
  -alveococal, 284
  -body, healthy, 4, 503
  -crystallization, 17
  -destruction, 5, 10, 107, 111, 140, 257, 301
  -devitalized, 403
  -exposing, 3
  -fibrous, 353, 501
  -frozen, 166
  -interstitial, 352
  -living, 5, 105, 419
  -necrosis, 433
  -normal, 351
  -parasitic, 284, 286, 288
  -pathological, 3,4

  -specificity, 5
  -surrounding, 95, 177, 212, 284
  -surrounding, soft, 427
  -swelling, 3
  -volum, 73
Tongue, 475, 485, 486
Tracheostomy, 317
Treatment
  -adjuvant, 419
  -anorectal disorders, 319
  -baldness, 503
  -bone tumors, 424
  -Bowen's disease, 320
  -cutaneous lesion, 165
  -hemorrhoidal disease, 319, 329
  -initial, 320
  -lesion, 10, 487
  -nevus Ota, 446
  -option, 21, 137
  -pancreatic disease, 137
  -rectal polyp, 319
  -session, 165, 189, 445
  -surgical, 211
  -wart, 166
Trocar, 3, 4, 10, 101, 273, 276
Tumor
  -benign 172, 303
  -bronchial, 303
  -bronchiogenic, 303
  -carcinoid, 311
  -cavity, 424–429
  -cell, 235, 419, 424
  -cryonecrotized, 251, 252, 299
  -destruction, 484
  -harbor, 425
  -liver metastatic, 237
  -mass, 4, 86, 87, 95, 98–100, 102, 236, 250, 299, 341, 359, 367, 394, 484, 509
  -periocular, 166
  -recurrence, 137
  -region, 235
  -residual, 267
  -skin, 10, 86, 168
  -tibial, 431
  -unresectable, 319
  -untreated, 304
  -vascular, 269, 271

U Ulcer, 339
  -varicous, 204
Ulceration, 206, 216, 339, 391, 500
Ulcus rodens, 198
Ultrasonography, 403

Ultrasound
  -examination, 274, 411
  -images, 11, 344–350
  -images, intraoperative, 11, 111–113, 249, 274, 407, 411
  -intraluminal, 339
  -machine, 410
  -monitoring, 98, 143, 236, 256, 257, 301, 411
Ureter, 414
Urine leakage, 403

Varicectomy, 489
Vascular
  -congestion, 166, 352, 353
  -damage, 351
  -endothelium, 114
Vena
Ventricular aneurism, 501
  -cava, 114, 261, 284
  -cava inferior, 114
Ventriculotomy, 501
Vulgaris verruca, 180

Vulva, 499, 500
Vulvar region, 499

Warts
  -chin, 183
  -finger, 179
  -plantar, 178
Wound
  -drain, 437
  -superficial, 165, 445
  -full-thickness, 165, 445
  -oozing, 223, 224, 226, 227
  -dehiscence, 420

Xanthelasma, 185

Yag-laser, 316

Zone
  -border, 501
  -necrosis, 114
  -peripheral, 353

SpringerMedicine

Nikolai N. Korpan (ed.)

Basics of Cryosurgery

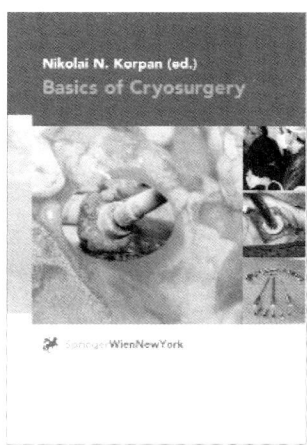

2001. Approx. 500 pages. Approx. 600 figures, mostly in colour.
57 tables and diagrams.
Hardcover DM 255,–, öS 1790,–, as of Jan. 2002 EUR 130,–
Subscription price, valid until 3 months after publication:
DM 204,–, öS 1432,–, as of Jan. 2002 EUR 104,–
(Recommended retail prices)
All prices are net-prices subject to local VAT.
ISBN 3-211-83701-9

"Basics of Cryosurgery" is the first publication specialising in the fundamentals of modern cryosurgery. It is dedicated to surgeons and all doctors and specialists throughout the world – especially those working in cryosurgery and cryotechnology, who, in their devotion to advancing medical science, are helping patients in their fight against malignant tumours. This book presents what is currently known in modern cryosurgery and is the first on the subject to appear at the start of the third millennium. It aims to contribute to the further development of this branch of medicine, which is set to become indispensable in treating patients.

"Basics of Cryosurgery" is a unique contribution – no previous work has compiled in one source all available scientific data on the theoretical, experimental, and clinical investigations that have been undertaken in the field of cryosurgery. The chapters were written by authorities in the field who have not only experienced the triumphs but have learnt from their own and others' failures, and how to avoid these, and who have helped many patients to escape what had previously seemed an inevitable outcome.

SpringerSurgery

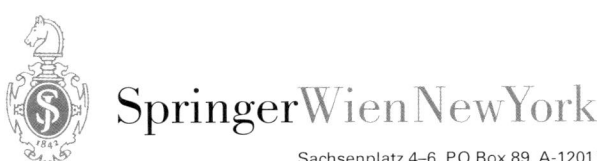

Sachsenplatz 4–6, P.O.Box 89, A-1201 Wien, Fax +43-1-330 24 26, e-mail: books@springer.at, Internet: www.springer.at
New York, NY 10010, 175 Fifth Avenue • D-14197 Berlin, Heidelberger Platz 3 •Tokyo 113, 3–13, Hongo 3-chome, Bunkyo-ku

SpringerMedicine

Manfred Frey (ed.)

Endoscopy and Microsurgery

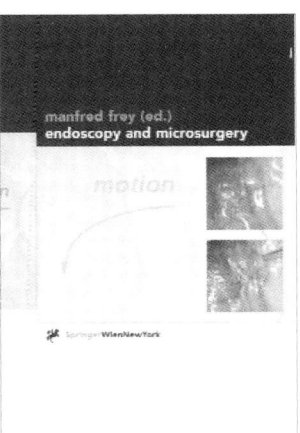

2001. XXII, 134 pages. 115 figures, partly in colour.
Hardcover DM 228,–, öS 1596,–, as of Jan. 2002 EUR 115,90
(Recommended retail prices)
All prices are net-prices subject to local VAT.
ISBN 3-211-83439-7
Update in Plastic Surgery

Endoscopic microsurgery is a developing technique in plastic surgery. There are many advantages over traditional methods: improved access to difficult and hidden areas, better mobility, one optical instrument for endoscopic dissection and the microsurgical part, reduced overall costs, and a possibility to develop new procedures supported by the use of the endoscope.

In the first volume of the series "Update in Plastic Surgery" internationally acknowledged experts give an up-to-date view of the clinical possibilities in plastic surgery which result from video-assisted microsurgery with the endoscope. Advantages and disadvantages are discussed, and reasons are presented why it can be assumed that this technique will be the standard in plastic surgery within a few years.

SpringerSurgery

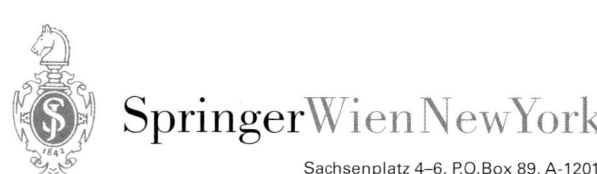

Sachsenplatz 4–6, P.O.Box 89, A-1201 Wien, Fax +43-1-330 24 26, e-mail: books@springer.at, Internet: www.springer.at
New York, NY 10010, 175 Fifth Avenue • D-14197 Berlin, Heidelberger Platz 3 • Tokyo 113, 3–13, Hongo 3-chome, Bunkyo-ku

SpringerMedicine

Mario Campanacci

Bone and Soft Tissue Tumors

Clinical Features, Imaging, Pathology and Treatment

Foreword by William F. Enneking.
Second, completely revised edition.
1999. XX, 1319 pages. 1120 figures.
Hardcover DM 632,–, öS 4421,–, as of Jan. 2002 EUR 321,–
(Recommended retail prices)
All prices are net-prices subject to local VAT.
(Distribution rights: worldwide except Italy.
Jointly published with Piccin Nuova Libraria, Padova)
ISBN 3-211-83235-1

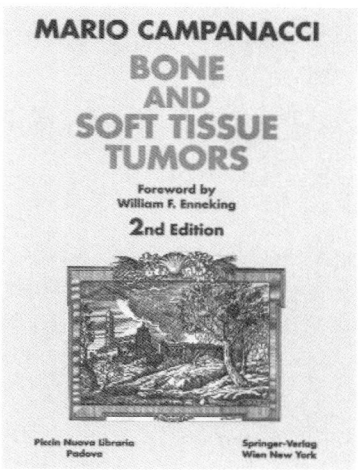

"This is an extraordinary book by an extraordinary author. Dr. Campanacci brings to the readers the vast experience in musculoskeletal oncology of the Rizzoli Orthopaedic Institute in Bologna. As such, he has had at his disposal the patient records, radiographs and pathologic material dating back to 1905. The wealth of clinical material that has been accumulated at the Rizzoli Institute, with exquisite documentation and maintenance is a unique resource and testimonial to not only the author but his predecessors. This book brings to the reader an almost unparalleled experience from one of the leading centers of musculoskeletal oncology in the world.
From the Foreword of William F. Enneking

This second english edition is an entirely new book. It has been thoroughly rewritten, from the first to the last word. About 30% of the pictures are new. The new book incorporates the accumulated personal experience of the author, covering over 20.000 inpatients and many more outpatients, the perusal of the literature of the last 10 years, the recent developments in imaging (particularly MRI), microscopic diagnosis (especially immunohistochemistry and electron microscopy) and the ultimate progress in surgical and non-surgical treatment modalities.
Mario Campanacci (1932–1999) was an orthopaedic surgeon and a pathologist with 40 years of experience (started in 1958 in the Laboratory of Pathology and Tumor Center of the Rizzoli Orthopaedic Institute) focused on musculoskeletal oncology. He was Professor of Orthopaedic Surgery and Pathology, University of Bologna, Director of the 1st Orthopaedic Clinic and of the Tumor Centre, Rizzoli Orthopaedic Institute, Bologna and Director of the Graduate School of Orthopaedics, University of Bologna.

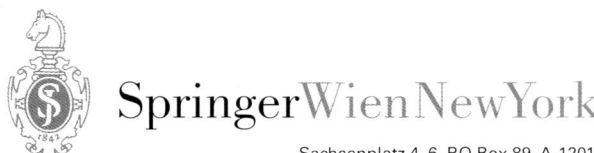

Sachsenplatz 4–6, P.O.Box 89, A-1201 Wien, Fax +43-1-330 24 26, e-mail: books@springer.at, Internet: www.springer.at
New York, NY 10010, 175 Fifth Avenue • D-14197 Berlin, Heidelberger Platz 3 • Tokyo 113, 3–13, Hongo 3-chome, Bunkyo-ku

*Springer-Verlag
and the Environment*

We at Springer-Verlag firmly believe that an international science publisher has a special obligation to the environment, and our corporate policies consistently reflect this conviction.

We also expect our business partners – printers, paper mills, packaging manufacturers, etc. – to commit themselves to using environmentally friendly materials and production processes.

The paper in this book is made from no-chlorine pulp and is acid free, in conformance with international standards for paper permanency.